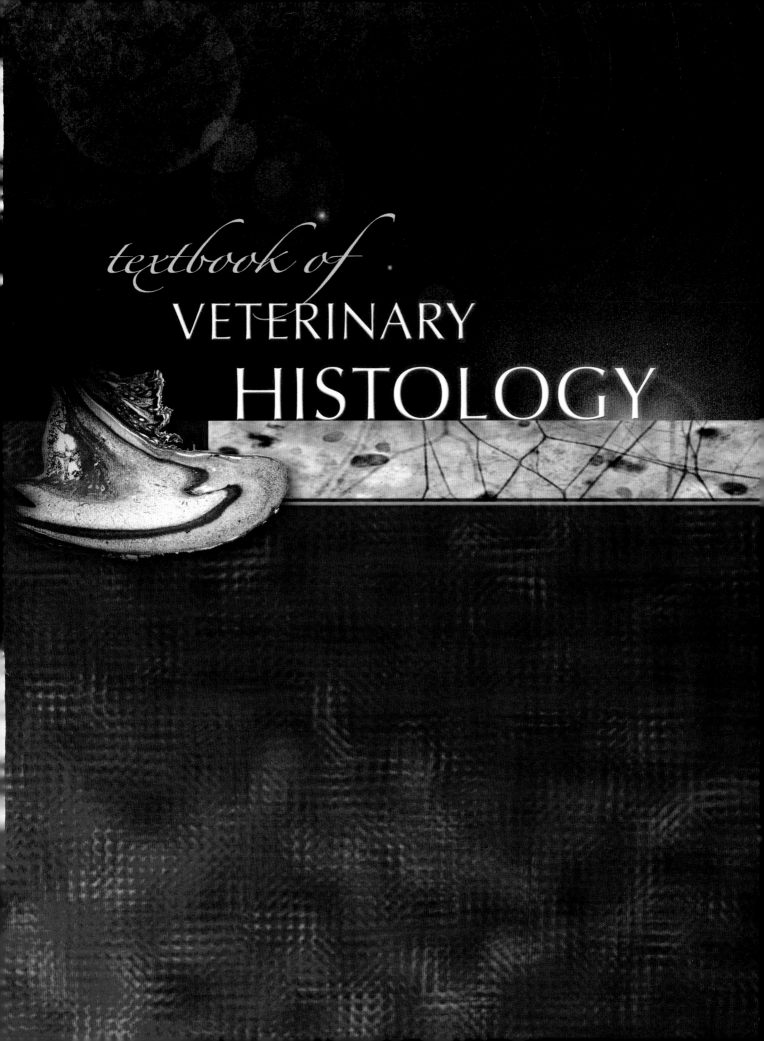

textbook of
VETERINARY
HISTOLOGY

textbook of VETERINARY HISTOLOGY

DON A. SAMUELSON, PhD, MS

Professor, Anatomist, and Visual Scientist
Department of Small Animal Clinical Sciences
College of Veterinary Medicine
University of Florida
Gainesville, Florida

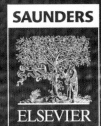

SAUNDERS

ELSEVIER

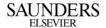

SAUNDERS
ELSEVIER

11830 Westline Industrial Drive
St. Louis, Missouri 63146

TEXTBOOK OF VETERINARY HISTOLOGY

ISBN-13: 978-0-7216-8174-0
ISBN-10: 0-7216-8174-3

Copyright © 2007 by Saunders, an imprint of Elsevier Inc.

ISBN-13: 978-0-7216-8174-0
ISBN-10: 0-7216-8174-3

Publishing Director: Linda L. Duncan
Publisher: Penny Rudolph
Managing Editor: Teri Merchant
Publishing Services Manager: Patricia Tannian
Senior Project Manager: Anne Altepeter
Design Direction: Bill Drone

Printed in China

Last digit is the print number: 9 8 7 6 5 4 3 2 1

Working together to grow
libraries in developing countries

www.elsevier.com | www.bookaid.org | www.sabre.org

ELSEVIER   BOOK AID International   Sabre Foundation

*To the students whom I have taught for the past 25 years;
many of them have become dear friends and have allowed me
to learn from them as well.*

*I especially dedicate this work to my wife, my two sons,
and my mother and father.*

Preface

Histology is a subject that focuses on the interrelationship and integration of molecular and physiological activities within the body to specific anatomical structures and, as a result, requires much visual conceptualization. Although illustrations and diagrams convey a substantial amount of information and certainly help one appreciate key features of cells and tissues and their assemblage into organs, learning histology relies primarily on using the light microscope to understand these features. For this reason, this book liberally uses light micrographs so that students are able to develop as much as possible an appreciation of histological interpretation.

In addition to the many images found within, the book makes extensive use of full color, which is a vast improvement over the traditional black and white images presented in many histology textbooks. Color images allow readers to draw histological impressions immediately rather than requiring them to refer to an atlas and microscope concomitantly. In this way, the laboratory experience becomes one of reinforcement rather than an initial learning event.

Legends for the micrographic images used throughout the book include original magnifications so that students can appreciate the appropriate magnification needed to examine cellular, tissue, and organ components of the body. Also, by noting the corresponding stain applied for each image, students are able to understand the usefulness of color reactions as they reveal important features of these different components.

Because this is a textbook of veterinary histology, comparative aspects are drawn upon continuously, with emphasis placed primarily on differences observed among domestic animals. However, from time to time, examples are offered from other sometimes exotic animals, to demonstrate the strong similarities among many tissues, regardless of the species.

In the course of learning about histology, many correlations are made between structure and function of the wide variety of tissues and organs that make up the body. Because different species are considered here, additional variations occur as well. To ensure that students appreciate and understand the numerous correlations and variations that exist, each chapter contains compilation tables. The tables are designed to give readers a ready resource of information that can also be used for review when needed. In addition to the tables and in concert with them, relevant words within the body of the text are highlighted in boldface type. Overall the book is designed to enhance the experience of learning veterinary histology for students who have had little or no previous exposure.

Don A. Samuelson

Acknowledgments

Illustrations and enhanced micrographs were contributed in part by Peter Samuelson. Members of my faculty provided recommendations for other images. I am especially indebted to Drs. Rosanne Marsella and Colin Burrows for their reviews of the chapters on the integument and digestive system, respectively. I also thank Drs. John Harvey, Gary Butcher, and Roger Reep for specimens for the chapters on blood, the female reproductive tract, and the nervous system. Special thanks to Drs. Kirk Gelatt and Elliott Jacobson for their encouragement and advice.

And finally, much gratitude is owed to the project team at Elsevier, headed by Teri Merchant, managing editor, and Anne Altepeter, senior project manager.

Don A. Samuelson

Contents

Chapter 20
Eye and Ear, 487

Histotechniques

Veterinary histology is the science that focuses on the detailed morphology of domestic animals and correlates specific structures with function. As a component of structural biology, veterinary histology, which is synonymous with veterinary microanatomy, involves the examination and description of the microscopic anatomy of normal cells of the body and all of their contents and products.

As cell types become recognized, an appreciation of their grouping and organization can be made—the identification of tissues. The orientation and composition of the different tissues, in turn, provide the basic construct for the organs and organ systems of the body. And it is important to understand clearly the functional relationship of each bodily structure, whether it be cell, tissue, or organ, in an inclusive manner. To that end this textbook incorporates useful information from the other sciences that directly reveal function, including physiology, biochemistry, cell biology, and, occasionally, pathology.

PRESERVATION

Cells and tissues to be examined structurally, in a traditional manner (by light microscopy and/or electron microscopy) need to be preserved. Otherwise, cells can undergo autolysis (self-digestion) and be invaded by opportunistic organisms such as rapidly multiplying bacteria. Adequate preservation or fixation should cease the putrefaction and autolysis that

accompany postmortem changes and keep the tissue in a state that is as close as possible to the living condition. Most fixations are performed chemically using a variety of agents that render materials within cells to relatively insoluble states and, in effect, allow them to remain insoluble during subsequent treatments such as dehydration and embedding. In this way, a useful fixative minimizes distortion and shrinkage. The right fixative also permits good staining and allows the observer to recognize the necessary elements that distinguish cells and tissues from one another.

Fixation is usually performed by exposing tissues to chemical preservatives such as formaldehyde. Mechanically speaking, exposure can be active or passive. The active process of fixation involves replacing body fluids with a perfusate such as saline wash, which is followed by the fixative of choice, 10% buffered formalin for example. This process, which is called *perfusion fixation*, involves introducing the perfusates, saline and then the fixative, into one or more major arteries by the use of a pressure pump or simply by gravity. Perfusion fixation may require large volumes of perfusates, depending on the size of the animal or region of the body to be preserved. It has the advantage of preserving a large mass thoroughly and relatively evenly. Overall, perfusion fixation is the preferred method for sampling most animal tissues.

By comparison, passive fixation involves placing the tissue in the preservative, again such as formalin, and relies on gradual diffusion of the fixative to replace the natural fluids. This process, which is called *immersion fixation*, is restricted by the fixative's ability to penetrate the specimen and consequently is most effective for comparatively small amounts of tissues (2 cm or less in thickness). Immersion fixation, which is also called *passive fixation*, requires a volume of fixative that should exceed that of the specimen by at least 5:1 and the replenishment of fresh fixative several hours after initial immersion. Passive infiltration is a longer process than the perfusion process and can require several days to 1 month or more to become effective.

Once preserved, specimens can be stored at room temperature or refrigeration indefinitely as long as an adequate amount of fixative (at least four times the volume of the specimen) is present. However, if specimens are kept too long in relatively strong or "harsh" preservatives, which are osmotically quite high, the tissues can become hard and shriveled. As a result, embedding is difficult and staining is greatly weakened (Table 1-1). Harsh or strong fixatives can be useful for shortening preservation times and effectively holding certain biological materials that are not necessarily kept by other less severe or less hypertonic fixatives. Specimens preserved in strong fixatives should be processed expeditiously.

There are times when the preservation of tissues is performed in a "gentle" manner, involving fixatives that are slightly hypertonic to the specimen. Preservation of this type is used for close examination of cells at very high magnification. Typically, a fixative such as glutaraldehyde (a dialdehyde vs. formaldehyde, a monaldehyde) preserves cells in a way that allows subcellular structures to retain an appearance that is closer to the living state than that preserved by a monaldehyde.

PROCESSING AND EMBEDDING

Tissues that have been preserved or pretreated can be processed for sectioning in a number of ways. Certain tissues, such as brain specimens, for example, can be sectioned directly using cold temperatures (dry ice or cryostat) to maintain firmness. Most tissues benefit from the use of a supporting matrix, that is, an embedding medium. Paraffin, which consists of a true nonsynthetic wax, is the most common embedding medium for creating standard histological sections. It can have a hard or soft consistency, depending on the temperature used for embedding (50°-55° C for soft media; 56°-68° C for hard media). When thinner sections (5-6 µm thickness or less) are desired, which is usually the case, hard paraffin is preferred.

Because paraffin is not miscible with water, tissues need to be thoroughly dehydrated before embedding in a graded manner using alcohol (ethanol) or some other water-miscible substance that will remove water. Most alcohols will not dissolve or mix with molten paraffin. Consequently, an intermediate step is needed that results in placing the specimens in a fluid that is miscible with both paraffin and alcohol before infiltration of the embedding matrix is possible. This intermediate step is usually referred to as "clearing" because dehydrated tissues often become clear or more transparent than previously.

Tissues to be examined at very high magnifications by transmission electron microscopy (TEM) undergo similar dehydration, but have to be embedded in a supporting matrix that will withstand the rigors of a strong vacuum (10^{-5} torr) and an intense electron beam that is generated from a power supply of 75,000 volts or more. Plastics are routinely used for these

TABLE 1-1	Problems Encountered during Histological Preparation of Specimens		
PROBLEM	**CAUSE**	**RESULT**	**CORRECTION**
Inadequate fixation	Improper fixative; specimen size is too large	Uneven embedding; hypotonic solution will swell specimen; hypertonic solution will shrink specimen; improper staining	Reduce specimen size and/or deliver fixative by perfusion; readjust fixative strength for best tonicity
Improper embedding	Inadequate fixation and/or dehydration; inadequate embedding medium	Specimens section unevenly; presence of holes within sections	Improve fixation; use appropriate embedding medium
Irregular sections	Improper embedding; dull knife edge; faulty microtome	Compression marks; tears throughout specimen	Resolve fixation and/or embedding problems; use fresh disposable blades or sharpen knives; service microtome
Inadequate staining	Inadequate fixation; old stains or dyes	Little to no color imparted by the stain or dye	Improve fixation; make fresh stains and dye solutions

reasons. **Plastic embedding** also can be used for light microscopic observations of small samples of tissues (usually less than 1 cm in width) and compared with paraffin-embedded samples of the same tissue. Shrinkage and expansion artifacts of the samples and their sections are greatly reduced in plastic embedded preparations. Unfortunately, plastic embedding has several major limitations, including difficulty of infiltrating the tissues, interference with the traditional histological stains, and costs. It is largely for these reasons that paraffin embedding is more commonly used for histology and histopathology than plastic embedding.

SECTIONING AND STAINING

Sectioning involves cutting tissues into even pieces that are thin enough to be examined by a microscope. The microtome, which is the standard tool for sectioning, can vary in its ability to cut a range of thicknesses (Figure 1-1). The vibratome, for example, produces thick sections (50-200 nm), whereas the ultramicrotome used for TEM, in contrast, can produce very thin sections (50-100 nm). It is important to keep in mind that the quality of sectioning has a considerable effect on subsequent staining results. Thus, it is essential to obtain the best sections possible. Artifacts that can be generated from sectioning include compression lines (chatter), knife marks or tears, and uneven thickness, to mention a few (Figure 1-2). These and other problems may be the result of improper fixation, inadequate embedding, and dulled knives.

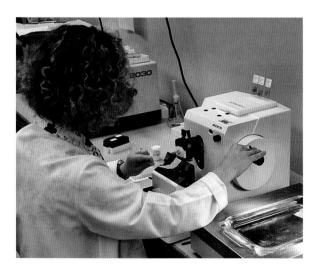

Figure 1-1. Using a microtome with a sharpened blade, the histotechnologist produces a series of sections in the form of a ribbon from a paraffin-embedded block.

For most paraffin-embedded specimens, sections are cut at 5- to 6-nm thickness and maintained in a ribbon, which is then placed on a warm-water bath. Once on the water bath, the sections expand. If left on too long, the sections will spread too far and create large artifactual spaces between tissues, cells, and extracellular fibers.

Individual sections or perhaps a small ribbon of section is collected on glass slides. The paraffin is first removed and then the sections on the slides are rehydrated before stained. Most tissues in unstained sections lack sufficient contrast to be viewed light microscopically. Consequently, a stain or dye is applied to reveal cellular and extracellular components, which are normally transparent, by their color reactions. In instances in which components cannot be readily stained, dark field, phase, and fluorescent microscopy have been often employed (Figure 1-3). Fortunately, most components of tissues do react to various dyes and reagents and thus permit their identification by standard, reproducible techniques. Hundreds of stains are available, and from these stains thousands of techniques have been derived. For most histological purposes, only a small number of stains are routinely used, such as hematoxylin and eosin (H&E) (Table 1-2).

Staining reactions of tissues may be purely a passive event involving diffusion along a concentration gradient, or it may be active as in vital staining, when living cells and their physiological processes are involved. Most often, staining reactions involve bonding interactions in which dye-tissue or reagent-tissue affinities occur. The most common of these is electrostatic bonding or salt linkage. Other interactions include hydrophobic bonding (grouping of hydrophobic chains), van der Waal forces, and covalent bonding.

For transmission electron microscopy, tissues within ultrathin sections are exposed to solutions that contain fairly high concentrations of a particular heavy metal salt, such as lead, uranium, iron, silver, or bismuth. Salt linkage in this instance occurs within specific cellular and extracellular components. The heavy metals are sufficiently dense enough to block the electrons of the electron beam that otherwise would pass through the tissue unimpeded.

SPECIALIZED HISTOTECHNIQUES

The interpretation of structures that have been prepared for light microscopy and electron microscopy continues to be a challenge for both novice and experienced observers, but, of course, on different levels. To interpret structures in a meaningful way, an

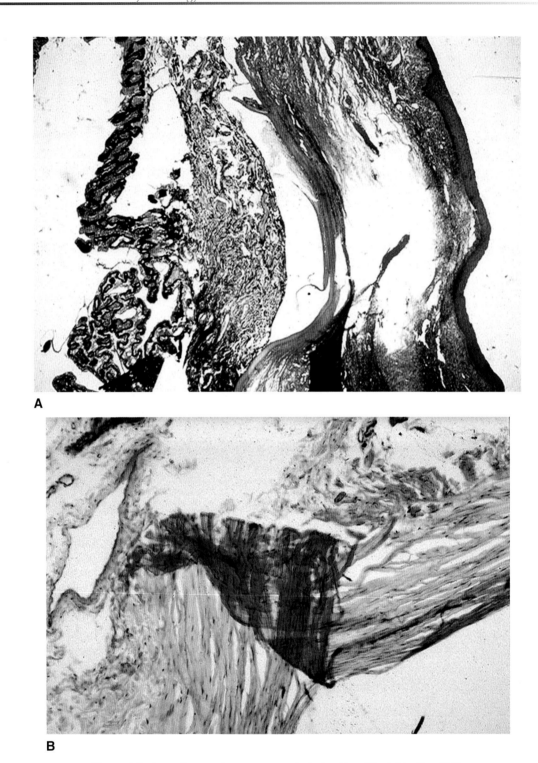

A

B

Figure 1-2. Imperfect sections can contain holes (**A,** ×20), folds (**B,** ×100),

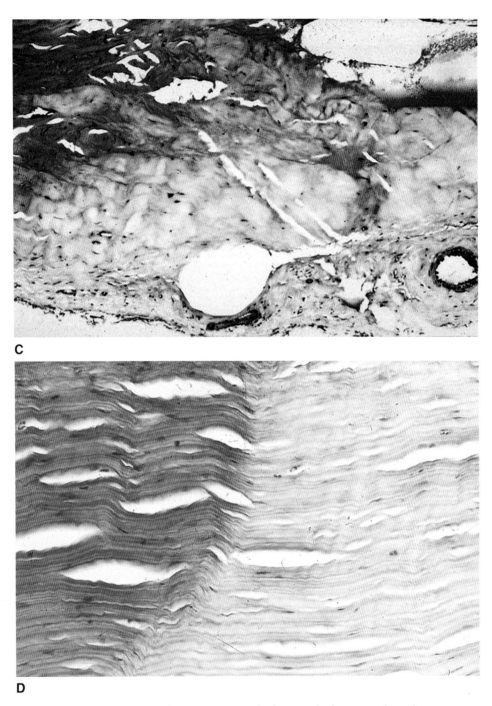

C

D

Figure 1-2, cont'd knife marks (**C,** ×100), and uneven section thickness, which can result in changes in staining intensity (**D,** ×200).

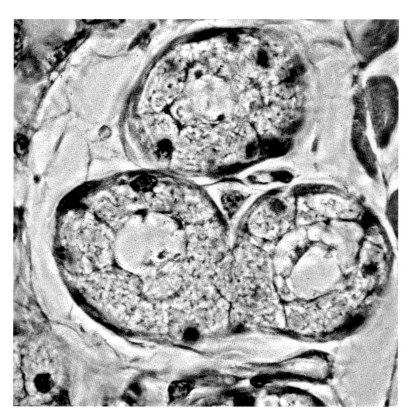

Figure 1-3. Viewing of histological specimens can be aided by supplemental imaging techniques, such as phase microscopy as seen in this light micrograph of an eccrine gland of a horse. (×625.)

TABLE 1-2	Commonly Used Histological Stains and Their Reactions	
STAIN	**APPLICATION**	**REACTION**
Hematoxylin and eosin	Cellular tissues	Nuclei, blue; cytoplasm, various shades of pink
Trichrome (Masson)	Connective tissues (and cellular tissues to some extent)	Collagen, blue; nuclei, black; cytoplasm, keratin, and muscle fibers, red
Periodic acid–Schiff (PAS)	Carbohydrates	Basement membrane, glycogen, mucin, and amyloid deposits—purplish red/fuchsia
Alcian blue	Proteoglycans (mucosubstances) within extracellular matrices (ECM)	ECM—light to dark blue (reaction can vary by pH)

understanding of their functions is needed, and an excellent method to learn structure-function relationships is to locate molecular components that comprise cells and their surrounding environment. A variety of histologically related techniques have evolved that allow observers to explore tissues in ways that far exceed the simple viewing of structure. These techniques, which are largely directed toward being able to identify the chemical makeup of each ingredient within a tissue, include histochemistry, cytochemistry, immunohistochemistry and immuno-cytochemistry, in situ hybridization, autoradiography, and energy-dispersive x-ray microanalysis.

Histochemistry and cytochemistry involve the identification and localization of specific chemical components within a tissue and cell, respectively. A component can be general or specific. An excellent example of localizing a general component is staining for polysaccharides, which is most commonly achieved by generating the periodic acid–Schiff (PAS) reaction. Glucose-rich components are predisposed by periodate, causing 1,2 glycol groups on glucose molecules to be oxidized to aldehydes, which in turn react with the Schiff reagent and result in a purple fuchsin colorization of most polysaccharides (Figure 1-4). However, if greater selectivity of poly-

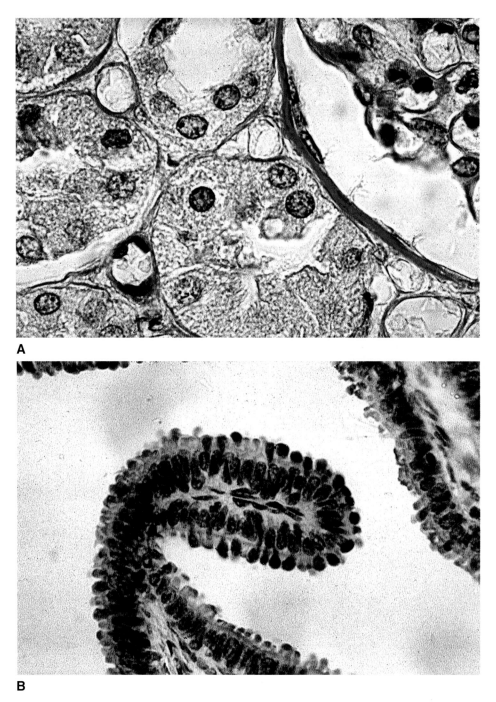

A

B

Figure 1-4. Many special stains are used to reveal specific histological features, including one of the most commonly used special stains, periodic acid–Schiff (PAS), which reveals carbohydrate-laden components, such as basement membranes, by its fuchsin reaction in the canine kidney (**A,** ×1000), and mucin-filled goblet cells of the small intestine (**B,** ×400).

saccharides is desired, other histochemical procedures can be used such as enzyme degradation, in which a solution containing a specific enzyme (amylase for glycogen identification, for example) is placed on the section before staining, or lectin labeling, which involves applying a proteinaceous material (mostly derived from plants) that has specific affinities for selected polysaccharides such as galactosyls, fructosyls, and so on (Figure 1-5).

In some instances, the fixation process does not adequately preserve a compound being held by the cell, and, as a result, the subsequent treatment steps—

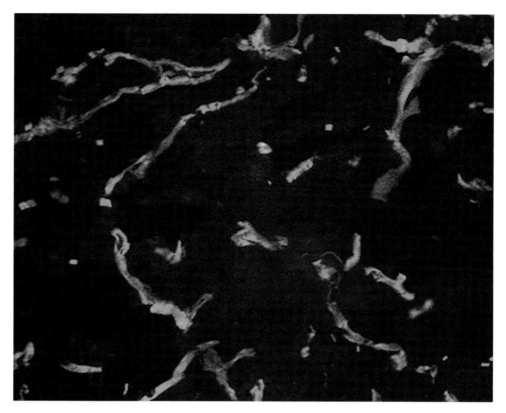

Figure 1-5. Although specific stains are generally not used routinely, they offer considerable information. Lectins reveal the presence of specific polysaccharides, such as wheat germ agglutinin (WGA) seen in this micrograph reacting with meningeal components of nervous tissue in the dog. (×125.)

dehydration and embedding—remove or alter the compound in a way that prevents its visualization. In these instances, the tissue sample can be frozen and sectioned in that state prior to staining. Lipids and lipid-rich materials are examples of compounds that are best revealed through the use of frozen sections and subsequent appropriate stains, such as Sudan black or Nile blue (Figure 1-6).

Immunohistochemistry and immunocytochemistry comprise another technique that detects specific materials, especially those proteinaceous in nature, within tissues and cells, respectively. The precision of this technique, which employs antibody labeling, makes it an exciting and powerful tool that is being used increasingly by clinicians (Figure 1-7). With this method pathologists can diagnose certain diseases. Immunohistochemistry and immunocytochemistry in-volve the coupling of antibodies (derived from other species) to specific antigens (an enzyme, cytokine, or some other molecule). The antibodies, in turn, are typically labeled with a color marker for light microscopy or an electron-dense tag for TEM (Figure 1-8).

In situ hybridization is a different localization technique that selectively labels deoxyribonucleic acid (DNA) and ribonucleic acid (RNA) sequences within cells. With the recent development of recombinant DNA technology, hybridization techniques can be performed on tissue sections and consequently reveal specific DNA or RNA sequences among a large variety of different cell populations. Using the process known as *gene cleaving*, a sequence of DNA is able to be amplified in a host (usually bacteria) by a vector (plasmid or bacteriophage). Probes of DNA and RNA can then be made during their synthesis by using labeled nucleotides. The labels can be radioactive (tritium) or nonradioactive (biotin or digoxigenin). Hybridization is subsequently performed whereby complementary strands of DNA:DNA, DNA:RNA, or copy RNA (cRNA):RNA are allowed to join.

Autoradiography is a technique that relies on the incorporation of radiolabeled precursors or substrates in cells. The precursors, such as a tritium-labeled proline for collagen synthesis or tritium-labeled thymidine for DNA replication, are given to living tissue samples or cell cultures for a period of time

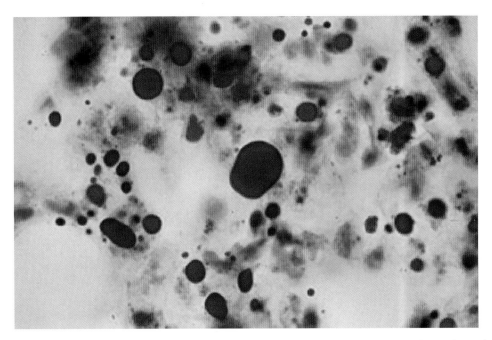

Figure 1-6. Some components of the cell can be best seen by frozen preparations, rather than the traditional methods that include dehydration and paraffin embedding. Such is the case for lipids, which are revealed here by the stain oil red O. (×400.) *(Courtesy E. Jacobson.)*

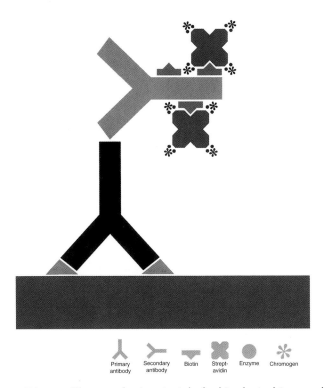

| Primary antibody | Secondary antibody | Biotin | Strept-avidin | Enzyme | Chromogen |

Figure 1-7. Diagram illustrates basic principle for histological immunolabeling.

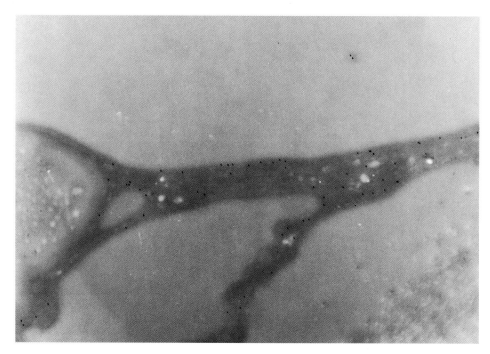

Figure 1-8. The transmission electron micrograph shows the presence of colloidal-gold immunolabel that is adhered to specific receptors for endothelin-1, a potent vasoconstrictor. (×20,000.)

before being processed (preserved, embedded, and so on) for light microscopic or ultrastructural observation. Sections that now have the radiolabel incorporated within the tissue are developed in a manner similar to that performed for photographic film. Slides with sections are coated with a photographic emulsion and stored in light-proof boxes until sufficient radioactive decay occurs, which causes the reduction of the silver bromide crystals within the film emulsion. The slides are then "developed" like sheets of film, removing the unexposed silver. This technique has allowed investigators to understand the dynamics involved in the production and breakdown of many materials formed by the cell and which organelles play a role in the dynamics.

SUGGESTED READINGS

Hayat MA: *Principles and techniques of electron microscopy: biological applications,* ed 3, Boca Raton, Fla, 1989, CRC Press.

Humason GL: *Animal tissue techniques,* ed 3, San Francisco, 1972, WH Freeman.

Maunsbach AB, Afzelius BA: *Biomedical electron microscopy: illustrated methods and interpretations,* San Diego, 1999, Academic Press.

Sheehan DC, Hrapchak BB: *Theory and practice of histotechnology,* ed 2, Columbus, Ohio, 1987, Battelle Press.

Slayter EM, Slayter HS: *Light and electron microscopy,* Cambridge, UK, 1997, Cambridge University Press.

The Cell

One could suppose that each cell has the potential to carry out an independent existence. During the process of evolution, as unicellular organisms progressed to multicellular states, cell differentiation developed, giving rise to specialized cells. Specialized cells collectively performed specific functions with greater efficiency. In vertebrates, numerous functions are performed by specialized cells including motility (muscle cell); conductivity of an electrical signal (nerve cell); synthesis and secretions of enzymes, mucous materials, steroids, and so on (pancreatic acinar cells, mucous gland cells, gonadal cells, etc.); ion transport (cells of kidney); clearance of debris and foreign materials (inflammatory cells); transformation of external and internal stimuli into nervous impulses (sensory cells); and nutrient absorption (cells of gastrointestinal tract). As the diversity of function has grown with time, there has been a concomitant development of morphological diversity, having resulted in an enormous range of cell size and shape (Figure 2-1).

Chemically, a cell consists chiefly of water, ranging from 60% to 95% of the total volume of the cell. Other components of the cell include protein, carbohydrate, fat, nucleic acids, and inorganic substances such as sodium, potassium, chloride, bicarbonate, phosphate, and ascorbate.

a double-unit membrane. Contents of the eukaryotic cell are referred to as the *protoplasm*, which is enclosed by a cell membrane. The protoplasm is subdivided into the karyoplasm, components of the nucleus, and the cytoplasm, being all cell material other than the nucleus (Figure 2-2). The cytoplasm contains a variety of distinctive and highly ordered organelles such as mitochondria, lysosomes, Golgi apparatus, smooth and rough endoplasmic reticulum, ribosomes, centrioles, microtubules, and filaments (Table 2-1). Organelles should never be thought of as static structures. They are dynamic components that can increase or decrease in size, number, and metabolic activity. In fact, their morphology can reflect the relative age and health of a given cell and corresponding tissue. Organelles are often in a state of flux, being broken down and removed, and concomitantly regenerated.

In addition to the structural parts of the cell, both the nucleus and the cytoplasm contain an amorphous ground matrix known as the **nucleoplasm** and **cytosol,** respectively. Although the terms *nucleoplasm* and *cytosol* are not clearly definable morphological entities as once thought by investigators who had only light microscopy available, they do refer to ground substances that surround the structural components of the cell.

EUKARYOTIC CELL

Eukaryotes comprise protozoa and higher forms, having true organelles, including a nucleus bounded by

NUCLEUS

The **nucleus** is the main or fundamental component of the cell, guiding the cell structurally and

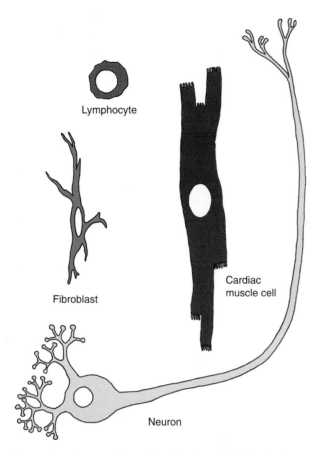

Figure 2-1. Among domestic animals, cells of the body have enormous variations in size and shape. The typical white blood cell is round and comparatively small, approximately 5 to 10 μm in diameter. The usual fibrocyte is also fairly small, but thin and relatively short at 15 to 30 μm, with short irregularly branching processes. The cardiac muscle cell, or myocyte, also has branches but they occur at each end of this cylindrically shaped cell, which can attain lengths up to 60 μm or more. The nerve cell or neuron, by comparison, possesses thin processes that have polarity and surround a round to oval cell body, where most metabolic activities occur. This cell can reach enormous lengths, up to 1 m or more in many large species.

functionally. The genetic material that it holds, deoxyribonucleic acid (DNA), directs synthesis of proteins and polypeptides through the process known as transcription. Even though the genetic information is the same throughout all cells within a single organism, it is the variation of this direction that is responsible for cell differentiation. Another equally important activity of DNA is replication, thus ensuring transcriptional activity for each new cell after division.

The interphase or somatic nucleus, which is found in the nondividing cell, consists of several structures that include chromatin, nucleoplasm, and one or more nucleoli (Figure 2-3). Light microscopically, chromatin consists of irregular clumps that have affinity for basic dyes (Figure 2-4). The chromatin actually represents tangled masses of very long slender threads of chromosomes. Electron microscopically, chromatin is arranged either in dense aggregates and referred to as **heterochromatin,** being relatively coiled chromatin, or in less tightly packed and extended configuration, forming translucent regions of the nucleus known as **euchromatin** (Figure 2-5; see also Figure 2-3). The amount of heterochromatin or lack of it may be an index to cellular activity. Cells with extensive amounts of condensed chromatin tend to be either largely inert or involved in only a major metabolic activity. In cells of female individuals, one of the sex chromosomes is clustered throughout interphase and is known as the **Barr body,** or sex chromatin (Figure 2-6). In mammalian females the Barr body is one of the X chromosomes that remain heterochromatic throughout interphase. As DNA becomes uncoiled and invisible to traditional microscopic observations, that is to say it is euchromatic, it is able to serve as a template for the three types of ribonucleic acid (RNA): messenger (mRNA), transfer (tRNA), and ribosomal (rRNA). In nuclei that are primarily euchromatic, small amounts of heterochromatin may still occur, lying next to the nuclear envelope.

The nucleus in most cell types is round to ovoid. In certain cells, however, such as mammalian leukocytes, the nucleus can be highly lobulated or in macrophages, often kidney shaped. Certain cell types may also have more than one nucleus per cell. The multinucleated condition is most familiar in skeletal muscle and is found in renal tubular cells, osteoclasts, and older hepatocytes (Figure 2-7). Although the roles that multinucleated cells play vary, they generally have a common thread in that they tend to be very active metabolically.

Within the nucleus the most discrete intranuclear structure is the **nucleolus** (see Figures 2-3, 2-5, and 2-6). The nucleolus is composed mostly of protein and RNA and a small amount of DNA (nucleolar-associated chromatin, which is involved in the transcription of ribosomal RNA). The primary function of the nucleolus is to synthesize the major components of the ribosomes (ribosomal RNA). Nucleoli are usually round and sometimes quite prominent, one micron or more in diameter. By transmission electron microscopy (TEM), two regions, the pars fibrosa, which consists of extremely fine filaments in which nucleolar chromatin is being transcribed, and the pars granulosa, which consists of granular material where ribosomal subunits are constructed, are distinguished in the nucleolus. Both regions contain ribonucleoprotein

Text continued on p. 17

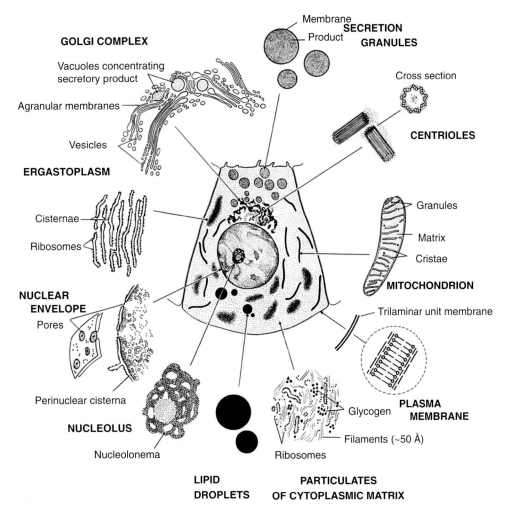

Figure 2-2. Within the cytoplasm of each mammalian cell, a complement of organelles and inclusion bodies (illustrated in this figure) is formed at some time within its life cycle. In most instances, these structures are not fully resolved by light microscopy as portrayed by the cell in the center and thus are most effectively examined with the assistance of electron microscopy. *(From Bloom W, Fawcett DW:* A textbook of histology, *ed 11, Philadelphia, 1986, Saunders.)*

TABLE 2-1	Organelles of the Cytoplasm			
TYPES OF STRUCTURES	NUCLEIC ACID ASSOCIATION	MEMBRANE ASSOCIATION	SHAPE/SIZE (DIAMETER)	FUNCTION
Ribosome	RNA (rRNA, tRNA, mRNA)	ER (rER) or unbound (polysome)	Pear-shaped; 15 × 25 nm	Polypeptide and protein synthesis
Rough endoplasmic reticulum (rER)	RNA (see ribosome)	Possesses single membrane; associated with nuclear envelope, sER	Highly variable	Polypeptide and protein synthesis with some glycosylation
Smooth endoplasmic reticulum (sER)	None	Possesses single membrane; associated with outer nuclear envelope, cell membrane, rER	Highly variable	Steroid synthesis; lipid synthesis; detoxification; calcium storage
Golgi apparatus	None	Possesses single membrane; associated with sER (from rER), vesicles (secretory and transition)	Convex-concave stack of flattened saccules of variable diameters (often 1 μm or so)	Carbohydrate synthesis; protein glycosylation (and deglycosylation) phosphorylation, and sulfation
Primary lysosome	None	Possesses single membrane; associated with Golgi apparatus, phagosomes, pinosomes, cell membrane	Round; 50 nm (and greater) in diameter	Stores hydrolytic enzymes for intracellular digestion and extracellular lysis
Peroxisome	None	Possesses single membrane; associated with sER	Approximately 500 nm (and smaller) in diameter	Stores oxidizing enzymes, especially those regulating peroxide metabolism
Mitochondrion	RNA (rRNA, tRNA, mRNA); DNA	Possesses double membranes; not directly associated with membranous organelles	Oval to cylindrical, but can be round; variable in length	Produces energy for the cell (in the form of the high-energy-bond molecules, ATP)
Melanosome	None	Possesses single membrane; associated with Golgi apparatus	Round to oval, but can be tubular; 100-500 × 500-2000 nm	Absorbs light (UV); and can function as cation exchange polymer
Centriole	DNA	No direct association	Short cylindrical; 100 × 300 nm	Microtubule organizing center for: spindle apparatus during nuclear division; and axoneme of flagella and cilia

ATP, Adenosine triphosphate; *DNA,* deoxyribonucleic acid; *ER,* endoplasmic reticulum; *RNA,* ribonucleic acid; *mRNA,* messenger ribonucleic acid; *rRNA,* ribosomal ribonucleic acid; *tRNA,* transfer ribonucleic acid; *UV,* ultraviolet.

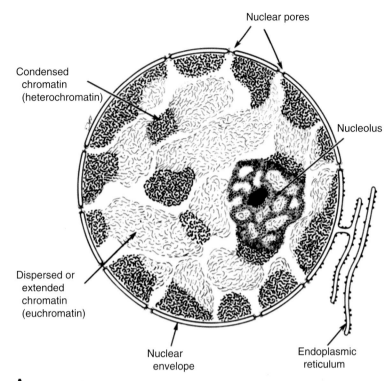

Nuclear pores

Condensed chromatin (heterochromatin)

Nucleolus

Dispersed or extended chromatin (euchromatin)

Nuclear envelope

Endoplasmic reticulum

A

Figure 2-3. Nuclei of many cells contain a combination of coiled or condensed chromatin known as *heterochromatin* (Hc) and uncoiled or extended chromatin known as *euchromatin* (Ec) **A,** Illustration of a nucleus with substantial amounts of both euchromatin and heterochromatin plus a nucleolus, which together are enclosed by a nuclear envelope. **B,** Transmission electron micrograph of a nucleus similar to that drawn in **A.** (×12,000.) Note the prominent nucleolus (Nu), which is the site of synthesis for the ribosomal subunits. *(A From Bloom W, Fawcett DW: A textbook of histology, ed 11, Philadelphia, 1986, Saunders.)*

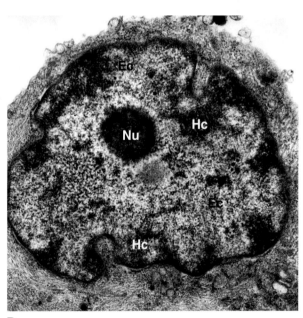

B

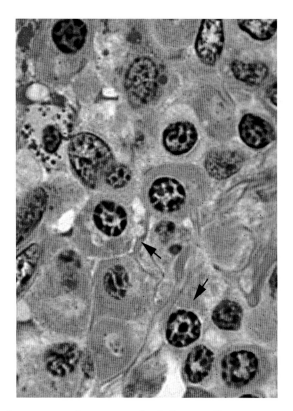

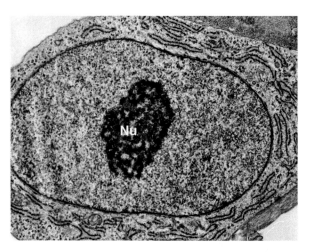

Figure 2-5. Transmission electron micrograph of a developing fibroblast and its euchromatic nucleus. The nucleus has no recognizable condensed chromatin, having instead dispersed chromatin and a prominent nucleolus (Nu), both indicators of strong metabolic activity. (×8000.)

Figure 2-4. Light micrograph of plasma cells *(arrows)* within the small intestine, with distinct round nucleoli (small nuclei) placed centrally within their nuclei. One-micron plastic section stained with H&E. (×1000.)

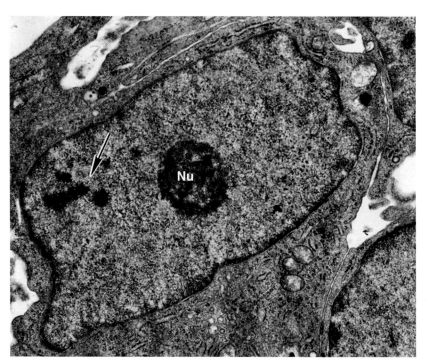

Figure 2-6. In this transmission electron micrograph taken from a female dog, the euchromatic nucleus with its central, round nucleolus (Nu) has a single area of condensed chromatin *(arrow)*, representing the second uncoiled X chromosome, also known as the *Barr body*. (×10,000.)

The nuclear envelope does not form a complete morphologic barrier between the nucleus and cytoplasm because there are numerous channels interconnecting the two regions. These channels are areas in which the inner and outer nuclear membranes fuse and are referred to as *nuclear pores* (see Figure 2-8).

The margins of nuclear pores are thickened, resulting in an octagonally arranged annulus. The annulus is closed by a thin diaphragm-like structure, which contains a central granule. The pores are primarily the passageways that allow the transport of substances between the nucleus and cytoplasm, such as the transport of RNA (mRNA and ribosomal subunits), for example. During the induction of cell division, the nuclear envelope eventually disappears, but will be reconstituted at the completion of mitosis.

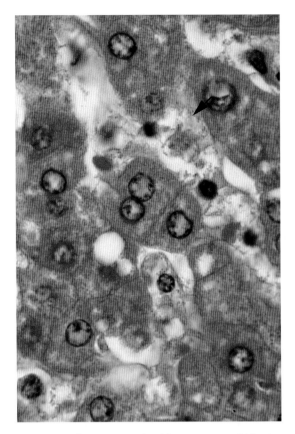

Figure 2-7. Light micrograph of hepatocytes within the liver, some binucleated *(arrow)*. One-micron plastic section stained with H&E. (×1000.)

CYTOPLASM

The cytoplasm surrounds the nucleus and is encased by the cell membrane. It is that region of the cell involved in energy formation and release, protein synthesis, growth, motility, and phagocytosis. It is dependent on the nucleus for direction, renewal, and regeneration.

The volume of the cytoplasm in proportion to the nucleus—the nuclear/cytoplasmic ratio—is variable from one cell type to another and changes during cell development. This ratio can be used as an indicator of a cell's stage of development, or lack thereof, or changes associated within disease.

The cytoplasm can be subdivided into regions or zones based on the general location of organelles and consistency (Figure 2-9). The cytoplasm next to the nucleus is named the **cytocentrum** and consists of a narrow, gelatinous region, which is generally void of organelles except for endoplasmic reticulum attached to the nuclear envelope, a pair of centrioles, and cytoskeletal elements (see Figure 2-8). Adjacent to the cytocentrum is the **endoplasm,** the largest region of the cytoplasm. The endoplasm is less viscous and houses most of the structural components of the cytoplasm. Active cytoplasmic streaming occurs here, as well as most metabolic activities. External to the endoplasm and adjacent to the cell or plasma membrane is a very narrow band called the **ectoplasm.** As in the cytocentrum this region has few organelles and is jelly-like. In motile cells (wandering histiocytes) numerous microfilaments may be found here. The ectoplasm typically plays a very integral role with the cell membrane. The general nature of the cytoplasm with all of its subcomponents can show the relative health of the cell(s) and tissue. Each cell type has its

precursors of future ribosomes, which are eventually assembled in the cytoplasm, and together form a distinct network with its moth-eaten appearance that is sometimes called the **nucleolonema.**

The somatic nucleus is separated from the cytoplasm by a double membrane structure, the nuclear envelope (Figure 2-8). Each membrane is approximately 70 Å in thickness and separated by a perinuclear space or cistern of 150 Å or more. The inner membrane is lined by a filamentous mat known as the *nuclear lamina.* This mat most likely serves as scaffolding for chromatin and associated proteins. The outer nuclear membrane is often continuous with a system of membranous sheets known as the *endo-plasmic reticulum,* particularly **rough endoplasmic reticulum** (rER). As the rER extends from the outer membrane of the nuclear envelope, the cisterns of the rER and the nuclear envelope are contiguous. The close association of the nuclear envelope with the endoplasmic reticulum system is further supported by the role the endoplasmic reticulum plays during reformation of the nuclear envelope during mitotic or meiotic telophase as segments of the endoplasmic reticulum line-up around the reconstituted nuclear mass.

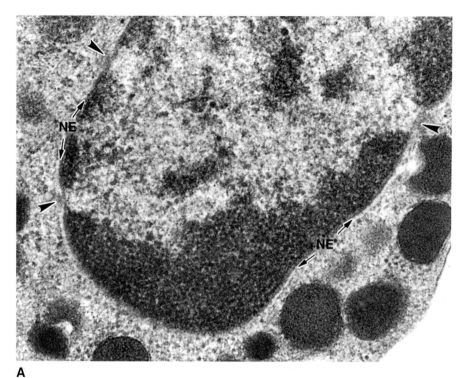

A

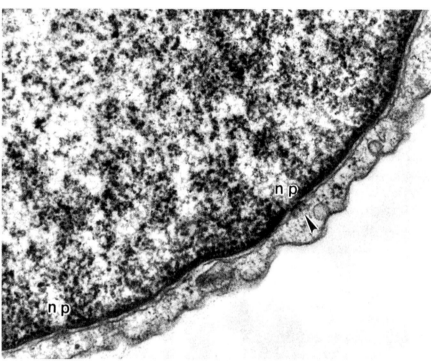

B

Figure 2-8. Nuclear envelope. **A,** Transmission electron micrograph of a nucleus and surrounding nuclear envelope (NE) of a mast cell. (×30,000.) The nuclear pores *(arrowheads)* occur in regions where euchromatin exists. **B,** In this transmission electron micrograph, two nuclear pores (np) are visible, one of which has cytoplasmic subunits *(arrowhead).* (×50,000)

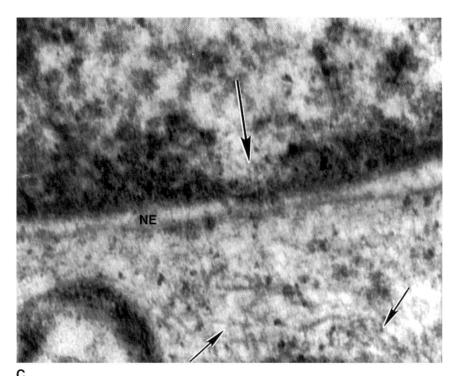

C

Figure 2-8, cont'd C, Transmission electron micrograph of the nuclear envelope *(NE),* with the peripheral edge of a nuclear pore and its nucleoplasmic subunits *(large arrow)* next to the inner membrane, which is lined by the nuclear lamina and associated condensed chromatin. Note the presence of fine filaments *(small arrows)* within the cytoplasm next to the outer membrane of the nuclear envelope. (×120,000.) **D,** Transmission electron micrograph of a tangential section of a nucleus *(N)* reveals the round shape of nuclear pores *(arrows)* as viewed face-on. (×25,000.)

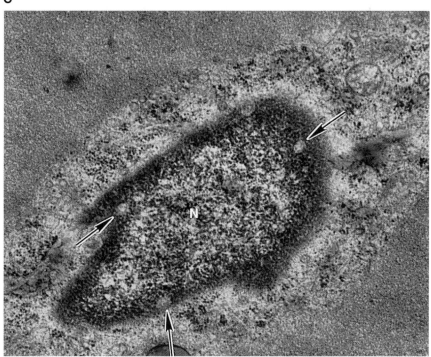

D

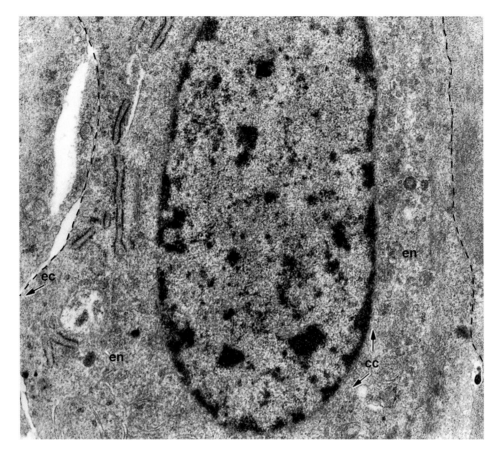

Figure 2-9. Transmission electron micrograph of a cell and its cytoplasm and centrally placed nucleus. Immediately surrounding the nucleus is a thin region called the *cytocentrum (cc)*, which is composed mostly of filaments and microtubules. Most of the organelles lie outside the cytocentrum in the endoplasm *(en)*. Next to the cell membrane *(dotted line)* is another thin layer of cytoskeletal elements known as the *ectoplasm (ec)*. (×12,000.)

own cytoplasmic makeup or composition, and it is imperative that we recognize the traits of healthy cells and tissues so that signs of stress and disease become recognizable.

Endoplasmic Reticulum

The **endoplasmic reticulum** is a cytoplasmic structure that is closely associated with the nuclear envelope, being often continuous with the outer nuclear membrane as previously described. This organelle is composed of a system of membrane-lined tubules, vesicles, and sacs or cisternae. Development and amount of endoplasmic reticulum within the cytoplasm depends on cell type, age, and region within the cell. It is typically the most common organelle in any given cell. Two types have been characterized structurally and functionally and are referred to as *smooth* and *rough*. **Smooth endoplasmic reticulum** (sER) has a variety of functions, including steroid hormone production, storage and delivery of high levels of calcium,

carbohydrate synthesis, detoxification, and lipid complexing from fatty acids. Ultrastructurally, sER consists of an often convoluted arrangement of membranous tubules (Figure 2-10). Certain cells such as muscle fibers and hormone-producing cells are amply endowed with this organelle, comprising much of the cell's total volume. It is possible to visualize sER light microscopically by using a variation of the silver impregnation technique. In most cells sER amounts to a very small portion of the total cytoplasm and is most commonly found at areas where rER gives rise to vesicles, many (transfer vesicles) of which are moved to another organelle, the Golgi apparatus.

rER is similar to sER, with the additional presence of ribosomes (Figure 2-11). Morphologically, rER, which is sometimes called *granular ER* (sER being agranular), consists of interconnecting membrane-bound flattened sacs that are lined by ribosomes. Functionally, rER synthesizes protein and further assembles protein into larger molecules, which are usually packaged and eventually released as secretory

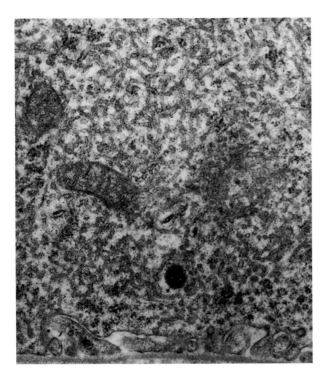

Figure 2-10. Transmission electron micrograph of sheep pigment epithelium shows an extensive system of smooth endoplasmic reticulum with numerous membranous tubules. (×20,000.)

vesicles directly or from the Golgi apparatus. The actual synthesis of protein is performed by the ribosome.

Ribosomes

Ribosomes are extremely minute structures, being beyond the limit of resolution of the light microscope. However, clusters of ribosomes can be detected by basic stains because of the presence of RNA. This is particularly true for a mat or layer of rER, which is referred to as an *ergastoplasm*. In certain cells such as neurons, the presence of stained rER and ribosomes (Nissl bodies) is used to identify specific portions (dendrites, soma) of the cell. In active B lymphocytes the cytoplasm, which becomes filled with ribosomes, characteristically stains basophilically and is readily identified for that property. At high magnification, a bipartite, pear-shaped structure is revealed, measuring 15×25 nm. Each part or subunit consists of RNA, derived from the nucleolus, and protein. The subunits lie separate from each other in the cytosol until they become associated with a strand of mRNA at which time they will become bound together. Ribosomes are responsible for the formation of polypeptides. Polypeptide synthesis will not occur until they are linked with mRNA. The smaller of the two subunits binds mRNA (Figure 2-12). After this linkage occurs the ribosomes receive amino acid constituents by tRNA. As the ribosomes go along a thread of mRNA, amino acids are being added to the base of the ribosomal complex at the larger subunit. The larger subunit also forms part of the tRNA binding site, catalyzes the peptidyl transfer, holds the growing polypeptide chain and attaches the ribosome to the endoplasmic reticulum. The transient attachment of the ribosomes to endoplasmic reticulum is due to the presence of proteinaceous receptors called *ribophorins*. The smaller unit is also needed for the binding site of tRNA. Ribosomal translation can equally occur freely in the cytoplasm without endoplasmic reticulum association. Chains of ribosomes, which move along single strands of the mRNA template unassociated with endoplasmic reticulum, are called **polysomes** (see Figure 2-11, *D*). Ribosomes and rER are most highly developed in young growing cells and mature cells (glandular cells, plasma cells, neurons, fibroblasts) that are actively secreting.

Golgi Apparatus

The **Golgi apparatus,** or **Golgi complex,** is an organelle that is intimately associated with the endoplasmic reticulum system. The Golgi apparatus within a cell consists of clusters of stacks of flattened membranous sacs that are involved in carbohydrate synthesis (see Figure 2-2). Unless impregnated with a heavy metal, such as silver salts, the Golgi apparatus is difficult to observe histologically. Using traditional stains (hematoxylin and eosin [H&E]), its presence can be implied by its weak staining reaction, which results in a negative Golgi image. Each cluster may be referred to as a *dictyosome*, and neighboring dictyosomes are usually interconnected by a system of sER (Figure 2-13). The convex or proximal face of the dictyosome is the forming face (cis-face), which is either directly connected to rER through sER or indirectly through the transfer vesicles that outpocket from the rER and eventually fuse with the forming face of what will become a saccule (Figure 2-14). Within each dictyosome the stack of parallel saccules is interconnected by a network of tubules. It is within the cisternal lumen of each saccule that protein becomes glycosylated, phosphorylated, sulfated and so on. As the modifications come to completion, the protein enters the final saccule, which forms the distal face of the Golgi apparatus. The distal, or concave, face is the maturing side (trans-face) from which **secretory vesicles** are formed. The membranes of the maturing face are slightly thicker than the forming face and may be related to the processing and pack-

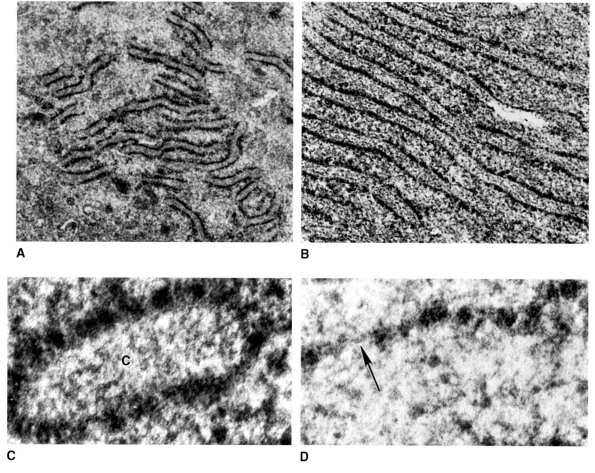

Figure 2-11. Rough endoplasmic reticulum and ribosomes. **A,** In this transmission electron micrograph, the rough endoplasmic reticulum is arranged interconnecting layers of flattened membranous sacs. (×15,000.) **B,** At higher magnification, individual ribosomes can be distinguished along each sac. (×25,000.) **C,** Outline of a sac seen in cross section at high magnification. C, Cisterna. (×200,000.) **D,** Ribosomes can also be arranged in chains called *polysomes* as seen in this transmission electron micrograph. Arrow points to the strand of mRNA to which the ribosomes have become attached. (×180,000.)

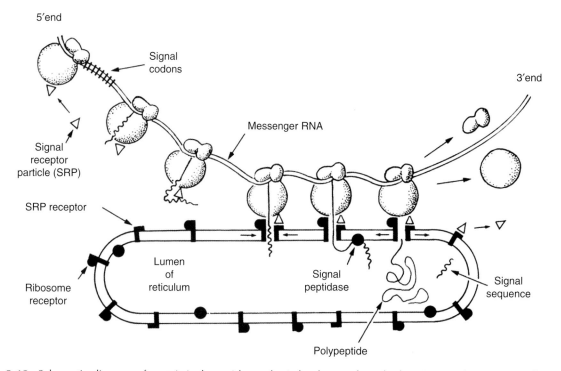

Figure 2-12. Schematic diagram of protein/polypeptide synthesis by the rough endoplasmic reticulum. *(From Bloom W, Fawcett DW: A textbook of histology, ed 11, Philadelphia, 1986, Saunders.)*

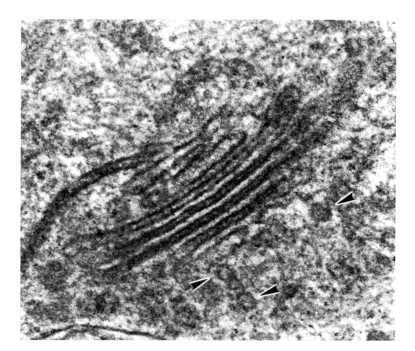

Figure 2-13. Transmission electron micrograph of a portion of the Golgi apparatus in a secreting cell. Arrowheads point to transitional vesicles that arise from rER and fuse with the convex forming face. (×60,000.)

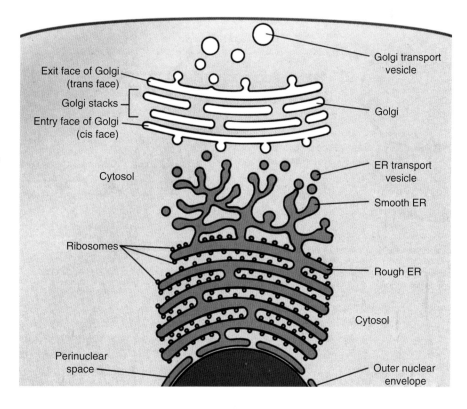

Figure 2-14. Schematic diagram of the membranous interrelationships between rER, sER, and the Golgi apparatus within the cell. *ER, Endoplasmic reticulum. (From Bergman RA, Afifi AK, Heidger PM Jr: Histology, Philadelphia, 1996, Saunders.)*

Labels in figure: Exit face of Golgi (trans face); Golgi stacks; Entry face of Golgi (cis face); Cytosol; Ribosomes; Perinuclear space; Golgi transport vesicle; Golgi; ER transport vesicle; Smooth ER; Rough ER; Cytosol; Outer nuclear envelope

aging of proteins, lipids, and carbohydrates that will be subsequently secreted.

Secretory proteins that are stored before secretion form precursor structures known as condensing vacuoles or vesicles. Secretory vesicles may be stored for some time before they are released or they may migrate quickly to the cell surface, where they are released from the cell by a process called *exocytosis.* Exocytosis involves the fusion of the vesicle's membrane with the cell's limiting membrane. When this fusion occurs, an opening to extracellular environment is formed and the contents of the secretory vesicle are released. The size and development of the Golgi apparatus within a cell depend largely on the metabolic activity and type of activity of the cell. As one might guess, Golgi apparatuses are most prominent in glandular cells, for example. With the assistance of radioactive-labeling experiments, it has been shown in active glandular cells that only 1 to 2 hours are required for newly synthesized protein to be modified, packaged, and secreted through the Golgi apparatus.

Lysosomes

Lysosomes comprise a class of membrane-bound vesicles that hold a variety of lytic enzymes. Under normal circumstances the lytic enzymes, which include acid phosphatase, acid hydrolase, lysozyme, and so on, will not permeate the vesicle's membrane and cause considerable metabolic disruption. These organelles, which may be present in all types of cells at some point in time, are extremely abundant in phagocytic cells (macrophages and eosinophils, for example). Lysosomes, which function basically as the digestive system of the cell, are formed mostly as coated vesicles that originate from the transmost face of a Golgi complex. These vesicles shed their coat of clathrin and become smooth vesicles—the **primary lysosomes**—that fuse with either phagosomes or pinosomes to form **secondary lysosomes** in which intracellular digestion will then occur. Recent classification has distinguished the lysosome as one component of the acid vesicle system, which requires an acid environment for lytic enzymes to be active. To that end, lysosomal membranes usually possess proton pumps (H$^+$-adenosine triphosphatase [ATPase]) that ensures an effective low pH. Approximately 40 acid hydrolase enzymes are known to occur in lysosomes, each involved in the digestion of carbohydrates, proteins, or lipids as well as their derivatives.

A phagosome is a membrane-bound vesicle, resulting from cellular ingestion of particulate matter such as a bacterium by invagination of the cell membrane **(heterophagosome)** or from the segregation of old or damaged organelles by joining segments of smooth endoplasmic reticulum **(autophagosome)** (Figure 2-15). A pinosome, or endosome is a membrane-bound vesicle that was formed from the cellular ingestion of fluid matter by a process referred to as **endocytosis.** All pinosomes are not phagocytized. Many, in fact, are involved in the normal transferance of substances into the cell **(transcytosis)** that otherwise cannot pass through the cell membrane. Catabolites will diffuse from the secondary lysosomes and enter the cytoplasm, and any material that cannot be broken down will be retained in the vesicle, now referred to as a

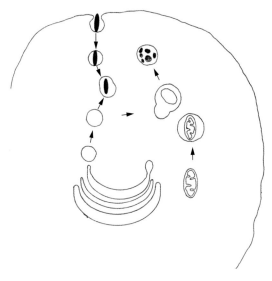

Figure 2-15. Lysosomal system. Derived from the Golgi apparatus, lysosomes can degrade either old or damaged organelles or substances taken into the cell by either phagocytosis or pinocytosis.

residual body, and either immediately expelled from the cell or lie freely for some time in the cytoplasm. A high number of lysosomes in a cell that usually possesses few or none at all often indicate stress and disease. As cells grow older, especially during aging, a buildup of residual bodies known as **lipofuscin** occurs. This gradual buildup is particularly true in nervous tissue and is considered to be a normal aging process. Malfunction of lysosomes can lead to a number of disorders, generally known as *lysosomal storage disease*. One of the most important lysosomal storage diseases of animals is **mannosidosis,** which is the result of either a deficiency or an inhibition of alpha mannosides. Deficiency is usually hereditary, whereas inhibition is nutritional resulting from the ingestion of certain plants including locoweeds (*Astragalus* and *Oxytropis*) that contain indolizidine alkaloids.

Peroxisome

The **peroxisome,** or **microbody,** is a spherical or oval membrane-bound vesicle, up to 0.5 μm in diameter, that contains a variety of oxidizing enzymes, including catalase, peroxidase, uric acid, and amino acid oxidases, and those involved in μ-oxidation breakdown of long chain fatty acids to acetyl-coenzyme A (CoA). These enzymes, particularly catalase and peroxidase, are involved in the regulation of H$_2$O$_2$ metabolism, which are associated with various oxidative reactions such as the electron transport system of the mitochondrion. Specifically, hydrogen peroxide is hydrolyzed to oxygen and water. Peroxisomes are formed directly from the endoplasmic reticulum and have been classified based on various inclusion bodies that have been observed by TEM within these vesicles. These bodies, which are dense or crystalline in appearance, are called **nucleoids** and are species specific (Figure 2-16). Peroxisomes are typically found in certain cell types such as a liver cell (hepatocyte) and the kidney (epithelium of proximal convoluted tubules). Their numbers can be influenced by changes in age, diet, hormones, and drugs. In most cells they are infrequent and difficult to distinguish unless cytochemically stained (for peroxidase activity).

Mitochondria

Second to the nucleus, the **mitochondrion** is the most essential organelle in the eukaryotic cell, being present in all cells except erythrocytes of blood, mature lens fibers of the eye, and terminal keratinocytes of the skin's epidermis. It is this structure that provides energy for the rest of the cell. Most cells rely on the glycolytic and citric acid pathways for their major sources of energy. Enzymes for the citric acid pathway, as well as those for oxidative phosphorylation, reside in the mitochondrion. Mitochondria are generally tubular (cigar shaped) in form (see Figure 2-2). However, this organelle can be quite pleomorphic,

being twisted or bent or even spindly and branched (*mitos*, Greek for thread). Early microanatomists recognized mitochondria as elementary components of the cell. In more recent times, mitochondria have been proposed to be of prokaryote origin because of a variety of characteristics including the presence of nucleoid-like circular DNA, their own RNA, ribosome-associated protein, and their ability to divide independently from the rest of the cell. Ultrastructurally, they are a double membranous structure, with the outer membrane being smooth and thin, approximately 6.0 to 6.5 nm thick (Figure 2-17). The outer membrane contains many multipass transmembrane proteins called **porins** that form portals for water-soluble molecules of considerable size to move through. Because of the relatively leaky nature of the outer membrane, it is not unusual to observe ultrastructurally fairly wide spaces between the inner and outer membranes of mitochondria that can be exaggerated by disease. The inner membrane is folded into cristae, having a slightly narrower thickness. This membrane contrasts sharply with the outer membrane in a number of ways. The membrane lacks porins and instead contains **cardiolipin,** a phospholipid that makes the inner membrane very tight and nearly impermeable to all materials. Within the inner

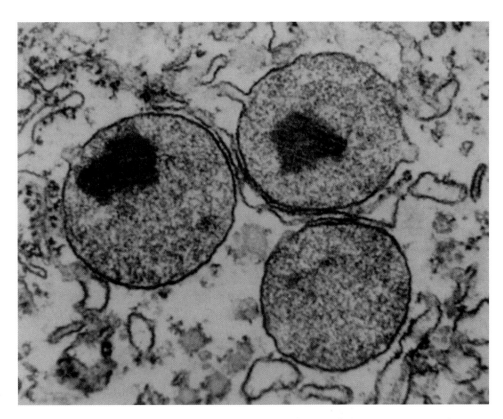

Figure 2-16. Transmission electron micrograph of three peroxisomes from rat hepatocytes. *(From Bloom W, Fawcett DW: A textbook of histology, ed 11, Philadelphia, 1986, Saunders.)*

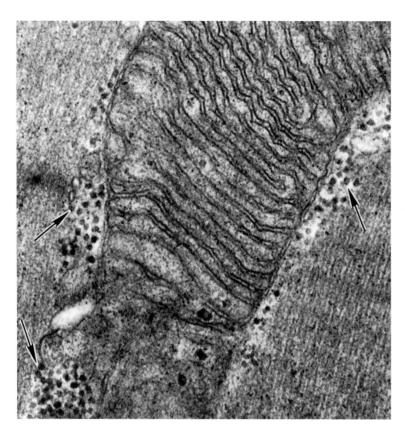

Figure 2-17. Transmission electron micrograph of a mitochondrion from canine skeletal muscle. The cristae are tightly packed, and within the matrix there are occasional granules. Arrows point to the glycogen that surrounds the mitochondrion. (×75,000.)

membrane, including the cristae, are particles that represent sites of adenosine triphosphate (ATP) synthase complexes. In between these complexes are enzymes responsible for electron transport and thus form the electron transport chain (Figure 2-18).

Most of the volume of the mitochondrion consists of the matrix, which houses the enzymes needed for aerobic respiration (Krebs cycle). The ATP that is ultimately formed is either used by the organelle or moved into the cytosol through an adenosine diphosphate (ADP)-ATP antiport system. Throughout the catabolic process involving glycolysis and the Krebs cycle, 1 molecule of glucose will result in the production of 36 molecules of ATP. Glucose metabolism will not always yield high amounts of ATP. There are instances in which oxidation is not coupled with phosphorylation, resulting in heat rather than high-energy molecules. This uncoupling requires a proton shunt, consisting of **thermogenin,** which is not able to produce ATP but does resemble ATP synthase.

Within the matrix are granules that possess divalent cation binding sites (see Figure 2-17). These granules increase in number and size as cation concentrations within the cell are raised above apparent critical levels. Thus there are two organelles—

the mitochondrion and smooth endoplasmic reticulum—within the cell that are able to play a role in the regulation of certain cation levels within the cell.

STORAGE STRUCTURES OF THE CELL

Many cells have the capability to store compounds as potential energy reserves that can be used at a later time for catabolic activity. Specifically, glucose is stored in the form of **glycogen,** and triglycerides are stored as **lipids.** Glycogen appears ultrastructurally as clusters of small opaque particles that individually measure from 15 to 30 nm in diameter (see Figure 2-17). The presence of this storage structure is common in muscle cells, especially striated forms, and hepatocytes of liver. Histologically, they can be revealed by employing the periodic acid–Schiff stain for carbohydrates (see Figure 1-4). Lipids, however, are seen as round, vacuole-like bodies, whose contents can only be revealed when properly prepared (see Figure 1-6). The solvents normally used for histological processing and embedding extract the triglycerides and leave transparent lipid droplets, or locules.

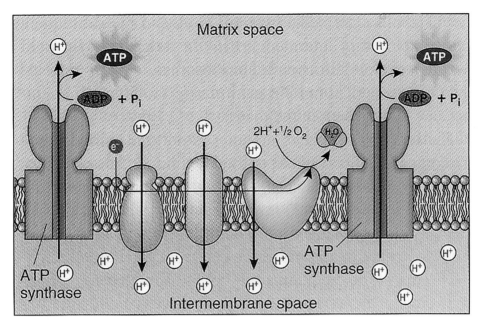

Figure 2-18. Diagram displays a functional portion of a crista, including two ATP synthase complexes and three of the five members of the electron transport chain that also function to pump protons from the matrix into the intermembrane space. *(From Gartner LP, Hiatt JL:* Color textbook of histology, *Philadelphia, 1997, Saunders.)*

CYTOSKELETON OF THE CELL

The cell possesses an infrastructural support system that consists of filaments (solid protein rod-line components) and microtubules. These structures are largely responsible for the overall shape of the cell, its movement, its division, and intracellular transportation of most cytoplasmic materials. Although all cells are equipped with some kind of cytoskeleton, being primarily located within the ectoplasm and to a lesser degree within the cytocentrum, certain cell types, including muscle fibers, fibroblasts, neurons, glial cells, and keratinizing epithelial cells, have especially well-developed cytoskeletons.

Filaments are traditionally divided into three types or categories: microfilaments, intermediate filaments, and myosin filaments.

COMPONENTS OF THE CYTOSKELETON

Microfilaments, or thin filaments, are long, thin threads or strands that supply structural support for the cytoplasm, being mostly deposited beneath the cell membrane and around the nucleus (Figures 2-19 and 2-20). **Actin** is the major type of microfilament, being approximately 6 nm in diameter and up to 1 μm in

length. Actin is especially well developed in cells involved in pino- and phagocytosis, motility (by ameboid action), movement of materials (presence of microvilli), and production of certain extracellular substances (glycosaminoglycans). Although most cells are usually well equipped with these microfilaments, in certain cells, smooth and striated muscle, they comprise the largest body of subcellular structures and are better known as **actin myofilaments** (α-actin). In addition to α-actin, there are also two other forms of actin (β-actin and γ-actin), both occurring in non-muscle cells.

Intermediate filaments comprise a heterogeneous group of filaments that are approximately 8 to 10 nm in diameter and noncontractile in function. At least five major classes have been determined based on their protein composition, including **cytokeratin** (prekeratin and tonofilament), **desmin, glial filaments** (glial fibrillary acidic protein), **neurofilament,** and **vimentin** (Figure 2-21). Construction of intermediate filaments, in general, consists of helically arrayed tetramers of proteinaceous rods.

Tonofilaments, which are members of the cytokeratin class, are one of the more common or ubiquitous members of intermediate filaments, consisting of strands 8 nm in diameter that are primarily involved in junctional complex structural elements, that is, **desmosomes. Desmin** filaments are associated with

Figure 2-19. Transmission electron micrograph of numerous microfilaments within a canine fibroblast. (×60,000.)

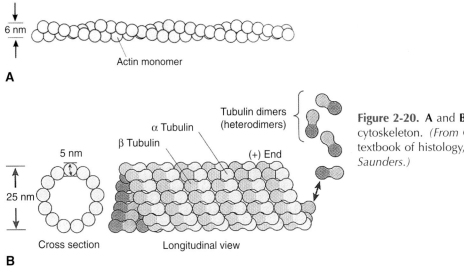

Figure 2-20. A and **B,** Diagram of elements of the cytoskeleton. *(From Gartner LP, Hiatt JL: Color textbook of histology, Philadelphia, 1997, Saunders.)*

cells that are able to contract, the **myocytes** of muscle. These filaments help maintain the organization of the contractile filaments within these cells. Like desmin, glial filaments and neurofilaments are less common than actin, occurring in glial cells **(astrocytes)** and **neurons,** respectively.

Myosin myofilament comprises a third and largest (with regard to size) class of microfilaments, being approximately 12 to 15 nm in diameter. Myosin filaments were once thought to be found only in cells modified for contractile purposes (muscle and myoepithelial cells) and in direct contact with actin myofilaments. Myosin is, in fact, found in most cells and may move only actin filaments (myosin-II) or actin and a variety of other cytoplasmic structures, including vesicles (myosin-I).

Microtubules are the largest component of the cytoskeletal system, comprised of tubulin (see Figure 2-20), that are helically arranged to form a hollow cylinder, approximately 24 nm in diameter or about twice the diameter of a myosin filament. Whereas microfilaments offer elasticity, connectivity, and con-

tractibility, microtubules provide true cytostructural support. Other functions include intracellular transport, motility, and cell division. Cytoplasmic microtubules and those within cilia are relatively stable, whereas microtubules associated with the mitotic apparatus are easily assembled and disassembled. Construction of a microtubule consists of the assembly or disassembly of heterodimers of this structural protein (tubulin α and β), which are arranged spirally, forming 13 parallel protofilaments.

CELL MEMBRANE

The cell or **plasma membrane,** also known as the **plasmalemma,** is possibly the most dynamic component of the cell, continually undergoing changes due to both external and internal influences. The cell membrane, which provides a semipermeable boundary, is approximately 8 to 11 nm thick and is not visible light microscopically. When viewed by the electron microscope, the cell membrane and all other protoplasmic membranes, for example, those comprising the various organelles, consist of a trilaminar structure with two thin opaque layers or bands encompassing a single transparent layer (Figure 2-22). Biochemically, membranes consist of roughly two thirds protein, one third lipid (phospholipid and cholesterol), and 5% or less carbohydrate. Consequently, the lamellated structure led scientists to believe that protoplasmic membranes were composed of a basic phospholipid leaflet with hydrophobic groups (fatty acid chains facing each other) directed toward the middle and hydrophilic (polar head) groups directed toward the outside, with this bimolecular leaflet encased by single layers of protein. With the advent of a technique known as *freeze-fracture* in which cells are

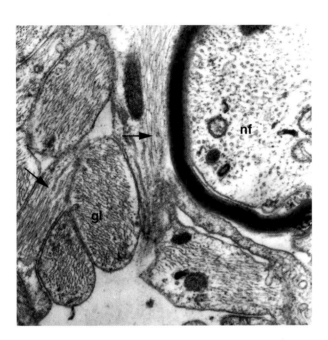

Figure 2-21. In this transmission electron micrograph intermediate filaments *(arrows)* heavily populate the cytoplasm of the supporting glial cells *(gl)* that surround nerve fibers *(nf)* within the canine central nervous system. (×5000.)

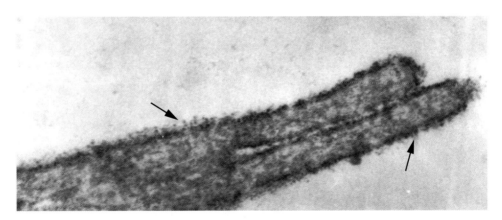

Figure 2-22. Transmission electron micrograph of the cell membrane of a vascular endothelial cell. Arrows point to the carbohydrate moieties associated with the external surface of the cell membrane, referred to as the *glycocalyx*. The glycocalyx has been revealed by using a special localization technique with colloidal iron. (×110,000.)

directly frozen in liquid nitrogen and then cleaved, artifacts that could arise as a result of standard preparatory procedures for TEM, including protein denaturation, were avoided and the model of the "unit" membrane was revised. The more recent model rejects the idea of protein naturally forming layers over the phospholipid and instead places the protein within the lipid leaflet. Protein bodies can completely cross the lipid leaflet, some of which are believed to provide channels for water-soluble materials (Figure 2-23). Proteins located within the cell membrane are **integral proteins,** and those that span the entire thickness are **transmembrane proteins.** Keep in mind, the bodies of protein are not thought to be fixed in position, but lie adrift in a sea of lipid, influenced by external and internal factors. Other proteins lying adjacent to the lipid leaflet are **peripheral proteins,** which may be associated with polysaccharides (cell coat) as well (see Figure 2-22). In all, at least five categories of proteins can be associated functionally with the cell membrane (Table 2-2):

1. Channel proteins, which permit movement of ions and small molecules in and out of the cell, for example, gap junctions
2. Carrier proteins, which transport substances across the cell membrane in a binding-unbinding process

TABLE 2-2	Cell Membrane Protein
TYPE	**FUNCTION**
Channel proteins	Provide conduits or pores for ions such as Ca^+, Na^+, K^+, H^+ and Cl^-. Move in and out of the cell at a rate similar to that of diffusion, or from one cell to another as in the case of gap junctions. If they can be opened or closed in response to signals, they are referred to as *gated channels*.
Carrier proteins	Bind site-specific substances that are then transported across the cell membrane in a binding-unbinding process.
Enzymes	As a form of carrier proteins, specific enzymes such as Na^+/K^+- ATPase, are used for active transport and involve specific binding, using energy from ATP hydrolysis.
Receptors	Bind specifically to external signaling molecules for the purpose of transmitting and transducing information into the cell. Examples of external signaling molecules include hormones and neurotransmitters. Receptors can, in turn, open and close ligand-gated channels or activate and inactivate ligand-dependent enzyme activity.
Structural proteins	Form cell-to-cell connections or junctions, such as the zonula occludens (tight junction) that forms a morphological barrier between adjacent cells.

ATP, Adenosine triphosphate; *ATPase,* adenosine triphosphatase.

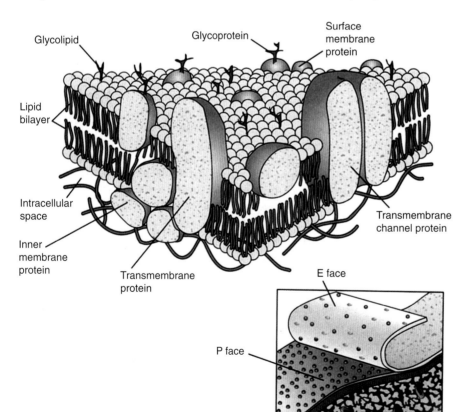

Figure 2-23. Diagram of the fluid mosaic model of cell membrane. *(From Bergman RA, Afifi AK, Heidger PM Jr: Histology, Philadelphia, 1996, Saunders.)*

Glycolipid

Glycoprotein

Surface membrane protein

Lipid bilayer

Intracellular space

Inner membrane protein

Transmembrane protein

Transmembrane channel protein

E face

P face

3. Enzymes, such as ATPase, which work as pumps that actively transport selective ions such as sodium
4. Receptor proteins, which recognize and bind specific substances (ligands) to the cell membrane
5. Structural proteins, which are involved in the formation of certain cell junctions such as tight junctions (see Chapter 3)

CELL CYCLE

Cells periodically undergo a cycle that alternates between **mitosis,** or cell division, which consists of a sequence of events involving the division of the nucleus and the cytoplasm, and **interphase,** which in many cell types span a considerably longer time frame than mitosis and include metabolic activities inherent for the growth and maturation of each cell and subsequent replication of genetic material before the next cell division. In some instances cells lose the ability to divide any further—they become terminally differentiated, as in the case of neurons and muscle cells and a variety of other types of cells located in different tissues of the body. These cell types have essentially left the cell cycle and remain in a **resting stage.**

Cells that continue to self-replicate at some later time have an interphase that is subdivided into three periods or phases: the **gap ($G)_1$ phase, G_2 phase,** and **synthetic (S) phase.** Cells derived from mitosis enter the G_1 phase, which involves the reestablishment of metabolic activities including RNA and protein syntheses, some of which are essential for the replication of DNA. The cell volume, which had been previously reduced in half by the division of the cytoplasm (referred to as **cytokinesis**) at the end of mitosis, is replenished during this phase. Proteins (protein kinases and cyclins) that can initiate another mitosis are most likely manufactured during this period of the cell cycle. The failure to produce these proteins results

in the cessation of cell cycle renewal, and the cell has ended in a resting phase also known as the G_0 **phase.**

In the presence of the appropriate kinases and cyclins, the cell enters the **S phase,** which involves duplication of the cell's genome, including both DNA and associated nucleoprotein. From the S phase, the cell enters the G_2 **phase,** and its activity becomes focused on the production of the protein, including tubulin for microtubule assembly and RNA necessary for mitosis to occur.

At the end of the G_2 phase, the cell is ready to divide and enter the **mitosis (M) phase,** consisting of both nuclear and cytoplasmic division. Mitotic events occur sequentially, with each event given a specific name: prophase, prometaphase, metaphase, anaphase, telophase, and cytokinesis. **Prophase** is indicated by concomitant changes in the cell body and its nucleus. The cell, which has become already appreciably enlarged, loses any previously formed processes, and the chromosomes become visible microscopically as each condenses into parallel pairs of identical (sister) chromatids, which are joined at the **centromere.** The centriole-containing region next to the nucleus, the **centrosome,** has divided and moves to opposite poles of the cell. During this process, each pair of centrioles establishes a **microtubule-organizing center** (MTOC) from which the **mitotic spindle apparatus** with its astral rays and spindle fibers is made (Figure 2-24). Some of the microtubules associated with this apparatus from opposite poles will attach to each centromere. Concomitantly, cytoplasmic microtubules are disassembled.

At this point, the nuclear envelope begins to disappear and the nucleolus disintegrates. The stage known as **prometaphase** has now begun. Within the inner lining of the nuclear envelope, the nuclear lamina undergoes phosphorylation, which contributes to the disappearance of the bimembrane structure. Within each centromere a kinetochore is formed to which **mitotic spindle microtubules** of the

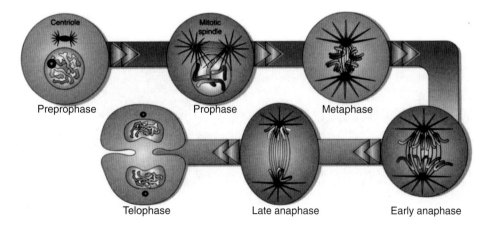

Figure 2-24. Stages of mitosis. A schematic series demonstrates the sequence of stages that occur during mitosis. *(From Bergman RA, Afifi AK, Heidger PM Jr: Histology, Philadelphia, 1996, Saunders.)*

Preprophase　　Prophase　　Metaphase

Telophase　　Late anaphase　　Early anaphase

MTOC become attached. These microtubules form the spindle fibers that facilitate the migration of the sister chromosomes to the opposite poles. Other microtubules not involved in this process are called **polar microtubules,** which undoubtedly contributes to the overall structural organization of the mitotic spindle apparatus and spacing of chromosomes during mitosis.

At **metaphase,** chromosomes become fully condensed and are aligned in a single row, defining the equator of the mitotic spindle (see Figure 2-24). The "arms" of each chromosome are now bent in the direction of the pole that they will be moving to.

As the kinetochore of each chromosome splits, the sister chromatids pull apart and migrate to each pole. Nuclear division has now entered **anaphase,** and each complement of chromosomes for their respective new cells can be distinguished. Spindle microtubules are believed to be depolymerized at the kinetochore in a manner similar to that occurring during cytoplasmic streaming. At the same time, polar microtubules lengthen further, causing the spindle poles to be pushed at greater distance from one another. Near the end of this phase, early events of cytokinesis can be observed, including the initiation of the cleavage furrow with the invagination of the cell membrane.

With the end of the chromosomal migration, **telophase,** the final phase of karyokinesis, begins (see Figure 2-24). The spindle apparatus breaks down and the nuclear envelope is reconstituted. The chromosomes uncoil into euchromatin and heterochromatin that are characteristic for that cell type during interphase. The nucleolus is concomitantly reestablished as well.

MEIOSIS

In reproductive organs, germ cells for each gender are produced with half of the diploid set of chromosomes that typically exist in most somatic cells. This amount of DNA is known as the *haploid* number of chromosomes that are carried by ova and spermatozoa and, when combined, ensures the recombination of genetic information. Nuclear division that reduces the diploid condition to the haploid one is referred to as *meiosis*, which will be covered later (see Chapters 18 and 19).

CELL DEATH

A substantial change in an individual cell's activities, especially resulting from a significant insult and subsequent damage, can often lead to its death. When observing cell death morphologically within mammalian tissues, one of two processes usually occurs: necrosis or apoptosis. These processes were initially recognized by ultrastructural observations and can be seen with careful scrutiny with a light microscope. Both processes consist of a sequence of morphological events.

NECROSIS

In many instances of necrosis, cellular injury and subsequent death progress gradually. For that reason, morphological abnormalities can be observed with some frequency. Early events include cytosolic swelling and blebbing (Figure 2-25). Mitochondria become dilated and the cristae are fewer and less noticeable than the normal condition. Cisternae of smooth and rough endoplasmic reticula as well as that of the nuclear envelope may swell considerably. Chromatin within the nucleus aggregates or clumps more than usual. As the cell approaches death, the swelling of the organelles increases with a concomitant loss of ribosomes, rER, sER, and Golgi apparatus. Ruptures and dissolution of the cell membrane occur. Other membranes within the cell, including those of the endoplasmic reticulum and the nuclear envelope, partially dissolve. The clumping of the chromatin continues to a point at which less condensed or coiled chromatin is reduced substantially and may altogether disappear, especially when viewed light microscopically.

APOPTOSIS

The events associated with apoptosis differ sharply for the most part from those associated with necrosis. Microscopically, the early stages involve changes that occur within the nucleus. The chromatin aggregates in a discrete manner. Rather than clumping in an irregular and random fashion as seen during necrosis, the chromatin condenses in distinct masses next to the inner membrane of the nuclear envelope. The cytoplasm undergoes condensation, which can result in protrusion and possible blebbing of the cell surface. As apoptosis continues, portions of the cell bleb away from the main body. These portions are referred to as *apoptotic bodies*, which are frequently engulfed by resident cells that are not undergoing apoptosis, as well as inflammatory cells, such as macrophages. The events of apoptosis advance at a more rapid pace than those of necrosis. The disintegration of a cell into a cluster of apoptotic bodies can transpire in just minutes, whereas necrotic events take hours and days. In addition, cells undergoing apoptosis tend to be iso-

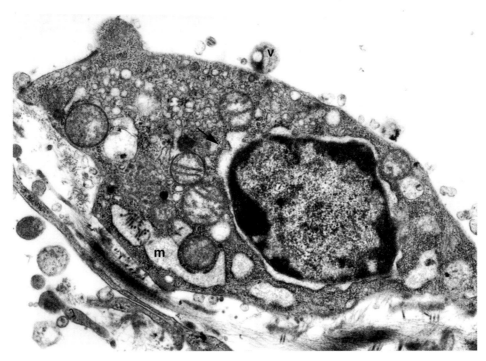

Figure 2-25. Cell injury frequently leads to necrosis, as seen ultrastructurally in this canine endothelial cell. Note the swelling of the mitochondria *(m)*, exocytotic-like blebbing of vesicles *(v)* with breaks in the cell membrane, and expanded separation of the two membranes of the nuclear envelope *(arrow)*. (×15,000.)

lated from one another in a general population. By comparison, cells undergoing necrosis often adjoin each other and frequently occur as groups rather than individually.

SUGGESTED READINGS

Bergman RA, Afifi AK, Heidger PM, Jr: *Histology,* Philadelphia, 1996, Saunders.

Bershadsky AD, Vasiliev JM: *Cytoskeleton,* New York, 1988, Plenum Publishing.

Fawcett DW: *The cell,* Philadelphia, 1981, Saunders.

Fawcett DW: *Bloom and Fawcett: a textbook of histology,* ed 12, Philadelphia, 1994, Saunders.

Hermo L, Green H, Clermont Y: Golgi apparatus of epithelial principal cells of the ependymal initial segment of the rat: structure, relationship with endoplasmic reticulum, and role in the formation of secretory vesicles, *Anat Rec* 229:159, 1991.

Holtzman E: *Lysosomes,* New York, 1989, Plenum Publishing.

Junqueira LC, Carneiro J, Kelley RO: *Basic histology,* ed 7, Norwalk, Conn, 1992, Appleton & Lang.

Kerr JF, Gobe GC, Winterford CM, Harmon BV: Anatomical methods in cell death. In Schwartz LM, Osborne BA, editors: *Methods in cell biology,* vol 46, San Diego, 1995, Academic Press.

Lane MD, Pedersen PL, Mildvan AS: The mitochondrion updated, *Science* 234:526, 1986.

Miething A: Intercellular bridges between germ cells in immature golden hamster testis: evidence for clonal and nonclonal mode of proliferation, *Cell Tissue Res* 262:559, 1990.

Miller M, Park MK, Hanover JA: Nuclear pore complex: structure, function, and regulation, *Physiol Rev* 71(3):909, 1991.

The Epithelium

KEY CHARACTERISTICS

- Polar orientation: one side facing lumen/free space, other side attached to another tissue
- Classified according to cell shape and number (one or more) layers of cells
- Very little extracellular space between adjacent cells
- Can have well-developed apical modifications
- Forms basement membrane

The epithelium is the tissue that covers all free surfaces of the body. *Epithelium* is a term derived from Greek; it literally means "tissue grows" (*theleo*) "upon another" (*epi*). Epithelia generally consist of sheets of closely packed cells that lie typically in apposition over the surfaces of the body or organs. This tissue is chiefly characterized by having high cellular density with very little intercellular space and lacks direct vascular supply (except for blood vessels). It is most commonly associated with connective tissue and is attached to the latter by the basement membrane. Because epithelia are concomitantly exposed to free space on one side, the apex, and anchored to another tissue on the other side, the base, inherent polarity is along the apical-basal axis of each epithelium. However, in certain instances, epithelia that are involved in endocrine secretion have lost free surface associations but remain tightly aggregated and epithelial-like or epithelioid. In epithelioid tissues the apical-basal orientation is largely lost.

Functions of epithelia include protection of external surfaces and body orifices, absorption and secretion of materials into and away from lumens or cavities, surface transport of substances by cilia, and sensory reception as in gustation and olfaction.

Although epithelia had been traditionally described to be derived from the ectoderm, this tissue is in fact derived from all three primary germ layers: ectodermal—epithelia lining the body surface; endodermal—epithelia lining the digestive and pulmonary tracts; and mesodermal—epithelia lining the heart, blood vessels, lymphatics, and coelomic spaces.

CLASSIFICATION

Epithelial classification has little regard for location or function (except for that being glandular) and is based primarily on cell shape and arrangement of cells into one or more sheets or layers (Table 3-1) (Figure 3-1). Single layered epithelia are called *simple*, whereas epithelia with more than one layer are referred to as *stratified*. Epithelia are further subdivided into squamous, cuboidal, and columnar types by the shape of the cells that face the free space. In stratified epithelia the cells form the outermost (apical) layer. The squamous shape is the condition in which the width and depth of the cell exceed the height. Usually the difference between the height and width or depth

TABLE 3-1 Morphology, Function, and Location of Epithelia

TYPE	SURFACE CELL SHAPE	FUNCTION	LOCATION
Single Layered			
Simple squamous	Flattened	Selective fluid and gaseous exchange (limiting membrane); frictionless surface	Lining: blood and lymphatic vessels; alveoli of the lung; pleural and peritoneal cavities; parietal layer of Bowman's layer and loop of Henle in the kidney
Simple cuboidal	Cuboidal	Secretion; absorption; providing conduit; protection	Convoluted tubules of kidney; ducts and secretory portions of many glands; surface epithelium of the ovary; pigment epithelia of the eye
Simple columnar	Columnar	Absorption; secretion; protection; transportation; providing conduit	Lining: glandular stomach; small and large intestine; uterus and uterine tubes; second-degree bronchi; ductal and secretory portion of glands
Pseudostratified	Columnar (not all cells are exposed to the surface)	Transportation; secretion; absorption; protection	Lining: trachea, first- and second-degree bronchi; lacrimal sac and nasal cavity; epididymis and ductus deferens
Multilayered			
Stratified squamous (noncornified)	Flattened (with nuclei)	Protection	Lining: oral, esophageal and anal portions of gastrointestinal (GI) tract; cornea and conjunctiva; larynx; portions of female and male reproductive tracts
Stratified squamous (cornified)	Flattened (without nuclei)	Protection	Lining: general body surface; buccal cavity and esophagus in ruminants; ruminant forestomach
Stratified cuboidal	Cuboidal	Providing conduit; absorption; secretion	Lining: larger ducts of compound glands and ducts of sweat glands; areas between simple or pseudostratified epithelia and stratified squamous epithelia
Stratified columnar	Columnar	Providing conduit; absorption; secretion; protection	Lining: larger ducts of some compound glands; conjunctivae of eyelids; areas between simple or pseudostratified epithelia and stratified squamous epithelia
Transitional	Cuboidal (relaxed), flattened (distended)	Protection; distensible capability	Lining: urinary tract

is well defined, but in some instances height and width appear nearly identical; however, as the cells age, the width and depth broaden considerably, whereas the height shortens (Figure 3-2). The cuboidal shape among epithelia is defined as when the cells' height, width and depth are approximately identical. Subtle variations occur in which the height might exceed the width and depth by 50% or vice versa, and these variations are often the results of increased metabolic activity or the lack thereof. To be accurate, observers could describe such tissues as cuboidal to columnar (or low columnar) or cuboidal to squamous, but for the sake of classification these tissues are generally called *cuboidal*. Columnar epithelia possess cells facing free space that have heights that are distinctly greater than their widths and depths.

In multilayered epithelia it is the shape of the surface cells that categorizes and identifies the type of epithelium that is being observed. This is an important concept to remember because in most stratified epithelia the morphology of the cells can vary considerably from one layer to another.

Simple squamous epithelium is composed of a single layer of plate- or scalelike cells (Figure 3-3). The sheet of flattened cells is kept intact by cell processes or interdigitations which line the lateral surface of each cell (Figure 3-4). Simple squamous epithelium is best suited for the transport of substances

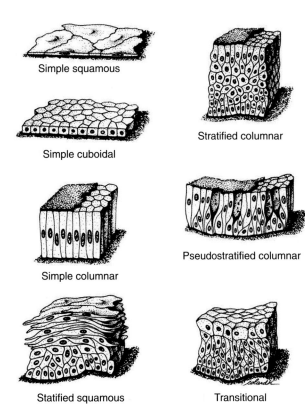

Simple squamous

Simple cuboidal

Simple columnar

Statified squamous

Stratified columnar

Pseudostratified columnar

Transitional

Figure 3-1. Illustration of seven of the eight types of epithelia that occur in domestic species. *(From Fawcett DW: Bloom and Fawcett: a textbook of histology, ed 11, Philadelphia, 1986, Saunders.)*

across the cytoplasm. Consequently, it mostly lines moist, internal surfaces such as blood vessels and distal pathways of the lung (Figure 3-5). The simple squamous epithelium that lines these regions of the body is often referred to as an *endothelium*. Simple squamous epithelia also form part of the serous lining of cavities—the pericardium, pleura, and peritoneum—between organs. This epithelium is often called a *mesothelium*.

Simple cuboidal epithelium consists of a single layer of cells that generally are cube shaped. Because these cells have heights that match their widths, they possess a polarized arrangement of organelles (Figure 3-6). This tissue is usually associated with secretion and/or absorption and is found in the thyroid, kidney, lung, ovary, and ducts and secretory portions of many glands (Figure 3-7). In organs that have undergone a period of production and storage of secretory materials, such as the thyroid, this epithelium may become less cuboidal (more squamous) and concomitantly less physiologically active (Figure 3-8).

Simple columnar epithelium is a third type of a single-layered epithelium in which the heights of

individual cells easily exceed their widths. As in simple cuboidal epithelia, this tissue is associated with secretion and absorption. Simple columnar epithelial cells represent the major cell type for many exocrine glands, that is, they are secretory in nature and highly polarized cytoplasmically (Figure 3-9). They are also common as absorptive cells in the intestine, female reproductive tract, and lung (Figure 3-10). The nuclei in these cells reside roughly at the same level or levels, which in most instances is near the cell base. The free, or luminal surface, of the tissue, and to a lesser extent of simple cuboidal epithelium, often possesses a variety of cell modifications (microvilli, cilia, glycocalyx, etc.).

A fourth category of single-layered epithelia is **pseudostratified columnar epithelium,** which is usually characterized by the irregular positioning of nuclei (not being oriented in one level), giving the impression of a multilayered tissue (Figure 3-11). All cells in fact form a uniform basal boundary that is attached to a common basement membrane (Figure 3-12). However, some cells do not reach the luminal surface. Often several cell types can be defined, including basal, columnar, and goblet cells. This tissue is mostly found along the trachea and bronchi of the respiratory tract and epididymis and vas deferens of the male reproductive tract and functions largely in secretion and movement of particles along the tubular organs (Figure 3-13). The key difference between pseudostratified columnar epithelium and simple columnar epithelium is the presence of undifferentiated, germinative cells (basal cells) in the former. These basal cells do not form a solid, continuous layer, but can vary considerably in number: frequent along the respiratory tract (see Figure 3-12) and few within the male reproductive tract (see Figure 3-13).

As in single-layered epithelia, multilayered epithelia are classified according to shape. All multilayered epithelia possess a continuous basal layer that has proliferative capabilities.

Stratified squamous epithelium is the most common of the multilayered epithelia, covering most external body parts. It functions primarily to protect underlying tissues and prevent their desiccation. Epithelium that is not immediately exposed to the external environment but remains moist, as that found in the mouth, esophagus, conjunctiva, cornea, and vagina, has a basal layer of cuboidal cells, and several layers of polygonal cells that become progressively more squamous (Figure 3-14). This epithelium is sometimes called nonkeratinized stratified squamous epithelium, which is actually a misnomer because some keratinization can occur in this tissue. Keratinized stratified squamous epithelium is distinctly layered, forming the outer covering of skin, the

Text continued on p. 40

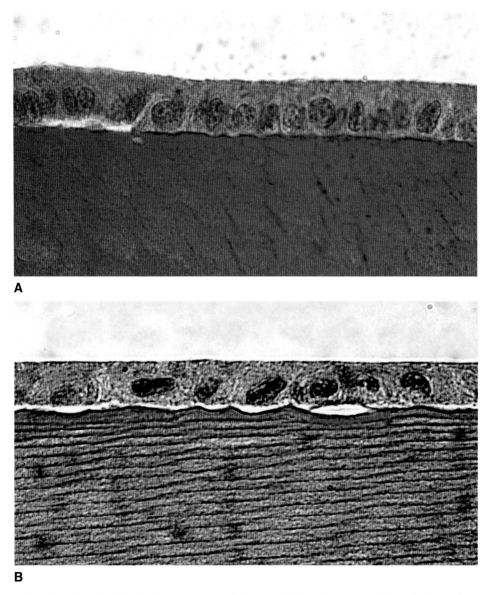

A

B

Figure 3-2. Simple and stratified epithelia change in morphology with development and age. In these photomicrographs, the anterior epithelium, **A,** of a young (3-month-old) canine lens appears slightly columnar, but that of an adult (2-year-old), **B,** has become more cuboidal, with the cells less densely populated (note fewer nuclei) than when younger. (×1000.)

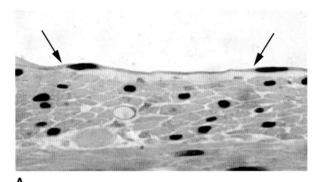

A

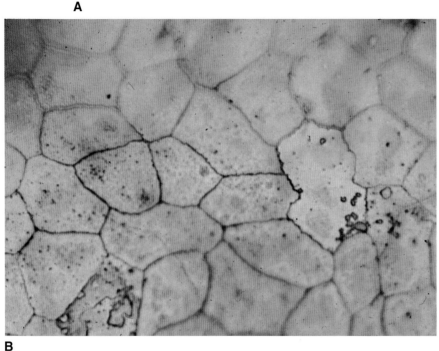

B

Figure 3-3. A, Light micrograph of simple squamous epithelium *(arrows)* of the serosa of the small intestine seen cross sectionally. (Plastic section stained with hematoxylin and eosin stain; ×400.) **B,** Simple squamous epithelium seen face-on from a flat mount of mesentery that was treated with a silver stain to reveal cell boundaries. (×400.)

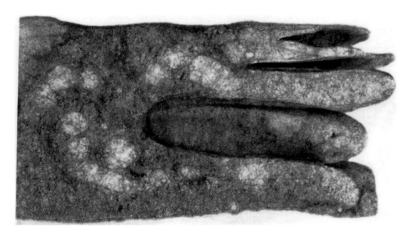

Figure 3-4. The end of a simple squamous epithelial cell possesses interdigitating processes. These processes allow adjacent cells to interact greatly with one another and form an excellent environment for barrier and transport proteins within the cell membrane. (Layered transmission electron micrograph; ×25,000.)

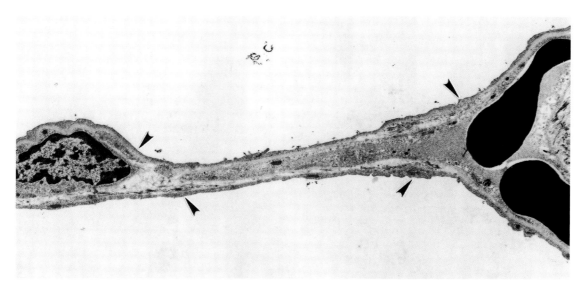

Figure 3-5. Air sacs, or alveoli, of the lung are lined by simple squamous epithelia *(arrowheads)* that can be extraordinarily thin, permitting suitable gas exchange. The enclosed capillary with a flattened red blood cell also is lined by a very thin simple squamous epithelium. (Transmission electron micrograph; ×5000.)

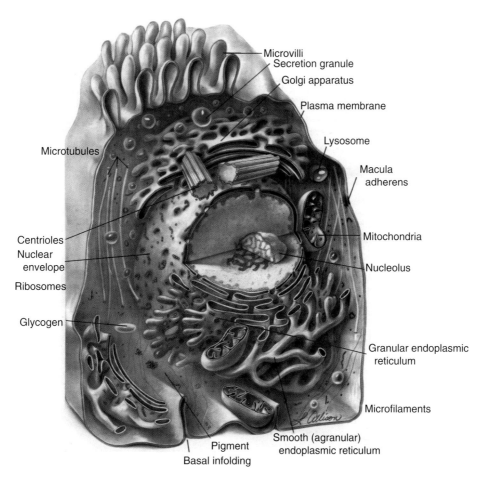

Figure 3-6. Cells of simple cuboidal epithelia possess organelles that are arranged with distinct polarity. *(From Leeson CR, Leeson TS, Paparo AA: Atlas of histology, Philadelphia, 1985, Saunders.)*

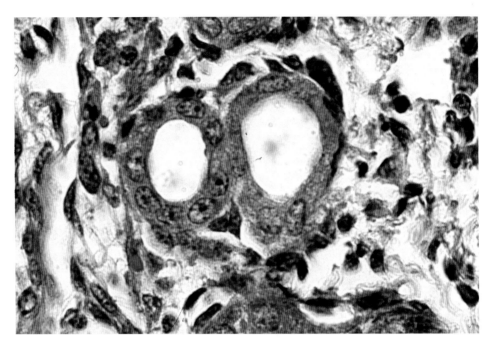

Figure 3-7. As seen in this light micrograph, tubules within the porcine kidney (seen cross sectionally) are lined by simple cuboidal epithelia. (Hematoxylin and eosin stain; ×1000.)

epidermis. The process of keratinization is complete in this tissue and leads to the subsequent death of each involved cell. As a result, this tissue consists of both living and dead cells and is generally subdivided into several groups of layers: the basal stratum (stratum basale) single layer of cuboidal to columnar cells, also the proliferative or germinative layer; stratum spinosum—two or more layers of cells with spiny processes; stratum granulosum external to the stratum spinosum and similar to the stratum spinosum but containing detectable granules of keratin material; stratum lucidum—thin, translucent layer next to stratum granulosum, involving cell death; and stratum corneum—most superficial layer, composed of many layers of dead, scalelike cells lacking nuclei (Figure 3-15).

Stratified cuboidal epithelium can be found as a tissue between simple and stratified epithelia along different regions of the body including the anal canal, female urethra, and proximal respiratory tract. This tissue also occurs as a bilayered epithelium that lines the ducts of sweat and salivary glands (Figure 3-16). Similarly, bilayered **stratified columnar epithelium** occurs between simple and stratified epithelia and lines the large ducts of salivary glands, having usually a basal layer of small cuboidal cells and an apical layer of cuboidal to columnar cells (often species specific) that do not reach the basement membrane (Figure 3-17).

A fourth type of multilayered epithelium is the **transitional epithelium,** found only in the urogenital system. The urinary tract is subject to marked variations of internal pressure and capacity and consequently is lined by this special type of epithelium that can alter its shape. The transitional epithelium has an appearance that changes between stratified squamous and stratified cuboidal epithelium. In a relaxed state the apical or surface cells are cuboidal to columnar in appearance as they bulge into the lumen (Figure 3-18). However, in a stretched state the thickness of the epithelium is greatly reduced and the apical cells become markedly flattened (Figure 3-19). Without knowing where this tissue came from, a less experienced observer can mistakenly identify it as a stratified squamous or cuboidal epithelium, depending on how relaxed the surface cells are. However, some of the surface cells are binucleated, and this characteristic can be useful for distinguishing this type of epithelium from the other stratified types.

SURFACE MODIFICATIONS

Modifications or specializations of the free or luminal surfaces of epithelial cells can be found among the different forms of epithelia and are most pronounced in simple columnar and pseudostratified

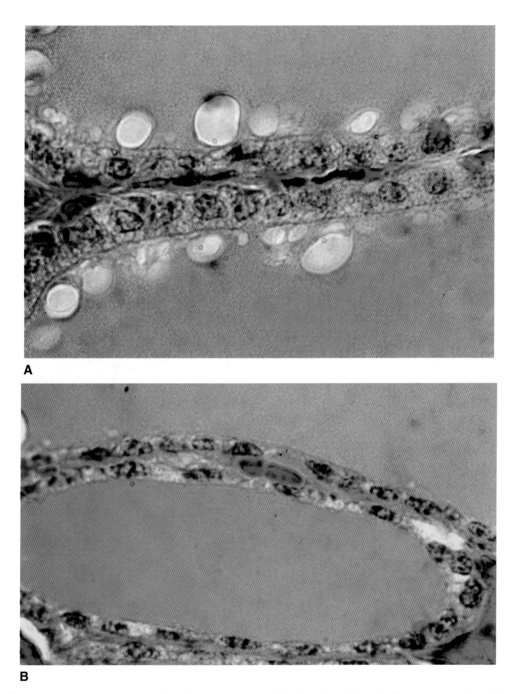

A

B

Figure 3-8. The state of metabolism can alter the appearance of simple cuboidal epithelia as seen in these light micrographs. In the equine thyroid, active follicular cells **(A)** are distinctly cuboidal. By comparison, inactive or quiescent follicles are lined by epithelial cells **(B)** that appear more squamous than cuboidal. (×1000.)

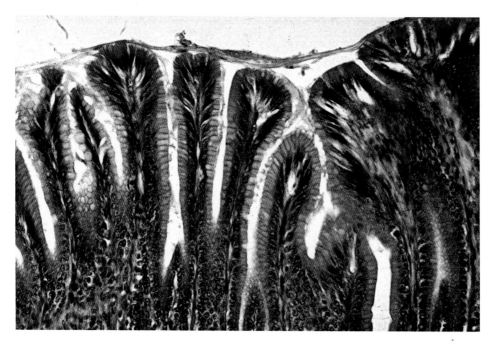

Figure 3-9. The gastric mucosa of the feline stomach possesses a simple columnar epithelium that actively secretes. (Hematoxylin and eosin stain; ×250.)

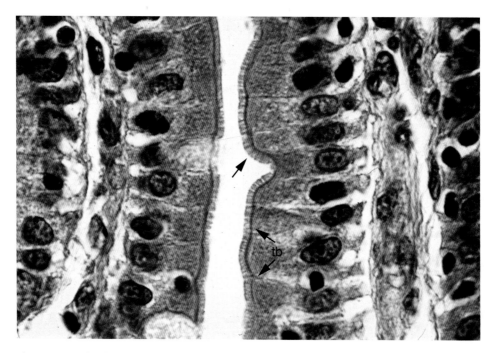

Figure 3-10. Light micrograph of the mucosa of the small intestine. The intestine is lined by a simple columnar epithelium that functions primarily to absorb as indicated by the presence of a striated border *(arrow)*, a surface modification that amplifies the surface area greatly. The striated border is subtended by a terminal bar *(tb)*. (Hematoxylin and eosin stain; ×1000.)

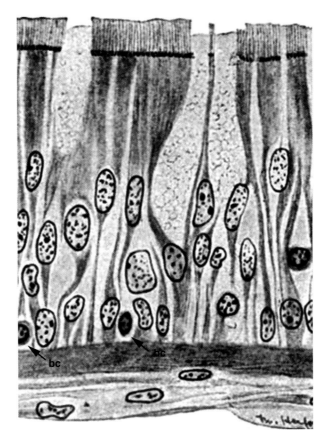

Figure 3-11. Illustration of a pseudostratified columnar epithelium. The hallmark feature of this type of epithelium is the presence of scattered stem cells known as *basal cells (bc) (arrows). (Modified from Greep RO:* Histology, *New York, 1954, Blakiston.)*

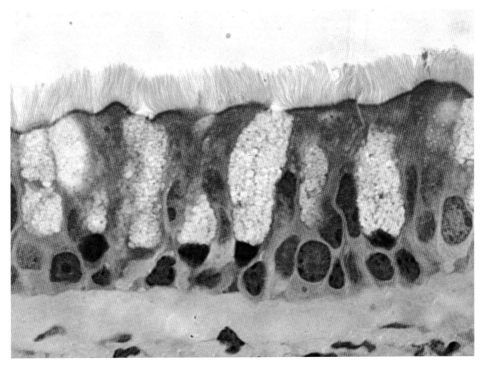

Figure 3-12. Photomicrograph of pseudostratified columnar epithelium that occurs within the proximal portion of the pulmonary tract as seen here in the trachea. (Plastic section, hematoxylin and eosin stain; ×600.)

columnar epithelia (Box 3-1). In these particular tissues the apical portion of columnar cells possesses a variety of modifications that assist in the breakdown, digestion, and movement of particulate materials.

Microvilli are slender, cylindrical cytoplasmic processes, which are approximately 0.1 μm in diameter and mostly 0.5 to 2.0 μm in length. They possess a central filamentous core of actin that extends well into the apical cytoplasm and is anchored in the terminal web (Figure 3-20). The actin is linked to the cell membrane of each microvillus by **myosin-I** and **calmodulin,** giving support to the microvillus. The **terminal web** consists of a network of microfilaments that lie horizontally just beneath the apex of the cell. Microvilli are found mostly on absorptive and transport cells in columnar and cuboidal epithelia and frequently are referred to as being a **brush border** (kidney) or **striated border** (intestine) (see Figure 3-10).

They function to increase the surface area for absorption (up to 10,000 times in the small intestine) and can contain enzymes for the hydrolyzation of sugar as shown in biochemical analysis of striated borders isolated from intestinal epithelium. Along the proximal convoluted tubules of the kidney, microvilli can extend up to 5 μm in length (Figure 3-21). Using the traditional formalin/paraffin preparation, light microscopic observations of these structures reveal a matted form—the brush border—that is similar to a moistened artist's brush. In non- or less-absorbing cells that possess these structures, microvilli are generally fewer and may lack an actin core altogether (uterine glands).

Glycocalyx is essentially a glycoprotein surface coat that covers the entire cell (of all cells of the body) and is prominent in intestinal cells with microvilli (Figure 3-22). There is a close association of the glycocalyx and microvilli, as the former with its gel-like rigidity offers additional support for the latter.

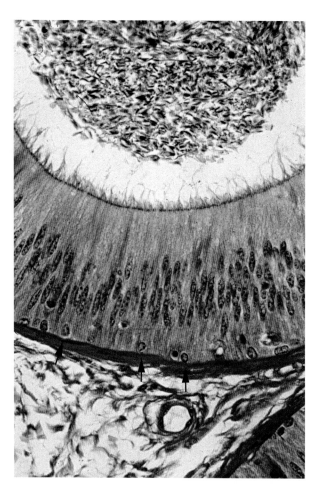

Figure 3-13. Light micrograph of the epididymis of a horse. Epididymis is lined by a tall pseudostratified columnar epithelium, consisting of tall columnar cells and scattered short basal cells *(arrows)*. (Hematoxylin and eosin stain; ×400.)

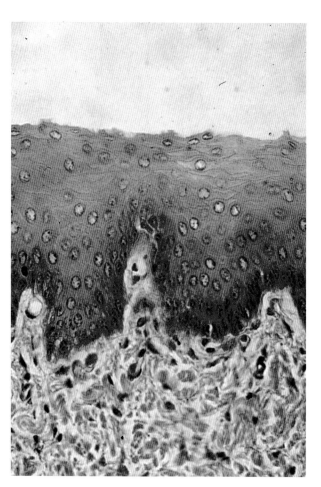

Figure 3-14. Light micrograph of the esophagus of a pig. The esophagus is lined by a moistened stratified squamous epithelium. (Hematoxylin and eosin stain; ×400.)

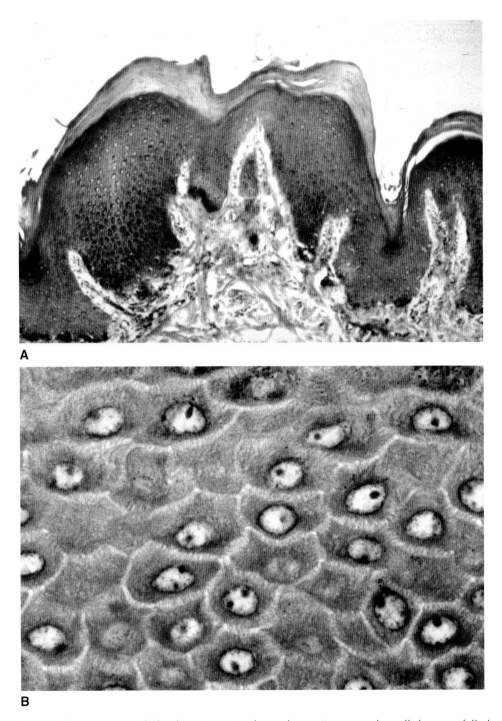

A

B

Figure 3-15. In stratified squamous epithelia that are exposed to a dry environment, the cells become fully keratinized. In certain areas of the integument among domestic animals this type of epithelium can be well developed, such as along the nares of the nose. **A,** Light micrograph (×100) of the entire thickness of the stratified squamous epithelium that forms the epidermis of a canine naris. **B,** Light micrograph (×1000) of the stratum spinosum.   *Continued*

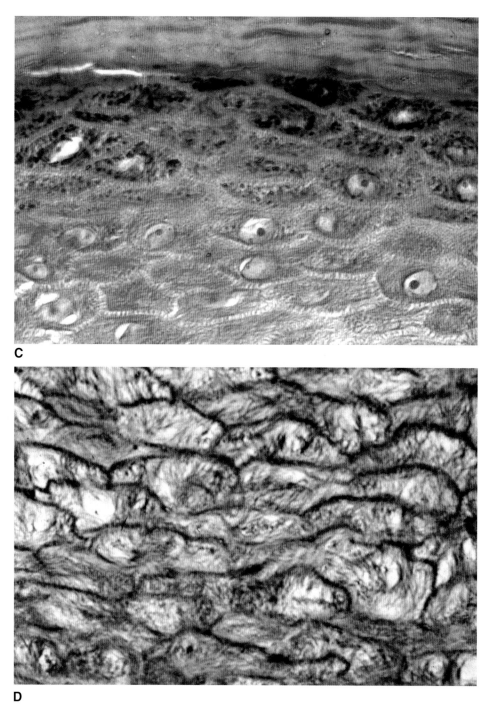

C

D

Figure 3-15, cont'd C, Light micrograph (×1000) of the stratum granulosum. **D,** Light micrograph (×1000) of the stratum corneum. (All micrographs were stained with hematoxylin and eosin.)

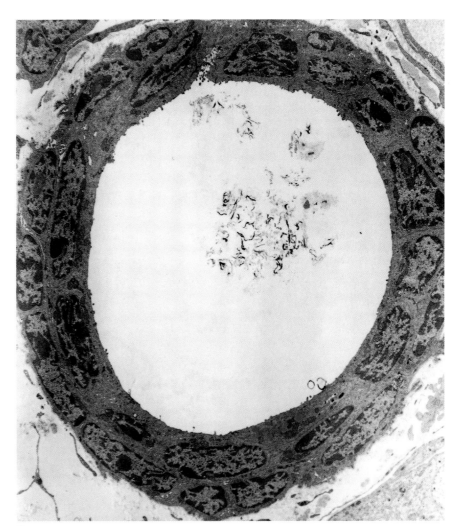

Figure 3-16. Stratified cuboidal epithelia. **A,** Transmission electron micrograph (×4200) of a duct within a canine parotid gland. **B,** Light micrograph (×400) of the stratified cuboidal epithelium seen in Figure 3-16, *A.* (Hematoxylin and eosin stain.)

A

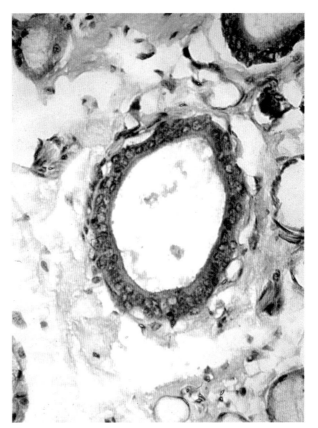

B

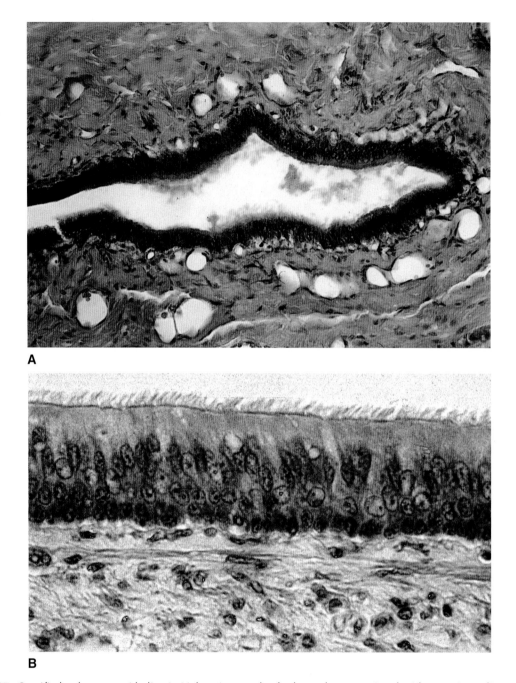

A

B

Figure 3-17. Stratified columnar epithelia. **A,** Light micrograph of a large duct associated with a canine salivary gland. (Hematoxylin and eosin stain; ×200.) **B,** Light micrograph (×400) of the epithelium along the larynx of a pig.

This carbohydrate-rich coat also offers protection so that only dissolved substances will penetrate between microvilli. The carbohydrate residues that form the bulk of the glycocalyx are attached to the transmembrane proteins of the cell membrane.

Stereocilia are very long microvilli that can measure up to 10 μm in length and line the luminal surface of certain columnar cells (e.g., those lining the epididymis and vas deferens of the male reproductive tract and associated with sensory hair cells of the inner ear, cochlea; Figure 3-23). At high magnification they are seen to be thin cilium-like structures. However, stereocilia are considerably narrower than true cilia (kinocilia) and are nonmotile, possessing actin cores. Although their function is not well established, they most likely promote absorption through amplification

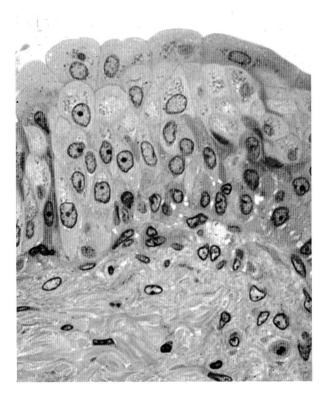

Figure 3-18. Photomicrograph of the transitional epithelium lining the urinary bladder in a relaxed state as demonstrated by the swollen, cuboidal-like apical cells. (Plastic section, hematoxylin and eosin stain; ×400.)

Box 3-1 Cells with Apical Modifications

Microvilli (striated border, brush border) can occur sparsely along the surface of most epithelia and are most prevalent along the following:

   Absorptive columnar epithelia, especially small intestinal epithelium
   Proximal convoluted tubule within the urinary system
   Follicular cells of the thyroid, especially when stimulated with thyroid-stimulating hormone (TSH)
   Proximal portions of the respiratory tract
   Simple gustatory neuroepithelium
   Pigment epithelium of the retina

Stereocilia (long microvilli):

   Epididymis of the male reproductive tract
   Vestibular receptor of the vestibular sense organ along the semicircular canals, utricle and saccule of the inner ear.

Cilia (kinocilia):

   Proximal portions of the respiratory tract
   Concha and sinuses
   Naso- and oropharynx (above soft palate)
   Larynx
   Trachea
   Bronchi
   Bronchioles
   Uterine tube (oviduct) of female reproductive tract
   Olfactory cells of the olfactory epithelium

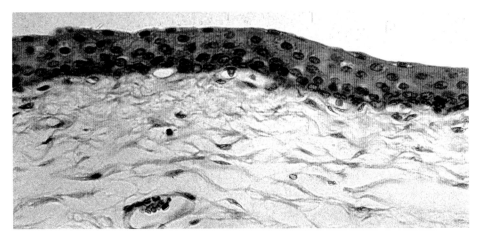

Figure 3-19. Light micrograph of the transitional epithelium lining the urinary bladder of a cow in a stretched state. The apical cells appear flattened and squamous-like. (Hematoxylin and eosin stain; ×200.)

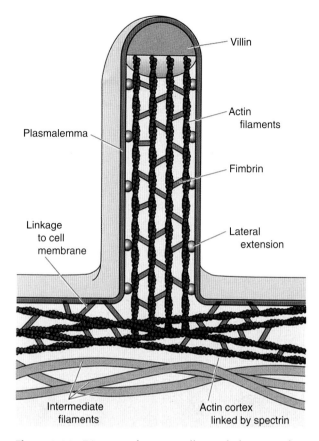

Figure 3-20. Diagram of a microvillus and elements of its construction. *(From Gartner LP, Hiatt JL: Color textbook of histology, Philadelphia, 1997, Saunders.)*

of the cell surface in the male reproductive tract and generate signals in the ear.

Cilia or **kinocilia,** as opposed to stereocilia and microvilli, are curly motile cell processes. Each cilium possesses an internal microtubular substructure designed for contractility. The cilium—5.0 to 10.0 μm in length and 0.2 μm in diameter—is within resolution of the light microscope (Figure 3-24). Ciliated cells are most common in the respiratory tract, oviduct, and uterus, moving mucus and other substances by **metachronal rhythm,** whereby successive cilia in each row begin their beat in sequence resulting in each cilium being slightly more advanced in its stroke than the preceding one. The core of a cilium is the axoneme, which consists of a nine doublet plus two singlet arrangements of microtubules (Figure 3-25).

BASEMENT MEMBRANE

Another specialization of cell surfaces of epithelia is the presence of a **basement membrane,** occurring as the name indicates at the base (away from the face or luminal end) of the cell. The basement membrane is made up of a mixture of mucopolysaccharides and proteins immediately adjacent to the basal surface of the epithelium. It functions primarily to anchor each type of epithelium to adjacent tissue as well as provide

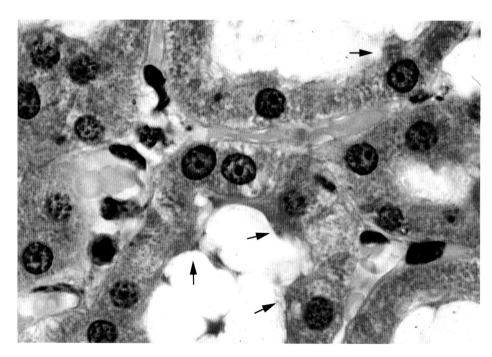

Figure 3-21. Light micrograph (×1000) of brush borders *(arrows)* extending into the lumen of proximal convoluted tubules.

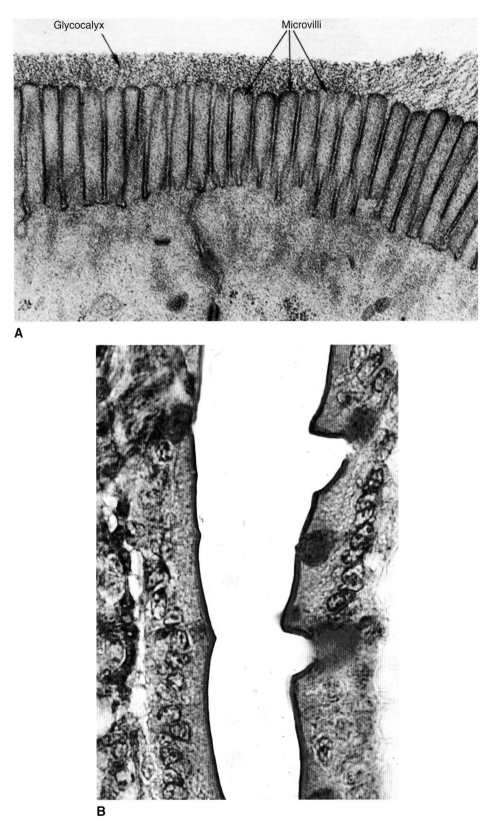

Glycocalyx   Microvilli

A

B

Figure 3-22. Glycocalyx. **A,** Transmission electron micrograph of microvilli surrounded and protected by a well-developed glycocalyx. **B,** Along the mucosal lining of the canine small intestine, the glycocalyx has been revealed by periodic acid–Schiff. (×1000.) *(A from Fawcett DW:* Bloom and Fawcett: a textbook of histology, *ed 11, Philadelphia, 1986, Saunders.)*

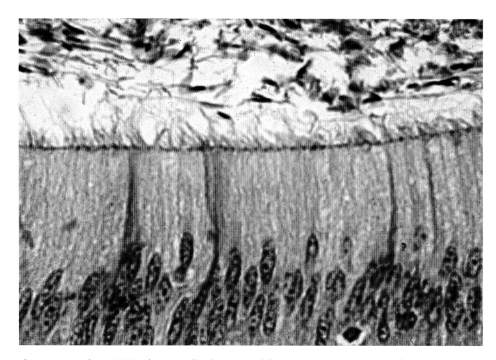

Figure 3-23. Light micrograph (×1000) of stereocilia that extend from the columnar cells of the epididymis within the male reproductive tract.

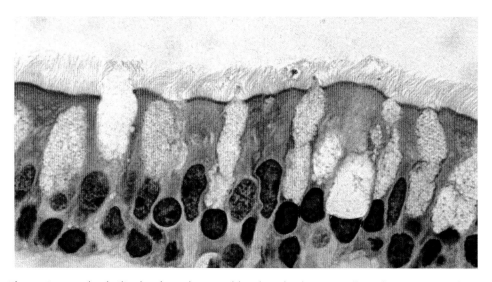

Figure 3-24. Photomicrograph of cilia that form the apical border of columnar cells within most pseudostratified columnar epithelia. (Hematoxylin and eosin stain; ×1000.)

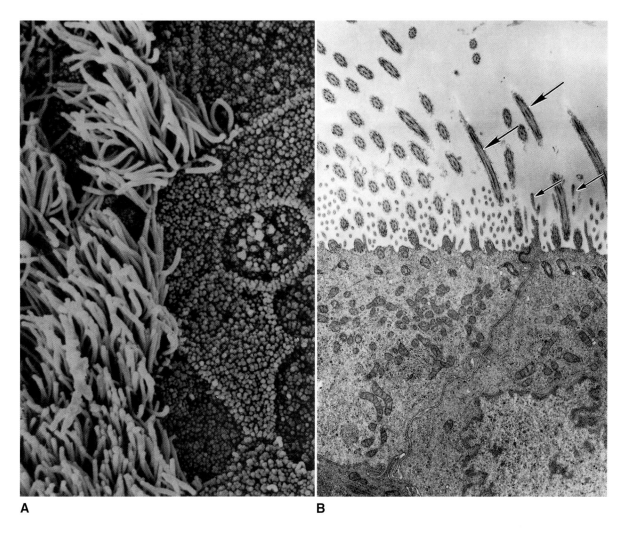

A   **B**

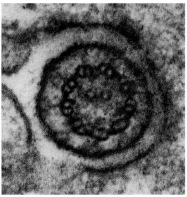

C

Figure 3-25. Cilia. **A,** Scanning electron micrograph (×6000) of cilia along a ferret trachea. Some cells lack cilia, having microvilli, which by comparison protrude only a short distance into the airway. **B,** Transmission electron micrograph (×10,000) of this same tissue reveals the difference in size between the cilia *(large arrows)* and microvilli *(small arrows)*. **C,** Transmission electron micrograph (×100,000) of an individual cilium with an axoneme of microtubules seen in cross section.

additional protection and serve as a semipermeable barrier. Most basement membranes consist of two layers: a **basal lamina** that lies next to the cell membrane of the basal epithelial cell and is made solely by the overlying epithelial cells; and a **reticular lamina** that consists of small irregular bundles of small collagen fibrils within a layer of ground substance and is made by both epithelium and adjacent tissue (Figure 3-26). The amount of reticular lamina varies from tissue to tissue, and is especially well developed by simple squamous epithelia in the kidney and the eye (Figure 3-27; see also Figure 1-4).

CELLULAR ATTACHMENTS

The remaining specializations of the epithelial cell surface are concerned with those at the lateral surface, primarily cell junctions or attachments.

Macula adherens, commonly referred to as a **desmosome,** is a cell junction that significantly increases adhesion between epithelial cells. This type of junction is often randomly placed along the lateral sides of epithelial cells and is particularly well developed in the stratum spinosum of the epidermis (see Figure 3-15). Light microscopically, desmosomes appear as small, round, dense thickenings or dots along the cell boundaries. At higher magnification they are found to consist of bipartite structures lining a narrow intercellular space with a faint intermediate line (Figure 3-28). The bipartite plaques are constructed of dense intracellular sheets that lie against the cell membrane, and are areas where densely packed tonofilaments insert. The tonofilaments, which most likely dissipate physical forces throughout the cell, are believed to be held by transmembrane linkers that penetrate the cell membrane, form hairpin loops going through adjacent hairpin loops of the apposing cell, and reenter the cell. Desmosomes are thus sites of cystoskeletal attachment to the cell membrane and its surface as well as of cell-cell adhesion. Desmosomes are never continuous, but are round (as the Latin name *macula* suggests), acting as spot weldings. In addition to being scattered laterally over the cell surface, they can occur at discrete locations. In simple columnar epithelium they will often form an uneven row below the zonula adherens.

Zonula adherens, another cell junction that functions to bind adjacent epithelial cells, forms an apical boundary of a transverse zone of microfilaments, the terminal web. This cell junction occurs as a band or zone that encompasses the entire apical perimeter of the cell in columnar and cuboidal epithelia (those epithelia that possess a great deal of cytoplasmic polar-

ity) (Figure 3-29). Although the cytoplasm next to the contact region is densely granular, distinct plaques and an intermediate line between adjacent cells (found in desmosomes) are lacking. Still, apposed cell membranes are separated by a regular extracellular space in the contact zone.

Zonula occludens, or **tight junction,** is a cell junction that forms a morphological barrier between the intercellular spaces of adjacent cells. Along the lateral sides of two apposing cells, the cell membrane of each cell protrudes to the other and forms a network of contacts that can be fully appreciated when seen face-on (Figures 3-30 and 3-31). This cell junction is formed in epithelia, such as simple squamous epithelia, that require luminal materials to be transported selectively through cells. In simple cuboidal and columnar epithelia the tight junction is located apically, forming the outermost component of a **junctional complex** that typically consists of three components, the zonula occludens, zonula adherens, and macula adherens, with the zonula occludens located most apically (luminally), followed by the zonula adherens and then the macular adherens (see Figure 3-31). The zonula adherens and desmosome together serve to keep the tight junction intact. Light microscopically these junctions and the terminal web are seen collectively as dense bars, referred to as *terminal bars* (see Figure 3-10). Tight junctions, however, were first discovered ultrastructurally, viewed at several points where adjacent cell membranes would meet with no intercellular space between. With the advent of the freeze-fracture technique, this junction was found to be an anastomosing network of membrane ridges entirely surrounding the apical border.

Nexus, or **gap, junction** is a specialized platelike junction that mediates the flow of current from one cell to another. This junction is located on the deeper lateral surfaces of apposing cells, and typically hundreds if not thousands of these structures connect one cell to another. Minute gaps, approximately 20 Å wide, link adjacent cell membranes, permitting electronic coupling. The use of selective stains (uranyl acetate) and specific tracers (lanthanum) revealed the presence of hexagonally arranged subunits, which form these junctions as they interconnect cells, most likely for the direct passage of small ions (Figure 3-32). The subunits are referred to as *connexins,* consisting largely of protein. Before the use of the selective stains, the subunits had often been mistaken for tight junctions.

The cell junctions associated with different epithelia are not restricted to epithelia but, in fact, have been found in all four major tissues (nerve, muscle, connective, and epithelia).

Text continued on p. 59

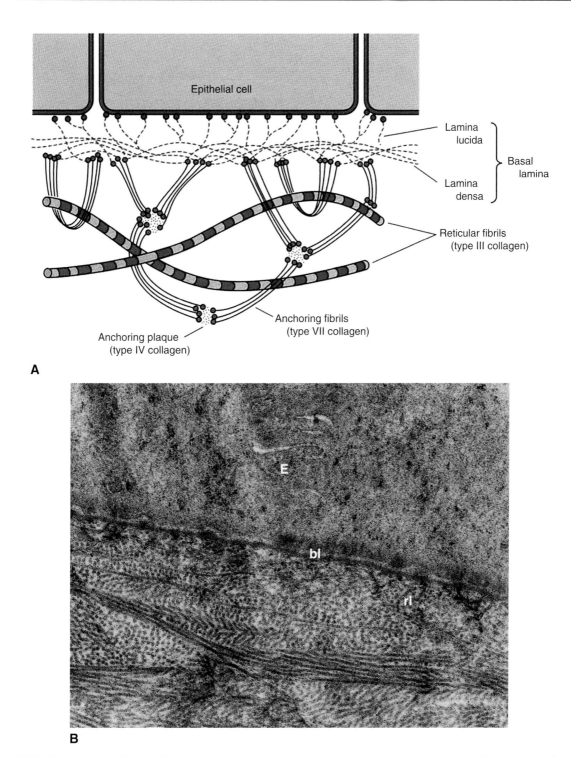

A

B

Figure 3-26. Basement membrane. **A,** Diagram of a basement membrane showing the interrelationship between the basal lamina and the reticular fibers of the reticular lamina **B,** Transmission electron micrograph (×15,000) of the basal lamina *(bl)* and reticular lamina *(rl)* associated with a canine epithelium *(E). (**A** from Gartner LP, Hiatt JL: Color textbook of histology, Philadelphia, 1997, Saunders.)*

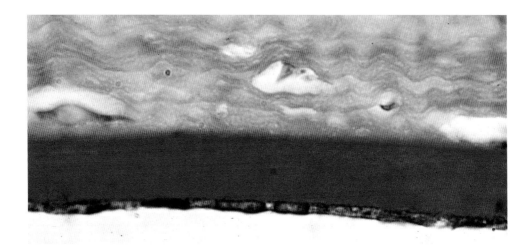

Figure 3-27. Light micrograph of the prominent basement membrane produced by the simple squamous epithelium that internally lines the cornea. (Periodic acid–Schiff stain; ×1000.)

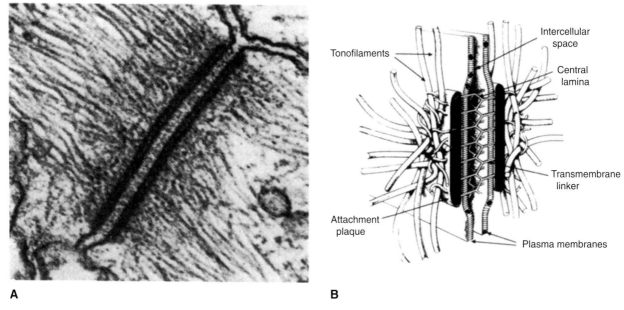

A   **B**

Figure 3-28. Macular adherens (desmosome). Transmission electron micrograph, **A,** and illustration, **B,** of this cell junction, which provides points of firm attachment between adjacent cells resulting from the combination of the tonofilaments that are cemented within dense plaques along with transmembrane linkers. *(From Fawcett DW: Bloom and Fawcett: a textbook of histology, ed 11, Philadelphia, 1986, Saunders.)*

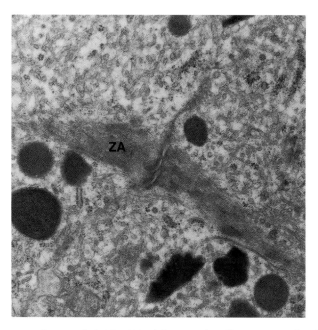

Figure 3-29. Transmission electron micrograph (×20,000) of the zonula adherens *(ZA)* that forms a perimeter zone of attachment within a simple cuboidal epithelium of a sheep.

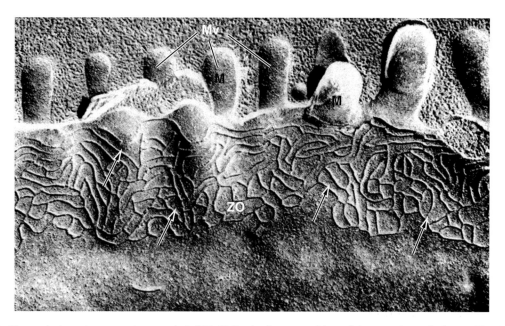

Figure 3-30. Transmission electron micrograph (×100,000) of a freeze-etching of the zonula occludens *(ZO)*. Arrows point to the network of membranous ridges that form a morphological barrier beneath the microvilli *(M)* of this absorbing cell. *(Modified from Ross MH, Reith EJ, Romrell LJ:* Histology: a text and atlas, *ed 2, Baltimore, 1989, Williams & Wilkins.)*

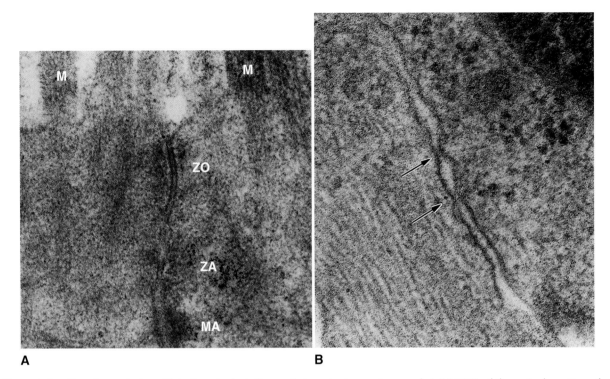

A   **B**

Figure 3-31. Zonula occludens (tight junction). **A,** Transmission electron micrograph (×60,000) of the apical portion of adjacent columnar cells along the intestinal mucosa of a rat. The zonula occludens *(ZO)* forms the luminal-most cell junction of a junctional complex that includes the zonula adherens *(ZA)* and macula adherents *(MA)*. *M,* Microvilli. **B,** Transmission electron micrograph (×100,000) of the zonula occludens within the vascular endothelium of a dog. Arrows point to projections of the cell membrane between adjacent cells.

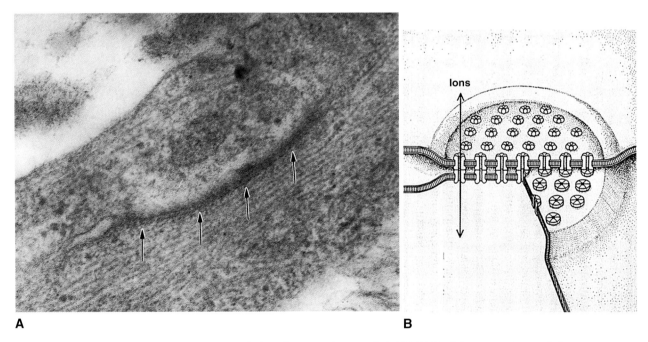

A   **B**

Figure 3-32. Nexus (gap junction). **A,** Transmission electron micrograph (×100,000) of the nexus *(arrows)* that occurs between adjacent cells. **B,** Illustration reveals the presence of numerous channels for ionic flow and communication between one cell and another. *(Modified from Junqueira LC, Carneiro J, Long JA:* Basic histology, *ed 5, Los Altos, Calif, 1986, Lange Medical Publications.)*

REGENERATION

Epithelial regeneration occurs along many regions of the body but is most pronounced on exposed body surfaces, holocrine glands, the intestinal tract, and the female genital tract. In epithelia, which possess a layer of basal cells (stratified squamous epithelium), regenerative action is usually constant. Other epithelia as in the alimentary tract have undifferentiated cells along intestinal crypts and necks of gastric glands. Epithelia that form the lining of vessels can regenerate from stem cells in connective tissues. All in all, epithelia have strong regenerative capabilities that weaken with age.

SUGGESTED READINGS

Bergman RA, Afifi AK, Heidger PM Jr: *Histology,* Philadelphia, 1996, Saunders.

Farquhar MG, Palade GE: Junctional complexes in various epithelia, *J Cell Biol* 17:375, 1963.

Fawcett DW: *The cell,* Philadelphia, 1981, Saunders.

Fawcett DW: *Bloom and Fawcett: a textbook of histology,* ed 11, Philadelphia, 1986, Saunders.

Gartner LP, Hiatt JL: *Color textbook of histology,* Philadelphia, 1997, Saunders.

Goyal H: Morphology of the bovine epididymis, *Am J Anat* 172:155, 1985.

Junqueira LC, Carneiro J, Kelley RO: *Basic histology,* ed 7, Norwalk, Conn, 1992, Appleton & Lang.

Matter K, Balda MS: Signaling to and from tight junctions, *Nat Rev Molec Cell Biol* 4:225, 2003.

Mayhew TM: Striated brush-border of intestinal absorptive epithelial cells: stereological studies on microvillus morphology in different adaptive states, *J Electron Microsc Tech* 16:45, 1990.

Roperto F, Langella M, Oliva G, et al: Ultrastructural and freeze fracture cilia morphology of trachea epithelium in apparently healthy small ruminants, *J Submicrosc Cytol Path* 30:65, 1998.

Simon AM, Goodenough DA: Diverse function of vertebrate gap junctions, *Trends Cell Biol* 8:477, 1998.

Taylor KA, Robertson JD: Analysis of the 3-dimensinsal structure of the urinary-bladder epithelial-cell membranes, *J Ultrastruct Res* 87:23, 1984.

Glands

- Secretory in function
- Organelles within cells are strongly polar
- Classified according to:
    cell number; secretion into a lumen/free space or into vasculature; single duct versus multiple ducts; shape of adenomere; type of secretion—serous versus mucous; mode of secretion

Epithelial cells and associations of epithelial cells specialized primarily for secretions are known as glands. Unlike the eight types of epithelia previously described and from which they are derived, glands can be classified a number of ways, including method of secretory distribution, cell numbers, form, type of secretory material, and manner by which secretions are released.

METHOD OF SECRETORY DISTRIBUTION

Being able to secrete the product to a luminal or free surface either directly or by a secretory duct system is known as being **exocrine.** Glands that lack a duct system and have lost their connections to external or internal surfaces are referred to as being **endocrine.** Endocrine glands are essentially involved in hormone synthesis. Hormones constitute various cell secretions that are directed to specific target organs by the bloodstream. Consequently, endocrine glands are always found to be in proximity to blood vessels. The secretions of the endocrine cells typically pass through the basement membrane of that tissue. By comparison, exocrine cells release their secretions distally or apically, either directly to the epithelial surface of which they are a part or by way of one or more ducts, which facilitates movements of these substances to the epithelial surface. Interestingly, both exocrine and endocrine glands originate the same way—proliferation of epithelial tissue into subjacent tissue, followed by secretory cell differentiation (Figure 4-1). In exocrine glands, epithelial cells can be transformed into assorted elaborations of ducts, which along with the secretory cells, comprise the **parenchyma** of the gland. Adjacent connective tissue supporting the parenchyma constitutes the **stroma.** However, the parenchyma of endocrine glands consists only of the secretory cells as the cells that once connected the secretory cells to parent epithelium degenerate and disappear by the end of development. Histological and cytological diversity of endocrine glands further inhibits their classification along general morphological lines. Exocrine glands, however, are readily subdivided by morphological criteria into a variety of categories. Table 4-1 lists the different exocrine glands that can be found throughout the bodies of domestic animals.

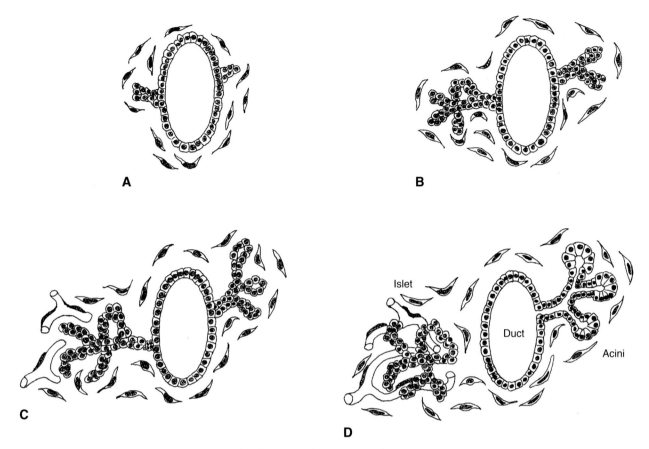

Figure 4-1. Illustration of the concomitant development of exocrine and endocrine glands within the pancreas. **A,** Epithelial buds invaginate into adjacent mesenchyme from the developing endoderm. **B,** While the epithelial buds grow, they are initially connected to the surface epithelium. **C** and **D,** Within the exocrine portion, the connection is transformed into ducts that lead to individual acini; in the endocrine portion, the connection disintegrates and disappears as blood vessels become closely associated with the glandular cells.

NUMBER OF CELLS

Segregation of exocrine glands can be made into unicellular and multicellular types. **Unicellular glands** consist of either mucus or goblet cells scattered among columnar cells of simple columnar and pseudostratified columnar epithelia (Figure 4-2 see also Figure 3-24). The name of this cell type, *goblet*, is derived from its shape, which is best seen in the tracheal lining of many species. Cytoplasmically these cells are characterized by the presence of groups of secretory droplets that coalesce apically and eventually fuse with the plasma membrane (Figure 4-3).

Multicellular glands have a variety of forms ranging from a sheet of cells as found along the surface epithelium of the gastric mucosa (see Figure 3-9) to different systems of tubular and rounded invaginations, which comprise most of the multicellular types. It is important to keep in mind that the secretory cells of multicellular glands act, especially those which form distinct clusters, as collective entities rather than

individually. The organization of the clusters of the secretory cells into a single functional unit is referred to as an **adenomere** and each adenomere empties its secretions into a duct. Multicellular glands are further subdivided or classified into **simple** and **compound** categories based on the presence of one or more ducts.

SIMPLE GLANDS

The simple gland consists of a cluster of secretory cells (the adenomere, or secretory endpiece) that is connected to the surface by an unbranched duct. The configuration and the actual shape of the adenomere are the two principal characters for classifying simple glands (Figures 4-4 and 4-5). The shape of the endpieces is typically either **tubular** or **acinar** (rounded), which is also called **alveolar**. The endpieces may be branched or unbranched. In those that are simple tubular glands, the adenomeres can be subdivided further based on their configuration—whether the endpiece is **straight** or **coiled.**

TABLE 4-1   Exocrine Glands of the Body

TYPE	SHAPE	EXOCRINE GLANDS PRODUCT	METHOD OF SECRETION	LOCATION
Single Cell				
Goblet cell	Goblet	Mucus	Merocrine	Epithelium lining digestive, respiratory, and reproductive tracts
Multicellular				
Simple				
Sweat gland	Tubular, coiled	Salts; albuminoids; serum globulins; urea (horse)	Merocrine; apocrine (predominant in domestic animals)	Skin, foot pads (carnivores)
Sebaceous gland	Alveolar branched	Lipids	Holocrine	Skin
Anal sac gland (carnivores, rodents)	Tubular	Salts and lipids (cats)	Apocrine; holocrine	Perianal sinuses
Labial (submucosal) gland	Tubuloalveolar, branched	Mucus (small ruminants and carnivores); mixed	Merocrine	Lips
Buccal glands	Tubuloalveolar, branched	Serous; mucus; mixed	Merocrine	Cheeks
Cardiac and fundic glands	Tubular, coiled, branched	Mucus	Merocrine	Stomach
Pyloric	Tubular (short), ± branched	Mucus	Merocrine	Stomach
Intestinal crypts	Tubular, branched	Serous, mucus	Merocrine	Small intestine
Colonic glands	Tubular	Mucus	Merocrine	Large intestine
Anal gland	Tubuloalveolar	Lipids (dog); mucus (pig)	Holocrine; merocrine	Anal canal
Uterine glands	Tubular, ± branched, coiled (especially during pregnancy)	Serous, mucus, lipids	Merocrine	Uterus
Vestibular glands, minor	Tubular, branched	Mucus	Merocrine	Vulva
Seminiferous tubules	Tubular branched	Spermatids	Holocrine; apocrine (swine)	Testes
Respiratory submucosal glands	Tubuloalveolar, branched	Mucus, serous, mixed	Merocrine	Nasopharynx
Respiratory submucosal glands	Tubuloalveolar, branched	Mucus (serous and mixed canivores)	Merocrine	Larynx
Multicellular				
Compound				
Bronchial glands	Tubuloalveolar	Mixed	Merocrine	Primary and secondary bronchi, tertiary in cats
Tracheal glands	Tubuloalveolar	Mixed	Merocrine	Trachea
Meibomian gland (tarsal)	Alveolar	Lipid	Holocrine	Eyelids
Vomeronasal glands		Mixed	Merocrine	Vomeronasal organ
Salivary glands in general	Tubuloalveolar	Serous, mucus, mixed	Merocrine	Buccal cavity

TABLE 4-1 Exocrine Glands of the Body—cont'd

TYPE	SHAPE	EXOCRINE GLANDS PRODUCT	METHOD OF SECRETION	LOCATION
Specific major types				
Parotid	Tubuloalveolar	Serous; slightly mixed in carnivores	Merocrine	Buccal cavity
Mandibular		Mucus (carnivores); serous (rodents); mixed (horses, ruminants)		
Sublingual		Mucus (ruminants, swine, rodents); mixed (small carnivores, horses)		
Specific minor types				
Labial	Tubuloalveolar	Mucus (small ruminant and carnivores); serous (large ungulates)	Merocrine	Buccal cavity
Lingual		Mucus (carnivores and sheep); mixed (large ruminants and horses)		
Gustatory		Serous		
Dorsal buccal glands		Mucus (large ungulates, carnivores)		
Ventral buccal glands		Serous (large ungulates, carnivores)		
Exocrine pancreas	Aveolar; tubuloalveolar	Serous	Merocrine	Pancreas
Accessory genital glands				
Ampullary glands	Tubular; tubuloalveolar branched	Serous	Merocrine	Male reproductive tract; ampulla
Vesicular glands (seminal vesicle)	Tubular; tubuloalveolar	Serous, mucus, lipid	Merocrine	Male reproductive tract
Prostate	Tubuloalveolar	Serous, mucus, lipid	Merocrine	Male reproductive tract
Bulbourethral gland	Tubular	Serous, lipid	Merocrine	Male urethra
Vestibular glands, major	Tubuloalveolar	Mucus	Merocrine	Female reproductive tract; vestibule
Mammary glands	Tubuloalveolar	Lipid, serous	Aprocrine; merocrine	

COMPOUND GLANDS

Compound glands are those whose adenomeres empty into more than one duct. The classification of compound glands can then be thought of as consisting of a variable number of simple glands at the ends of a branching system of ducts. Adenomeres can be all of one kind or mixed as in compound tubuloalveolar-salivary glands (Figure 4-6). Larger glands are further described according to basic histological organization, which involves condensation of connective tissue. These glands can then be separated into parenchyma and stroma. Parenchyma is traditionally subdivided into aggregates of secretory units according to natural boundaries formed by stroma, going from lobes to lobules to microlobules to tubules or acini (Figures 4-7 and 4-8). The system of ducts is similarly subdivided, going from the main duct to lobar, interlobar, intralobar (which can be several orders), and eventually to intercalary ducts. When viewing histological sections of most compound glands one is limited to a two-dimensional view or plane. Frequently, the cross-section of the tubular portions appears identical to that of the alveolar portions, and thus these glands can best be described by three-dimensional reconstructions of serial sections.

TYPE OF SECRETORY PRODUCT

The type of secretory product is a further way to classify glands. Glands that form a clear, watery fluid are termed **serous,** whereas those that produce a more viscid fluid are termed **mucous.** Glands that produce a mixture of serous and mucous fluids are referred to as **mixed.** Serous secretory cells are overall smaller than mucus-secreting cells and have centrally positioned nuclei that lie next to the base (Figure 4-9, A). The secretory product is high in enzyme content; the

Text continued on p. 68

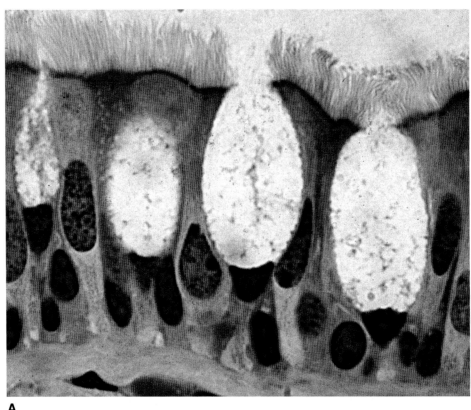

A

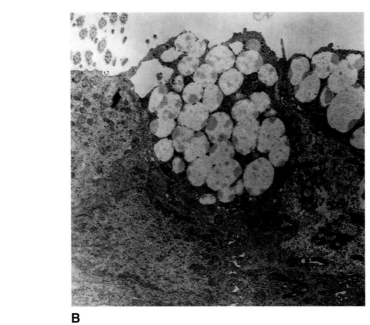

B

Figure 4-2. Goblet cell. **A,** Photomicrograph of goblet cells within a pseudostratified columnar epithelium. (×1000.)
B, Transmission electron micrograph of a goblet cell *(G)* reveals the compact nature of the secretory droplets interspersed
occasionally by mitochondria and other elements of the cytoplasm. (×4000.)

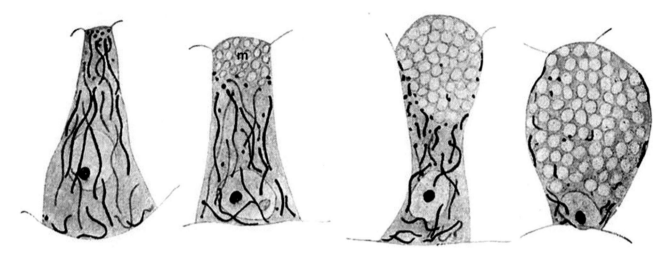

Figure 4-3. Illustration of the development of mucus-bearing *(m)* secretory droplets within the goblet cell. *(Modified from Greep RO:* Histology, *New York, 1954, Blakiston.)*

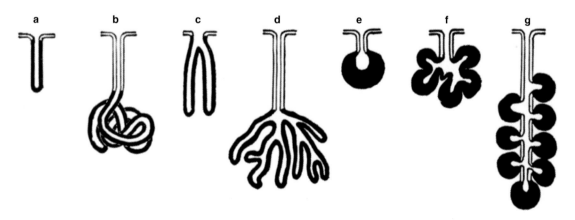

Figure 4-4. Diagram of the different shapes of simple glands: *a,* simple tubular; *b,* simple coiled tubular; *c* and *d,* simple branched tubular; *e,* simple acinar; *f* and *g,* simple branched acinar. Blackened secretory portions empty into the double-contoured ducts. *(From Fawcett DW:* Bloom and Fawcett: a textbook of histology, *ed 11, Philadelphia, 1986, Saunders.)*

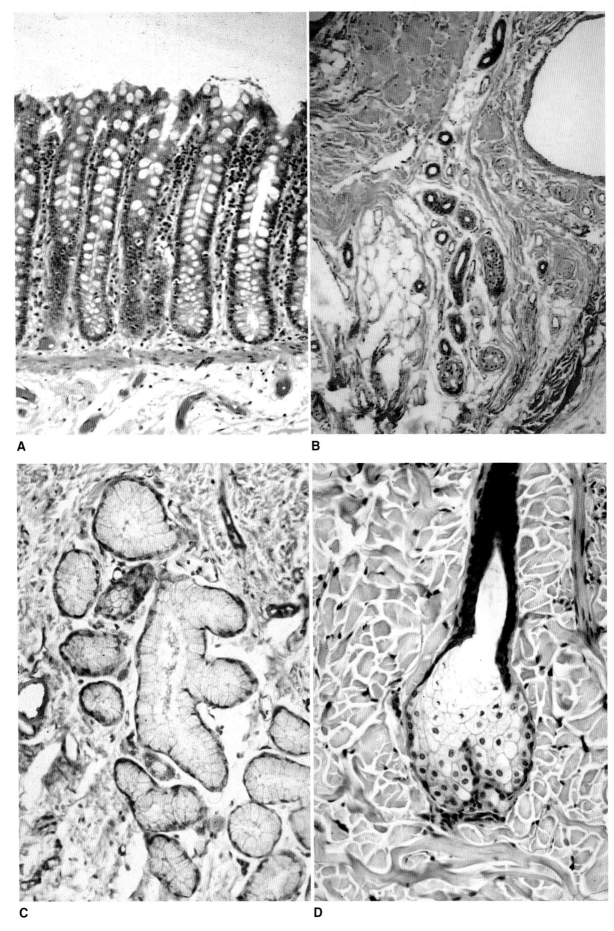

A

B

C

D

Figure 4-5. For legend see opposite page.

Figure 4-5. Simple glands. **A,** Light micrograph of simple tubules within the large intestine. (Hematoxylin and eosin [H&E] stain; ×25.) **B,** Light micrograph of a simple coiled tubule (sweat gland) within the dermis of skin. (H&E stain; ×200.) **C,** Light micrograph of simple branched tubules within the esophagus. (H&E stain; ×200.) **D,** Light micrograph of simple branched acini (sebaceous glands) within the dermis of skin. (H&E stain; ×200.)

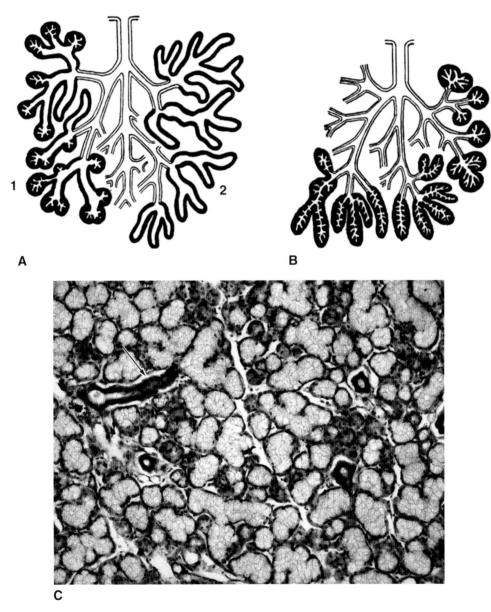

Figure 4-6. A, Diagram of the examples of compound glands: *1,* compound tubuloacinar (left portion) and *2,* tubular (right portion). **B,** Compound acinar with some variation in the shape of the acini. Blackened secretory portions empty into the double-contoured ducts. **C,** Light micrograph of a compound tubuloacinar gland (canine salivary gland). The arrow points to a duct that collects the secretions of several secretory units to the right of it. (Hematoxylin and eosin stain; ×100.) *(A and B from Fawcett DW: Bloom and Fawcett: a textbook of histology, ed 11, Philadelphia, 1986, Saunders.)*

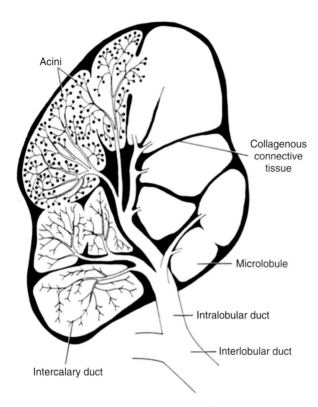

Figure 4-7. Diagram showing the organization of the secretory units and associated system of ducts within the stroma of a lobular portion of a compound gland. *(From Fawcett DW: Bloom and Fawcett: a textbook of histology, ed 11, Philadelphia, 1986, Saunders.)*

best examples of serous secreting cells can be found in the salivary glands and the exocrine pancreas.

Mucus secretory cells present a strong contrast to serous secretory cells because they are often filled with mucigen droplets, and as a result have a pale, vacuolated (foamy) appearance (Figure 4-9, B). The nucleus is characteristically displaced against the base of the cell to the point of appearing disklike. The secretory product in mucus cells is rich in sugars, containing richly glycosylated proteins that easily bind water and can act as a lubricant and protective coat. An excellent example of a mucus secretory cell is the goblet cell (see Figures 4-2 and 4-3). Mucus secretory cells are also well populated throughout much of the digestive tract and upper respiratory tract. In adenomeres possessing both types of cells, such as in the salivary glands, the **demilunes** (crescent-shaped bodies of serous cells) frequently lie outside the mucus cells (see Figure 4-9, B). Their secretions enter small channels, canaliculi, between the much larger mucus cells.

MODE OF SECRETION

This classification is based on the manner by which secretory cells of exocrine glands secrete their products (Figure 4-10).

Merocrine glands possess secretory cells that release their products by exocytosis, where the cell product is delivered through the cell membrane in

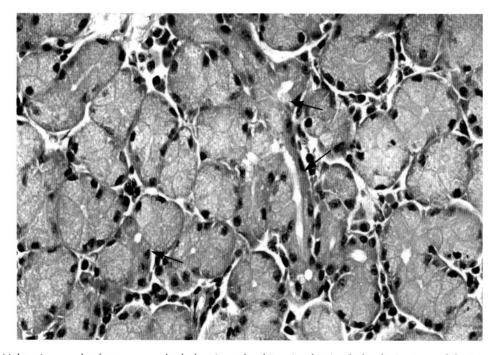

Figure 4-8. Light micrograph of a compound tubuloacinar gland (equine lacrimal gland). Portions of the intercalary ducts *(arrows)* can consist of both nonsecretory cells (duct cells) and secretory cells. (Hematoxylin and eosin stain; ×400.)

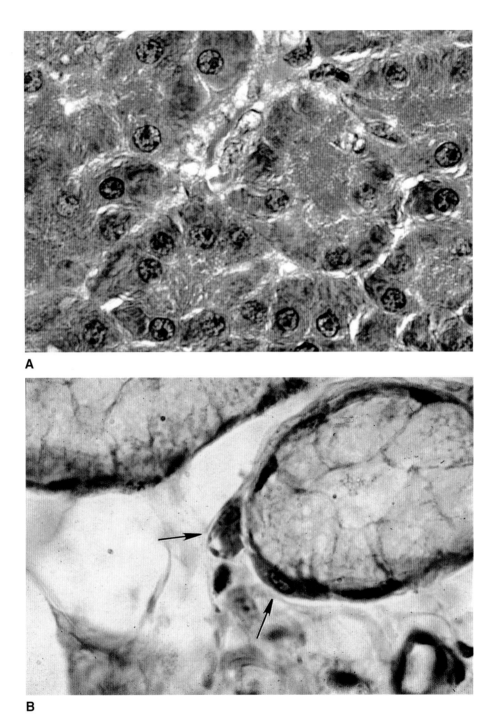

Figure 4-9. Light micrographs of **A,** serous-secreting cells within the equine pancreas and, **B,** mucus-secreting cells within the canine parotid gland demonstrate contrasting appearances in size, shape, and staining reaction to hematoxylin and eosin. Arrows point to the serous-secreting demilunes that envelop portions of mucus secretory units. (×1000.)

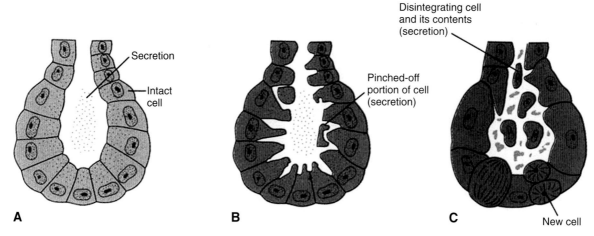

Figure 4-10. Mode of secretion in exocrine glands. **A,** Merocrine gland (e.g., salivary gland). **B,** Apocrine gland (e.g., sweat gland). **C,** Holocrine gland (e.g., sebaceous gland). *(From Bergman RA, Afifi AK, Heidger PM Jr:* Histology, *Philadelphia, 1996, Saunders.)*

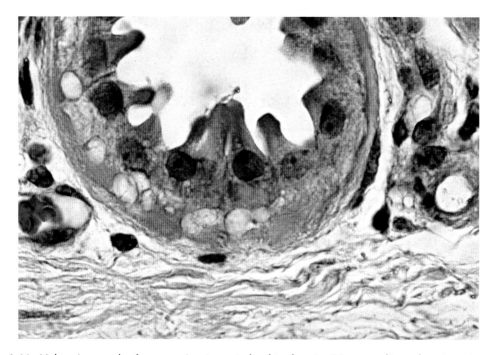

Figure 4-11. Light micrograph of an apocrine (sweat) gland in the pig. (Hematoxylin and eosin stain; ×1000.)

membrane-bound vesicles that are fused with the cell membrane and in this manner keeps the cell membrane intact. Thus there is no loss of cellular material during this process other than the secretory material. The majority of glands are merocrine, and examples are many, including the pancreas and the rest associated with the digestive system.

In **apocrine** glands part of the apical cytoplasm is discharged along with the secretory product. Electron microscopy has revealed that this process is not as likely as once believed and that many glands that were previously termed apocrine may be truly merocrine. Still, close inspection of secretory release in mammary

glands has revealed some loss of the cell membrane and a thin rim of cytoplasm. Among domestic animals sweat glands are primarily apocrine (Figure 4-11).

Glands with **holocrine** secretion involve cell detachment and subsequent death. As a result the entire content of the cell contributes to the secretory product. The principal example is the sebaceous gland of the integument (Figure 4-12).

ANCILLARY TISSUE

Secretory cells of epithelial origin are closely associated with adjacent connective tissue elements,

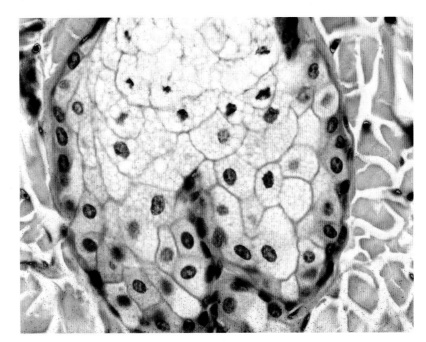

Figure 4-12. Light micrograph of a holocrine (sebaceous) gland in the cat. (Hematoxylin and eosin stain; ×400.)

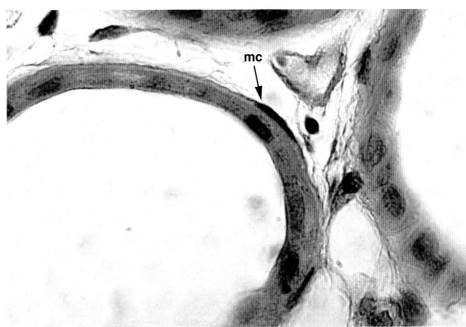

mc

Figure 4-13. Light micrograph (×1000) of a myoepithelial cell *(mc)* lining in an inactive sweat gland of a pig.

which are largely vascular. Efferent terminations of nervous tissue are also frequently involved with glands, both with regard to production and release of the secretions. In conjunction with these ancillary tissues, many exocrine glands contain specialized epithelial cells that have contractile capability, the **myoepithelial cell,** which are tightly woven as a single intermittent layer around the periphery of each adenomere (and in some instances small ducts), but inside (and contributing to) the basement membrane of the gland (Figure 4-13). Myoepithelial cells share a similar cytoplasm of the smooth muscle cell but differ primarily from the latter in having branched cellular processes.

SUGGESTED READINGS

Bergman RA, Afifi AK, Heidger PM Jr: *Histology,* Philadelphia, 1996, Saunders.

Fawcett DW: *Bloom and Fawcett: a textbook of histology,* ed 11, Philadelphia, 1986, Saunders.

Gesase AP, Satoh Y: Apocrine secretory mechanism: recent findings and unresolved problems, *Histol Histopathol* 18:597, 2003.

Ito M, Motoyoshi K, Tanizawa M, et al: The holocrine secretion of sebaceous glands—a histochemical and ultrastructural study, *J Invest Derm* 80:375, 1983.

Vidic B: Structure and cytochemistry of acinar cell in rat maxillary gland, *Am J Anat* 137:103, 1973.

Connective Tissue

CHAPTER 5

KEY CHARACTERISTICS

- Presence of extracellular matrix (ECM)
- Provides attachment, support, defense and protection for other tissues
- Classified according to:
  ECM organization: connective tissue proper
  Specialized forms: blood, cartilage, bone

Connective tissue, as the name implies, connects and holds other tissues together. This tissue consists of a three-dimensional framework supporting epithelial and other tissues and plays a major role in heat regulation, storage, defense, protection, and repair. Connective tissue is mostly mesodermal in origin and is composed of free and fixed (nonmotile) cells that are surrounded by an extensive extracellular matrix of proteinaceous fibers, amorphous ground substance, and tissue fluid (Figure 5-1). It is the presence of these extracellular components that easily distinguishes connective tissue from the other major tissue types (epithelia, muscles, and nerve). Connective tissue represents a fairly heterogeneous collection of subtypes including connective tissue proper (loose and dense), bone, cartilage, and hematopoietic types (leukocytes, erythrocytes, bone marrow, and lymph). For the most part, connective tissue proper develops from mesenchyme (embryonic connective tissue). Many of the cell types associated with connective tissue migrate into the connective tissue from other sources such as bone marrow and neural crest.

Types of cells in connective tissue vary considerably. The types described are most commonly observed in connective tissue proper, especially loose connective tissue, and consist of those that either remain fixed in place (resident cells of connective tissues) or those that migrate into the tissue (transient cells of connective tissues).

RESIDENT CELLS

FIBROBLAST AND FIBROCYTE

The **fibroblast** forms the foundation for all connective tissue proper. It functions primarily to create the extracellular matrix that characterizes this tissue. Fibroblasts are fixed cells that are typically stellate to spindle shaped, with cellular processes that extend to adjacent cells and possess ovoid nuclei (see Figure 5-1). Cytologically, this cell type is quite active, containing much rough endoplasmic reticulum (rER) and a well-developed Golgi apparatus (Figure 5-2). The fibroblast originates from the mesenchymal cell, which is pleuripotential and can give rise to other cell types in connective tissues (Figure 5-3). In mature tissue, the fibroblasts become considerably less active than during development. The cell body is reduced gradually in size, being more spindly and less stellate

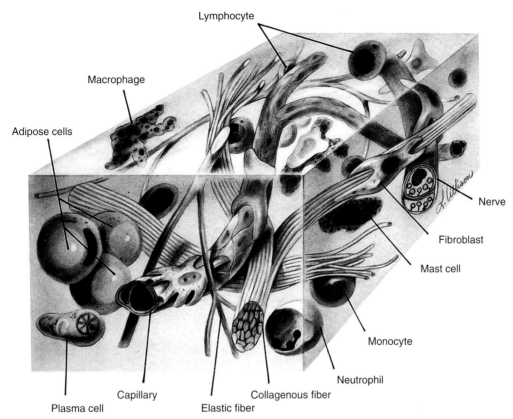

Figure 5-1. Illustration of cells and extracellular components of connective tissues. *(From Leeson CR, Leeson TS, Paparo AA:* Atlas of histology, *Philadelphia, 1985, Saunders.)*

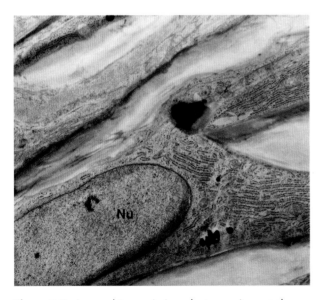

Figure 5-2. Layered transmission electron micrograph (×25,000) of a fibroblast with a euchromatic nucleus *(Nu)* and well-developed rough endoplasmic reticulum.

than before with smaller amounts of cytoplasm and a smaller, darker (more heterochromatic) nucleus. The less active cell is called the **fibrocyte** and is normally surrounded by an abundance of extracellular fibers and ground substances (Figure 5-4). The fibrocyte can be microenvironmentally stimulated to return to a more metabolically active state and become fibroblastic in appearance, but not necessarily to the extent that it was originally. Consequently, the histological distinction between fibrocytic and fibroblastic states can be challenging, particularly to the less experienced individual. In many instances the terms are used interchangeably.

PERICYTE

A cell similar in morphology to the fibroblast/ fibrocyte is the **pericyte,** which likewise is derived from the mesenchymal cell. Pericytes retain the small size of the mesenchymal cell and are closely associated with small blood vessels (capillaries), lying immediately adjacent to the endothelial cells that line the blood vessels. They share endothelial and smooth muscle cell characteristics including the formation of

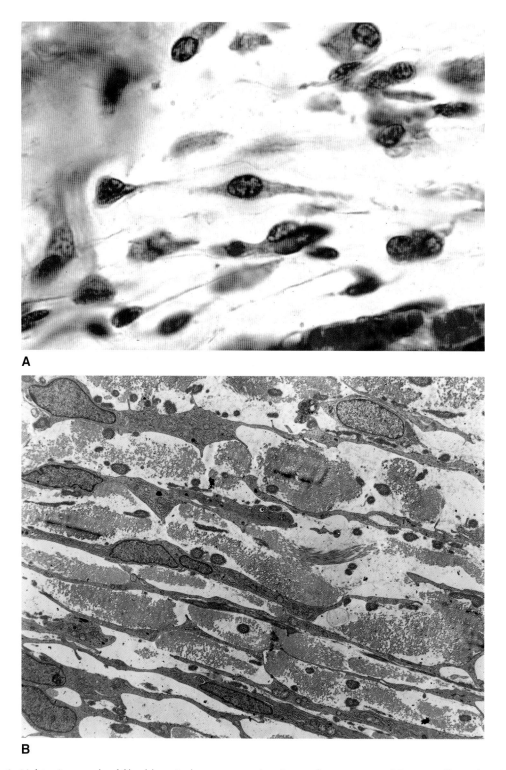

A

B

Figure 5-3. A, Light micrograph of fibroblasts in loose connective tissue of a young cat. (Hematoxylin and eosin stain; ×400.) **B,** Transmission electron micrograph (×5000) of developing fibroblasts in canine sclera.

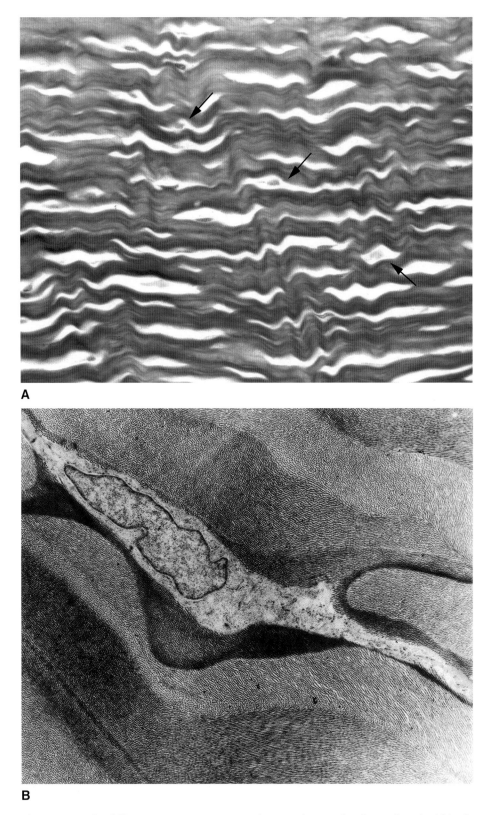

A

B

Figure 5-4. A, Light micrograph of fibrocytes *(arrows)* scattered among layers of collagen found within the corneal stroma of a horse. (Masson trichrome stain; ×200.) **B,** Layered transmission electron micrograph (×10,000) of a canine fibrocyte within a regular dense connective tissue environment shows most of the shape of this relatively quiescent cell.

its own basal lamina and contractile elements (Figure 5-5). The function of the pericyte has not been fully revealed. Some speculation has been given to the possibility that this cell type can further differentiate into vascular smooth muscle cells or endothelial cells upon injury to blood vessels.

MYOFIBROBLAST

The **myofibroblast** is, as the name suggests, part fibroblastic and part muscle-like, having a contractile apparatus similar to the smooth muscle cell. Histologically this cell type is nearly identical to the fibroblast and can be distinguished best by immunohistochemical or ultrastructural verification. Myofibroblasts have been associated with injury repair after wounding, periodontal ligaments and tooth eruption, and aqueous humor removal apparatus of the eye.

MACROPHAGE

A cell occasionally seen in connective tissue is the **macrophage.** Macrophages play an important role in protection (defense) of the body by ingestion of foreign materials. Their precursors are **monocytes,** which originate from bone marrow and pass into the connective tissue from the vasculature (part of the mononuclear phagocyte system). After monocytes have entered a tissue, such as loose connective tissue, they are referred to as *macrophages* or *histiocytes.* These cells are either fixed (resident) or migrating (elicited). If the latter is occurring, they move to a site of potential activity by ameboid movement (Figure 5-6). The presence of chemotactic substances such as potential pathogens or cytokines released by other cells stimulate the macrophage to pseudopodially move into place. By comparison, fixed, inactive macrophages are somewhat spindle shaped and may be occasionally mistaken for fibroblasts. The elicited macrophage is thus more easily distinguished than the resident macrophage because of the presence of numerous short, thick pseudopodia (Figure 5-7; see also Figure 5-6). Furthermore, these cells tend to be more active in phagocytosis and consequently have the usual complement of cellular structures involved in the ingestion and breakdown of foreign materials—primary and secondary lysosomes, phagosomes, residual bodies and peroxisomes, as well as a well-developed Golgi apparatus and rER (see Figure 5-7). The nucleus can be distinctive, being often indented on one side and resultantly kidney shaped. Fixed and migrating macrophages are different phases of the same cell. Their potential mobility makes these cells most suitable for the defense of the organism, as well as removal of debris from damaged tissue. In situations in which tissues are exposed to foreign bodies over an extended period, macrophages may coalesce and form a **foreign body giant cell.** These cells can be comparatively large and have several or more nuclei (Figure 5-8). Keep in mind that the main function of the macrophage is

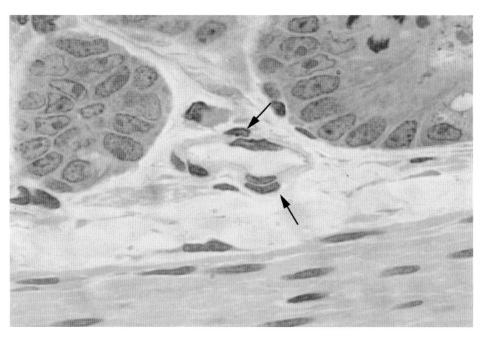

Figure 5-5. Light micrograph of pericytes *(arrows)* that are associated with a small blood vessel within the small intestine of a rat. (Plastic section stained with hematoxylin and eosin; ×1000.)

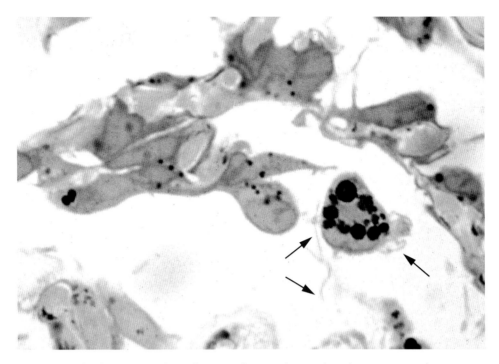

Figure 5-6. Light micrograph of an active (elicited) macrophage with pseudopodia *(arrows)* and numerous secondary lysosomes. (Plastic section stained with toluidine blue; ×1000.)

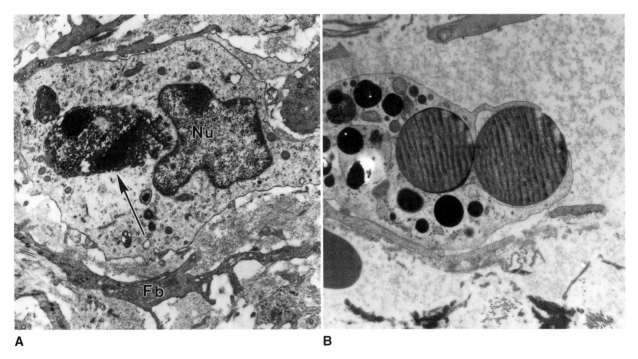

A   **B**

Figure 5-7. Transmission electron micrographs of different active canine macrophages. **A,** The macrophage is removing and breaking down damaged extracellular matrix seen in the large secondary lysosome *(arrow)* that lies next to an indented nucleus *(Nu)*. Note the proximity of adjacent fibrocytes *(Fb)* (×12,000.) **B,** A macrophage is ingesting plastic microspheres up to 3 μm in diameter in addition to other foreign substances. As a result of this activity, numerous opaque secondary lysosomes fill the cytoplasm of this cell. (×10,000.)

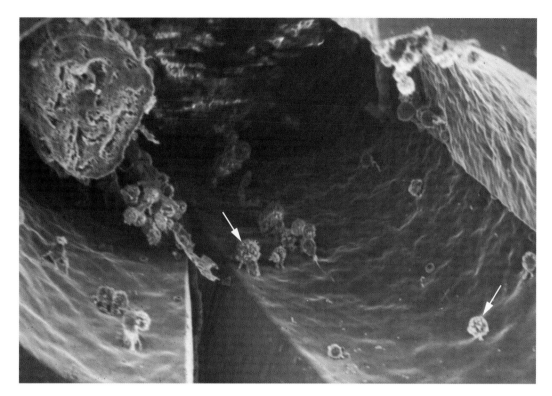

Figure 5-8. Scanning electron micrograph (×800) of macrophages and foreign-body giant cells *(arrows)* that have attacked a plastic valve implanted within a dog.

phagocytosis during either active defense or cleanup of debris.

The "phage" is also involved in immune reactions by making foreign cells or proteins antigenic.

Other monocyte/macrophage cells of the mononuclear phagocytic system include the Kupffer cell (liver), alveolar macrophage (lung), osteoclast (bone), microglia (central nervous system), and Langerhans cell (epidermis) (Table 5-1).

MAST CELL

The **mast cell** is a more common cell type than the macrophage in connective tissue, being most often found near blood vessels within loose connective tissue. Mast cells are somewhat ovoid and can be larger than macrophages, with diameters of 20 to 30 μm and greater. The presence of numerous basophilically stained secretory granules distinguishes their cytoplasm, which also contains scattered mitochondria, rER, polysomes, and Golgi apparatus. These granules surround an often centrally located spherical-to-oval nucleus (Figure 5-9). The granules, which are membrane bound, contain a variety of substances including the sulfated glycosaminoglycan heparin, which reacts metachromatically with certain stains

such as toluidine blue. The presence of these cells can be best revealed by ultrastructural and immunohisto-chemical light microscopic observations (Figure 5-10). Electron microscopy demonstrates small variations among the granules in the size and consistency, especially among mast cells that appear to be in the process of releasing their contents. The substances within the granules are water soluble and can function to promote localized inflammation. In addition to heparin, which acts as an anticoagulant, the granules contain histamine, which induces increased dilation and permeability of capillaries and small venules (edema), slow-reacting substance of anaphylaxis (SRS-A), eosinophil chemotactic factor of anaphylaxis (ECF-A), and neutral proteases. The mast cells can also be involved in allergic responses and anaphylaxis and participate in conditions such as asthma, drug sensitization, hay fever, and anaphylactic shock.

The surface of the mast cell has specific receptor antibodies sensitive to antigens that have invaded the body and are possibly circulating throughout it. When an antigen becomes attached to the receptor *(cell-surface Fc receptor)*, the granules are released or extruded by an active catabolic process, exocytosis (Figure 5-11, A). The receptors are not produced by mast cells but, in fact, originate from plasma cells and

TABLE 5-1 Cells of the Monocyte-Macrophage System throughout the Body

TYPE	LOCATION	FUNCTION
Pluripotent stem cell	Bone marrow	Gives rise to variety of blood cell progenitors including monoblasts
Monoblast	Bone marrow	Differentiates into monocyte
Monocyte	Peripheral blood	Along with the macrophage and the neutrophil, this cell provides first line of defense against infection
Histiocyte/resident macrophage	Connective tissues	Positioned in different connective tissues of the body; this cell becomes elicited and is able to move quickly to sites of potential infection
Kupffer cell	Liver	Lines sinusoids and breaks down debris including old erythrocytes
Langerhans cell	Skin, esophagus	Antigen-presenting cells that process foreign antigens, presenting their isotopes to T lymphocytes
Microglia	Central nervous system	Clear debris and damaged portions of the central nervous system
Dust cell/alveolar macrophage	Lung	Clear particles and bacteria from the pulmonary epithelium of distal airways, maintaining a pathogen-free environment
Osteoclast	Bone	Resorption of bone for continued development and remodeling
Foreign-body giant cell	Site of chronic inflammation	Joined (fused) macrophages engulf large structure to be degraded

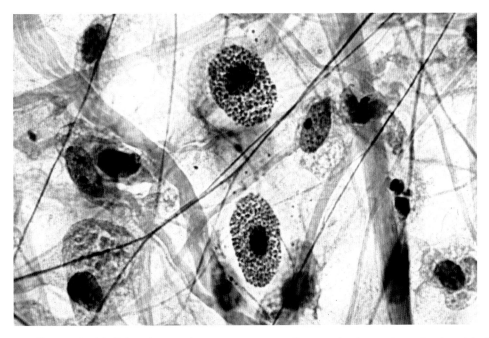

Figure 5-9. Mast cells seen in this light micrograph possess many small, even-sized granules stained positively by azocarmine. (×1000.) Taken from a flat mount preparation of mesentery tissue.

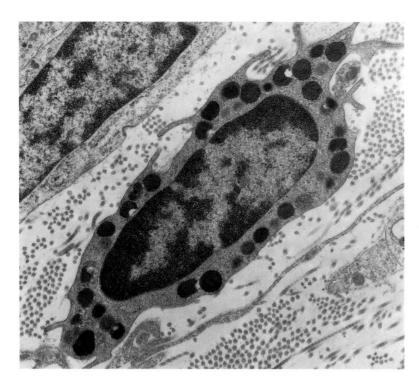

Figure 5-10. Transmission electron micrograph (×8000) of a feline mast cell reveals the presence of numerous, even-sized granules and pseudopodia. The pseudopodia suggest the possibility that these cells have good motile capability.

consist of immunoglobulins of the immunoglobulin E (IgE) class, which were formed previously in response to an earlier presence of an antigen (Figure 5-11, *B*). When infiltration of the antigen recurs, the antigen complexes with the attached sensitive-specific IgE and trigger host cell granule release of primary and secondary mediators, which causes edema of surrounding tissues. With repeated exposure to a particular antigen, mast cells develop increased sensitivity, which can lead to a hypersensitive response and possibly anaphylaxis.

Mast cells are unevenly distributed throughout the body, being well populated within the integument and lung on one hand but nonexistent within the central nervous system except for the outer connective tissue coat, the meninges, on the other. The life of the cell is determinate, lasting only for several months and replenished by new cells that originate most likely from stem cells of the bone marrow. The mast cell is similar to another cell type, the basophil, which is found in the vasculature and comprises about 1% of circulating leukocytes. Like the mast cell, the basophil contains basophilic granules within its cytoplasm that hold some of the same substances as the mast cell's granules. Basophils, however, have a segmented nucleus as opposed to the large and nonsegmented nucleus of the mast cell.

MELANOCYTE

Melanocytes are cells of connective tissue that provide the pigment **melanin,** to the skin, primarily the epidermis, but they exist in other portions of the body, too, including the eye, the liver of certain reptiles, and developmentally within tracts of the central nervous system (CNS). In the skin and eyes, melanin helps shield the skin from too much exposure of ultraviolet light of the sun through its absorption as well as scattering of light. In tissues not exposed to light, melanin probably provides one or more of a variety of functions, including electron exchange, metal ion binding, and free radical scavenging. Melanocytes are fiber-like cells that when associated with the epidermis of skin are often semirounded with long irregular extensions (Figure 5-12, *A* and *B*). They are most commonly observed beneath or between cells of the basal layer and upper layers of the epidermis, with the extensions branching toward the body's surface. These cells have fairly well-developed rER and Golgi apparatus organelles that are involved in melanin synthesis. The derivation of melanin from its precursor, tyrosine, occurs in the organelle referred to as the **melanosome,** which is believed to be a modified component of the lysosomal system. When melanin synthesis has ceased in these bodies they are often

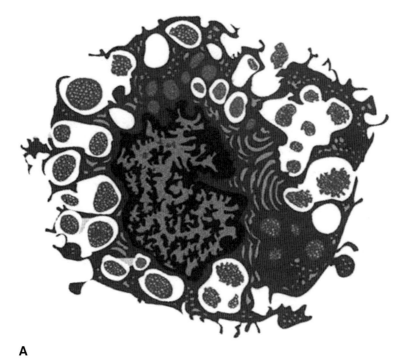

A

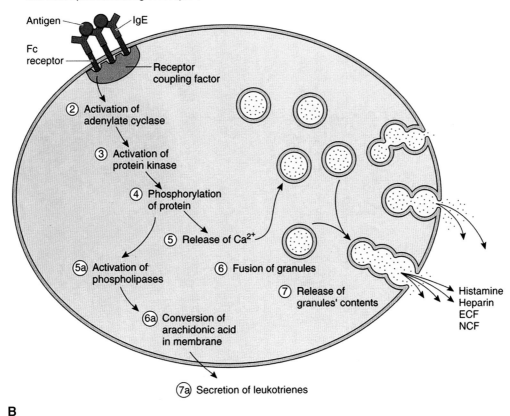

① Binding of antigen to IgE-receptor complex causes cross-linking of IgE and consequent clustering of receptors

Antigen — IgE

Fc receptor —

Receptor coupling factor

② Activation of adenylate cyclase

③ Activation of protein kinase

④ Phosphorylation of protein

⑤ Release of Ca²⁺

⑤a Activation of phospholipases

⑥ Fusion of granules

⑦ Release of granules' contents

Histamine
Heparin
ECF
NCF

⑥a Conversion of arachidonic acid in membrane

⑦a Secretion of leukotrienes

B

Figure 5-11. Illustrations of a mast cell. **A,** When given the signal to exocytose, all granules are actively released at the same time. **B,** The mast cell has a close relationship with plasma cells and the antibodies that they secrete, which attach to Fc receptors within the mast cell's cell membrane. *ECF,* Eosinophil chemotactic factor; *NCF,* neutrophil chemotactic factor. *(A from Bergman RA, Afifi AK, Heidger PM Jr: Histology, Philadelphia, 1996, Saunders; B from Gartner LP, Hiatt JL: Color textbook of histology, Philadelphia, 1997, Saunders.)*

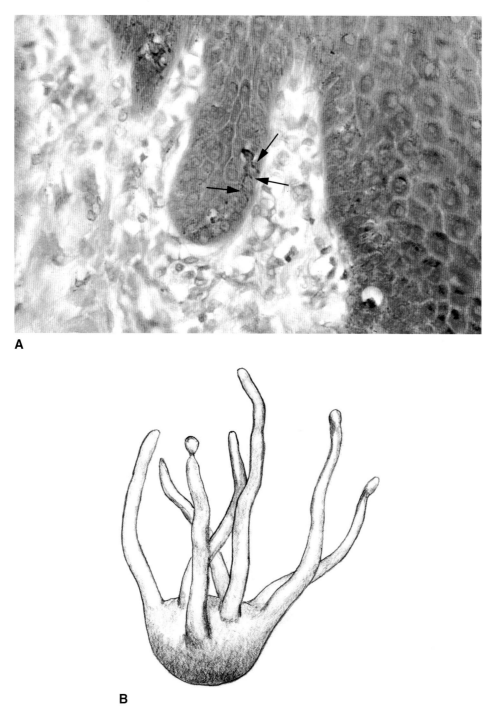

A

B

Figure 5-12. A, Photomicrograph of a melanocyte within the basal cell layer of the epidermis of the canine nose. Note the presence of several processes *(arrows)* that extend from the melanocyte. (Hematoxylin and eosin stain; ×1000.) **B,** Illustration of an epidermal melanocyte, such as the one seen in Figure 5-12, *A,* with its tentacle-like processes that function to insert melanin granules into adjacent cells.

referred to as **melanin granules,** which migrate into the long finger-like cellular extensions and eventually are transferred to cells of the basal stratum and stratum spinosum. Unlike other cells of connective tissue, melanocytes originate from the neural crest. When fully differentiated, melanocytes do not normally undergo cell division, but their capacity to produce melanin is sustained throughout the life of the individual.

ADIPOCYTE

Fat cells, adipose cells, or **adipocytes** form another resident cell type of connective tissue. Although they may be isolated or clustered in small groups within connective tissue, these cells are generally found in large numbers, forming adipose tissue. Like many cells of the body (neuron, muscle cell, osteocyte, melanocyte, etc.), once an adipocyte has formed, it loses its ability to further replicate **(terminal differentiation).** Adipocytes function simply to manufacture and store triglycerides. In this capacity adipose tissue can store energy, control body temperature, and provide in a manner of speaking "shock absorption." Adipose tissue is traditionally subdivided into two types based on cell structure, localization, color, and function and is discussed at further length later in this chapter. **Unilocular** (common, yellow) adipose cells at maturity possess a single, large central droplet of lipid (Figure 5-13). The color of the unilocular form may vary from white to dark yellow because it is influenced by the presence of carotenoids dissolved in the fat droplets. This tissue is the most common type of fat in adult animals. The nucleus is flattened and considerably displaced to one side. The lipids forming the large droplet are mostly triglycerides (esters of fatty acids and glycerol), and a unilocular droplet can easily exceed 100 µm in diameter (see Figure 5-13). The dynamics of triglyceride storage and release are illustrated in Figure 5-14. Fat that is digested within the small intestine is enzymatically separated into glycerol and fatty acids by lipase that was formed in the pancreas and released within the duodenum. As the intestinal mucosa absorbs the glycerol and fatty acids they become reesterified to triglycerides within the smooth endoplasmic reticulum (sER) of the absorbing cells of the epithelium, **enterocytes.** The triglycerides are enveloped by proteins and become **chylomicrons,** which are transported to the bloodstream and general circulation via lymph channels. At the site of adipose tissue the chylomicrons or triglyceride droplets are dissembled once more into glycerol and fatty acids by lipoprotein lipase secreted from the adipocytes before diffusing into the fat cells and reassembling into triglycerides. Concomitantly, glucose that is circulating in the bloodstream can also readily diffuse into the adipocyte, where it can be converted into triglycerides as well.

Multilocular (brown) adipose tissue is composed of cells with numerous small fat droplets (Figure 5-15). Cytoplasmically, these cells contain more mitochondria than their unilocular counterpart. The brown coloration is due to the presence of the numerous mitochondria. Multilocular fat is more highly innervated and vascularized than unilocular fat. This is in part directly related to its function, which is to heat

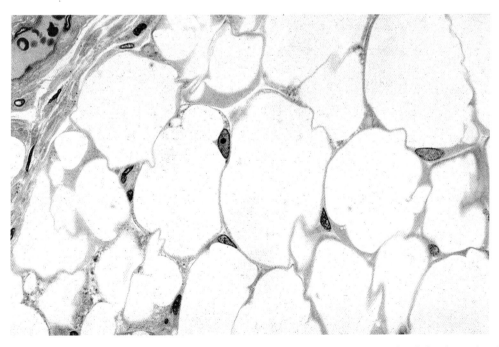

Figure 5-13. Light micrograph of unilocular adipocytes, each cell possessing a prominent lipid droplet or locule. When in the plane of the section, the nucleus is fairly distinct. (Plastic section stained with hematoxylin and eosin; ×400.)

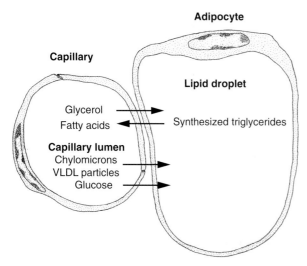

Figure 5-14. Diagram of the relationship between a unilocular adipocyte and neighboring bloodstream. Within the bloodstream (capillary), lipid is transported in the form of very low-density lipoproteins (VLDL) and chylomicrons from the liver and small intestine, respectively. The adipocyte is able to secrete lipase, which enters the capillary and hydrolyzes the lipid (triglycerides) to fatty acids and glycerol. The fatty acids and glycerol diffuse into the adipocyte and are reesterified into triglycerides. In addition, glucose can diffuse from the capillary into the fat cell and be used to form lipid. At another time, the stored triglycerides may be hydrolyzed into glycerol and fatty acids by a hormone-sensitive lipase and reenter the bloodstream.

blood that flows through it and consequently raise the body temperature. By comparison, white or unilocular fat functions primarily to provide a source of potential energy reserve. Multilocular fat forms prenatally, being much more confined than unilocular fat. It is also found in certain hibernating mammals (e.g., hibernating rodents). The placement of adipose cells as a cell type within connective tissue has been debated for some time. Some histologists have proposed that it be assigned as a separate tissue. The adipose cell is the only cell type in connective tissue that forms its own basement membrane. Still, the fact that these cells can arise singly in connective tissue and are most likely derived from progenitors which give rise to fibroblasts greatly strengthens their placement within connective tissue as a form of it.

TRANSIENT CELLS

PLASMA CELL

The **plasma cell** is another cell type that participates in host tissue defense. These cells typically migrate into connective tissues, especially specific regions that are subjected to continual invasion of bacteria and foreign proteins (for example, intestinal mucosa, female genital tract, lymphoid organs and bone marrow, and areas of inflammation). Otherwise

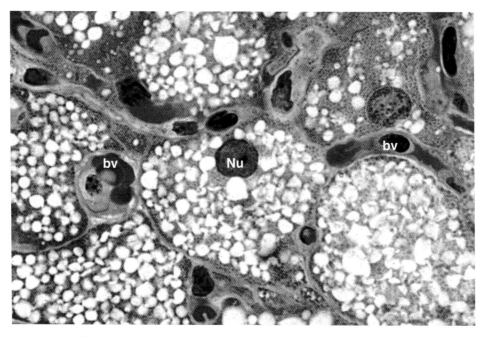

Figure 5-15. Light micrograph of multilocular adipocytes, which possess round nuclei *(Nu)* and have close associations with many small blood vessels *(bv)*. (Plastic section stained with hematoxylin and eosin; ×400.)

in most connective tissues these cells are generally sparse to nonexistent. Plasma cells, like other transient cells of connective tissue, are derived from progenitors that are housed in bone marrow. Plasma cells are histologically characterized by the eccentrically placed cartwheel (distinctly heterochromatic) nuclei within round to ovoid cells (Figure 5-16, A and B). When viewed by electron microscopy (EM) the bulk of the cytoplasm is composed mostly of stacks of rER and a notable Golgi apparatus (Figure 5-17). Light

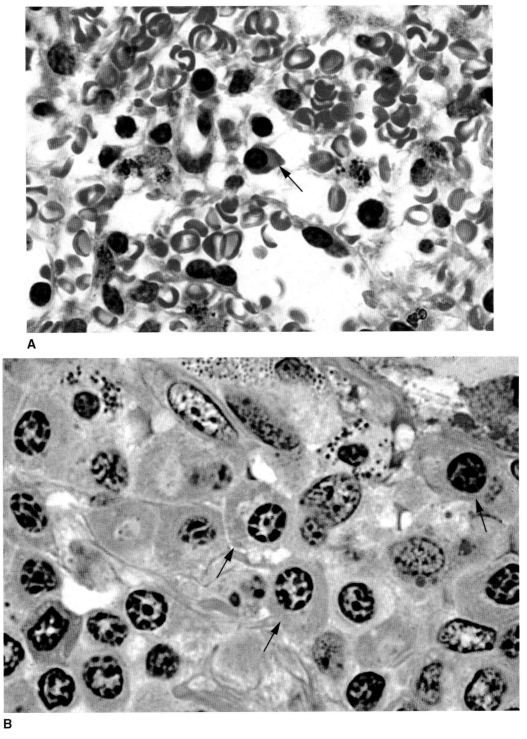

Figure 5-16. Plasma cell. **A,** Light micrograph of a plasma cell *(arrow)* with bluish staining regions within its cytoplasm. Spleen of a horse. (Hematoxylin and eosin stain; ×1000.) **B,** Light micrograph of a number of plasma cells *(arrows),* each possessing a distinctive cartwheel nucleus. (Plastic section stained with hematoxylin and eosin; ×1000.)

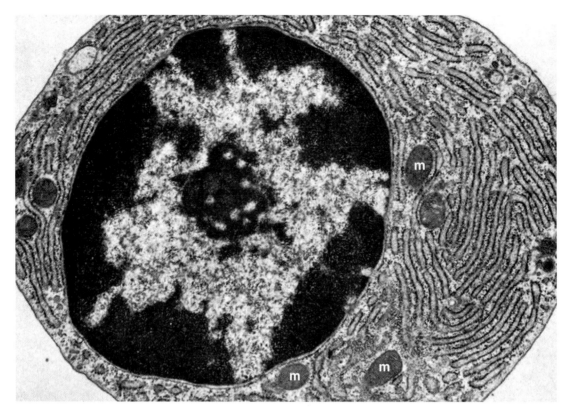

Figure 5-17. Transmission electron micrograph of a plasma cell reveals extensive rough endoplasmic reticulum *(rER)* with scattered mitochondria *(m)*. *(From Fawcett DW:* Bloom and Fawcett: a textbook of histology, *ed 11, Philadelphia, 1986, Saunders.)*

microscopically, the large amount of rER and associated nucleic acid (transfer RNA [t-RNA] and messenger RNA [m-RNA]) cause the cytoplasm to react basophically to stains. The rER in the plasma cells is responsible for the synthesis of antibodies that are released into the bloodstream (antibodies are specific globulins that are produced in response to specific antigens) Certain antigens need to contact macrophages first, making them immunogenic, so that plasma cells can then produce antibodies in response. Other antigens act directly on the precursors of plasma cells, B lymphocytes.

LYMPHOCYTE

The B lymphocyte system is characterized by a remarkable variety of immunoglobulins (humoral antibodies) having virtually all conceivable antigenic specificities (see Chapter 12). The system is designed suitably to deal with unpredictable and unforeseen microbial and toxic agents. T (thymus-derived) lymphocytes, which will not be covered here, seem to be precommitted to make only one type of antibody, which is cell bound. These cells can be intimately

associated with macrophages, responding to antigens attached to the phages.

Within connective tissue, lymphocytes comprise the smallest of the free cells with a diameter that typically lies within a range of 5 to 9 µm, as compared, for example, with the plasma cell, which measures approximately 20 µm in diameter. There are essentially two functional cell types: T lymphocytes and B lymphocytes. T lymphocytes tend to have long life spans, whereas B lymphocytes vary in their longevity, having the ability to divide several times and mature into plasma cells, which have short life spans (2-3 days).

LEUKOCYTES

Leukocytes comprise the white blood cells that circulate throughout the vasculature and provide active defense to regions of the body that are being invaded by foreign matter, including pathogens. Thus all leukocytes are capable of becoming transient components of connective tissue. Monocytes, which are referred to as macrophages after entering connective tissue, and lymphocytes constitute a portion of the leukocytes. The remainder consists of the granule-bearing cells **(granulocytes)** of inflammation: **neutrophils,** which ingest and break down bacteria; **eosinophils,** which defend against parasites; **basophils;** and **heterophils,** which exist in nonmammalian blood and are neutrophil-like in function. Leukocytes are described in detail in Chapter 7.

EXTRACELLULAR COMPONENTS—FIBERS AND GROUND SUBSTANCE

The bulk of connective tissue is made of its extracellular components or **extracellular matrix** (ECM). It is through the construction of the ECM that each type of connective tissue is given its characteristics. In connective tissue proper the extracellular environment is composed of fibers and ground substance.

COLLAGEN

The most common fiber in connective tissue is **collagen.** Collagen fibers impart both strength and flexibility to connective tissue and are often aggregated into branching bundles. The fibers, in turn, are composed of smaller subunits, **fibrils,** which are banded structures (Figure 5-18) when viewed ultrastructurally. The fibril itself is made up of laminated filaments, **tropocollagen** subunits (Figure 5-19). Tropocollagen units are 280 nm long and are spaced in a stairstep pattern every 67 nm. It is the spacing that is responsible for the staining pattern seen by transmission electron microscopy (TEM) because heavy metals such as lead and silver can readily fill the spaces between the tropocollagen. Each tropocollagen unit is composed of three polypeptide chains (α-chains) helically coiled about each other in a right-hand fashion. The molecular weight of each chain is 95,000 daltons and is composed of nearly 1000 amino acids, most of which are glycine (30%) and proline (20%) and the hydroxylated amino acids, hydroxyproline and hydroxylysine, the latter being a rare amino acid of the body. Chains of polypeptides are synthesized on polysomes attached to the ER of collagen-secreting cells. Hydroxylysine and hydroxyproline are hydroxylated in the cisternae of rER and then transported to dictyosomes. The hydroxylation of the early forming chains is critical for the subsequent assembly of the chains and their eventual extracellular transport. Also within the rER, the **procollagen** molecule becomes

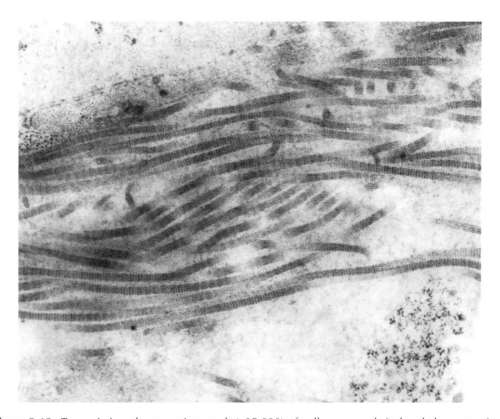

Figure 5-18. Transmission electron micrograph (×25,000) of collagen reveals its banded construction.

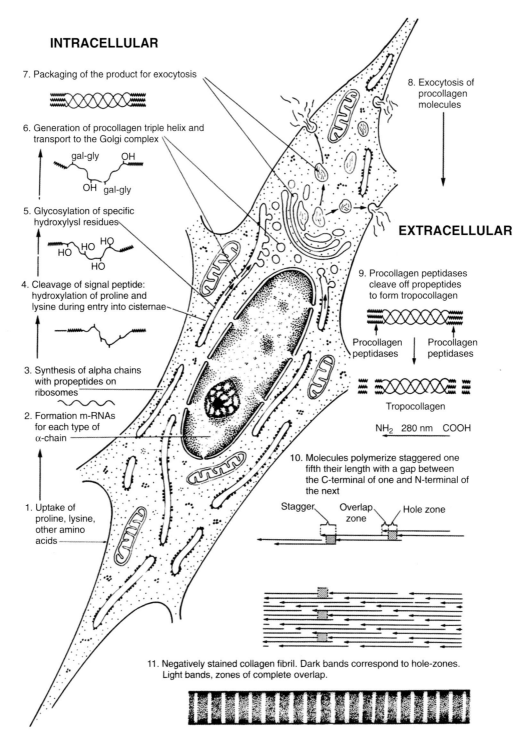

INTRACELLULAR

7. Packaging of the product for exocytosis

6. Generation of procollagen triple helix and transport to the Golgi complex

gal-gly   OH

OH   gal-gly

5. Glycosylation of specific hydroxylysl residues

HO   HO
HO
HO

4. Cleavage of signal peptide: hydroxylation of proline and lysine during entry into cisternae

3. Synthesis of alpha chains with propeptides on ribosomes

2. Formation m-RNAs for each type of α-chain

1. Uptake of proline, lysine, other amino acids

8. Exocytosis of procollagen molecules

EXTRACELLULAR

9. Procollagen peptidases cleave off propeptides to form tropocollagen

Procollagen   Procollagen
peptidases   peptidases

Tropocollagen

NH₂ 280 nm COOH

10. Molecules polymerize staggered one fifth their length with a gap between the C-terminal of one and N-terminal of the next

Stagger   Overlap   Hole zone
            zone

11. Negatively stained collagen fibril. Dark bands correspond to hole-zones. Light bands, zones of complete overlap.

Figure 5-19. Diagram of both the intracellular association of collagen with the fibroblast with regard to its synthesis and its extracellular construction just outside of the cell. *(From Fawcett DW: Bloom and Fawcett: a textbook of histology, ed 11, Philadelphia, 1986, Saunders.)*

assembled and to some extent glycosylated. The ordered procollagen molecules become coiled into right-handed helices and are transported then to the Golgi apparatus by transfer vesicles. Variable amounts of glycosylation can continue within the Golgi appa-ratus. Glycosylation helps further strengthen the sta-bility of the helically oriented chains of the collagen macromolecule as well as assists in its transport and release at the cell surface (Figure 5-20; see also Figure 5-19). Procollagen is subsequently converted to

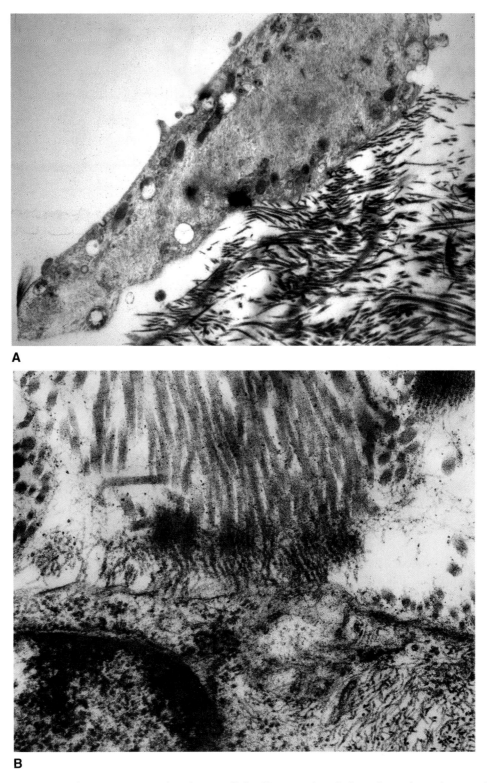

A

B

Figure 5-20. Transmission electron micrographs of extracellular fibers produced along the surface of canine fibroblasts. **A,** Individual collagen fibrils are formed at discrete sites along the cell membrane. (×25,000.) **B,** At certain times collagen synthesis is stopped and elastic fiber synthesis proceeds. (×50,000.)

tropocollagen by the enzyme **procollagen peptidase,** which lies on the surface of the cell. Procollagen peptidase, which is secreted along with procollagen, actually consists of two forms, procollagen carboxylase, which cleaves the C-terminal peptide, and procollagen aminopeptidase, which removes the N-terminal peptide. These enzymes remove most of the nonhelical extensions that are present on each end of the procollagen molecule. With much of the nonhelical extensions removed, the collagen molecule, which is now referred to as **tropocollagen,** can be assembled into a fibril with its characteristic banded appearance. Collagen fibrils can vary greatly in diameter, typically ranging from 20 to 200 nm. The stepwise cross linkage of tropocollagen that results in the formation of fibrils is made possible by the enzyme lysyl oxidase, which forms aldehydes through its oxidative deamination of lysyl and hydroxylysyl residues between the remaining portions of the nonhelical extensions.

Collagen has been chemically subdivided into numerous types in different species. Table 5-2 lists the four major types of collagen and where they have been found throughout the body of different animals. Although fibroblasts are the principal cells involved in collagen synthesis, especially collagen fibers, many other cells of the body have the capability of producing this extracellular material, including chondroblasts, osteoblasts, epithelial cells, myoblasts, and glioblasts (developing support cells of nervous tissue). The predominant form of collagen in the body is **type I,** which is produced mostly by fibroblasts and osteoblasts. Type I consists of two chains being the same (α_1) and one different (α_2). This ubiquitous type occurs in skin, bone, tendon, ligaments, and teeth, as well as the fascia and connective tissue proper of virtually all other organs. It functions to provide resistance to force, tension, and stretch. **Type II** consists of chains that are identical (3 α_1), having more glycosylated hydroxylysine. This type is found primarily in hyaline and elastic cartilage. The fibers, which are relatively short, function to provide resistance primarily to pressure. Type II collagen reacts differently to histological stains than type I, or type III for that matter, being considerably less acidophilic and as a result poorly revealed by eosin. **Type III** also consists of three identical chains (3 α_1) but differs from type II by having 12 tripeptide units shorter than that of type II. Type III is now known to be reticular fibers, which are characteristically small and contribute to loose connective tissues. The first three types of collagen are typically assembled into discrete fibers that are visible with the appropriate stain light microscopically.

Of the remaining collagen types (types IV, VI, and up), many are not assembled into fibrils. **Type IV** is found only in basal laminae of epithelia, muscle, and glial cells of nervous tissue and is not produced by fibroblasts or their progenitors, the mesenchyme. It is like type I in that the tropocollagen consists of two different α chains (type IV). It functions primarily to provide support and a filtration barrier and is sometimes referred to as the *basement membrane collagen.* **Type V** has also two chains that are the same (α_1 V) and one different (α_2 V) and is found in placental and other (interstitial) tissues, being associated with type I. Like types I through III, type V is assembled into recognizable banded fibrils when observed ultrastructurally. **Type VI,** like types I, IV, and V, consists of different α chains and can be found in locations where type I exists. At present, there are approximately 12 other types of collagen that have been discovered in recent times. Some of these other types (see Table 5-2) are less common or ubiquitous than the first three types and comprise only a small fraction of the total

TABLE 5-2 Collagen Types I through IV

Collagen consists of three helically intertwined polypeptide chains. For each type of collagen the composition of each chain may be the same or differ as indicated by α_1, α_2, and so on.

TYPE	COMPOSITION	FUNCTION	LOCATION
I	$\alpha_1(I)_2\ \alpha_2(I)$	Provides resistance against tension, force, and stretch	Dermis of skin, organ capsules and fascia, ligament, tendon, dentin
II	$\alpha_1(II)_3$	Provides resistance to pressure	Hyaline and elastic cartilage, intervertebral disk
III	$\alpha_1(III)_3$	Provides structural support for cell mobility	Connective tissues associated with blood vessels, nerve bundles, secretory units of glands, ducts, and stromal elements of cellular organs (spleen, liver, etc.)
IV	$\alpha_1(IV)_2\ \alpha_2(IV)$	Provides structural support and filtration barrier	Basal laminae of epithelia, muscle cells, and neural glia

collagen within the body. Some, such as **types IX** and **XII,** bind to the surface of fibrillar collagen and may play a role in fibril organization and interaction with ground substance.

Reticular fibers are none other than collagen type III, having the same substructural periodic structure seen in most fibrillar collagen. In terms of their biochemistry, they differ principally from the other collagens by the presence of more carbohydrate residues. Consequently, reticular fibers are best detected by selective **argyrophilic** (silver loving) stains that detect polysaccharides (e.g., silver-staining techniques) (Figure 5-21). Reticular fibers represent the collagen associated with loose connective tissue, being most abundant within the framework of hematopoietic organs (e.g., lymph nodes) and form a reticulate network around cells of epithelial organs, such as endocrine glands. They also help comprise the connective tissue next to small blood vessels, adipose, nerve bundles, and muscle cells. These fibers can be extremely fine and do not form bundles that are characteristic of type I.

ELASTIC FIBERS

Elastic fibers are typically more spread out from one another, not usually forming bundles as seen in collagen (Figure 5-22). These fibers can be thin and long, with the capability to be stretched one and one-half times their normal length. As one might expect,

elastic fibers occur where flexibility is needed: in mesentery and around blood vessels, for example. They also are found in dense connective tissues with abundant amounts of collagen that nevertheless require some degree of distensibility (Figure 5-23, A). These fibers can also be a part of certain cartilage and ligaments. Elastic fibers are poorly distinguished from collagen (type I) by hematoxylin and eosin (H&E). The fibers react with eosin more intensely than collagen does, but the distinction is often too difficult to make. Thus, selective methods (the use of stains: resorcin-fuchsin or orcein) are needed to reveal them. When observed by TEM, elastic fibers lack the banding seen in collagen and reticular fibers (Figure 5-23, B; see also Figure 5-20, B). Instead, they consist of an amorphous central region, **elastin,** which in turn is enveloped by small fibrils **(microfibrils)** approximately 10 to 12 nm in diameter and consisting of the glycoprotein **fibrillin.** The relationship between the two components, elastin and microfibrils, is not truly understood. The microfibrils, undoubtedly, offer structural support as a framework of glycoprotein for elastin as an amorphous mass to be deposited onto and concomitantly provide the fiber directionality. Grossly, elastic fibers that are fresh and great in quantity usually have a yellow appearance. Elastin's composition is similar to that of collagen in that it is rich in glycine and proline, but still differs substantially, having little of the hydroxylated amino acids that comprise collagen such as hydroxyproline.

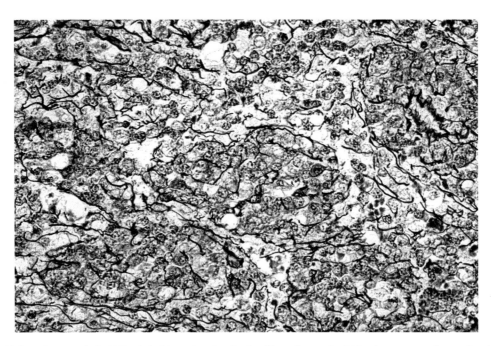

Figure 5-21. Light micrograph (×400) of darkly stained reticular fibers located within the stroma of a canine lymph node.

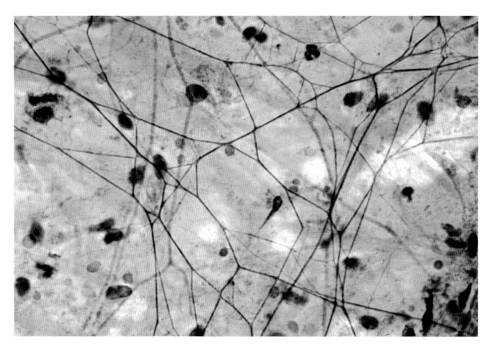

Figure 5-22. Light micrograph of darkly stained elastic fibers that form a delicate weblike network within the loose connective tissue of a flat-mounted mesentery, which was stained by Verhoeff-orange safranin. (×400.)

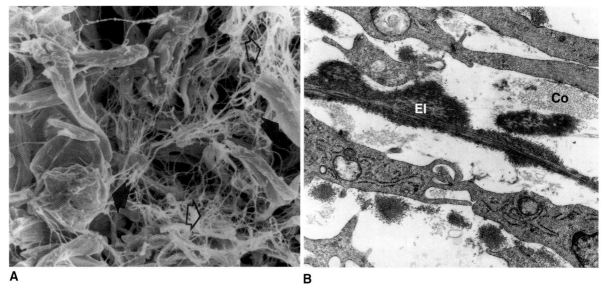

A   B

Figure 5-23. Ultrastructural observations of collagen and elastic fibers. **A,** Scanning electron micrograph of the dermis of feline skin shows the sharp difference that can occur with regard to the size and close association of the two types of fibers, being considerably more robust in collagen *(closed arrows)* than the elastic fibers *(open arrows).* **B,** Transmission electron micrograph of collagen *(Co)* and elastic *(El)* fibers in the canine eye. (×10,000.)

GROUND SUBSTANCE

Ground substance is the colorless, transparent, and homogeneous component of the extracellular environment of connective tissue. Chemically, the amorphous intercellular ground substance is composed mainly of **glycosaminoglycans (GAGS),** also known as *acid mucopolysaccharides*, and forms the major portion of **proteoglycans** (Figure 5-24). Most GAGS in connective tissue possess a characteristic repeating disaccharide unit consisting of uronic acid (gly-couronic acid) and hexosamine (glycosamine or galactosamine). These molecules form the substantially larger molecules, proteoglycans, through further association with protein cores. Specifically, the GAGS are arranged in a bristle-like manner around a protein strand, covalently bound to the protein (see Figure 5-24). In this arrangement, types of GAGS are restricted in their location and aggregated one from another. The large proteoglycan molecules are attached also covalently to long chains of hyaluronic acid (hyaluronans), which is a nonsulfated glycosaminoglycan.

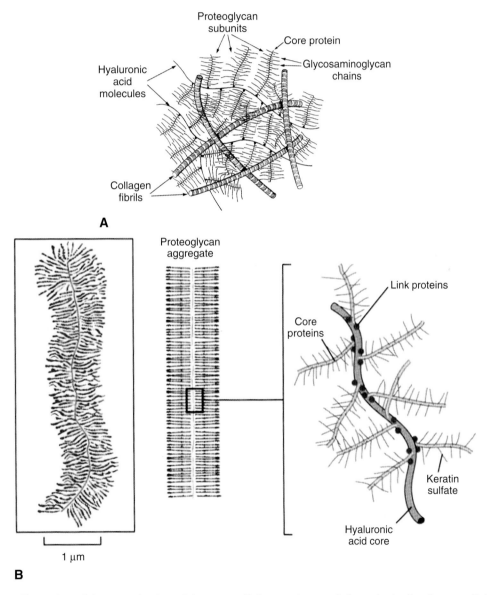

Figure 5-24. A, Illustration of the organization of the extracellular matrix, consisting principally of extracellular fibers (collagen fibrils) surrounded by proteoglycans attached to strands of hyaluronans, which collectively form molecular or proteoglycan aggregates, also known as *aggregans.* **B,** The proteoglycan aggregate shown from electron-microscopic observation and schematically. *(A from Fawcett DW: Bloom and Fawcett: a textbook of histology, ed 11, Philadelphia, 1986, Saunders; B from Bergman RA, Afifi AK, Heidger PM Jr: Histology, Philadelphia, 1996, Saunders.)*

These large macromolecules of proteoglycans attached to hyaluronans are sometimes referred as **aggrecan** (a proteoglycan aggregate), which is specifically associated with cartilage. In general, proteoglycan aggregates have great affinity for water and function as extremely efficient space fillers, forming a viscous gel that metabolites and nutrients must diffuse through before interacting with the different cells of this tissue. By varying the polymerization of glycosaminoglycans with regard to both types and amounts, the viscosity of the ground substance can be controlled. In addition to being space fillers, GAGS function in a number of other ways including regulating cell growth; alterating mitotic rate of cell replication; providing cellular adhesive qualities; mediating cell-cell communication; and shielding of surface receptors. In short, GAGS mediate many receptor-ligand interactions at the cell surface and consequently play a critical role in wounding and repair, as well as development. In many ways the GAGs that are produced by the resident cells of a particular connective tissue establish the environment for the rest of the components (extracellular fibers, glycoproteins, and other cells) of that connective tissue to coexist. The visualization of proteoglycans and their GAGS by light microscopy is difficult unless special stains are used, such as alcian blue. However, GAGS that are highly sulfated, such as chondroitin sulfate and keratosulfate, are pale blue when stained by H&E (Figure 5-25).

CLASSIFICATION OF CONNECTIVE TISSUE PROPER

LOOSE CONNECTIVE TISSUE

In connective tissue proper there are two types: loose and dense. **Loose connective tissue** or **areolar connective tissue** is the more common of the two, found subcutaneously and interstitially within most organ systems, between muscle fibers and sheaths, and around bundles of peripheral nerve fibers, adipose tissue, and lymphatic and blood vessels (Figure 5-26; see also Figure 5-22). Loose connective tissue serves to connect one tissue to another (such as epithelium to muscle) and concomitantly holds adjacent tissues together during motile activity of an organ. This tissue also provides an appropriate domain for transient cells of defense and wound repair and is especially well developed in those regions where transient cells are often called into action such as the small intestine. This tissue is chiefly characterized by the abundant amount of amorphous ground material (GAGS) within the intercellular space. When compared with other forms of connective tissue (dense connective tissue, cartilage, and bone), loose connective tissue is moderately cellular, having a variety of cell types previously described. The extracellular fibers (collagen, reticular, and elastic) are "loosely" arranged in this

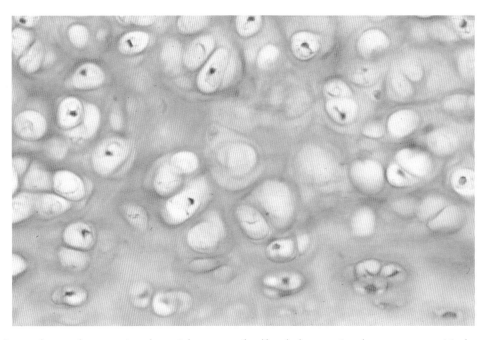

Figure 5-25. Proteoglycans that contain substantial amount of sulfated glycosaminoglycans react positively to hematoxylin as seen in the light micrograph of the interterritorial matrix of hyaline cartilage in canine tracheal rings. (Hematoxylin and eosin stain; ×400.)

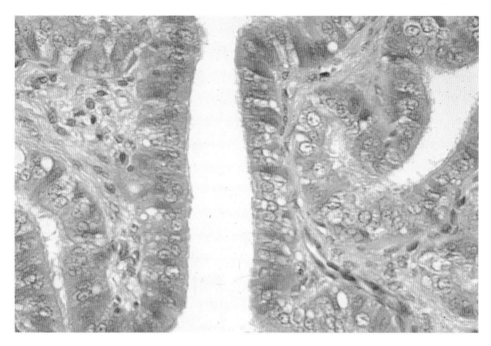

Figure 5-26. Light micrograph of the loose connective tissue that subtends the epithelium lining the uterine tube of the dog. (Hematoxylin and eosin stain; ×400.)

tissue, and for the most part widely spaced. The fibers only aggregate to any extent where the connective tissue meets other structures (blood vessels, nerve bundles, muscle, epithelium, etc.).

DENSE CONNECTIVE TISSUE

Dense connective tissue essentially is composed of the same elements that make up loose connective tissue. But in this type of connective tissue there is a marked predominance of extracellular fibers with considerably less amorphous ground substance. Moreover, the fibroblast/fibrocyte is by far the most common cell type in this tissue. Dense connective tissue is considerably less flexible and more resistant to stress than loose connective tissue. Dense connective tissue is subdivided into two forms: irregular and regular. **Dense irregular connective tissue** is readily distinguished by the presence of numerous collagen fibers that are closely packed and irregularly arranged. These bundles of collagen in fact form a three-dimensional network that can provide resistance to stress from most directions, and thus prevent "overstretching." An excellent example of this multidirectional network of fibers can be seen in the dermis of skin (Figure 5-27). Often, however, the fibers of fascia and capsules in the body can be more unidirectional than that of tissue like the dermis with most of the fibers running circumferentially around a specific organ. But because some of the fibers interweave radially, this type of dense connective tissue is classified as irregular. Dense irregular connective tissue light microscopically has a very wavy appearance as the bundles of collagen bend in a random manner. This tissue occurs most frequently in capsules of organs, fasciae, pericardium, dermis of skin, and periosteum of bone (Table 5-3).

Dense regular connective tissue is delineated by the presence of closely packed extracellular fibers that are arranged in a highly organized manner. Light microscopically the fibers are seen to be oriented in a single direction, forming definitive sheets or layers of collagen with interspersed elastic fibers that are oriented in the plane. Examples of regular dense connective tissue include tendons, ligaments, and cornea (Figure 5-28; see also Figure 5-4). It is important to note that the fibers run parallel to each other and do not interweave as in the irregular form.

Although most tissues of this type contain predominantly collagen, elastic fibers can be arranged into thick, parallel bundles, as in the yellow ligaments of the vertebral column, and can be referred to as **dense regular elastic connective tissue** (Figure 5-29).

ADIPOSE TISSUE

Adipocytes can exist in almost any structure of the body. Their ubiquitous appearance, which at times can be unexpected, is a phenomenon that is still not

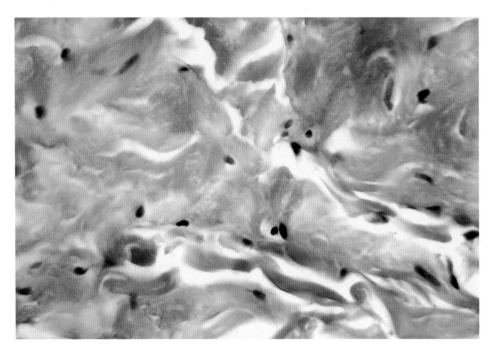

Figure 5-27. Light micrograph of the dense irregular connective tissue that comprises much of the dermis within the skin of the pig. (Hematoxylin and eosin stain; ×250.)

TABLE 5-3	Types of Connective Tissue Proper	
TYPE	LOCATION	FUNCTION
Loose (areolar) connective tissue	Immediately surrounding small blood vessels including vascular plexuses, lymph vessels, nerve bundles, ducts and glandular units, lamina propria along the digestive tract, stromal elements within parenchymatous organs (liver, pancreas, lung, spleen, thymus, thyroid, etc.)	Provides appropriate scaffolding for an existing cellular environment or one that could potentially be cellular
Dense irregular connective tissue	Dermis, capsules of many organs, fascia of heart and skeletal muscle, sheaths of nerves, sclera of the eye	Resist stress from various directions
Dense regular connective tissue	Ligaments, tendons, cornea	Withstand tensile strength (longitudinal stress)

truly understood. Although they can be found singly, these cells, for the most part, occur in clusters and can be referred to as a tissue. Within the deeper regions of skin, the hypodermis or subcutaneous layer, adipocytes can form a distinct layer referred to as the **panniculus adiposus,** which in many animals functions to thermally and mechanically insulate (Figure 5-30). The cells are also routinely associated with visceral organs and regions within the musculoskeletal system, such as the synovial membranes of joints and digital cushions of feet. In these instances, adipose tissue serves to absorb shock. Adipocytes are believed to be derived from undifferentiated mesenchyme, but evidence to substantiate their origin from a specific stem cell is

lacking. The presence of brown or multilocular fat cells, which forms fetal fat or primary fat, begins with the occurrence of epithelioid cells at discrete locations within the developing fetus. By comparison, white fat cells arise from fusiform-shaped mesenchymal cells near the end of fetal development. Whether these morphologically different lipoblasts share the same derivation or arise from two distinct cell lines remains to be discovered. It is interesting to note that while the neonate matures, the numerous locules in brown fat cells coalesce into a single droplet and take on a unilocular white fat cell appearance (Figure 5-31).

Although brown adipose tissue is a developmental form of fat in mammals and birds, it can be retained

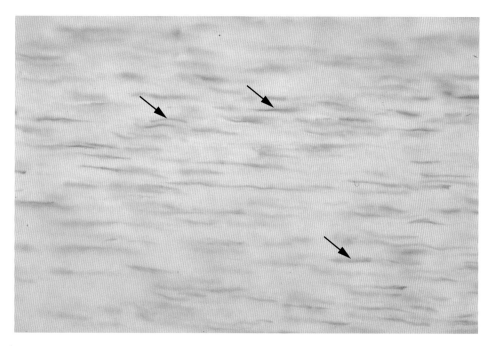

Figure 5-28. Light micrograph of dense regular connective tissue showing fibrocytes *(arrows)* interspersed between the layers of extracellular fibers of an equine ligament. (Hematoxylin and eosin stain; ×400.)

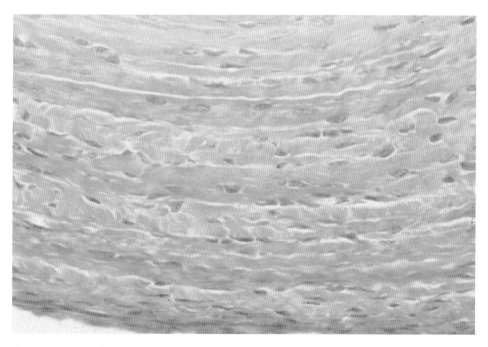

Figure 5-29. Light micrograph of dense regular elastic connective tissue that forms the yellow ligament between two adjacent canine vertebrae. (Hematoxylin and eosin stain; ×400.)

in the adult stage, especially in hibernating animals. These cells are equipped with the metabolic machinery, that is to say, the numerous mitochondria including the appropriate enzymes that allow fatty acids to be oxidized at much greater rates than that in uniloc-

ular adipose tissue. Moreover, the mitochondria of brown adipose fat cells primarily generate heat rather than adenosine triphosphate (ATP) and as a result can sustain the body heat during prolonged periods of cold. Like unilocular fat, the adipocytes are clustered

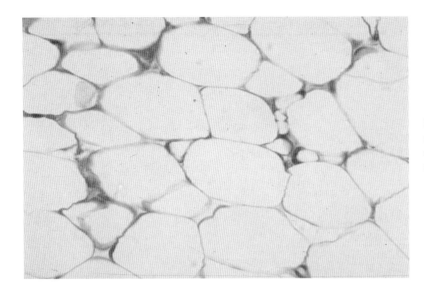

Figure 5-30. Light micrograph of unilocular adipose tissue that becomes a distinct layer subcutaneously in the sheep. (Hematoxylin and eosin stain; ×200.)

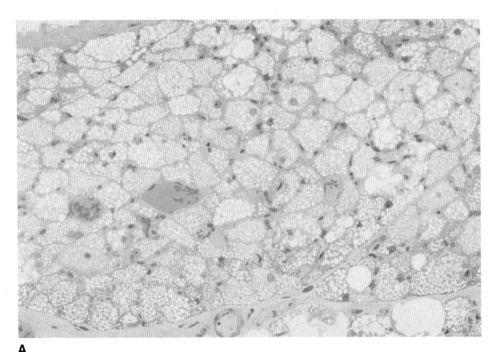

A

B

Figure 5-31. A, Light micrograph of multilocular adipose tissue near the trachea of a juvenile ferret. (Plastic section, hematoxylin and eosin stain; ×200.) **B,** Within multilocular adipose tissue an occasional adipocyte becomes unilocular as the small locules collect and fuse, as seen in this light micrograph. (Plastic section, hematoxylin and eosin stain; ×1000.)

into lobules, but these lobules are more richly vascularized and innervated than that in the former (see Figure 5-31). Cold nerve receptors located within the epithelial (epidermal) lining of skin are responsible for signaling the temperature-regulating center of the brain, which in turn directly innervates the multilocular adipocytes and results in fatty acid oxidation. Brown adipose tissue is formed principally in the axillary and intercapsular regions, in the mesenteries and mediastinum, and along the aorta and next to the kidney.

SUGGESTED READINGS

Bergman RA, Afifi AK, Heidger PM Jr: *Histology,* Philadelphia, 1996, Saunders.

Burke B, Lewis CE: *The macrophage,* New York, 2002, Oxford University Press.

Fawcett DW: *Bloom and Fawcett: a textbook of histology,* ed 11, Philadelphia, 1986, Saunders.

Gartner LP, Hiatt JL: *Color textbook of histology,* Philadelphia, 1997, Saunders.

Kuhn K: The classic collagens: types I, II, and III. In Mayne R, Burgeson RE, editors: *Structure and function of collagen types,* Orlando, Fla, 1987, Academic Press.

Leeson TS, Leeson CR: *A brief atlas of histology,* Philadelphia, 1979, Saunders.

Marone G, Lichtenstein LM, Galli SJ: *Mast cells and basophils,* San Diego, 2000, Academic Press.

Sutmuller M, Bruijn JA, de Heer E: Collagen types VIII and X, two non-fibrillar, short-chained collagens. Structure homologies, functions and involvement in pathology, *Histol Histopathol* 12:557, 1997.

Cartilage and Bone

KEY CHARACTERISTICS

- Highly specialized extracellular matrix (ECM)
- Provides support, protection and storage
- Cartilage:
  - classified according to prevailing fiber
  - cells rounded, isolated or in clusters ("nest")
  - noninnervated, avascular
- Bone:
  - classified according to prevalence and organization of ECM
  - highly mineralized and vascularized ECM
  - continuously remodeled

CARTILAGE

Cartilage is one of the specialized forms of connective tissue. It functions largely to support soft tissues, provide sliding areas for joints, and provide growth templates for long bone (pre- and postnatally). This tissue is neither innervated nor vascularized, lacking lymphatic and blood vessels of its own. Instead, cartilage is nourished by nearby vessels of adjacent connective tissue or by synovial fluid within the joint cavities. Blood vessels seen normally in cartilage are traversing it, not being involved in establishing any vascular bed within. Based on the frequency and type of fiber, cartilage is subdivided into three types: hyaline, elastic, and fibrous or fibrocartilage. Each cartilage has a single cell type, the **chondrocyte,** which is essentially a specialized fibrocyte that is involved in the production of an ECM that provides strong resistance to physical stress (Figure 6-1). Chondrocytes are referred to as **chondroblasts** during initial active production of the ground material. Chondroblasts are generally oval to round with rounded nuclei and basophilic cytoplasm filled with rough endoplasmic reticulum (rER), Golgi apparatus, secretory vesicles, and mitochondria. As chondroblasts become less active, having contributed greatly fibers and ground substance to the ECM, they are transformed into chondrocytes, which tend to have rounded to polyhedral shapes in the central regions of hyaline and elastic cartilage and to a lesser extent in fibrocartilage. As chondrocytes continue to add to the ECM and maintain it, they become more and more isolated from one another. Older chondrocytes have fewer of the organelles associated with ECM production previously described in the chondroblast, possessing instead occasional lipid droplets and glycogen. These cells, however senescent, have the ability to redivide under the proper conditions. Cellular replication may continue two or three times, resulting in **cell nests,** also called **isogenic cell groups** (Figure 6-

2). The matrix formed by these cells is approximately 40% collagen (dry weight), type II variety except for fibrocartilage, and 60% glycosaminoglycans (GAGS) (dry weight). The GAGS, here, consist of long molecules of hyaluronic acid from which numerous, short sulfated mucopolysaccharides radiate (chondroitin 4–sulfate, chondroitin 6–sulfate, keratan sulfate).

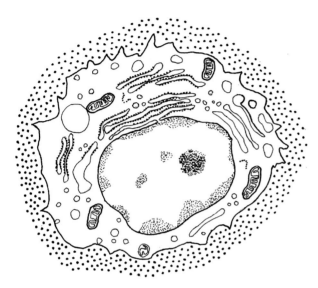

Figure 6-1. Illustration of the chondrocyte with its characteristic round cell body and short processes that are surrounded by its capsule.

HYALINE CARTILAGE

Hyaline cartilage has a bluish white glassy appearance when seen grossly and is the most common type of cartilage, occurring at most bone-forming sites, joint surfaces of articulating bones, tracheal rings, larynx, and nose. It is able to withstand a considerable amount of compression and tension. This ability to endure physical forces is largely due to the arrangement of the short collagen fibers that are of the type II variety and are arranged in accordance with the stress placed on the cartilage within the body. Within articular cartilage the fibers tend to form irregular bundles between the chondrocytes, whereas concomitantly near the surface they are oriented parallel to the surface. The bulk of the fibers and proteoglycans within the ECM of mature cartilage comprise the region called the **interterritorial matrix.** The proteoglycan-hyaluronan associations (**aggrecan composites**) in the ECM of cartilage can be large and richly sulfated, and as they pool in this region, a bluish color can result from hematoxylin and eosin (H&E) staining (Figure 6-3). Included within the ground substance of the interterritorial matrix are binding glycoproteins such as **chondronectin,** which assist in the attachment of collagen to the proteoglycans. In the absence of this basophilic reaction, the matrix will appear relatively clear due to the chromophobic properties of collagen type II and its similar refractive index to the ground substance. The ECM surrounding

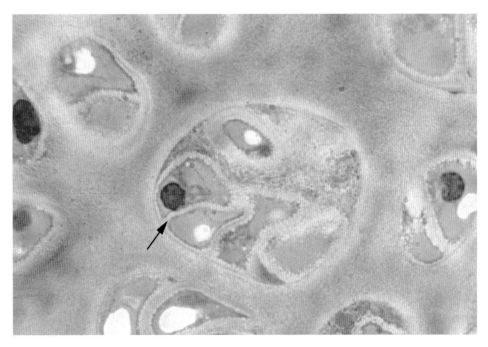

Figure 6-2. Light micrograph of chondrocytes in hyaline cartilage that are arranged in a nest. Recently divided cells initially share the same pericellular capsule *(arrow).* (Plastic section stained with hematoxylin and eosin; ×1000.)

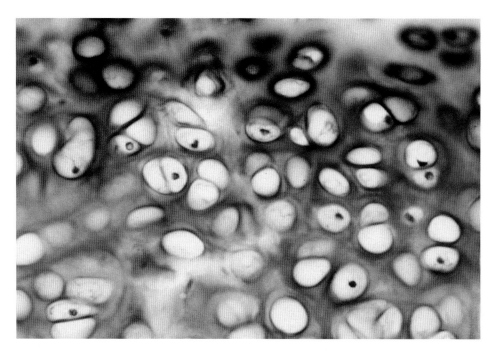

Figure 6-3. Light micrograph of hyaline cartilage that forms support rings within the canine trachea. The area between the cell nests, the interterritorial matrix, reacts positively (and basophilically) to hematoxylin. (Hematoxylin and eosin stain; ×200.)

the chondrocytes comprises the **territorial matrix,** having a different composition from the interterritorial matrix in that it consists of more chondroitin sulfate–rich proteoglycans and has less collagen type II, which is also smaller in size than that in the interterritorial matrix. Immediately adjacent to the chondrocyte is a thin (approximately 1-3 μm thick) region around the cell membrane that consists of ground substance with a fine meshwork of collagen fibrils. This zone or ring is called the **capsule** or **pericellular capsule** and is likewise basophilic when stained with H&E (also periodic acid–Schiff [PAS] positive) due to the high concentration of sulfated GAGS in this area (see Figures 6-2 and 6-3). The collagen in the pericellular capsule consists primarily of types III and IX through XI, and in articular cartilage type V above the tidemark. In most instances, there is little type II associated with the pericellular capsule. The cartilage cells occupy potential space known as **lacunae.** During routine processing practices for histological preparation, chondrocytes frequently shrink and pull away from their pericellular capsules, revealing their lacunae (Figure 6-4).

Along the external margins of the territorial matrix of hyaline cartilage, there is a sheath known as the **perichondrium** that encapsulates this tissue and forms an interface between the surrounding connective tissue and the body of the cartilage (Figure 6-5). The

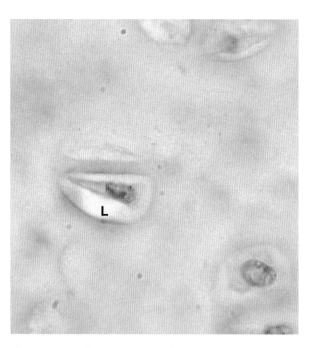

Figure 6-4. Light micrograph of a chondrocyte within hyaline cartilage. In formalin-fixed specimens, chondroblasts and chondrocytes often shrink away from the pericellular capsule, revealing some of the lacuna (*L*) that they occupy. (Hematoxylin and eosin stain; ×1000.)

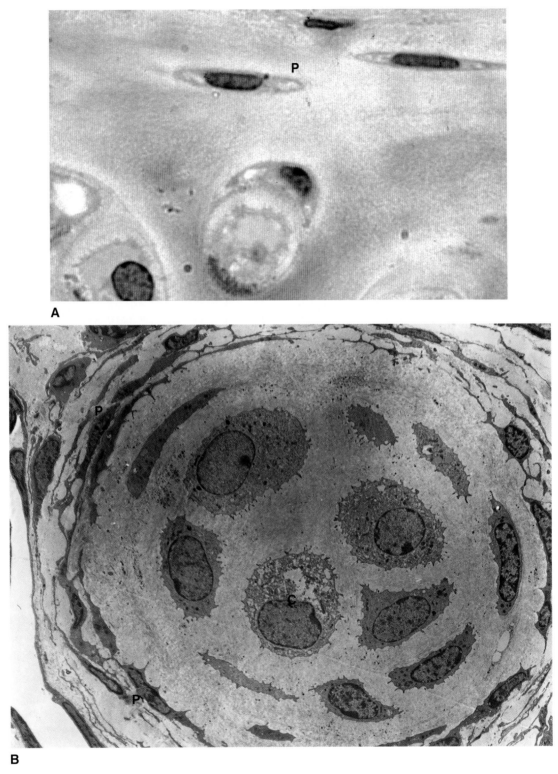

A

B

Figure 6-5. A, Light micrograph of the perichondrium *(P)* that surrounds the body of hyaline cartilage. (Plastic section of hyaline cartilage within the canine trachea stained with hematoxylin and eosin; ×1000.) **B,** Transmission electron micrograph (×3000) of hyaline cartilage within a canine bronchiole. Chondroblasts are created by appositional development from the surrounding perichondrium *(P)* with its fibroblasts and eventually transformed into round chondrocytes *(C)* seen centrally.

perichondrium is composed of fibroblasts (**perichondrial fibroblasts**) and bundles of collagen (type I), forming a thin fascia of dense connective tissue that in some ways is similar to a capsule or fascia that envelops many organs. The perichondrial fibroblasts next to the interterritorial matrix are believed to be chondrogenic, giving rise to chondroblasts. As chondroblasts mature and move away from the perichondrium, thus becoming chondrocytes, they contribute to both territorial and interterritorial matrices.

ELASTIC CARTILAGE

Elastic cartilage is yellowish and not nearly as common as the hyaline cartilage found in the external ear, external auditory canals, eustachian tubes, larynx, and epiglottis (Table 6-1). The major difference between this tissue and hyaline cartilage is the presence of a well-developed network of elastic fibers that imparts greater flexibility and distensibility than the other forms of cartilage. The elastic fibers are largely oriented within the territorial and interterritorial matrices in the same direction as the collagen fibers, varying in size as well, being most prominent in the territorial matrix (Figure 6-6). Although special stains are useful for revealing elastic fibers, in this type of cartilage the concentration of the elastic fibers is sufficient for the fibers to be readily seen by H&E (see Figure 6-6). By comparison, the perichondrium possesses little elastin even though it can be well developed, as seen in the epiglottis (see Figure 6-6). In mature tissue the chondrocytes can be large and appear foamy, housing a considerable number of lipid droplets.

FIBROCARTILAGE

Fibrocartilage is the least common of the three forms; it is found at intervertebral disks and certain ligamentous and tendinous attachments to bones (and menisci of stifle joints). Morphologically, this type of cartilage is the most different of the three types. Fibrocartilage does not possess a true perichondrium but develops directly from the mesenchyme (Figure 6-7). Although its matrix is basically similar to that of hyaline cartilage, the coarser type I collagen fibers predominate, making the matrix more acidophilic. These fibers, which form discrete bundles, enable this cartilage to withstand considerable force, especially along the longitudinal plane of the bundle, and at the same time remain resilient to deformation. Within the menisci of stifles and the tendinous and ligamentous attachments to bone, the bundles often assume a herringbone pattern as individual bundles crisscross each other in an interwoven V shape (Figure 6-8). Fibrocartilage is often associated with both dense connective tissue and hyaline cartilage, typically merging imperceptibly with them, and this tissue appears to be a cross between dense regular connective tissue and cartilage. The chondrocytes usually are aligned in rows, much like fibrocytes within tendons and ligaments. The chondrocytes, however, can form isogenic nests of cells, each having the characteristic rounded shape (see Figure 6-7).

TABLE 6-1	Cartilage Key Information			
TYPE	PREVAILING ECM FIBER	PERICHONDRIAL CHARACTERISTICS	MAJOR FEATURES	LOCATION
Hyaline	Collagen type II	Present except at growth plates and articular cartilage	Basophilic extracellular matrix (ECM), prominent isogenic nests of chondrocytes	Nose, larynx, proximal portion of lung, ends of long bones, ventral ends of ribs
Elastic	Elastic fiber and collagen type II	Present; well developed in large domestic species	Basophilic and acidophilic ECM	External and middle ear, epiglottis
Fibrocartilage	Collagen type I	Absent	Mildly acidophilic ECM; chondrocytes in small nests aligned in rows, associated with dense regular connective tissues and/or hyaline cartilage	Intervertebral disks, insertion of various ligaments and tendons

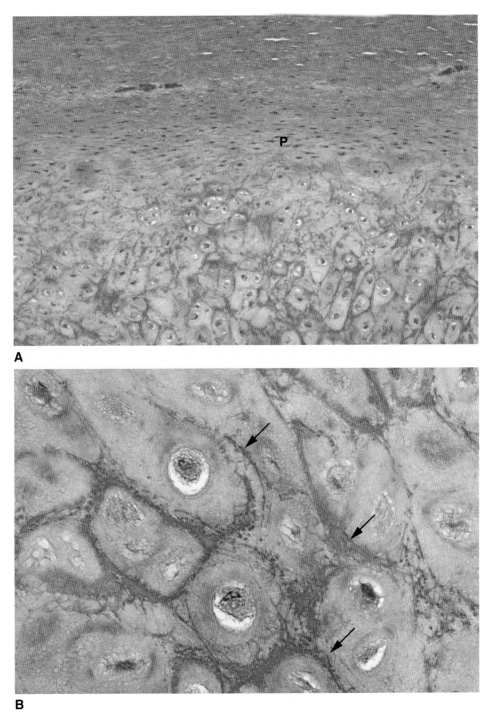

A

B

Figure 6-6. **A,** Light micrograph of elastic cartilage within the equine epiglottis. *P,* perichondrium. (Hematoxylin and eosin stain; ×100.) **B,** Light micrograph of the body of the elastic cartilage with its territorial and interterritorial matrices. The elastic fibers *(arrows)* are intensely stained by eosin and best developed within the interterritorial matrix. (Hematoxylin and eosin stain; ×1000.)

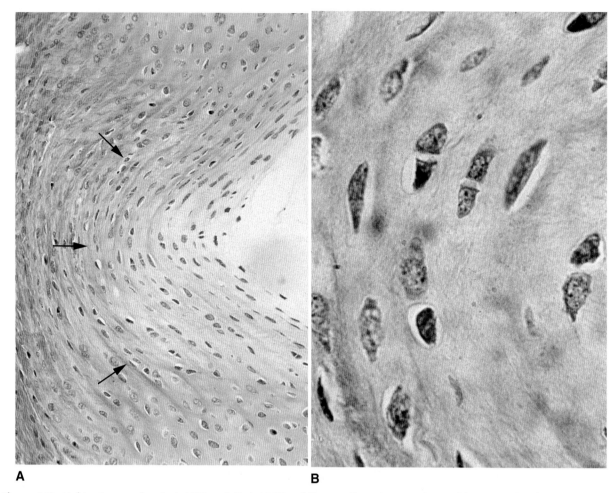

A

B

Figure 6-7. Light micrographs, **A,** (×400) and, **B,** (×1000), of fibrocartilage *(arrows)* located between developing canine vertebrae. In **B,** cell nests are aligned linearly. (Hematoxylin and eosin stain.)

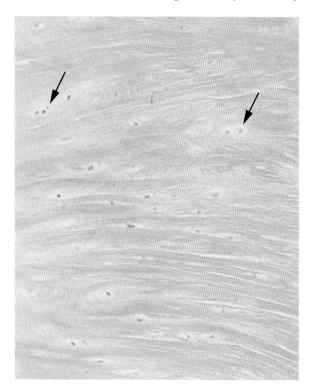

Figure 6-8. Light micrograph (×400) of fibrocartilage *(arrows)* within a canine tendinous attachment to bone.

HISTOGENESIS OF CARTILAGE

Cartilage initially develops from mesenchymal tissue as fibroblast-like cells "round up" and divide, giving rise to chondroblasts. These nests of cells are referred to as centers of chondrification. While the cells (chondrocytes by this time) are in the process of spreading apart, those located most superficially retain their fibroblastic nature and as a result comprise the perichondrium (in hyaline and elastic forms). Continued growth of cartilage from this point occurs two ways: **interstitially** and **appositionally** (see Figures 6-2 and 6-5). Interstitial growth involves the division of chondrocytes, which gives rise to isogenic groups that are surrounded by a condensation of mostly nonfibrous matrix (capsule). This type of cellular replication and growth is undoubtedly the hallmark feature that distinguishes cartilage from connective tissues. Appositional growth is chondrocytic differentiation from peripheral perichondrial cells (via chondroblasts) and occurs in hyaline and elastic cartilage (see Figure 6-5).

REPAIR AND AGING

It is important to keep in mind that the basic components of the different types of connective tissues (loose, dense, hyaline cartilage, etc.) vary little. Instead, it is the amount of the basic components (fibroblasts, elastin, collagen, chondroitin sulfates, etc.) that varies a good deal and as a result imparts specific qualities such as active defense, strength, elasticity, resiliency, and support that are essential for the functional relationship of that particular connective tissue within the body. These components become altered in all connective tissues during injury and subsequent repair and to a lesser extent during the aging process.

Cartilage is able to maintain itself through the normal physiological activities of the chondrocyte, which has the capacity to turn the ECM over on a gradual and regular basis. The life expectancy of chondrocytes is long in most instances except for those cells associated with bone-developing growth plates. Undoubtedly, older chondrocytes of the three different types of cartilage die infrequently and can be replaced interstitially by new cells that arise in recently formed isogenic nests. Once an individual reaches maturity, however, the ability to form new chondrocytes interstitially or appositionally from the perichondrium (in hyaline and elastic cartilage) becomes substantially reduced

During episodes of damage to adult hyaline and elastic cartilage, repair involves the presence of a "granulating" fibrous tissue that originates from the perichondrium and associated tissue. This tissue gradually becomes reconverted to cartilage. In the instance of fibrocartilage, which has a very limited vascular supply and lacks a perichondrium as well, successful repair is less likely to occur than in the other two types of cartilage. Because fibrocartilage protects against compression and shearing forces, surgical intervention may be required to attain the necessary repair.

BONE

Bone is a specialized hard connective tissue that serves for support, attachment, leverage, protection, and mineral storage. Consequently, this tissue is imparted with great strength and rigidity, having very limited elasticity. Bone is derived by direct connective tissue origin or by partial replacement of previously formed cartilage. The ability of this tissue to store minerals and especially calcium into mostly **hydroxyapatite** crystals is the principal characteristic that distinguishes bone from all other connective tissues, including cartilage. And unlike cartilage, bone is closely associated in its development and maintenance with the cardiovascular system, and has afferent associations with the nervous system. Except where bone ends in synovial articulations, it is externally surrounded by a tissue, known as the **periosteum,** that includes blood vessels, a variably thick layer of dense fibrous connective tissue (the capsule), and bone stem cells or **osteogenic cells,** which give rise to osteoblasts (Figure 6-9). Internal spaces within bone, including a central cavity, the **marrow cavity,** where the stem cells of blood are housed, are lined by a thinner tissue, the **endosteum,** which consists of the same cell types as those of the periosteum but within a loose connective tissue environment instead of the dense capsule that surrounds the periosteum (Figure 6-10).

Bone is composed of three major cell types: osteoblast, osteocyte, and osteoclast. The **osteoblast** is the cell responsible for the active synthesis of the organic components of bone, which is called **prebone,** or **osteoid,** and principally consists of collagen, proteoglycans, and glycoproteins. These cells, which can originate from nearby osteogenic cells, are positioned in a line along the surfaces of bone tissue. When metabolically active, osteoblasts tend to be cuboidal and basophilic, exhibiting many of the morphological characteristics seen in a secretory cell of epithelia (Figure 6-11). The cytoplasm contains a well-developed Golgi apparatus and rER that, along with mitochondria and other organelles, are aligned in an organized or polarized manner, resulting in a unidi-

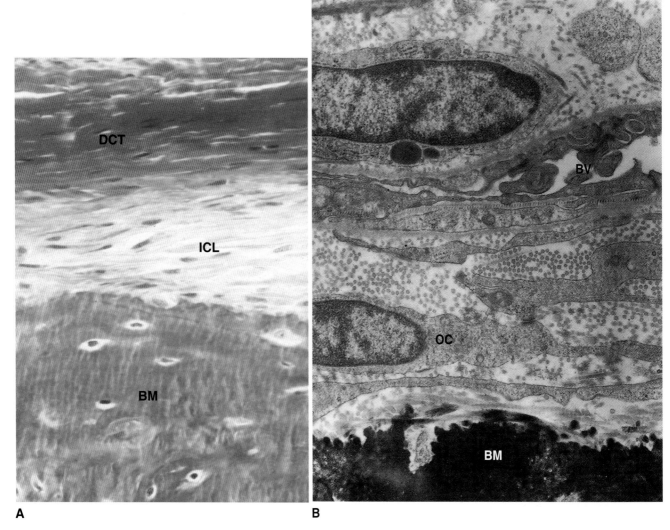

A   B

Figure 6-9. A, Light micrograph of the periosteum that externally lines a developing long bone in the rat, consisting of fibroblast-like cells with osteogenic potency, osteoblasts, and blood vessels. *DCT,* Dense connective tissue; *ICL,* inner cellular layer; *BM,* bone matrix. (Mallory-Azan stain; ×400.) **B,** Transmission electron micrograph (×10,000) of the periosteum of a developing flat bone in the pig. *BV,* Blood vessel, *OC,* osteogenic cells, *BM,* bone matrix.

rectional release of prebone material (Figure 6-12). When osteoblasts are less actively involved in prebone formation, they are flattened and less basophilic (Figure 6-13). During active osteoid synthesis, occasional osteoblasts become less actively involved and stop producing the prebone ECM secretions (see Figure 6-11, *B*). These cells become lodged within the osteoid that has been produced by adjacent active osteoblasts. Once an osteoblast has "entered" the bone matrix it is known as an **osteocyte.** The young osteocyte has not actually migrated into the bone matrix, but instead has been left behind. Thus, the osteocyte is in a sense a mature osteoblast, which soon becomes encapsulated within the mineralized matrix. These cells lie in oval-shaped cavities, or **lacunae,** in the matrix and from their bodies fine

filopodial cellular processes radiate to adjacent cells within small channels or **canaliculi** (Figure 6-14). The filopodial contacts, which includes the formation of gap junctions, function as "life support lines," allowing the passage of nutrients and metabolites from cell to cell. The cytoplasm of the osteocyte surrounding the nucleus is reduced in size when compared with the osteoblast, having few organelles associated with metabolic activity, such as rER, mitochondria and Golgi apparatus (see Figure 6-14). Although quiescent appearing, the role of the osteocyte continues to be examined as it facilitates the maintenance of the mineralized extracellular environment. It has recently been discovered that this cell is able to modulate signals from mechanical loading and subsequently direct bone tissue remodeling. When stimulated

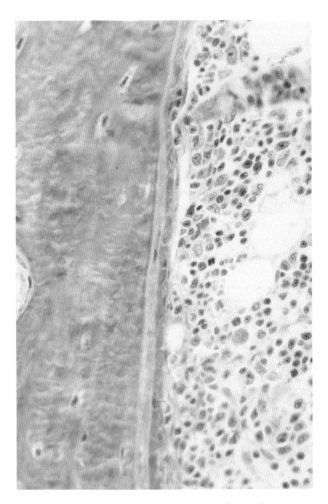

Figure 6-10. Light micrograph (×400) of the endosteum that internally lines a rat bone.

by the parathyroid hormone (PTH), the osteocyte is able to release minerals including calcium from the ECM surrounding its immediate vicinity by secreting different hydrolases. This process is known as **osteocytic osteolysis** and is important in producing the rapid phase of calcium release that is initiated by PTH.

The **osteoclast** is a multinucleated giant cell (6-50 or more nuclei) that is involved in the resorption and remodeling of bone tissue (Figure 6-15). These cells, which appear cytologically acidophilic, are lysosomally rich, having also numerous mitochondria and a well-developed Golgi apparatus (Figure 6-16). Although once traditionally thought to have been derived from osteoprogenitor cells, osteoclasts are now known to originate from the bone marrow, derived from coalescing monocytes. As bone develops and later is remodeled, it is being continually resorbed by these giant cells. The resorption of bone, which can be referred to as **osteoclasia,** is the result of the secretion of a variety of materials, including acids, such as

lactic and citric acids, that lower the pH and facilitate the dissolution of minerals, and strong hydrolytic enzymes (acid hydrolase, collagenase, etc.) that digest the extracellular matrix (ECM). Each osteoclast comes to lie within an enzymatically etched depression called **Howslip's lacuna,** or the **resorption bay** (see Figure 6-15). During active bone resorption, the region of the cell that directly contacts the bony matrix has many infoldings that collectively form a **ruffled border** subtended by the **vesicular zone,** consisting primarily of vesicles, most of which are filled with lysosomal enzymes (see Figure 6-16). Immediately peripheral to the ruffled border is a **clear zone,** an exaggerated ectoplasmic area laden with cytoskeletal elements, especially actin filaments, and free of most organelles. This portion of the cytoplasm may be involved in assisting the attachment of the osteoclast to the bony matrix along the perimeter of the resorption bay. The bulk of the osteoclast's cytoplasm, which houses most of the organelles and all of the nuclei, is called the **basal zone.** Osteoclasia is governed principally by components of the endocrine system: the thyroid, which secretes calcitonin; and the parathyroid, which secretes parathyroid hormone (Table 6-2).

BONE EXTRACELLULAR MATRIX

Most of the bone is composed of the extracellular matrix, which is approximately two thirds inorganic. The remainder of the ECM consists mostly of collagen fibers (type I) and a relatively small amount of amorphous ground substance. Of the inorganic material, calcium and phosphorus are particularly abundant, forming mostly **hydroxyapatite crystals** $(Ca_{10}[PO_4]_6[OH_2])$, which lie alongside the collagen. Calcium phosphate also exists in small amounts as well as magnesium, sodium, potassium, and various trace elements (copper, zinc, manganese, and others). The crystals of hydroxyapatite are arranged in an organized manner along the collagen fibrils and within their gap regions. Small proteoglycan molecules consisting chiefly of the sulfated glycosaminoglycans, chondroitin 4–sulfate, and keratan sulfate, attach to hyaluronans, forming aggrecan composites that line the hydroxyapatite crystals. In bone that is fully mineralized, which can take up to 1 year from the onset of mineralization, the amount of aggrecan composites is quite small, surrounding the free surface of the hydroxyapatite crystals. The proteoglycans within these composites are instrumental in initiating and inhibiting bone mineralization. As mineralization normally proceeds, the relative amount of proteoglycans within the ECM is decreased. Thus there is a reciprocal relationship in the amount of proteoglycans

Text continued on p. 115

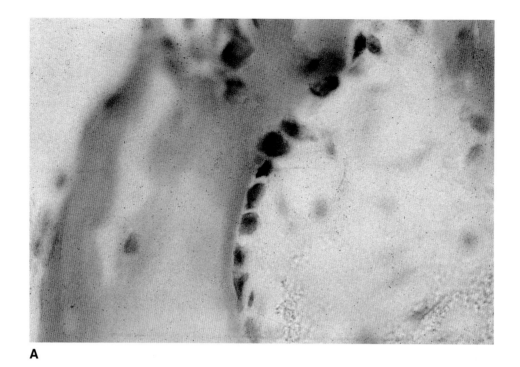

A

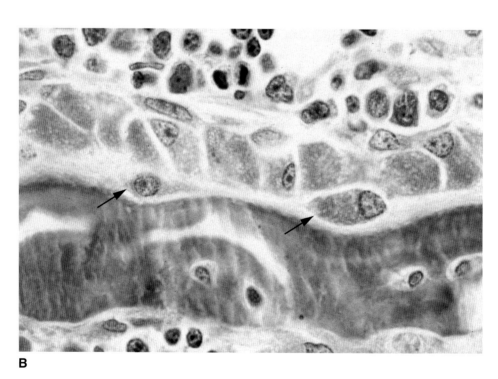

B

Figure 6-11. Light micrographs of active osteoblasts that form a cuboidal line of cells in the horse, **A** (×400), and the rat, **B** (×1000). Arrows point to newly formed osteocytes in **B.**

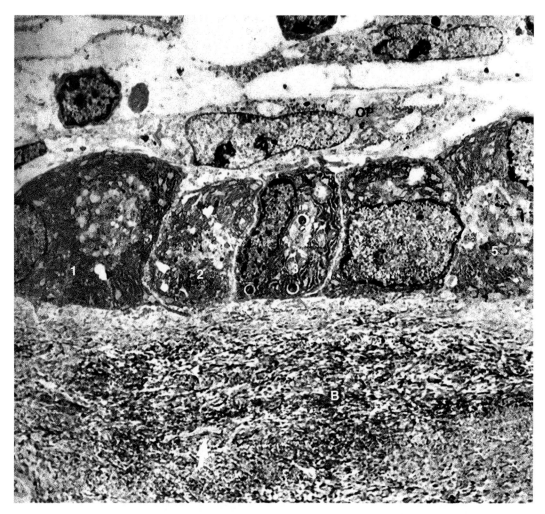

Figure 6-12. Transmission electron micrograph of an osteoprogenitor cell *(op)* and a row of osteoblasts actively secreting prebone material into bone *(B)*. Arrow points to a portion of an osteocyte's canaliculus. *(From Gartner LP, Hiatt JL:* Color textbook of histology, *Philadelphia, 1997, Saunders.)*

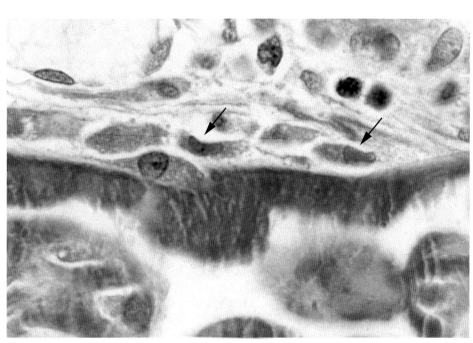

Figure 6-13. Light micrograph of osteoblasts *(arrows)* that are less active and consequently less cuboidal in appearance. (Mallory-Azan stain; ×1000.)

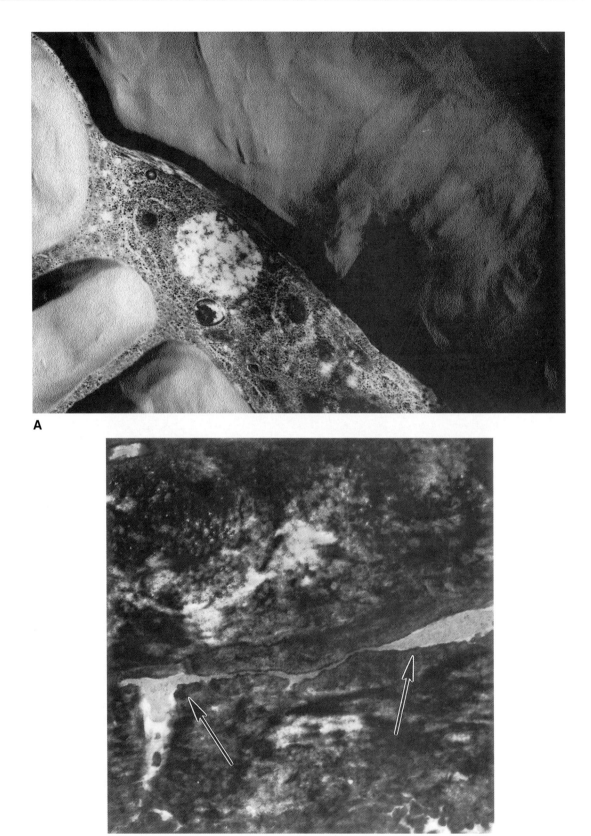

A

B

Figure 6-14. **A,** Layered transmission electron micrograph (×8000) of a revealed porcine osteocyte, showing some of its cell processes that travel toward adjacent cells. **B,** Transmission electron micrograph (×15,000) of an osteocyte process *(arrows),* branching and ramifying within the confines of the mineralized extracellular matrix.

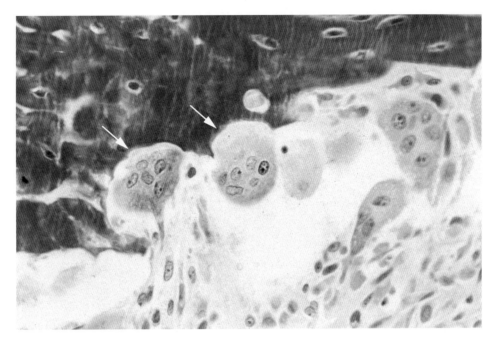

Figure 6-15. Light micrograph (×1000) of osteoclasts and their resorption bays *(arrows)* involved in the process of removing recently made bone.

TABLE 6-2	Various Factors Associated with Osteoclastic Activity	
SUBSTANCES	EFFECT OF OSTEOCLAST AND BONE DEVELOPMENT	CAUSE
Parathyroid hormone (released by parenchymal cells of the parathyroid)	Initiates secretion of osteoclast-stimulating factor by osteoblasts and subsequent bone resorption, resulting in the release of Ca^{++} into the bloodstream	Below normal levels of Ca^{++} (calcium deficiency); hyperparathyroidism
Calcitonin (released by parafollicular cells of the thyroid)	Inhibits osteoclasts from resorbing bone; causes disappearance of their ruffled border	Above normal levels of Ca^{++}
Cyclosporin A	Increases osteoclastic activity (osteoclasia) with concomitant reduction of bone formation at symphyseal sites	Drug administration
Irradiation	Initiates osteocytic osteolysis followed by osteoclasia	Cancer therapy

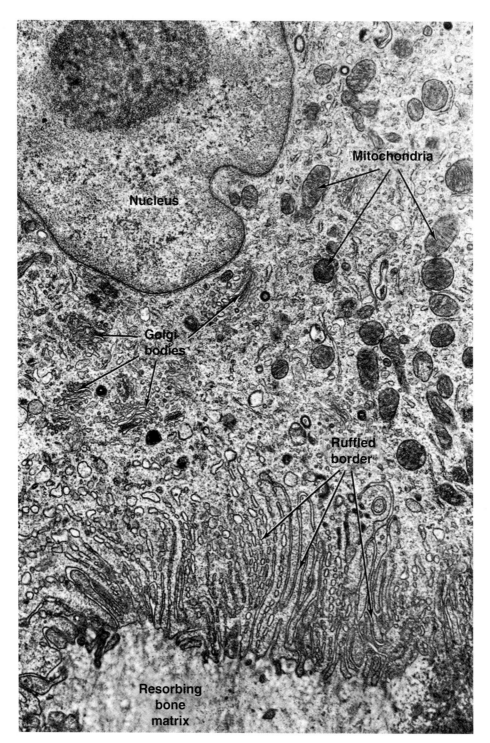

Figure 6-16. Transmission electron micrograph of the portion of an osteoclast with its ruffled border actively removing bone extracellular matrix (resorbing bone matrix). *(From Fawcett DW:* Bloom and Fawcett: a textbook of histology, *ed 11, Philadelphia, 1986, Saunders.)*

and the degree of mineralization in developing bone. The amorphous ground substance, which consists primarily of aggrecan composites, allows water to contact the crystals and ion exchange to occur. The total volume of water in mature bone is usually less than 10%. In addition to aggrecan composites, small amounts of glycoproteins and matrix proteins are present within the ECM's amorphous ground substance and play adhesive roles. The glycoproteins consist of **osteocalcin** and **osteopontin,** both of which bind to the crystals, the latter to other substances including **integrin,** the transmembrane protein associated with osteoblasts and osteocytes, as well as many other cell types, including fibroblasts. **Sialoprotein** is a matrix protein that also has adhesive qualities, being able to bind to the integrins of the bone-forming cells and the matrix components of bone.

The process of mineralization within the ECM of bone has not been fully determined. It undoubtedly involves the presence of matrix vesicles that are released into the osteoid by osteoblasts. The vesicles are filled with calcium and phosphate ions plus cyclic adenosine monophosphate (AMP), adenosine triphosphate (ATP), and adenosine triphosphatase (ATPase); two other enzymes, alkaline phosphatase and pyrophosphatase; and proteins that bind calcium. Moreover, the vesicles possess calcium pumps that allow further movement of this element into them. Thus it would appear that each vesicle is at some level an autonomous structure that is able to construct hydroxyapatite crystals outside the cytoplasm of the osteoblast and osteocyte and within the ECM prebone domain. As the crystals are released from the vesicles and deposited along the surface of nearby collagen molecules, they are believed to be microcenters of further calcification and mineralization over an extended period with the gradual removal of water.

HISTOGENESIS OF BONE

Bone originates normally by either intramembranous ossification (within a layer of connective tissue) or endochondral ossification (within a cartilaginous model). Development along either line results in bone tissue that is indistinguishable from how it had formed initially. The bone originally formed is **primary bone,** which is gradually and continuously replaced by **secondary bone.**

INTRAMEMBRANOUS OSSIFICATION

Intramembranous ossification originates in the mesenchyme as groups of cells form **bone blastemas** that become primary ossification centers (Figure 6-17). Initially the mesenchymal cells appear crowded and hyperplastic, forming **mesenchymal condensations.** These cells become more fibroblast-like, especially along the perimeter, secreting the early ECM, including collagen. Other mesenchymal cells differentiate into osteoblasts with osteoid synthesis and calcification following. The osteoblasts eventually form a line or "membrane" of cells and deposit their prebone secretions unidirectionally, trapping at the same time some cells that failed to join the line. These trapped osteoblasts become the first osteocytes that assist in osteonal development and its mineralization. The islands of early forming bone are called **spicules,** which subsequently fuse into **trabeculae,** giving the bone a spongy appearance (Figure 6-18). During this development, blood vessels form along the external boundaries, lying in proximity to the osteoblasts. Combined with the peripheral fibroblastic cells and neighboring undifferentiated cells that become osteoprogenitor cells, the periosteum is formed. The primary bone derived from intramembranous ossification appears spongy or woven and can be referred to as *spongy* or *woven* bone at this stage in development. As the bone matures, new bone is formed in layers, or *lamellae*, and the trabeculae disappear. Eventually only lamellar bone is left. Bones that offer protection, including the frontal and parietal bones of the skull, mandible, maxilla, and clavicle plus the periosteum of long bones, are all formed by this type of ossification.

ENDOCHONDRAL OSSIFICATION

Endochondral ossification takes place within previously formed hyaline cartilage. The shape of the cartilage is basically a model for the developing bone to follow, occurring during the formation of long and short bones (i.e., the weight-bearing bones of the body) (Figure 6-19). It is important to remember that this type of bone formation takes place within the cartilage model and requires several events to occur previously. Once the small hyaline cartilage has taken shape, blood vessels appear next to the perichondrium along the portion of the model that will become the shaft of the bone (see Figure 6-19). With the presence of these blood vessels, the chondrogenic cells of the perichondrium become osteogenic (i.e., the osteoprogenitor cells that will give rise to osteoblasts). Thus the lateral or midriff portion of the cartilage's perichondrium is transformed into the **subperiosteal bone collar,** and the first bone formed along the hyaline cartilage model is that produced by intramembranous ossification (see Figure 6-19).

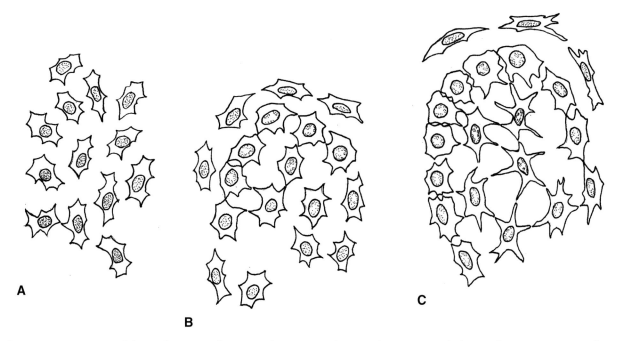

Figure 6-17. Diagram of the early stages of intramembranous ossification, beginning with the random arrangement of mesenchymal cells **(A)** that eventually form a rim or "membrane" of osteoprogenitor cells **(B).** This rim of cells **(C)** become the first osteoblasts, which along with cells inside the rim (the first osteocytes), secrete the bone matrix, resulting in the formation of a bone spicule.

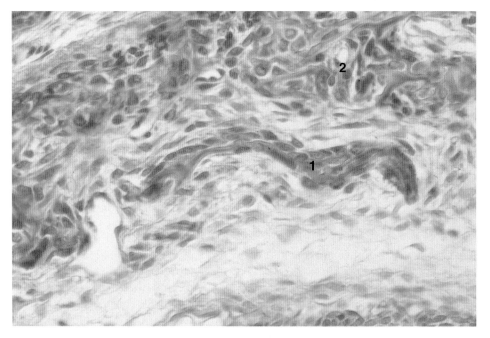

Figure 6-18. Light micrograph of intramembranous ossification occurring within the developing skull. A forming bone spicule *(1)* will soon unite with other nearby spicules *(2)*. (Masson trichrome stain; ×400.)

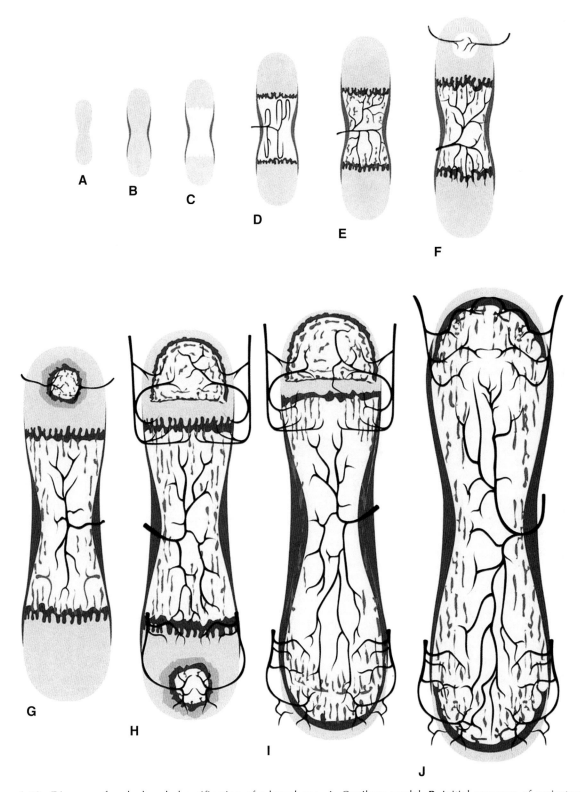

Figure 6-19. Diagram of endochondral ossification of a long bone. **A,** Cartilage model. **B,** Initial presence of periosteum and subsequent bone collar. **C,** Hypertrophy of adjacent chondrocytes and calcification of the matrix. **D and E,** Invasion of osteogenic tissue and vascular mesenchyme and subsequent removal of cartilage model along with the establishment of growth cartilaginous plates at opposite ends of the collar. **F,** Initiation of secondary centers of ossification within each end of the cartilage model. **G to I,** Continued development of the secondary centers, resulting in the formation of the epiphyses, and the primary center, resulting in the formation of the diaphysis with concomitant development of marrow within both centers. **J,** Growth plates disappear and the bone ceases to lengthen. *(From Bergman RA, Afifi AK, Heidger PM Jr:* Histology, *Philadelphia, 1996, Saunders.)*

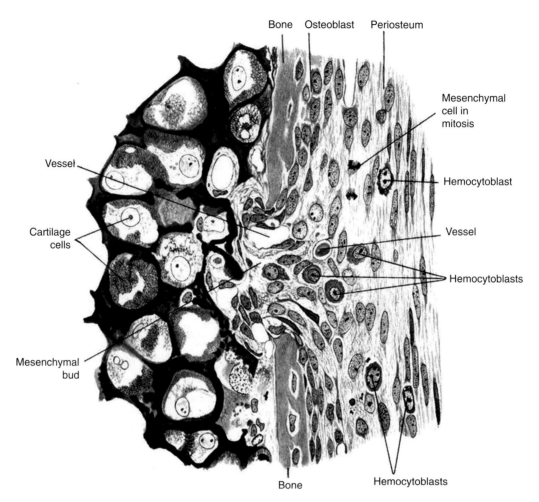

Bone Osteoblast Periosteum

Mesenchymal cell in mitosis

Hemocytoblast

Vessel

Vessel

Cartilage cells

Hemocytoblasts

Mesenchymal bud

Bone

Hemocytoblasts

Figure 6-20. Illustration of an osteogenic bud with cells of osteogenic potency and blood vessels as osteogenic tissue penetrates the recently formed bone collar. *(From Fawcett DW:* Bloom and Fawcett: a textbook of histology, *ed 11, Philadelphia, 1986, Saunders.)*

Subsequently, endochondral ossification occurs in a four-step process. Initially, the chondrocytes next to the developing bone collar enlarge or hypertrophy. As these chondrocytes grow in size, they concomitantly calcify their adjacent extracellular matrix. Second, as the bone collar takes shape and the ECM of the nearby chondrocytes is calcified, the chondrocytes have become self-entombed, losing all connection to nutrients and oxygen, and die, leaving empty lacunae surrounded by a now calcified cartilage matrix. Third, the formation of **osteogenic buds (periosteal buds),** consisting of osteogenic precursors and blood vessels, penetrate the degenerative spaces and make their residence within the cartilage template (Figure 6-20). And finally, osteoblasts line the septa of calcified cartilaginous matrices and secrete osteoid onto these supports for the beginning of ossification.

Near both ends of the cartilage model and immediately away from the developing bone collar, chondrocytes increase their activity in cell replication interstitially, but in a unidirectional manner (Figure 6-21). As a result, newly formed cells are produced in close synchrony, continually away from the developing shaft. These centers of replication are referred to as **zones of proliferation,** consisting of two for each developing bone (Figure 6-22). In a manner of speaking, as new cells are created, older cells become left behind, closer to site of endochondral ossification. These chondrocytes, which are now arranged isogenously in rows, mature and enlarge, storing glycogen at the expense of the ECM in the process and forming the region known as the **zone of hypertrophy** (see Figure 6-22). The oldest cells of this zone lie closest to the bone-forming tissue within the model (and far-

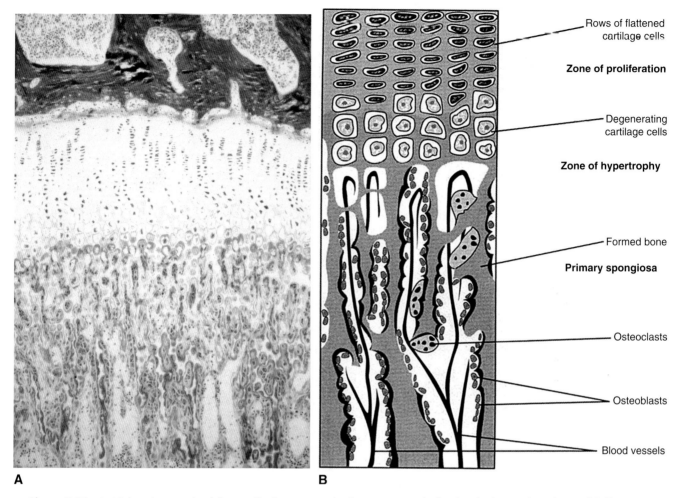

A   B

Figure 6-21. A, Light micrograph of the cartilaginous growth plate at one end of a developing rat long bone. (Mallory-Azan stain; ×100.) **B,** Diagram of the specific regions associated with the growth plate. *(Modified from Bergman RA, Afifi AK, Heidger PM Jr:* Histology, *Philadelphia, 1996, Saunders.)*

thest away from the proliferating zone) and calcify their surrounding ECM in much the same way as the original chondrocytes that lay next to the collar had previously done, forming the **zone of provisional calcification.** And as these cells die, osteogenic tissue penetrates the shell-like ECM, invades the lacunae, and establishes lines of osteoblasts that begin the bone-forming process along the most prominent remnants of the cartilage's ECM, with smaller remnants being absorbed by osteoclasts. The bone being formed on the cartilage model in this region has a channel-like appearance and can be called **cancellous,** a type of spongy bone arranged more in columns rather than in an irregular, woven manner. This bone, and the centers of calcified cartilage ECM that it surrounds, comprises the **primary spongiosa.** The bone-forming region immediately associated with the zone of provisional calcification (the primary spongiosa), is also

called the **zone of ossification,** and all of the described zones comprise the **growth plate** (see Figures 6-19, 6-21, and 6-22). Each long and short bone has two growth plates. Long bones are formed from cartilaginous models with dilated ends **(epiphyses)** on a central cylindric shaft **(diaphysis);** within the model endochondral bone continually replaces the matured cartilage of the **epiphyseal plates** (between the epiphyses and diaphysis), which represent the growth plates of long bones. The lengthwise expansion of newly formed long and short bones is primarily due to the interstitial growth occurring. However, widthwise expansion of these bones is due to appositional growth of new bone material along the periosteum. While the expansion of a long bone continues, a progressive process of remodeling involves selective sites of bone deposition and absorption that collectively results in forming the final shape (Figure 6-23).

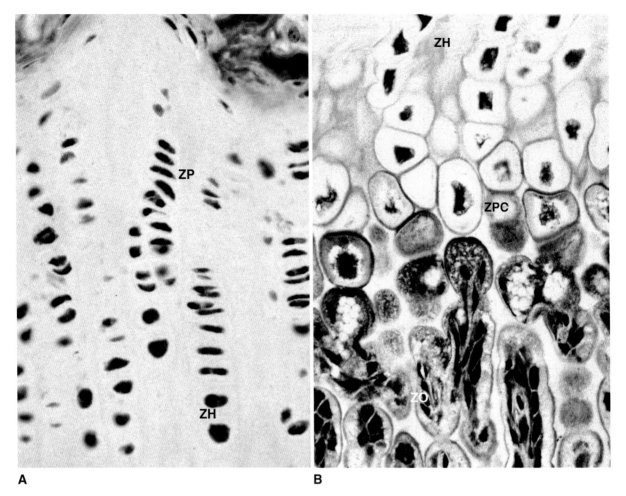

Figure 6-22. Organization within the cartilaginous growth plate. **A,** Light micrograph (×500) of the zones of proliferation *(ZP)* and hypertrophy *(ZH)*. **B,** Light micrograph (×500) of the zones of hypertrophy *(ZH)*, provisional calcification *(ZPC)*, and ossification *(ZO)*.

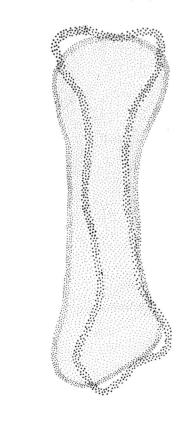

Figure 6-23. Illustration of the amount of surface remodeling that occurs during long bone development, resulting in marked changes in its shape as it grows in length and width. The overlaid shaded example represents the bone formed during fetal development and has been enlarged to approximately the same size as a nearly mature bone to demonstrate the extent of the remodeling.

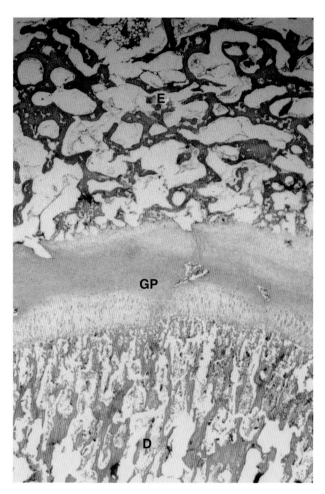

Figure 6-24. Light micrograph of an epiphysis *(E)* of a developing long bone of a horse containing woven spongy bone, appearing distinctly different from the cancellous spongy bone growing from the growth plate *(GP)* into the diaphysis *(D)*. (Hematoxylin and eosin stain; ×10.)

In bones with pronounced dilated ends (the epiphyses), **secondary centers of ossification** become established within each epiphysis (proximal and distal) (Figure 6-24; see also Figure 6-19). Secondary centers of ossification begin after the primary center of ossification has become established within the midriff portion of the cartilage model, which becomes the **diaphysis.** It is initiated differently from the primary center of ossification in that a bone collar is not required for the process to begin. Instead, at a few, discrete locations along the lateral sides of each epiphysis, blood vessels appear and the conversion process occurs as chondrogenic cells become osteoprogenitor cells and subsequent invasion proceeds into the cartilage template at each end of the model.

The chondrocytes within each epiphysis do not become organized in interstitial growth, but remain random in location. Consequently, osteogenesis results in the formation of bone that is woven or spongy in appearance, lacking directionality as opposed to the cancellous bone that is formed from the growth plates nearby (see Figure 6-24). While bone development continues in the fetus and after birth, the woven bone of the epiphyses increasingly thickens, providing the necessary strength to resist stress in these regions, and are readily distinguished from the small, newly formed "honeycomb" array of bone being formed from the growth plates.

BONE CLASSIFICATION

Classification of bone tissues is made on development, configuration, and organization. When using development as the basis, bone can be subdivided into immature and mature forms. **Immature bone** forms in the primary and secondary ossification centers of the fetus and primary spongiosa, postnatally. Within the cartilage model it consists initially of numerous cells with large lacunae that are scattered throughout a matrix that possesses randomly arranged collagen (thus not birefringent). Consequently, the first bone made during endochondral ossification is spongy. Similarly, the first bone made during the intramembranous ossification of flat bone creation is spongy even though it originated from the fusion of spicules. Eventually, immature bone is transformed to its mature form by the end of the development of the body. **Mature bone** is generally more compact than immature bone, consisting of orderly arranged matrices (birefringent) that are due to the helical deposition of collagen fibers.

Based on configuration, bone is broken down into spongy and compact types. Spongy bone, including cancellous bone, is tissue that generally has greater interosseous space than bone. As stated, this type of bone is often described as immature bone, especially in the developing portions of epiphyses and diaphysis of long bones (see Figure 6-24). In adults, however, it will also comprise mature bone but usually only a small portion of it. The area internally lining the compact bone of the shaft and in contact with the bone marrow is porous and spongy, having little of the organization seen in compact bone. Variable amounts of woven bone remain within the articular ends during adulthood of most species (see Figure 6-19). In birds, woven bone, which is lighter than compact bone, is more prevalent in adults than woven bone in adult mammals.

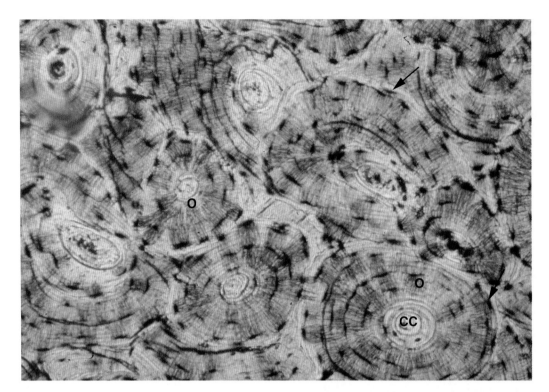

Figure 6-25. Light micrograph (×100) of compact bone oriented in cross section that has not been demineralized but instead ground to a thin wafer for histological observation. The principal feature of compact bone among domestic species is the presence of osteons *(O)*, each containing a central canal *(CC)* surrounded by rings of the lacunae and their associated canaliculi. Many osteons are bordered by cementing lines *(arrows)*.

In domestic animals **compact bone** comprises mostly mature bone and is characterized by the presence of more bone than interosseous space. Organizationally, compact bone is subdivided into lamellar and osteonal types. **Lamellar bone** consists of layers or lamellae of bone deposited as sheets from the periosteum externally and endosteum internally. And externally, the dense connective tissue elements of emerging tendons and ligaments—**Sharpey's fibers** or **perforating fibers**—intermingle with the outermost lamellae (see Figure 6-8). The internal and external lamellae, in turn, encompass another, much broader region of compact bone called **osteonal bone.** Osteonal bone consists of lamellae that are concentrically arranged to form a cylinder referred to as an **osteon** or **haversian system** (Figures 6-25 and 6-26). Within the center of each osteon is a central space, the **osteonal** or **haversian canal (central canal)** that contains blood vessels, vasomotor nerves, and cells of the cortical endosteum: osteoblasts and osteoprogenitor cells. An osteon or haversian system is composed then of a long, sometimes branching, cylinder of compact bone (running parallel to the diaphyses) surrounded often by a cementing substance **(cementing line).** Each osteonal canal is interconnected to adjacent osteonal canals by short communicating canals **(Volkmann's canals)** that are oriented at right angles to the longitudinal axes of the osteons (Figure 6-27). In this way, the close and necessary association between bone and blood (for calcium and oxygen delivery and so forth) is maintained. Osteons are formed along the perimeter of compact bone by the asymmetrical formation of interstitial lamellae around an individual blood vessel (Figure 6-28). Eventually the lamellae and adjacent osteogenic tissue surround the blood vessel and a young osteon is formed. Osteoblasts, which are now part of the endosteum, secrete the prebone matrix concentrically, and osteocytes become lodged in the bone matrix in the same manner. The size of the osteonal canal decreases to the point that allows a small amount of osteogenic tissue, nerve, and blood vessel to coexist.

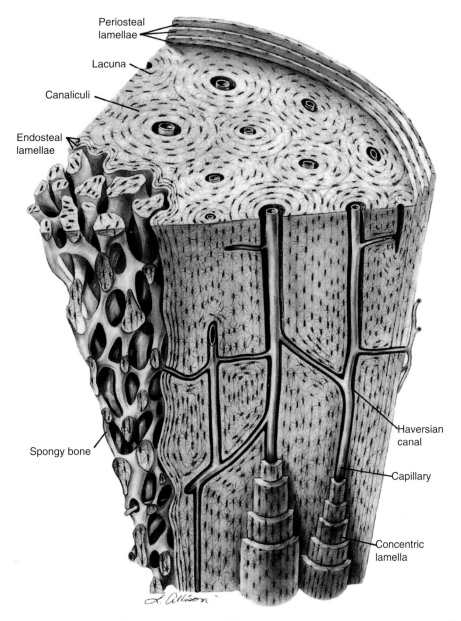

Periosteal lamellae

Lacuna

Canaliculi

Endosteal lamellae

Spongy bone

Haversian canal

Capillary

Concentric lamella

Figure 6-26. Illustration of the compact bone reveals its lamellar organization, which occurs concentrically within each osteon (Haversian system) and circumferentially (lamellae), inside the periosteum externally and endosteum internally. *(From Leeson CR, Leeson TS, Paparo AA:* Atlas of histology, *Philadelphia, 1985, Saunders).*

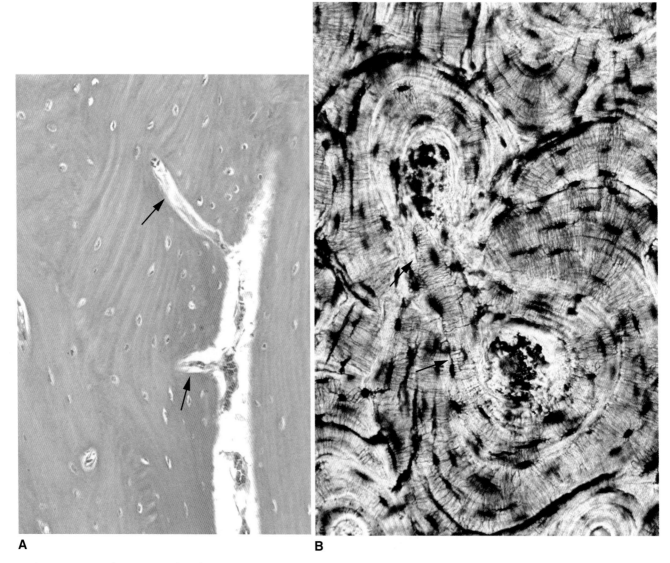

A   **B**

Figure 6-27. Light micrographs of communicating canals *(arrows)* that interconnect adjacent osteons. **A,** Longitudinal orientation of a demineralized canine diaphysis. (Hematoxylin and eosin stain; ×200.) **B,** Ground compact bone. The lamellae follow the course of the communicating canal, cutting across the concentric lamellae of the two adjacent osteons.

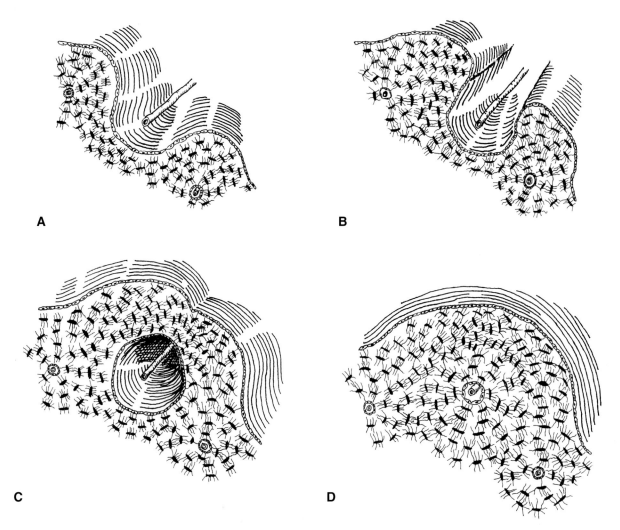

A

B

C

D

Figure 6-28. Diagram of osteonal formation along the periosteum of developing compact bone. Individual osteons arise by asymmetrical buildup of circumferential lamellae that surround blood vessels, which lie parallel to the longitudinal axis of the bone (diaphysis). In **(A)** a small blood vessel lies within the groove that resulted from two recently formed osteons. In **(B)** and **(C)**, lamellar bone grows eccentrically until surrounding and engulfing the blood vessel, producing a wide tunnel-like structure lined now by endosteal rather than periosteal tissue. In **(D)**, concentric lamellae are laid down by the endosteum, which lines what will become the central canal of a newly formed osteon.

BONE REMODELING AND REPAIR

All tissues undergo changes during development, and this process does not end with maturation but continues in a subtle manner and reduced pace as organelles within each cell, cells or portions of cell populations, and extracellular materials are gradually replenished. Bone tissue is no exception even though the remarkably mineralized environment would appear to provide a strong impediment for such a process to occur. Bone replenishment is an extension of the bone remodeling required during development.

While bones become formed, portions of them are remodeled at the same time. The cancellous bone that is created along the growth plate is not allowed to grow to the point of being compact, but instead is steadily removed by osteoclastic activity. In this way, there is sufficient bone in the region between the growth plate and the developing diaphysis, the **metaphysis,** to offer the needed structural support for this area. This support is especially important due to the pronounced shaping of the diaphysis at both distal and proximal metaphyseal regions where resorption occurs along the external surface (see Figure 6-23).

As the periosteum contributes new bone to the rest of the shaft externally, osteoclasts are active along the internal perimeter of the diaphysis, and resultantly increase the marrow's width, while preventing the collar from becoming too thick. Controlled osteoclasia, which is normally guided by physical stress and endocrine secretions, especially parathyroid hormone (see Table 6-2), and osteogenic activity together achieve **surface modeling** and are responsible for proper bone shaping.

At the end of the development of the body's skeleton, bone formation and resorption come into balance, occurring principally within the internal structure of each adult bone and, as a result, are known as **internal bone remodeling.** The remaining trabecular bone also is remodeled and at a faster rate than the remodeling of compact bone, but represents only a small volume of the total bone in adult mammals. The shift from modeling to remodeling ensures an appropriate turnover of old, dying osseous tissue. In addition to the removal of dead bone, other factors can promote remodeling, including extensive and prolonged episodes of physical (biomechanical) stress; nutritional influences such as deficiencies in vitamins, calcium, or other minerals; decrease in physical stress or even complete disuse such as during paralysis or fracture repair; and changes in endocrine secretions.

The osseous tissue, here, can consist of an osteonal unit that has become singled out for removal or be independent of specific osteons. When an area becomes resorbed, only a few osteoclasts are needed at first. As more surface area of the resorbing osteon is exposed, increasing numbers of osteoclasts are recruited and a **cutting zone** is in place (Figure 6-29). Subsequently, an **absorption cavity (resorption cavity)** is formed, which can exceed the original diameter of a primary osteon. In this way, a single osteon or a portion of one or two and some of the adjacent interstitial lamellae can be replaced. Within a short distance of the last line of osteoclasts a line of osteoblasts takes up residence, forming the **reversal line,** which seen longitudinally is cone shaped. The reversal line is much longer than that forming the cutting zone, because of the comparatively slow rate of bone formation versus bone resorption. For the reasons stated earlier, an increased activity of osteoclasts in compact bone will make it more porous as a result of too many absorption cavities.

Repair to bone often involves instances when trauma has occurred, such as a fracture to the midriff region of a long bone. At the site of a break, blood vessels have been ruptured and severed, resulting in a localized hemorrhage and blood clot that envelops the fracture zone and interrupts blood flow. With the disruption of the vasculature, nearby osteocytes soon die. The osteons and interstitial bone adjacent to the break weaken as more osteocytes perish, leaving empty canaliculi and lacunae. This process continues until routes for blood circulation within the bone and around it have become reestablished. Within a short time, the blood clot is transformed into granulation tissue as fibroblasts and small blood vessels invade it. Osteogenic cells of the periosteum and endosteum and multipotential cells of the bone marrow proliferate, forming a **callus** (Figure 6-30).

The osteogenic cells of the periosteum that are closest to the fracture site and next to newly formed blood vessels become osteoblastic and produce bony trabeculae, which collectively form a collar that attaches the opposing dead bone at the fracture site. Other proliferating osteogenic cells, lying outside the newly formed osteoblasts and growing at faster rates than adjacent blood vessels, become chondroblastic and produce hyaline cartilage within the external callus. And outside the developing cartilage are osteogenic cells that continue to divide, but remain osteogenic, having some capillaries. These three regions make up the **external callus.**

The osteogenic cells of the endosteum and multipotential cells of the marrow form an **internal callus,** consisting of proliferative tissue that can become osteoblastic and produce bony trabeculae as well. The internal and external calluses collectively form the callus and function together as a natural splint and have the capacity to form new bone that will attach the broken ends of the fracture site. The cartilage associated with the callus becomes transformed into bone by endochondral ossification. When the new bone becomes compact, subsequent remodeling further strengthens the old fracture site. In breaks that are "clean" (relatively even surfaces at the site) and held solidly in place by a bone fixator device, callus formation, particularly the external callus, can be reduced considerably and repair is able to proceed rapidly. But a fracture may be severe enough to prevent the successful formation of a useful callus and bony collar, and thus possibly require the intervention of other measures, including bone grafts.

JOINTS

When the ends of bones interconnect with each other they form joints that vary in construction according to the amount of movement normally allowed. Joints associated with little to no movement between adjacent bones are **synarthroses** and those

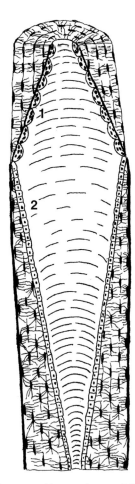

Figure 6-29. Diagram of internal remodeling of compact bone involving the removal of an old osteon by a line of osteoclasts *(1)* followed by a line of osteoblasts *(2)*, which build a new osteon.

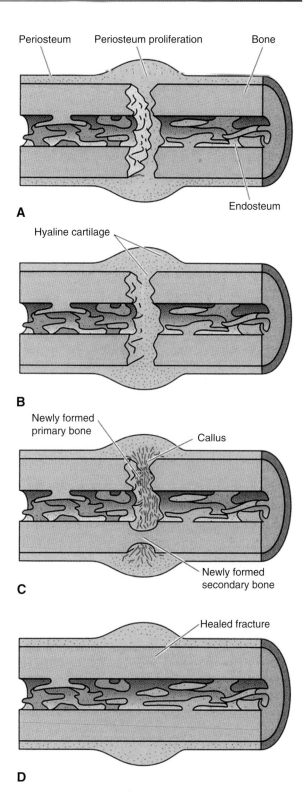

Figure 6-30. Diagram of the process of repair of a bone fracture. *(From Gartner LP, Hiatt JL:* Color textbook of histology, *Philadelphia, 1997, Saunders.)*

that function to articulate freely within the confines of a specific range of motion are **diarthroses** or **synovial joints.**

Synarthroses joints consist of three types, best exemplified by the junctions of bones that compose the skull. Adjoining bones, which are held together before maturation by dense connective tissue, are **syndesmoses.** Upon complete development of the skeletal system, the dense connective tissue is replaced by bone and the joints are now classified as **synostoses,** which prevent the occurrence of any movement. Another example of a syndesmosis joint is the pubic symphysis. In this instance, adjoining bones are connected by dense connective tissue as before, but with the assistance of fibrocartilage, which forms an attachment with the caps of hyaline cartilage at the ends of each bone. Intervertebral disks are another example of this type of joint. Here the caps of hyaline

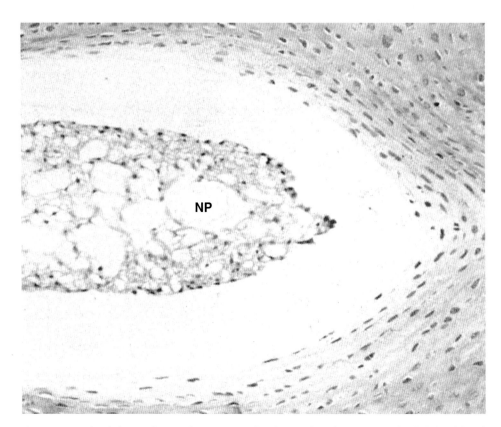

Figure 6-31. Light micrograph of the nucleus pulposus *(NP)* that lies within the intervertebral disk of the dog. (Hematoxylin and eosin stain; ×200.)

cartilage of adjacent vertebrae are joined by inner lamellae of fibrocartilage, whereas the bones are attached by outer lamellae of dense connective tissue, which together form the **annulus fibrosus** (see Figure 6-7). The center of the intervertebral disk contains a small cavity filled with a gelatinous material, **nucleus pulposus** (Figure 6-31). The nucleus pulposus recedes with age and can be calcified.

Synchondrosis represents a third type of synarthrosis joint and consists of adjacent bones that are connected by hyaline cartilage. An example of this joint is the growth plate within long bones (see Figures 6-21 and 6-24). A developmental joint, it will be replaced by synostosis as the bones of the epiphyses join the diaphysis.

Diarthroses comprise mostly joints of the extremities and serve to facilitate locomotion. Adjoining bones are lined by hyaline cartilage (**articular cartilage**) that normally persists throughout life. As a form of hyaline cartilage, it is unique in several ways. The cartilage lacks the usual perichondrium, but can still be subdivided into several zones: the **peripheral zone,**

the **middle zone,** and the **deep zone** (Figure 6-32). The zones are largely distinguished based on the arrangement of the cells and the collagen. In addition, a *tidemark* consists of a basophilic thin line that demarcates the border between the calcified and uncalcified layers of the deep zone. The articular cartilage of adjoining bones is surrounded by a **synovial cavity** filled with serous fluid (**synovial fluid**) and lined by the **synovial membrane,** which consists of a layer of synovial cells and a small amount of connective tissue with numerous small blood vessels. The synovial membrane is protected externally by a **fibrous layer** of dense connective tissue contiguous with the fibrous layer of the periosteum of both adjacent bones. The fibrous layer and synovial membrane constitute the **joint capsule.** The synovial fluid is plasma-like in its composition and possesses a high level of the glycosaminoglycan **hyaluronans,** and the glycoprotein **lubricin,** both of which are believed to be contributed by the synovial cells. The fluid acts to both nourish and lubricate the articular cartilage. If changes in the synovial fluid's composition

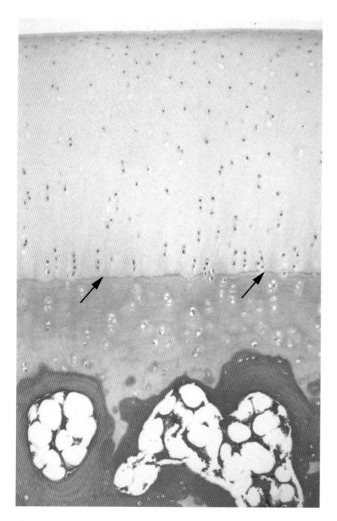

Figure 6-32. Light micrograph of the articular cartilage that externally lines an epiphysis of a canine bone. Arrows point to the tidemark within the deep zone. (Hematoxylin and eosin stain; ×200.)

occur, however, such as the result of inflammation, the health of the articular cartilage is very much at risk.

SUGGESTED READINGS

Aarden EM, Burger EH, Nijweide PJ: Function of osteocytes in bone, *J Cell Biochem* 55:287, 1994.

Bergman RA, Afifi AK, Heidger PM Jr: *Histology,* Philadelphia, 1996, Saunders.

Dambrain R, Raphael B, Dhem A, Lebeau J: Radiation osteitis of the clavicle following radiotherapy and radical neck dissection of head and neck cancer, *Bull Group Int Rech Sci Stomatol Odontol* 33:65, 1990.

Fawcett DW: *Bloom and Fawcett: a textbook of histology,* ed 11, Philadelphia, 1986, Saunders.

Fu E, Hsieh YD, Wikesjo UM, Liu D: Effects of cyclosporin A on alveolar bone: and experimental study in the rat, *Peridontol* 70:189, 1999.

Gartner LP, Hiatt JL: *Color textbook of histology,* Philadelphia, 1997, Saunders.

Ham AW, Cormack, DH: *Histology,* ed 8, Philadelphia, 1979, Lippincott.

Ham AW, Harris WR: Repair and transplantation of bone. In Bourne GH, editor: *The biochemistry and physiology of bone,* vol 3, New York, 1971, Academic Press.

Leeson CR, Leeson TS, Paparo AA: *Atlas of histology,* Philadelphia, 1985, Saunders.

Noble BS, Reeve J: Osteocyte function, osteocyte death and bone fracture resistance, *Mol Cell Endocrinol* 159:7, 2000.

Nunez EA, Krook L, Whalen JP: Effect of calcium depletion and subsequent repletion on parathyroids, parafollicular (C) cells and bone in growing pigs, *Cell Tissue Res* 13:373, 1976.

Poole CA, Wotton SF, Duance VC: Localization of type IX in chondrons isolated from porcine articular cartilage and rat chondrosarcoma, *Histochem J* 20:567, 1988.

Poole CA, Gilbert RT, Herbage D, Hartmann DJ: Immunolocalization of type IX collagen in normal and spontaneously osteoarthritic canine tibial cartilage and isolated chondrons, *Osteoarthritis Cartilage* 5:191, 1997.

Blood and Hemopoiesis

KEY CHARACTERISTICS

- Highly specialized connective tissue, with specialized cells but without usual extracellular matrix (ECM), involved in gaseous exchange, transport of nutrients, waste materials, and cells of defense.
- Erythrocytes:
  provide O_2, remove CO_2, pH buffer
- Leukocytes:
  cells of defense
  classified according to:
      shape of nucleus
      presence and staining reaction of granules

Blood is the circulating fluid connective tissue that supplies O_2 and nutrients and removes CO_2 and waste materials to all regions of the body as well as serving as a conduit for the distribution of heat, chemicals, and specialized cells, which are associated with exchange of respiratory gases and cellular and humoral defense. With its ability to incessantly move throughout the body, this tissue provides perhaps the body's greatest homeostatic force, especially with regard to the presence of various sensors that are able to detect changes in temperature, pH, hormone levels, and osmotic tension.

Blood is composed of the **formed elements,** the red blood cells, the white blood cells, and clotting cells or portions of them; platelets; and **plasma,** the intercellular liquid medium that constitutes blood's ECM. In terms of total volume of blood, the percentage of the formed elements is approximately 40% (30%-55% depending on the species) in normal individuals and can be viewed after the centrifugation of collected blood (pretreated with an anticoagulant), forming the two lowest layers—the **hematocrit** (Figure 7-1). The lowest layer is by far the largest, being viscous and red and consisting of red blood cells. The next layer is the **buffy coat,** which is thin and grayish white and consists of white blood cells and platelets that form nearly 1% of the total blood volume (Table 7-1). The highest layer is plasma, which is a clear, yellowish fluid, comprising 55% to 60% of the total blood volume. Blood accounts for 6% to 11% of the total body weight of most mammals, and is greatest in large animals.

The histological examination of blood can be a useful tool for the assessment of general health and disease, especially in diagnosing hematological diseases. This examination is best performed by creating **blood smears,** which involves placing one drop of blood pretreated with an anticoagulant such as ethylenediaminetetraacetic acid (EDTA) onto a glass slide and spreading and air-drying (and methanol preserving) the blood preparation evenly into a single layer.

TABLE 7-1 Averaged Blood Count for RBC among Domestic Mammals with Diameter Size in Parentheses and Averaged Blood Count for WBC with Percentage of Total WBC in Parentheses

ANIMAL	ERYTHROCYTES ($\times 10^6/\mu l$)	NEUTROPHILS* ($\times 10^3 \mu l$)	EOSINOPHILS ($\times 10^3/\mu l$)	BASOPHILS ($\times 10^3/\mu l$)	LYMPHOCYTES ($\times 10^3/\mu l$)	MONOCYTES ($\times 10^3/\mu l$)
Cat	7.5 (5.8 μm)	7.6 (59.5)	0.65 (5)	Rare (<0.5)	4.0 (32)	0.35 (3)
Dog	6.8 (7.0 μm)	7.1 (70.8)	0.55 (4)	Rare (<0.5)	2.8 (20)	0.75 (5)
Cow	7.0 (5.8 μm)	2.0 (28.5)	0.7 (9)	0.05 (0.5)	4.5 (58)	0.4 (4)
Horse	9.0 (5.5 μm)	4.8 (53.5)	0.3 (3.4)	0.05 (0.5)	3.5 (39)	0.39 (4.3)
Pig	6.5 (6.0 μm)	5.7 (38)	0.5 (3.5)	0.01 (0.5)	8.0 (53)	0.8 (5)

Modified from Jain NC: *Essentials of veterinary hematology,* Philadelphia, 1993, Lea & Febiger.
*Include banded form.

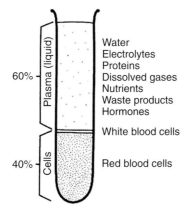

Figure 7-1. Illustration of anticoagulated blood that has been separated by centrifugation into three layers: the bottom red blood cell layer; the thin, middle white blood cell layer, also known as the *buffy coat,* which together with the red blood cell layer comprises the hematocrit; and the top, large plasma layer. *(From Cunningham JG: Textbook of veterinary physiology, ed 2, Philadelphia, 1997, Saunders).*

The blood is then stained with a mixture of two contrasting dyes that will reveal each cell's cytoplasm and nucleus (Table 7-2).

PLASMA

The formed elements are suspended in the liquid ECM known as **plasma.** Plasma not only provides fluidity for cell motility but also is a medium for electrolytes and organic compounds. Thus it consists primarily of water (93%) with most of the remainder being protein. Plasma proteins are formed in the liver and are released into its capillaries. Several primary proteins, including globulin and albumin, play roles in immune responses and transportation of hormones, metals and other materials, and fibrinogen, which promotes blood coagulation. Approximately 1% of plasma consists of electrolytes, nitrogenous compounds, gases, and nutrients. Among the electrolytes, Na^+, Cl^-, and HCO_3^- are the most common. The nitrogenous compounds are primarily associated with waste products such as creatine, uric acid, and urea nitrogen. Nutrients within blood plasma include glucose, lipids and lipoproteins, amino acids, and some vitamins. In addition to these substances, plasma carries minuscule amounts of hormones.

Most of the plasma easily diffuses from the lumen of the smallest blood vessels (capillaries) across the endothelial lining into adjacent tissues. However, some of the components, particularly the plasma proteins, often remain at much higher concentrations than in the tissues' fluids because they are not able to cross the capillary's endothelium. It should be kept in mind that certain tissues of the body have fenestrated blood vessels, such as the thyroid, and consequently, in these portions of the body there is very little difference in the composition of tissue fluid and plasma.

FORMED ELEMENTS

ERYTHROCYTE

Of the cells that are normally located in blood, the red blood cell, or **erythrocyte,** is by far most common,

TABLE 7-2 Hematologic Staining

STAIN—INGREDIENT	CELL REACTION	COMMENTS
Wright: Wright's powder w/methyl alcohol	Erythrocyte: yellowish red Nuclei: purple, deep blue Basophilic granules: deep purple Eosinophilic granules: pink to red-orange Neutrophilic granules: reddish brown to lilac Monocyte granules: azure Lymphocyte granules: reddish azure against sky blue cytoplasm Platelets: violet to purple	Most effective on thin films
Methylene blue, azure A, and eosin Y	Basophilic granules: deep blue with reddish cast Eosinophilic granules: bright red Neutrophilic granules: pale purple pink and indistinct Platelets: pale purple or lavender	Most effective on thick films
Wilcox method (Wright-Giesma): Giesma in glycerin, Wright staining solution	Erythrocyte: pink Nuclei: reddish purple Basophilic granules: deep purple Eosinophilic granules: pink to red-orange Neutrophilic granules: reddish brown to lilac Monocyte granules: azure Lymphocyte granules: reddish azure against sky blue cytoplasm Platelets: violet to purple	Effective on thick to thin films

having, for example, a density of 5000 to 8000 × 10³ cells/mL of blood in the dog or roughly 500 to 1000 times greater than cellular density of white blood cells. By comparison, platelets in the dog range approximately 200 to 600 × 10³ cells/mL. The erythrocyte is anucleated, disk shaped, and biconcave among mammals, ranging from 4 to 9 μm in diameter, greatest in dogs among domestic species, and less than 1 μm in its central thickness (Figure 7-2). By being biconcave, the erythrocyte retains a large surface area for gaseous exchange while remaining narrow and flexible for excellent fluidity, especially within the small lumen of capillaries. The mature erythrocyte lacks not only a nucleus but also the full complement of organelles found in most cells. At maturation, each red blood cell is equipped to perform its functions for a limited amount of time, having life expectancies that can range in domestic species from a little more than 2 months in cats to nearly 6 months in cattle. The biconcave shape of the cell is largely due to the filamentous arrangement of the contractile protein, **spectrin,** which is closely associated with the cell membrane.

Not all red blood cells of mammals are clearly biconcave. In ruminants and pigs erythrocytes have a tendency to be flat, lacking a central pallor seen in carnivores, horses, and primates. In some ruminants (deer and goats) the erythrocytes can even vary in shape, a condition known as **poikilocytosis.** More commonly, the size of individual red blood cells within an individual sample can vary considerably (Figure 7-3). And in members of the camel family, Camellidae, erythrocytes are elliptically shaped.

Immature erythrocytes occasionally appear in circulation under normal circumstances in some species, such as dogs and cats, but not in others (ruminants and horses). The immature erythrocyte seen in peripheral blood is called the **reticulocyte,** which is anucleated and polychromatic, reacting eosinophilically and basophilically (Figure 7-4). This cell still has some of the machinery for protein synthesis, including ribosomes, rough endoplasmic reticulum (rER), and mitochondria. In states of heightened erythropoietic activity these cells are observed in greater frequency and can serve as an indicator of increased red blood cell formation.

The principal function of the erythrocyte is to transport **hemoglobin,** the molecule responsible for carrying and exchanging the gases, oxygen, and carbon dioxide. During the normal development of each erythrocyte, hemoglobin is synthesized to a maximum level, which comprises nearly one third of its total volume. Hemoglobin is a large conjugated protein that possesses four polypeptide chains, each covalently bound to heme, an iron-binding porphyrin. Hemoglobin that carries oxygen is referred to as

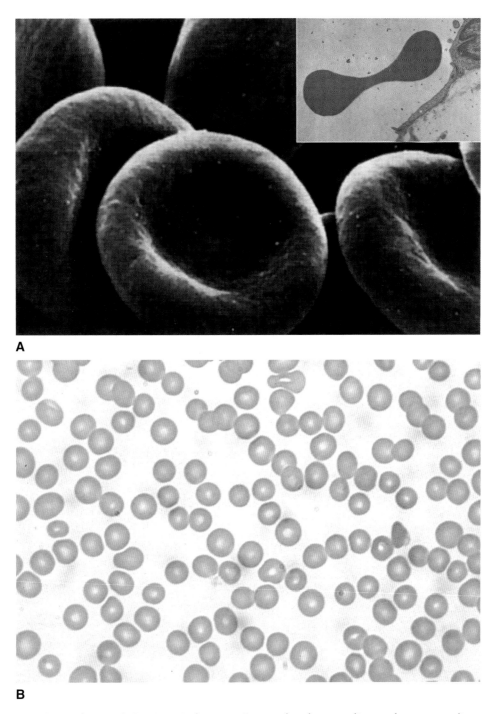

Figure 7-2. A, Scanning and transmission *(inset)* electron micrographs of mammalian erythrocytes or discocytes reveal their characteristic biconcavity. **B,** Light micrograph of feline erythrocytes with palely stained concaved centers. (Wright-Giemsa stain; ×1000.) *(A from Leeson TS, Leeson CR: A brief atlas of histology, Philadelphia, 1979, Saunders.)*

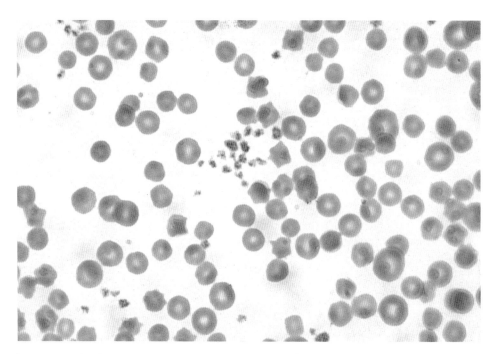

Figure 7-3. Light micrograph of bovine erythrocytes reveals considerable variation in their size (anisocytosis) and to a lesser extent in their shape (poikilocytosis). (Wright-Giemsa stain; ×1000.)

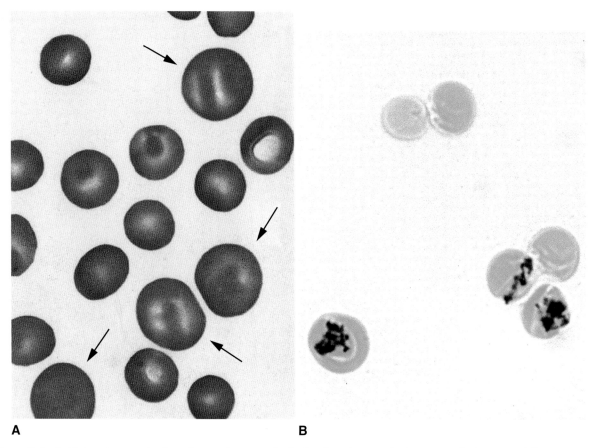

A   **B**

Figure 7-4. A, Light micrograph of canine erythrocytes, including four large reticulocytes (polychromatophilic erythrocytes) having additional basophilic reaction *(arrows)*. (Wright-Giemsa stain; ×1000.) **B,** Light micrograph (×1000) of reticulocytes revealed by the new methylene blue reticulocyte stain. *(From Harvey JW: Atlas of veterinary hematology: blood and bone marrow of domestic animals, Philadelphia, 2001, Saunders.)*

oxyhemoglobin, and that which carries carbon dioxide is **carboxyhemoglobin.**

The nondescript cytosol of the erythrocyte and its cell membrane contain other proteins that assist in its ability to exchange gases. One of the proteins is the enzyme **methemoglobin reductase,** which is able to convert methemoglobin with iron in the ferric form to the reduced hemoglobin with iron in the functional ferrous form, having now a greater affinity for O_2. Hemoglobin in its reduced state readily loads oxygen, but in oxygen-depleted tissues, O_2 is released and CO_2 is taken up by the globin moiety. The release of O_2 is further facilitated by the carbohydrate 2,3-diphosphoglyceride (2,3-DPG), which effectively causes a decrease in hemoglobin's affinity for O_2. Moreover, if the level of 2,3-DPG should increase within the cell, the level or amount of hemoglobin decreases. In localized hypoxic conditions within the body, tissues may release 2,3-DPG, thus promoting the further release of O_2.

Another of the proteins of the erythrocyte is the enzyme **carbonic anhydrase,** which combines CO_2 and H_2O to form carbonic acid, which readily dissociates into HCO_3^- (bicarbonate) and H^+. Enzymes associated with the glycolytic pathway and monophosphate shunt are present as well; they are necessary for the production of the high-energy compound, adenosine triphosphate (ATP), needed to maintain the activity of carbonic anhydrase and methemoglobin reductase. It is ironic that anaerobic pathways are used exclusively to perform the previously described activities in such an oxygen-enriched environment.

LEUKOCYTES

Under normal circumstances leukocytes, or white blood cells, comprise only a tiny fraction of the total number of blood cells circulating throughout the body (see Figure 7-1 and Table 7-1). As the central mechanism for the defense against the invasion of foreign materials, including pathogens, leukocytes use the circulatory system as a means to move to a particular site that has chemotactically attracted them. Within blood these cells assume a spherical shape, offering the least resistance to fluidity as possible. However, upon leaving the bloodstream by moving between adjacent endothelial cells (i.e., **diapedesis**), leukocytes become pleomorphic and can quickly reshape into any number of forms. Leukocytes can be subdivided into two fairly broad categories: cells that have segmented or distinctly lobed nuclei and granule-rich cytoplasms, **segmented leukocytes** or **granulocytes,** which consist of neutrophils, eosinophils, and basophils (Figure 7-5, A-C); and cells that possess nonsegmented nuclei and lack granules, **mononuclear leukocytes** or **agranulocytes,** which consist of monocytes and lymphocytes.

Neutrophil

The most common type of white blood cell in many species is the neutrophil, which receives its name of Latin (*neuter* = neither) and Greek (*philein* = to love) derivation from the general inability of its granules to be stained by either acidophilic or basophilic dyes and reagents. In dogs and cats the neutrophil, also known as the **polymorphonuclear leukocyte (PMN),** comprises the largest population of leukocytes (two thirds or more) that normally circulates in the bloodstream and functions to defend against microbial infection (Tables 7-3 and 7-4; see also Table 7-1). When observed in blood smears, the nucleus of this cell is heterochromatic and highly segmented, with distinct lobes that are attached to each other by thin threads of chromatin and nucleoplasm (Figure 7-6). In female animals an extra lobe in the shape of a small "drumstick," representing the **Barr body,** may be visible. The diameter of neutrophils ranges from 9 to 15 μm, being often smaller than the eosinophils but nearly the same size as basophils present in the blood smear being examined. The cytoplasm contains numerous granules interspersed with polysomes, Golgi apparatus, glycogen, and occasional mitochondria (Figure 7-7). Like the erythrocyte, the neutrophil uses anerobic metabolism for energy production.

Granules of the neutrophil are generally pale, but can be mildly eosinophilic, especially in some animals such as sheep and goats (Figure 7-8). Occasionally, large granules stain more intensely than smaller granules. In guinea pigs and rabbits, the large granules stain red, making the cytoplasm of these cells appear polychromatic. In those instances, the neutrophils are called **heterophils,** a term used more commonly for this cell type in nonmammals. In most species the granules are small (approximately 0.1 μm in diameter), especially in dogs, comprising the **specific granules,** which contain bactericidal enzymes and other substances needed to facilitate antimicrobial activity. Larger, less numerous granules, known as the **azurophilic granules,** are true primary lysosomes that also contain a variety of bactericidal substances including lysozyme, acid hydrolases, bactericidal permeability increasing (BPI) protein, myeloperoxidase, elastase, collagenase, and cathepsin G.

The neutrophil is one of the first cells to defend against the invasion of microorganisms and is particularly effective in combating bacteria. As these cells circulate throughout the body, they can be contacted by chemotactic agents, which direct their movement to the source of the invasion. At the site of an

Text continued on p. 140

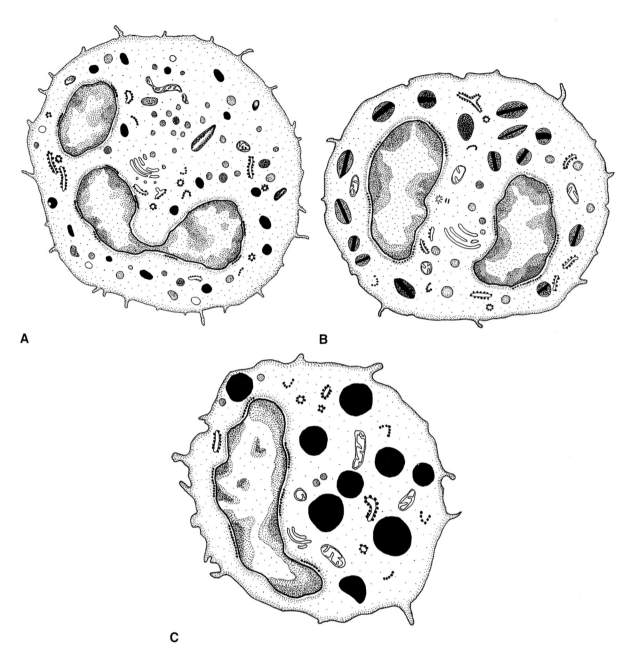

Figure 7-5. Illustration of examples of the category of leukocytes: the segmented leukocyte or granulocyte consisting of **A,** canine neutrophil; **B,** feline eosinophil; and **C,** equine basophil.

TABLE 7-3	White Blood Cell Histological Characteristics and Life Spans				
CELL TYPE	NUCLEUS	BACKGROUND CYTOPLASM	GRANULES	LIFE SPAN	COMMENTS
Neutrophil	Highly segmented at maturity, with distinct narrowing of nucleus between lobes; outline most scalloped/jagged in the horse; variably heterochromatic	Colorless at maturity	Secondary granules are numerous and nonreactive or mildly acidophilic in routine stains; primary granules in younger stages stain red-purple	Circulating half-life is 4 to 6 hours in the dog; 7-14 hours among different animals	Nonsegmented (banded) nuclei in normal animals vary in amount from less than 0.5% (ruminants) to nearly 3% (pig) and, when greater than normal, range can be clinically significant
Eosinophil	Distinctly segmented but less lobulated than neutrophils, often being bilobed; can be banded or less mature but generally of little clinical significance except for extreme eosinophilia	Stains faintly blue	Affinity for eosin in most species; often round but rod shaped in domestic cats; especially large in horses and small in ruminants	Circulating half-life is approximately 30 minutes in the dog	Eosinophils in dogs, especially greyhounds, can be vacuolated and misinterpreted as vacuolated neutrophils by inexperienced observation
Basophil	Often least segmented of the granulocytes; as in eosinophils, banded forms are mostly of little clinical significance except for extreme basophilia	Stains light blue to purple	Affinity for basic (blue) dyes of routine stains; size, number, and staining characteristics vary by species	Comparable to neutrophil	Granules are especially numerous in ruminants and pigs and least populated in the dog; in the cat the granules stain lavender
Monocyte	Nonsegmented but often variably shaped, being either round, indented, kidney shaped, band shaped, convoluted, or clover leaf–shaped; variably euchromatic	Stains blue-gray with variably sized vacuoles	Occasional pink to red-purple granules	Circulating half-life is approximately 2-3 days	Cells with banded nuclei can be confused with banded neutrophils if marked toxicity is present in the neutrophils; cells with rounded nuclei can be confused with large lymphocytes
Lymphocyte	Nonsegmented, round to oval; can be slightly indented and variable in size depending on the cell size; often heterochromatic	Clear to light blue staining, but can be darker blue in reactive cells	Often agranular, but some cells can have red- to purple-staining granules, usually within medium to large cells, which generally have more cytoplasm	Most cells are long-lived (few months to years), being mostly T cells; remainder are short-lived, few hours to 5 days, being B and T cells	Cells have high N (nucleus):C (cytoplasm) ratios, being highest in smaller cells; most cells being small to medium in size, but often larger in ruminants with more cytoplasm difficult to distinguish at times from monocytes

TABLE 7-4	Roles of Leukocytes and Correlation with Specific Morphological Features	
CELL TYPE	**ROLE**	**MORPHOLOGICAL CORRELATION**
Neutrophil	Ingestion and subsequent destruction and digestion of bacteria	Primary or azurophililic granules are formed initially, their number greatest in the promyelocyte stage; at maturity these granules are not usually revealed by routine blood film stains; weakly stained secondary or specific granules form later during myelocyte stage; lysosomes or tertiary granules form last; all granule types contain variety of hydrolytic enzymes
Eosinophil	Destruction, digestion, and control of metazoan parasites; ingestion of antigen-antibody complexes; contributes to regulation of allergic and acute inflammatory response	Presence of many azurophilic granules that can be large and either become transformed into crystalloid granules or remain homogeneous at maturity; in some species (horse and cow) the azurophilic granules remain homogeneous, whereas in others (cat and guinea pig) they become mostly crystalloid
Basophil	Elicitation of hypersensitive reaction through secretion of stored vasoactive mediators by degranulation; mediation of inflammatory responses	Like mast cell, presence of granules that store heparin, histamine (relatively low), ECF-A, NCF, and proteoglycans among other substances; basophil precursors may or may not contain metachromatic granules, which are generally homogeneous in appearance; at maturity granules may remain homogeneous (in rodents) or vary in appearance (by electron microscopy)
Monocyte	Precursors to macrophages; ingestion and presentation of antigens	Although cytoplasm may be comparatively abundant, granules are relatively few and azurophilic (red-purple); nucleus can assume most any form (ameboid); primary granules consist of sparsely populated lysosomes; blue staining of cytoplasm is largely due to abundance of rER and polysomes and associated RNA
Lymphocyte	Cell-mediated immune response (T cells); humorally mediated immune response (B cells)	Cytoplasm is least abundant among the leukocytes, especially sparse in small lymphocytes; occasional presence of few small azurophilic granules

ECF-A, Eosinophil chemotactic factor of anaphylaxis; *NCF,* neutrophil chemotactic factor of anaphylaxis; *rER,* rough endoplasmic reticulum; *RNA,* ribonucleic acid.

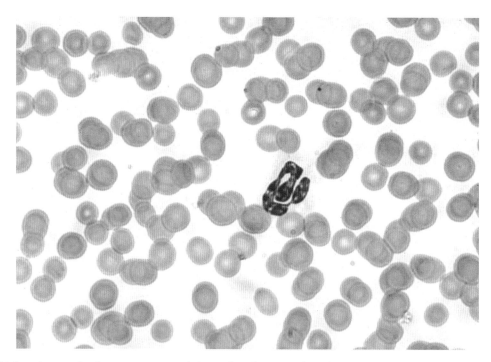

Figure 7-6. Light micrograph of a mature neutrophil in a female cat, with a characteristic narrowing of the nucleus between lobes. (Wright-Giemsa stain; ×1000.)

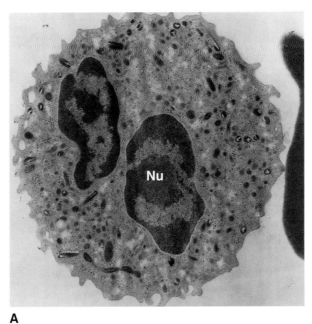

A

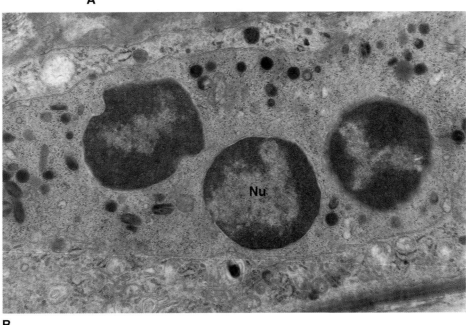

B

Figure 7-7. Transmission electron micrographs of a canine neutrophil. **A,** Taken from a blood sample, this neutrophil is seen with two segments of its nucleus *(Nu)* centrally positioned among the numerous granules, rough endoplasmic reticulum, and other elements of the cytoplasm. **B,** In small vasculature such as capillaries as seen here, the cell with three nuclear segments conforms to the luminal shape.

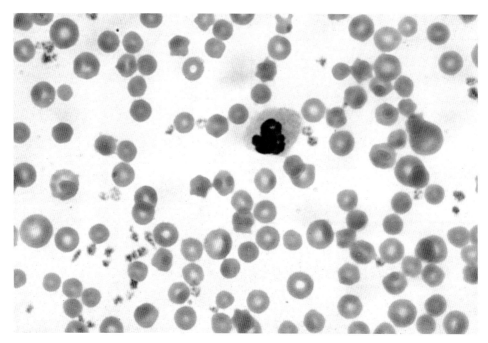

Figure 7-8. Light micrograph of a bovine neutrophil with a pale eosinophilic cytoplasm. (Wright-Giemsa stain; ×1000.)

infection, the neutrophil begins to phagocytize the foreign organisms and concomitantly release hydrolytic enzymes into the extracellular matrix. Engulfed microorganisms become fused with azurophilic granules and subsequently are destroyed. In addition to the lytic enzymes such as lysozyme and acid hydrolases held within the specific and azurophilic granules, other bactericidal substances come into play. For example, reactive oxygen compounds (superoxide, O_2^-; hydrogen peroxide, H_2O_2) are formed and released to the microorganisms as they are held within the secondary lysosomes. The protein **lactoferrin** is also released, which binds and chelates available iron, limiting certain bacteria that require this element for their growth. When a neutrophil has begun the process of engulfing and eradicating the invading microorganisms, it will soon die. The combination of destroyed foreign objects, dead and dying leukocytes, and damaged associated tissues produces **pus.** The combative process of these dying cells does not end with their death, but instead continues through the production and release of leukotrienes at their cell membranes, which in turn signals the call for more leukocytes.

Eosinophil

The **eosinophil** is the second most frequently observed leukocyte circulating in normal peripheral blood (Figures 7-9 and 7-10). This type of granulocyte com-

prises approximately 3% to 9% of the total leukocyte population and is primarily involved in either combating parasite infestation or regulating allergic and/or inflammatory processes (see Tables 7-1, 7-3, and 7-4). It possesses a polymorphous nucleus that is generally less heterochromatic and segmented than that of the neutrophil, being bilobed or to a lesser extent trilobed, but rarely more than that.

The granules in this leukocyte react eosinophilically in primates and many other species, and consequently this feature is used traditionally as the defining morphological characteristic for this cell type. Nevertheless, there is still some variation of staining among species. In ruminants and pigs the granules stain more orange than red. In most instances (the dog is the most notable exception) the granules within each cell are evenly sized and fairly interspersed between polysomes, rER, scattered mitochondria, and dictyosomes of the Golgi apparatus (see Figures 7-5 and 7-10). In canine eosinophils the granules tend to be less packed and more irregular in size and shape than those of other animals (see Figure 7-9). There is considerable variation in the size of the granules across different species (see Table 7-3 and Figures 7-9 and 7-10). As in neutrophils, the granules of eosinophils are lysosomes that consist of two types: specific granules and azurophilic granules. The azurophilic granules are present mostly during the cellular development within the bone marrow, and replaced as the cells mature by the specific granules. The specific granules can be

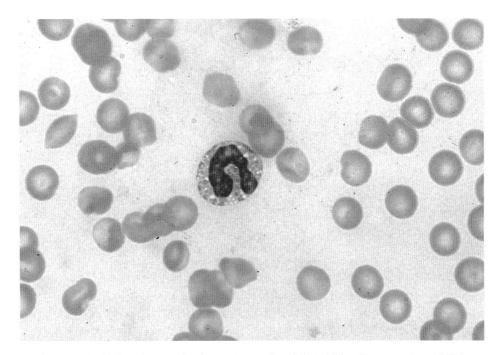

Figure 7-9. Light micrograph of a canine eosinophil. (Wright-Giemsa stain; ×1000.)

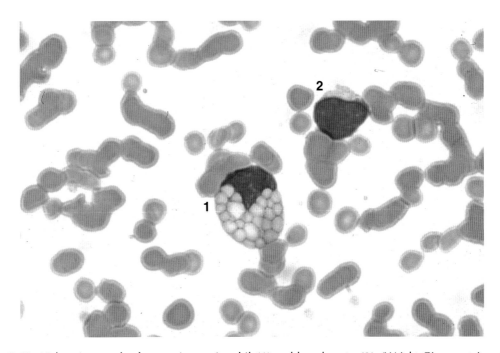

Figure 7-10. Light micrograph of an equine eosinophil *(1)* and lymphocyte *(2)*. (Wright-Giemsa stain; ×1000.)

round or oblong, depending on the species, and contain an electron-dense core when viewed ultrastructurally (see Figure 7-5).

The eosinophil is another phagocytically active cell that, too, depends on anerobic (glycolytic) respiration for its source of energy. Phagocytosis is not as prominent as in the neutrophil and is directed more toward the ingestion of antigen-antibody complexes than toward the ingestion and destruction of microorganisms. Eosinophils are not nearly equipped to deal with an invasion of microorganisms such as bacteria as neutrophils are. The lysosomes lack many of the bactericidal substances found in neutrophil granules. Instead, the granular contents of these cells possess

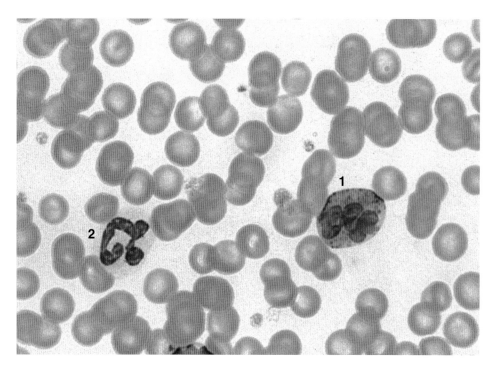

Figure 7-11. Light micrograph of a canine basophil *(1)* and nearby neutrophil *(2)*. (Wright-Giemsa stain; ×1000.)

cationic proteins that enable them to combat parasitic worms (helminths) effectively.

The cell membrane of the eosinophil is able to bind leukotrienes, histamine, and eosinophil chemotactic factor (ECF), which are factors that help guide this type of granulocyte to a specific location of a parasitic invasion, inflammation, or allergic reaction. Once at the location, they can either release cationic proteins, which will subsequently kill the parasitic worms, or ingest antigen-antibody complexes and release substances that will control the inflammatory response.

Basophil

In normal blood, the basophil is the least frequently observed leukocyte, representing 0% to 3% of the total blood cell population in circulation. The granules contained in this cell react positively to Giemsa, staining blue, and, as in neutrophils and eosinophils, consist of two types: **specific granules** and **azurophilic granules.** The specific granules are the predominant type, located throughout the cytoplasm between rER, Golgi apparatus, and mitochondria, and contain many of the substances found in the granules of mast cells, including heparin, histamine, and eosinophilic chemotactic factor (see Table 7-4 and Figure 7-5). The size, shape, number, and content of these gran-

ules vary according to the species. In dogs they are generally fewer in number and larger in size than those in other domestic animals, especially horses and cows (Figures 7-11 and 7-12). In cats, the granules are small and rod shaped and exhibit a lavender reaction when stained with Giemsa or Giemsa-Wright (Figure 7-13), whereas in pigs, the granules can be globose or dumbbell shaped.

The azurophilic granules, as in the other granulocytes, are lysosomes within the cytoplasm that reflect a similar phagocytic capability. Phagocytosis by basophils, however, is very limited. These cells appear primarily to play a role in directing inflammatory activities in a manner that is comparable with that performed by mast cells. Molecules of immunoglobulin E (IgE) derived from plasma cells become attached to the cell membrane of the basophil and form cell-surface Fc receptor sites in an identical fashion that occurs in mast cells. Likewise, the binding of antigens to these molecules results in the release of the granule's contents, which are water soluble and readily degranulate in the ECM, but occurs at a more gradual rate than those of mast cells.

The morphology of the nucleus of the basophil varies considerably, being strongly segmented in some instances and simply bilobed in other instances. In animals, such as the horse, that have darkly stained granules that fill the cytoplasm, the nucleus is often

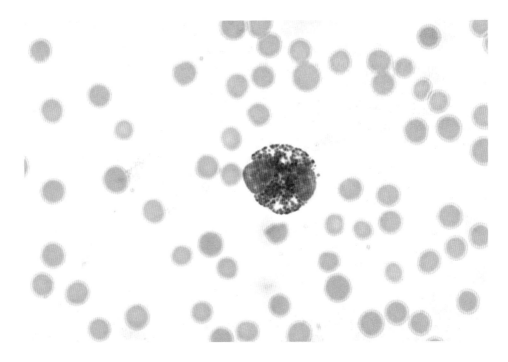

Figure 7-12. Light micrograph of an equine basophil. (Wright-Giemsa stain; ×1000.)

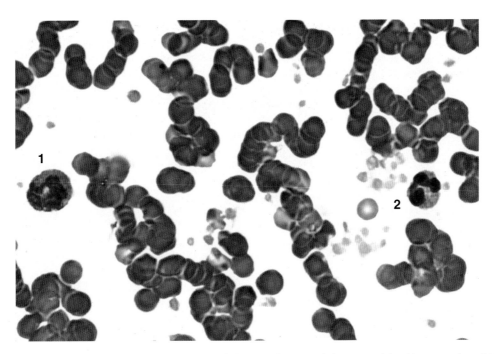

Figure 7-13. Light micrograph of a feline basophil *(1)* and eosinophil *(2)*. (Wright-Giemsa stain; ×1000.)

masked, making it difficult to determine the shape of the nucleus (see Figure 7-12).

Monocyte

The **monocyte,** typically the largest of the blood-borne cells (12-18 μm in diameter), possesses a nucleus that is often eccentrically positioned and variably shaped. When viewed in a smear, the nucleus can be either slightly indented, U shaped, kidney shaped, or trilobed in a cloverleaf manner (Figures 7-14 and 7-15). Although the cytoplasm lacks the distinguishing granules, that is, the specific granules that occur in the previously described white blood cells, it is comparatively large, having a grayish blue cast with azurophilic granules, and in an activated state is often interrupted by vacuole-like bodies that make it appear foamy. Ultrastructurally, the cytoplasm is found to have many lysosomes, often in different stages of activity (i.e., primary and secondary lysosomes), scattered rER, polysomes, mitochondria, and glycogen. At the periphery of the cell, filopodia may be present, particularly in active cells, along with an associated, well-developed outer rim of cytoskeletal elements (ectoplasm), including microtubules and microfilaments (Figure 7-16).

As one of the cells of defense, the monocyte is capable of phagocytic activity and, in fact, provides that capability more than any other function during a pathogenic invasion. The lysosomes (azurophilic granules) vary in size, shape, and number according to the extent of the attack. These cells usually stay in circulation within the bloodstream for only a few days, but when leaving peripheral blood and entering adjacent tissues as macrophages, they can survive for months (see Table 7-3). The blood-borne monocytes and tissue-held macrophages comprise the **mononuclear phagocyte system (MPS).** They function to engulf and break down intra- and extracellular foreign matter including bacteria; fungi; protozoans and viruses; dead, dying, or transformed cells; and cell debris. In addition, the MPS is able to make various cytokines (interleukin-1 and interleukin-3, and tumor necrosis factor) that can initiate the inflammatory response and assist in the proliferation of blood cells, specifically granulocytes and erythrocytes. Selected macrophages called **antigenic presenting cells** have the ability to ingest foreign materials and make them "antigenic." Having surface receptors for all immunoglobulins, the antigens taken in are processed and their most antigenic portions are now presented to lymphocytes (B or T), which in turn combat the impending threat.

Lymphocyte

The **lymphocyte** is the second most common leukocyte in many species and the predominant leukocyte

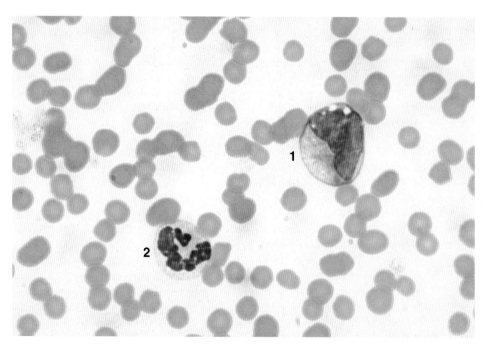

Figure 7-14. Light micrograph of an equine monocyte *(1)* in the presence of a neutrophil *(2)*. (Wright-Giemsa stain; ×1000.)

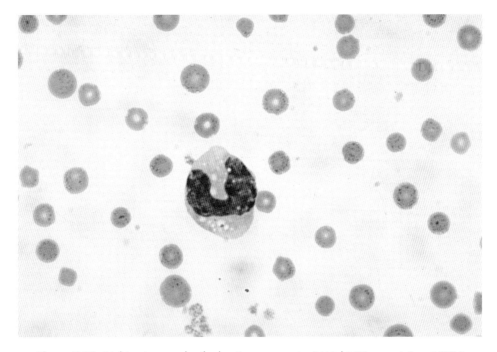

Figure 7-15. Light micrograph of a bovine monocyte. (Wright-Giemsa stain; ×1000.)

Figure 7-16. Transmission electron micrograph (×10,000), of a canine monocyte with its eccentrically placed nucleus *(Nu)* and long pseudopodial processes *(arrows)*.

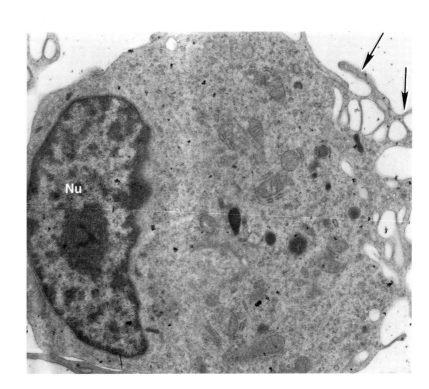

in swine and ruminants (see Table 7-1). Morphologically this cell type is the least pleomorphic of the circulating white blood cells, having a round, sometimes indented nucleus that occupies most of the cell's protoplasm (Figures 7-17 and 7-18). Lymphocytes can vary considerably in size and often are categorized as large (10-15 μm in diameter) and small (6-9 μm in

diameter) or large, medium, and small. When comparing the two size categories on the basis of their histology, the large lymphocyte often has several nucleoli within its nucleus, which may or may not be indented, and the cytoplasm tends to be more abundant and stain more evenly than small lymphocytes. By comparison, the small lymphocyte tends to have little

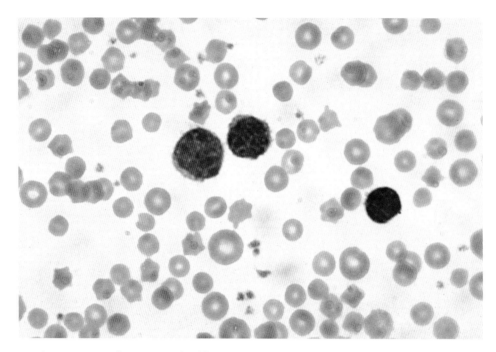

Figure 7-17. Light micrograph of bovine lymphocytes. (Wright-Giemsa stain; ×1000.)

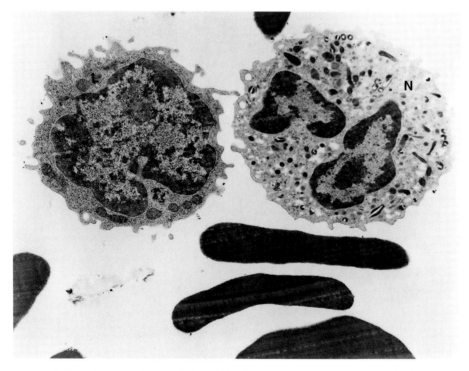

Figure 7-18. Transmission electron micrograph (×5000), of a canine lymphocyte *(L)* and adjacent neutrophil *(N)*.

cytoplasm, which can stain blue, surrounding the often round and quite basophilic nucleus. Small nonspecific, azurophilic granules or lysosomes may be observed. Of the two size groups, small lymphocytes are the most frequently encountered, especially in carnivores. Large lymphocytes are more often observed in ruminants than in carnivores (see Table 7-3).

Functionally the lymphocyte provides immunological defense for the body, as the principal cell type of the immune system. As in the case of the other cells of defense that circulate in the bloodstream, lymphocytes are principally active in the various tissues that they have migrated to after leaving the vasculature. On a functional basis, the lymphocyte can be categorized into three types: **B lymphocytes, T lymphocytes,** and **natural killer (NK) cells.** Histologically these cells are indistinguishable from one another. However, each type can be revealed by immunohistochemical methods that demonstrate differences of their surface receptors. Of the three types, the T lymphocyte is the most common, comprising 80% or so of the total population of lymphocytes circulating in the body. This cell type is involved in cellular or cell-mediated immunity and can become one of several subtypes when exposed to an antigen. B lymphocytes, however, give rise to plasma cells and provide humoral immunity, producing blood-borne antibodies. When antigenically stimulated, both T and B lymphocytes are able to further proliferate and subdivide into **effector** and **memory cells,** the former participating in an immune response and the latter awaiting activity at the next exposure to a specific antigen. In addition to T and B lymphocytes are natural killer cells, which are comparatively few in number and are able to destroy foreign cells directly (without the influence of T or B lymphocytes, lacking T or B cell markers) by cell-mediated cytotoxicity.

PLATELETS

Within the bloodstream, portions of cells or cell fragments that lack nuclei and occur between the erythrocytes and leukocytes and are called **platelets.** When viewing blood smears, platelets can vary in shape and size, being round (spherical), disc-shaped and elliptical and ranging from 1 to 5 μm in width (Figure 7-19). These structures are derived from a giant cell, the **megakaryocyte,** which is housed solely in bone marrow. Newly formed platelets have a fairly short lifespan, lasting less than 2 weeks in peripheral blood. The central area of each platelet, the **granulomere,** reacts positively to the traditionally used stains for blood smears, while the peripheral portion remains clear, the **hyalomere.** The hyalomere contains aggregates of microtubules that run parallel to

each other and the cell membrane (within the ectoplasm) and provide the appropriate infrastructure that is needed to maintain their shape (see Figure 7-19). The granulomere, however, contains scattered mitochondria, peroxisomes, lysosomes, glycogen, and granules of three types: α, δ (electron dense), and λ (lysosomal). The glycocalyx of platelets is well developed, forming an exterior coat that provides strong adhesive capability.

The platelet performs a central role in **hemostasis** and **blood clotting** or coagulation. During episodes when blood vessels are damaged, the pooling of blood outside the vessel is limited in part to the platelets' ability to aggregate and form a blood clot or **primary hemostatic plug.** Upon injury to a blood vessel, platelets contact and adhere to the endothelium and adjacent collagen at the wound site as well as to each other. These well-designed cell fragments, in fact, become activated and release their granules, which further enhances blood clotting, causing a larger clot or **secondary hemostatic plug** to form. Through a combination of plasma factors, platelet adhesion and the secretion of their blood clotting factors via the granules, and factors released by the injured endothelium, a successful clot is formed.

REPTILIAN AND AVIAN BLOOD

In nonmammalian blood a number of histological differences exist when compared with mammalian blood. The differences are, in fact, greatest when comparing erythrocyte morphology. Mature reptilian and avian **erythrocytes** are considerably larger than those in mammals, approximately 12 μm long, generally elliptical (sometimes referred to as **elliptocytes),** and nucleated (Figure 7-20). The nucleus can be equally elliptical or oval to round and heterochromatic. The cytoplasm typically is stained by eosin shades of pink to a pale orange.

The leukocytes of nonmammalian blood vary to some degree when compared with those of mammalian blood, especially with regard to the granulocytes, which tend to be smaller in diameter as a whole in nonmammalian blood. The most common granulocyte in reptilian and avian blood is the **heterophil,** which is the counterpart to the neutrophil in mammalian blood (Figure 7-21). The granules are usually rod shaped and often stain pink, but variably—some are reddish (in birds) and others hardly staining at all or containing darkly stained granules (in reptiles). The nucleus is polymorphous, particularly in birds, which can have as many as five lobes. In reptiles the degree of nuclear segmentation is generally less and often appears unilobular and pale staining.

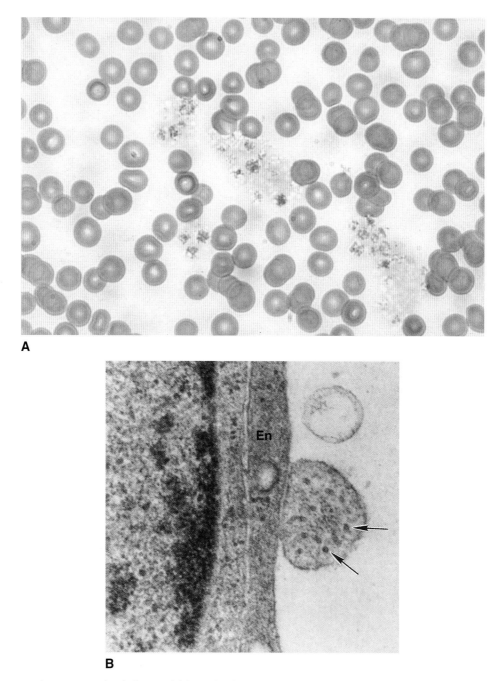

A

B

Figure 7-19. A, Light micrograph of clustered feline platelets. (Wright-Giemsa stain; ×1000.) **B,** Transmission electron micrograph (×50,000), of a canine hyalomere portion of a platelet next to the endothelial *(En)* lining of a blood vessel. Arrows point to microtubules, which provide cytoskeletal support to this structure.

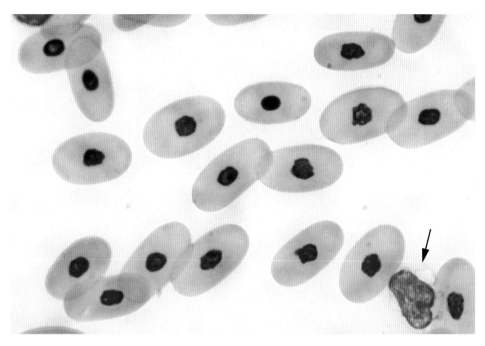

Figure 7-20. Light micrograph of nonmammalian (American alligator) erythrocytes. Arrow points to a thrombocyte. (Wright-Giemsa stain; ×1000.)

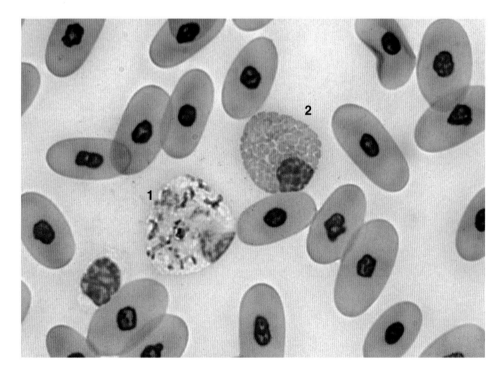

Figure 7-21. Light micrograph of a nonmammalian (American alligator) heterophil *(1)* and eosinophil *(2)*. (Wright-Giemsa stain; ×1000.)

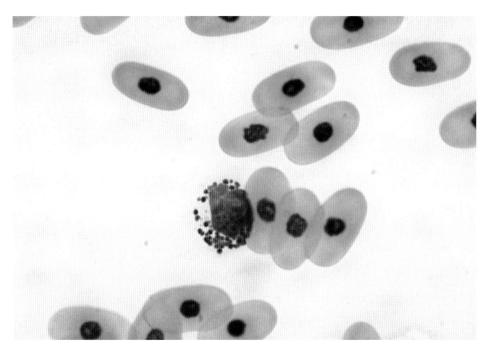

Figure 7-22. Light micrograph of a nonmammalian (American alligator) basophil. (Wright-Giemsa stain; ×1000.)

The **eosinophil** of nonmammalian animals is comparable with the mammalian eosinophil in general appearance and function and can be distinguished from heterophils within the same blood smear on the uniform eosinophilic staining of the granules and their round shape (see Figure 7-21). In birds, the nucleus of the eosinophil is less lobulated than the heterophil.

The nonmammalian **basophil** is also comparable with the mammalian basophil in general appearance and function, having same dark blue staining granules that easily separate these granulocytes from the other two types (Figure 7-22). The nucleus of the basophil, however, is not distinctly segmented or lobulated in avian or reptilian blood.

Lymphocytes of nonmammalian animals are nearly identical to mammalian lymphocytes and can have small and large types with round to slightly indented heterochromatic nuclei and small amounts of cytoplasm (Figures 7-23 and 7-24; see also Figure 7-17). On occasion, lymphocytes can be confused with another leukocyte that circulates within the nonmammalian bloodstream. As in mammals, large lymphocytes can be misconstrued for monocytes and vice versa. The nonmammalian **monocyte** can be the largest of all leukocytes. The nucleus varies to a moderate degree in shape, from round to elongated and sometimes indented, but this pleomorphism isn't nearly as marked as that seen in mammalian monocytes. Thus in those instances in which this cell is relatively inactive, the monocyte may be mistaken for a large lymphocyte. When the cytoplasm is vacuolated and foamy in appearance, the monocyte is more easily distinguished from the large lymphocyte.

The small nonmammalian lymphocyte may be confused with a different cell type within the bloodstream, the **thrombocyte.** The thrombocyte functions in the same capacity as the platelet, but it is a nucleated cell that is smaller in overall size than neighboring erythrocytes (see Figures 7-20, 7-23, and 7-24). The nucleus within each cell is usually round and can be irregular in outline. The cytoplasm often has a clear, foamy appearance or can stain a light blue with few to numerous vacuoles, which to some extent can depend on the degree of activation. In some avian species, such as the rosy flamingo, the thrombocyte can be spindle shaped, allowing one to easily recognize this cell type. Generally, the foamy characteristics of the cytoplasm, the somewhat irregular outline of the nucleus, and the clustering potential of these cells are the clues used for the observer to distinguish them from small lymphocytes.

HEMOPOIESIS AND BONE MARROW

The formation of blood cells before and after birth is called **hemopoiesis (hematopoiesis)** and occurs at different locations prenatally and within the bone marrow in birds and mammals postnatally. During fetal development, blood cells originate from the mes-

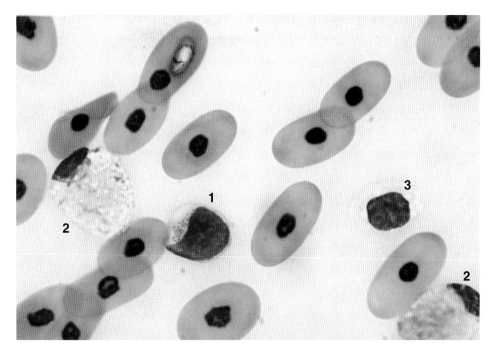

Figure 7-23. Light micrograph of a nonmammalian (American alligator) lymphocyte *(1)*, heterophils *(2)*, and thrombocyte *(3)*. (Wright-Giemsa stain; ×1000.)

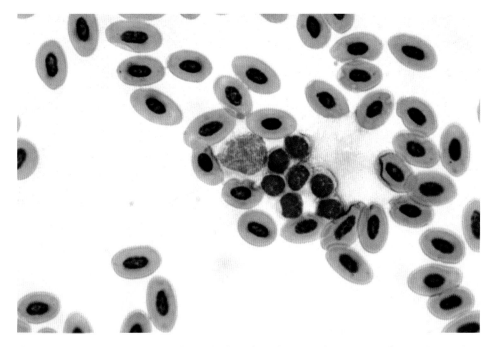

Figure 7-24. Light micrograph of a nonmammalian (chicken) lymphocyte adjacent to a cluster of thrombocytes. (Wright-Giemsa stain; ×1000.)

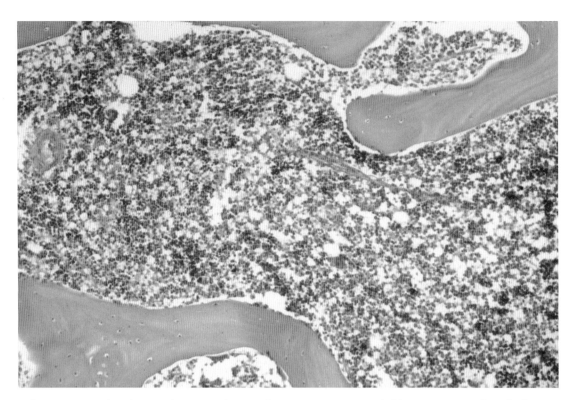

Figure 7-25. Light micrograph (×100) of canine bone marrow surrounded by spongy or trabecular bone.

enchyme of the yolk sac as small islands of erythroblastic cells. Subsequently, stem cells for blood cell formation migrate to the liver and eventually to the spleen, thymus, lymph nodes, and bone marrow. Shortly after birth, hemopoiesis within the liver and spleen is principally replaced by hemopoiesis within the bone marrow, especially regarding erythropoiesis and granulocytopoiesis. Even though the liver and spleen stop hemopoietic activity, they have the capacity to return to that activity if necessary. The marrow of the long bones, ribs, vertebrae, pelvis, skull, and sternum becomes the primary center of blood formation within the young, developing individual. With age, hemopoiesis becomes reduced in activity and the marrow of the bones changes from red **(red marrow)** to yellow **(yellow marrow)** as adipose tissue is added increasingly in these areas, particularly within the diaphyses of long bones.

During growth, **bone marrow** occupies most of the potential space in bones previously mentioned (long bones, ribs, etc.) and is separated from the bony matrices by the endosteum (Figure 7-25). In long bones this space consists primarily of the medullary cavity and the area or interstices between the trabeculae of woven or spongy, including cancellous, bone. These areas are interlaced with thin-walled sinusoids that

originate from branches of nutrient arteries that have entered the diaphysis through nutrient foramina. The sinusoids, in turn, drain into central veins that leave the marrow by the nutrient canal. Cells of hemopoiesis surround the sinusoids, and as new blood cells are generated, they eventually cross the sinusoid wall (consisting of a thin basal lamina and sparse adventitia with or without its own cells; **adventitial reticular cell),** and squeeze between adjacent endothelial cells that line the wall (Figure 7-26).

The bone marrow is then divided into two entities: the **vascular compartment,** which is composed of the arteries, veins, and sinusoids; and the **hemopoietic compartment,** which houses the hemopoietic cells and adventitia. The adventitia's reticular cells and small collagen (reticular) fiber provide the necessary support structure and appropriate environment for effective blood cell formation and development. In older bone marrow the adventitial reticular cells can become adipocytes. This phenomenon, which occurs first within the central portion of the medullary cavity and progresses toward the periphery, is inversely associated with the rate of blood formation and can be considered an aging event. Within the hemopoietic compartment, stem cells and the cells that they give rise to are regionalized to some degree according to

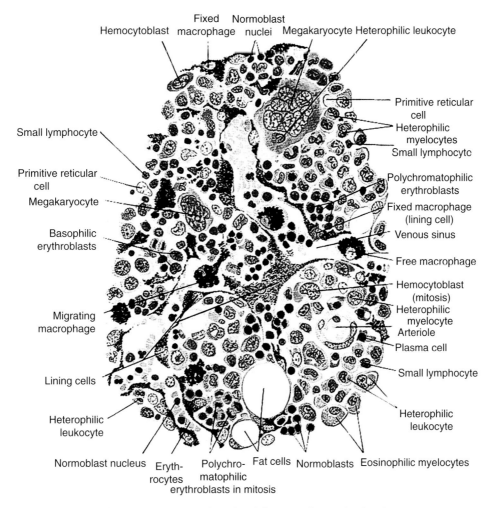

Fixed Normoblast
Hemocytoblast macrophage nuclei Megakaryocyte Heterophilic leukocyte

Small lymphocyte

Primitive reticular cell

Heterophilic myelocytes

Small lymphocyte

Primitive reticular cell

Megakaryocyte

Basophilic erythroblasts

Polychromatophilic erythroblasts

Fixed macrophage (lining cell)

Venous sinus

Free macrophage

Hemocytoblast (mitosis)

Heterophilic myelocyte

Migrating macrophage

Arteriole

Plasma cell

Lining cells

Small lymphocyte

Heterophilic leukocyte

Heterophilic leukocyte

Normoblast nucleus   Eryth-   Polychro-   Fat cells   Normoblasts   Eosinophilic myelocytes
                      rocytes   matophilic
                                    erythroblasts in mitosis

Figure 7-26. Illustration of rabbit bone marrow revealing the different cells involved in hemopoiesis. *(From Fawcett DW: Bloom and Fawcett: a textbook of histology, ed 11, Philadelphia, 1986, Saunders.)*

their proximal location to the sinusoids. The cells that generate new erythrocytes and megakaryocytes are situated next to the walls of the sinusoids, whereas those that produce new granulocytes are located away from the sinusoids. Most of the cells within the hemopoietic compartment are not stem cells and adventitial reticular cells, but rather immature blood cells that are in different stages of development (Figure 7-27). Active macrophages also are involved in the removal and breakdown of nuclei that have been recently extruded from developing red blood cells.

Formation of new blood cells requires multiple cell divisions that originate from individual stem cells. During the process of these cell divisions, progressive changes in cellular differentiation occur. Formation of the mature erythrocyte is referred to as **erythropoiesis.** Formation of granulocytes is called **granulocytopoiesis;** for monocytes the process is called **monocytopoiesis** and so forth. In each instance, the progenitor is the same—the **pluripotent hemopoietic**

stem cell. This stem cell gives rise to a second order of stem cells that, in turn, generate different progenies of cells. This second order of stem cells comprises the **multipotent hemopoietic stem cells** of which there are two types or populations (Figure 7-28). One type forms the progenitors for all lymphocytes and is called the *lymphoid stem cell,* or *colony-forming unit lymphocyte* (CFU-Ly). The other type is called the *myeloid stem cell,* or *colony-forming unit spleen* (CFU-S), and it gives rise to the rest of the blood cells. The cells immediately derived from multipotent hemopoietic stem cells comprise the **unipotent hemopoietic stem cells,** which are progenitor cells that produce only one type of blood cell, such as a B lymphocyte or a basophil. These progenitor cells are basically identical in appearance to one another as well as to the cells that formed them. They have little cytoplasm and what cytoplasm that does exist surrounds a round, fairly euchromatic nucleus. Except for the nuclear staining, hemopoietic stem cells have a lymphoid morphology.

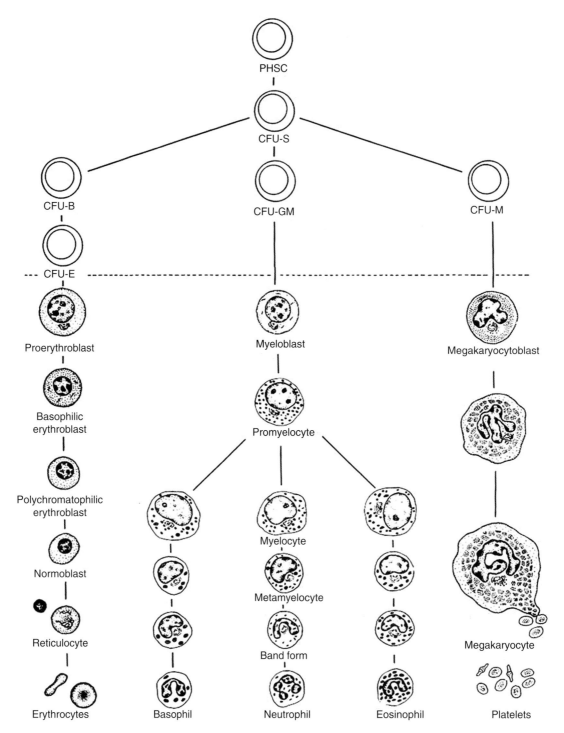

Figure 7-27. Diagram of the process of blood cell development within the bone marrow. (*Modified from Fawcett DW: Bloom and Fawcett: a textbook of histology, ed 11, Philadelphia, 1986, Saunders.*)

Consequently, these undifferentiated cells have high nuclear-to-cytoplasmic ratios (N:C), typical of undifferentiated cells in general.

The unipotent hemopoietic stem cells have specific names according to the cells they give rise to: for example, the progenitors for basophils are colony-forming unit basophil (CFU-B), erythrocyte progenitors are burst-forming unit erythroid (BFU-E), and so on. The proliferation of the different order of stem cells and their ultimate differentiation are guided

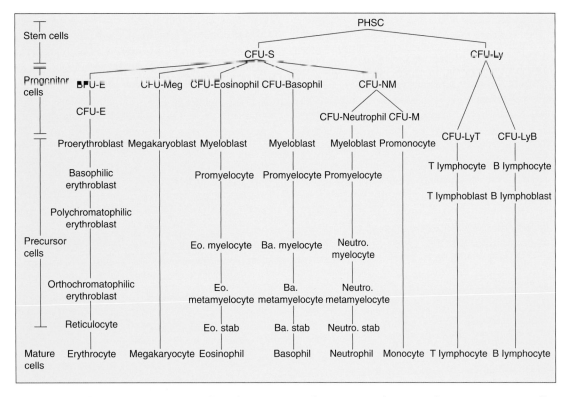

Figure 7-28. Cells of hemopoiesis. *CFU-S,* Colony-forming unit spleen; *PHSC,* pluripotent hemopoietic stem cell; *CFU-Ly,* colony-forming unit lymphocyte; *BFU-E,* burst-forming unit erythroid; *CFU-NM,* colony-forming unit neutrophil and monocyte; *CFU-E,* colony-forming unit erythroblast; *CFU-M,* colony-forming unit monoblast. *(From Gartner LP, Hiatt JL: Color textbook of histology, Philadelphia, 1997, Saunders.)*

largely by specific factors of local and systemic origin. The cytokine growth factors, *interleukin* 1 (IL-1), 3 (IL-3), and 6 (IL-6) together trigger mitotic activity of the pluripotent and multipotent hemopoietic stem cells. Separately, these growth factors can stimulate multipotent and unipotent hemopoietic stem cells or suppress their proliferation as seen in Figure 7-28. In addition, specific **colony-stimulating factors** (CSFs), such as erythropoietin and G-CSF, promote the mitosis and subsequent differentiation of unipotent cells.

With the cessation of mitotic activity by a specific unipotent stem cell, the resultant individual blood cells begin to mature and differentiate. The N:C ratio decreases in these cells as the cytoplasm continues to increase in amount. Eventually, the nucleus becomes heterochromatic and assumes a specific shape that is characteristic for a type of blood cell. The mature blood cell leaves the hemopoietic compartment and enters the vascular compartment by squeezing through small openings in sinusoid walls as mentioned. Undoubtedly, there are factors responsible for the timely release of mature blood cells. These factors have not yet been revealed, and the present understanding of blood cell release remains largely speculative.

ERYTHROPOIESIS

The formation of red blood cells is referred to as **erythropoiesis,** which is by far the most active component of hemopoiesis. Nearly, 1.5 trillion erythrocytes are produced weekly in a medium-sized dog, which is comparable to that made in humans, and this amount may increase substantially (four to eightfold) if situations demand it. Normally the rate of erythrocytes made should equal the rate being removed, but if this dynamic should fall out of balance, such as in anemia, an accelerated production of erythrocytes can be induced.

The first process of erythropoiesis begins with the proliferation and subsequent differentiation of the multipotent myeloid stem cell into **BFU-Es** or **CFU-Bs,** which continue to divide and form **CFU-Es** (see Figure 7-27). These latter cells form **rubriblasts (proerythroblasts)** that can be distinguished morphologically from their progenitors by their size (the largest of the erythrocyte lineage) and having a blue-stained cytoplasm and nucleus with observable nucleoli. As a rubriblast cell loses it nucleoli, it becomes the prorubricyte. Upon its subsequent division, the resultant cells, **basophilic rubricytes (basophilic**

erythroblast), are smaller in size with concomitant smaller nuclei that are more heterochromatic and surrounded by dark blue–stained cytoplasm. These cells further undergo division and become **polychromatic rubricytes (polychromatophilic erythroblasts),** which have very condensed nuclear chromatin that is now surrounded by yellowish orange cytoplasm. Initially, the cytoplasm of these cells has regions that react basophilically because of the presence of concentrations of ribonucleoprotein. As the polychromatic rubricytes further develop, the cytoplasm becomes progressively acidophilic with a concomitant increase in hemoglobin. Cell division ceases after this point. The cells become transformed into *metarubricytes* **(orthochromatophilic erythroblasts or acidophilic orthochromatic erythroblasts),** which have a reddish to pink cytoplasm that can be slightly polychromatic and surrounds a dark, pyknotic nucleus. The nuclei from metarubricytes are extruded, resulting in **reticulocytes** that when treated with a stain such as cresyl blue react diffusely basophilic because of the presence of clusters of ribosomes and mitochondria (see Figure 7-4, *B*). Most of the cytoplasm at this point is filled with hemoglobin. Eventually the remnant organelles disappear and only hemoglobin is contained within the cytoplasm. Differentiation is complete and the cell is now the **erythrocyte.**

In nonmammals, erythropoiesis is similar for most of the stages of development. The principal difference occurs during the development of the metarubricyte or acidophilic orthochromatic erythroblast. Rather than have nuclei that become uniformly basophilic or pyknotic and are eventually extruded, the nuclei of these cells change little, having irregular clumping of the chromatin. The cytoplasm when treated with cresyl blue has numerous granules, especially around the nucleus, that gradually become fewer and more dispersed.

GRANULOCYTOPOIESIS

The formation of white blood cells that form granules (i.e., granulocytes) is referred to as **granulocytopoiesis,** which under normal circumstances is not nearly as active a component of hemopoiesis as erythropoiesis. Granulocytes are derived from the multipotent myeloid stem cell, which gives rise to the unipotent stem cells: the colony-forming unit of eosinophil line of differentiation **(CFU-Eo);** the colony-forming unit of basophil line of differentiation **(CFU-Ba);** and the bipotent stem cells, which give rise to neutrophils and monocytes. The bipotent stem cells specifically form the colony-forming unit of granulocyte and monocyte differentiation **(CFU-GM or -NM),** consisting of their own colony-forming units (i.e., **CFU-G** and **CFU-M),** which create neutrophils and monocytes, respectively (see Figure 7-28). The pattern of proliferation and development within each unipotent stem cell line of the granulocytes is essentially identical. **Myeloblasts** are the first precursor cells formed by the unipotent stem cells and cannot be distinguished from one another (see Figure 7-27). In fact, there is the possibility that the myeloblast may be a multipotent stem cell that has the capacity to give rise to all of the granulocytic cell types. These cells are not too different in appearance from the rubriblast in that much of the protoplasm is occupied by a prominent, round nucleus. The cytoplasm, however, is stained a lighter blue than that of the rubriblast. Myeloblasts replicate and become **promyelocytes,** which have greater amounts of lighter stained cytoplasm than myeloblasts. Promyelocytes also divide and become transformed into myelocytes.

PLATELET FORMATION

Platelet formation begins with the development of the unipotential platelet progenitor, **CFU-M** or **CFU-Meg** (see Figures 7-27 and 7-28). This cell line produces the **megakaryoblast,** which can be large (40 μm in diameter and greater). The megakaryoblast has a lobulated nucleus that continues to increase in size and degree of lobulation through endomitosis (DNA replication without nuclear division), resulting in high ploidy levels of genetic material (up to 64N).

As the megakaryoblast continues to grow, it differentiates into the **megakaryocyte,** the platelet-forming cell that can attain diameters up to 100 μm. The nucleus, which has become highly lobulated, can appear multinucleated in thin sections (Figure 7-29). The cytoplasm of these cells is filled with anastomosing endoplasmic reticulum, primarily rER, a well-developed Golgi apparatus, and many lysosomes and mitochondria.

Positioned adjacent to sinusoids, each megakaryocyte is able to extend cytoplasmic processes into the vascular lumen. These processes become fragmented as the cell membrane forms narrowed invaginations called demarcation channels, causing clusters of **proplatelets** to be released. This activity can occur hundreds, if not several thousands, of times until much of the cytoplasm is exhausted and the lobulated nucleus and the remaining cytoplasm become engulfed and digested by nearby macrophages. The platelets then circulate throughout the vascular system, and are potentially useful for not much more than 1 week.

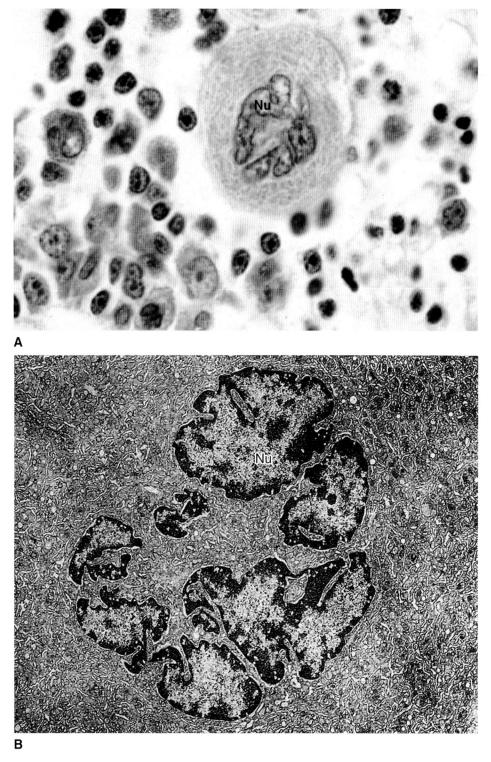

A

B

Figure 7-29. Megakaryocyte. **A,** Light micrograph of a megakaryocyte in the bone marrow of a rat. Its large lobulated single nucleus *(Nu)* and surrounding fragmenting cytoplasm stand out among the rest of the developing blood cells. (Hematoxylin and eosin stain; ×400.) **B,** Transmission electron micrograph reveals the extensive endoplasmic reticulum surrounding the highly lobulated nucleus *(Nu).* *(Modified from Gartner LP, Hiatt JL:* Color textbook of histology, *Philadelphia, 1997, Saunders.)*

SUGGESTED READINGS

Bergman RA, Afifi AK, Heidger PM Jr: *Histology,* Philadelphia, 1996, Saunders.

Cotter SM: *Hematology,* Jackson Hole, Wyo, 2001, Teton NewMedia.

From Cunningham JG: *Textbook of veterinary physiology,* ed 2, Philadelphia, 1997, Saunders.

Fawcett DW: *Bloom and Fawcett: a textbook of histology,* ed 11, Philadelphia, 1986, Saunders.

Gartner LP, Hiatt JL: *Color textbook of histology,* Philadelphia, 1997, Saunders.

Gurr E: *Staining animal tissues,* London, 1962, Leonard Hill.

Harvey JW: *Atlas of veterinary hematology: blood and bone marrow of domestic animals,* Philadelphia, 2001, Saunders.

Hawkey CM, Dennett TB: *A color atlas of comparative veterinary haematology,* London, 1989, Wolfe.

Humason GL: *Animal tissue techniques,* ed 3, San Francisco, 1972, Freeman.

Jain NC: *Essentials of veterinary hematology,* Philadelphia, 1993, Lea & Febiger.

Leeson TS, Leeson CR: *A brief atlas of histology,* Philadelphia, 1979, Saunders.

Williams WJ, Beutler E, Erslev AJ, Lichtman MA: *Hematology,* ed 4, New York, 1990, McGraw-Hill.

Muscle

KEY CHARACTERISTICS

- Highly cellular, vascularized, and innervated
- Cells specialized for contractility
- Subcellularly, highly differentiated with special terms associated for specific structures, including sarcoplasm, sarcolemma, sarcosome, sarcoplasmic reticulum, myofilament, myofibril

Movement in multicellular organs is accomplished by specialized cells called **muscle fibers, or myocytes.** Many cell types have contractile elements that permit the cell to move or change shape, but mostly in an individual and limited manner that is not usually coordinated with other cells. Muscle fibers are cells completely dedicated to the ability to change shape, mostly along their longitudinal axis, in a highly coordinated and rapid way. As a result, muscle tissue is responsible for body movements and is one of the most highly differentiated tissues of the body. Movement occurs by the ability of the muscle fibers to contract. Contraction, in turn, is mediated by the transformation of chemical energy into mechanical energy at the expense of adenosine triphosphate (ATP). Each of the three types of muscles—**smooth, skeletal,** and **cardiac**—can be distinguished from the others based on the shape and size of the muscle fiber, number and location of nuclei within, organization of contractile elements, and type of innervation. These muscles are derived mostly from mesoderm: somatic mesoderm giving rise to skeletal muscle; splanchnopleuric mesoderm giving rise to cardiac muscle; and somatic and splanchnic mesoderm, which give rise to smooth muscle. Exceptions do exist such as the iridal muscles of the eye, which consist of smooth muscle in mammals and skeletal muscle in nonmammals and in both instances are derived from the neuroectoderm.

From the early descriptions of muscle fibers and the cellular components within, a variety of terms have evolved, many of which are still used morphologically. The plasmalemma, or cell membrane, is often referred to as the **sarcolemma,** which can be highly developed in skeletal and cardiac muscle and envelopes the cytoplasm, also known as the **sarcoplasm.** Within each cell's sarcoplasm the principal contractile structures are **myofilaments,** which are organized to the point of forming bands or striations in skeletal and cardiac muscle—**striated muscle.** Myofilaments are closely associated with a well-formed smooth endoplasmic reticulum, which is usually called the **sarcoplasmic reticulum.** Mitochondria, which are essential for the production of ATP needed to drive the contraction, can be quite numerous and are referred to as **sarcosomes.**

SMOOTH MUSCLE

Smooth muscle tissue is the simplest or least differentiated form of muscle, consisting of narrow,

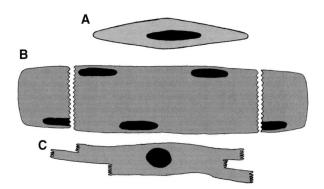

Figure 8-1. Illustration of the three different types of muscle cells or fibers. **A,** Smooth muscle; **B,** skeletal muscle; **C,** cardiac muscle.

spindle-shaped fibers that range from 20 to 200 μm or more in length, but only 5 to 8 μm at their greatest width (Figure 8-1). Histologically, this tissue has a fairly homogeneous appearance, being strongly acidophilic and staining a deep pink when reacted with eosin (Figure 8-2). Within each muscle fiber a single nucleus is positioned centrally, and when viewed in cross section these nuclei are viewed where the cells are at their broadest profiles (Figure 8-3). Because of their shape the fibers are arranged in a staggered manner so that the thickest region of one cell lies adjacent to the tapered ends of neighboring cells. Thus, when seen longitudinally, the nuclei tend to be grouped in stacks (see Figure 8-2). During contraction the elliptically shaped nucleus becomes coiled like a corkscrew (Figure 8-4). Each cell or muscle fiber is enveloped circumferentially by a loosely woven net of reticular fibers. The fibers, in turn, are closely associated with a basal lamina and contribute to the strong intercellular adhesive forces that exist in this tissue during different states of contraction and stretching.

FINE STRUCTURE OF SMOOTH MUSCLE

Cytologically, ribosomes, rough endoplasmic reticulum (rER), Golgi apparatus, mitochondria, and glycogen storage inclusions are concentrated perinuclearly around the poles of the nucleus within the sarcoplasm and immediately adjacent to the cell membrane (Figure 8-5). Smooth endoplasmic reticulum also is found in this region, but much of this organelle is intertwined with the contractile elements of the cell, forming the sarcoplasmic reticulum. The body of the cell is filled with the contractile elements (myofilaments) that consist primarily of actin interspersed by myosin. The myosin filaments are relatively

thick in diameter (15 nm) when compared with that of actin (7 nm) and possess **heavy meromyosin heads** projecting to the numerous actin filaments that envelop the myosin's entire length. As the heavy meromyosin heads function to repeatedly bind with the actin filaments during contraction, their even distribution enhances the potential for actin interaction and potentially results in sustained contractions. During contractions the myosin filaments are believed to slide by the actin at the expense of ATP. The interaction of the actin and myosin may be triggered to occur throughout the entire cell or in only a portion of it. Consequently, contractions may be rapid or gradual, depending on the amount of actin-myosin interaction.

The contractive process is facilitated by other filaments of intermediate size, **desmin,** and **vimentin.** These intermediate filaments provide additional cytoskeletal infrastructure, which is coordinated with actin-myosin interactions in a way that allows the cell to shorten its length (Figure 8-6). Desmin and vimentin occur in vascular smooth muscle, whereas only desmin is found in nonvascular smooth muscle. Both of the intermediate filaments are anchored in an amorphous structure called the **dense body.** Dense bodies consist of α-actinin and can be associated with the sarcolemma as well as located intermittently throughout the body of the myofilaments (see Figures 8-5 and 8-6). In addition to their association with desmin and vimentin, dense bodies provide attachment for actin, being analogous to Z lines in striated muscle and, in fact, contain other Z line–related proteins. Within the cell membrane, numerous vesicles called **caveoli** can be observed throughout the length of the muscle fiber (see Figure 8-6). These structures are believed to be involved largely in calcium sequestration and release.

CONTRACTION AND RELAXATION

Calcium plays an important role in the contraction of smooth muscle fibers. It is believed that when a muscle fiber contracts, calcium is released from the caveolae as ions that bind to the Ca^{2+}-modulating protein **(calmodulin),** which, in turn, activates the enzyme, myosin light-chain kinase. This enzyme slightly alters the composition of myosin by phosphorylating (via adenosine triphosphatase [ATPase]) one of its light chains, which causes a change in the shape of the filament, especially its light meromyosin moiety, and exposes its binding sites for the neighboring actin, resulting in the actin and myosin sliding by each other (i.e., contraction). As the myofilaments slide by each other, they influence directly the network of intermediate filaments and associated dense bodies, causing

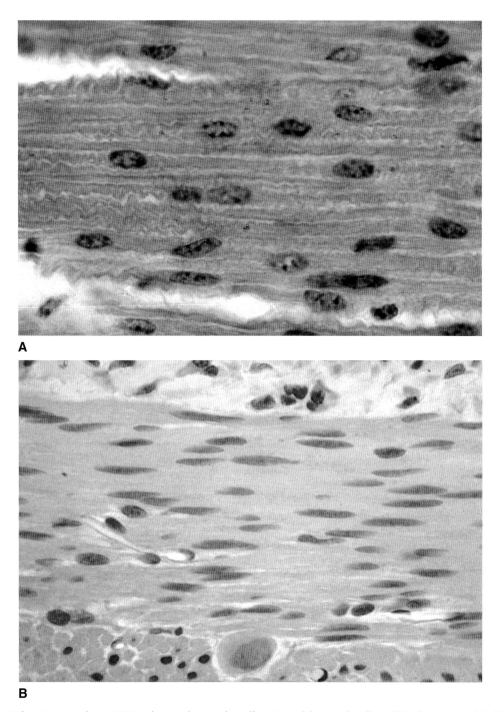

Figure 8-2. Light micrographs (×1000) of smooth muscle cells oriented longitudinally within the urinary bladder of the cow, **A** (paraffin section, H&E stain) and the small intestine of the rat, **B** (plastic section, H&E stain). Note the stacking of the nuclei.

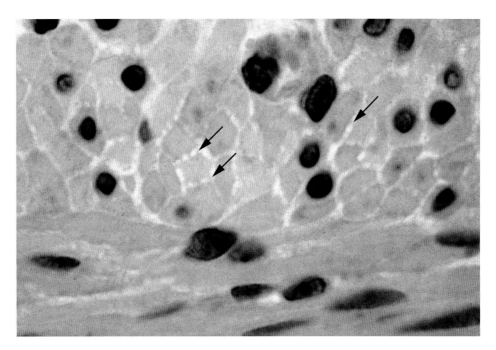

Figure 8-3. Light micrograph of smooth muscle cells oriented cross sectionally (inner layer of muscular tunic of the small intestine). Arrows point to the multiple attachments that link one adjacent cell to another. (Plastic section, hematoxylin and eosin stain; ×1000.)

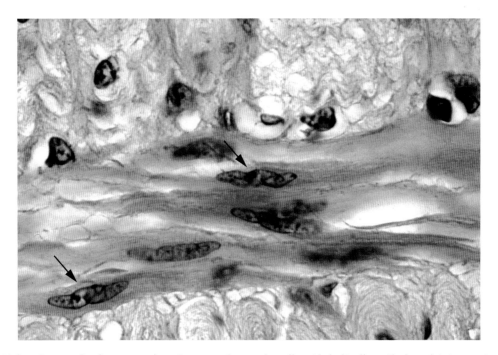

Figure 8-4. Light micrograph of contracted canine smooth muscle cells with helically coiled nuclei *(arrows)*. (Hematoxylin and eosin stain; ×1000.)

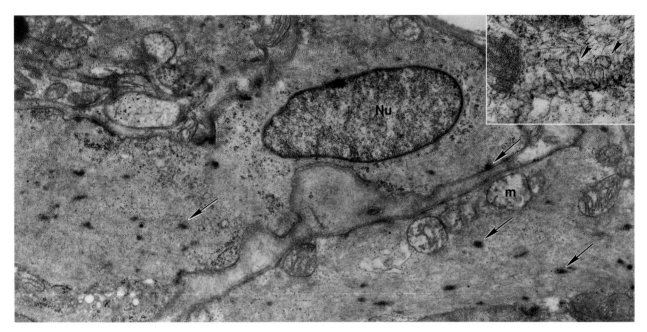

Figure 8-5. Transmission electron micrograph (×15,000) of canine smooth muscle cells. Mitochondria *(m)* and other organelles are located mostly along the perimeter surrounding the myofilaments, which are interspersed with dense bodies *(arrows)*. *Nu,* nucleus. Inset (×40,000) demonstrates presence of numerous caveoli *(arrowheads)* next to the cell membrane of a smooth muscle cell.

A

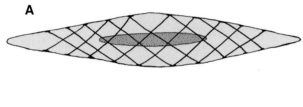

B

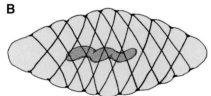

Figure 8-6. Diagram of smooth muscle and the relationship of the intermediate filaments that crisscross throughout the sarcoplasm and dense bodies and the sarcolemma during **(A)**, relaxed and **(B)**, contracted states.

the entire cell to become shorter and wider than when relaxed (see Figure 8-6). Eventually, the Ca^{2+}-calmodulin complexes dissociate or break apart and the light chains of the myosin are dephosphorylated, causing the actin-contact sites to be masked and allowing the actin and myosin filaments to return to a resting or stretched position.

INNERVATION

Adjacent muscle cells can be joined together by nexi or gap junctions and as a result spread excitation for the activation of the contractile mechanism. This arrangement is particularly well developed in muscle fibers that, for the most part, are not directly innervated, as in large sheets of smooth muscle (the walls of hollow viscera, i.e., forming an outer tunic or layer along digestive and reproductive tracts, especially intestines and uterus) and consequently may lead to either tonic or rhythmic contraction. These muscles can be referred to as **visceral smooth muscle** and may be stimulated humorally by agents such as oxytocin. In these instances, the sheets or layer of muscle are usually positioned at a right angle to an adjacent layer of muscle such as found in the small intestine, which has an inner circularly oriented layer surrounded by an outer longitudinally oriented layer (see Figure 8-3). Smooth muscle is **involuntary** in control, innervated by both sympathetic and parasympathetic nerves of the autonomic nervous system. In some instances the innervation is quite prevalent, such as within the vas deferens of the male reproductive tract and the iridal muscles of the eye and can be referred to as the **multi-unit type.** In addition to being found in tubular organs, smooth muscle can be either dispersed in con-

TABLE 8-1	Comparison of the Key Characteristics of the Three Muscle Types		
CHARACTERISTICS	SMOOTH	SKELETAL	CARDIAC
Length	20-200 μm	50 μm to 40 cm (and more)	60-100 μm
Shape	Spindle (fusiform)	Cylindrical	Cylindrical and branched
Nuclei	Single and centrally placed	Multiple (up to thousands) and peripherally placed	One or two and centrally placed
Myofilament organization	Myosin evenly dispersed and surrounded by actin	Myosin and actin interact as discrete bands	Myosin and actin interact as discrete bands
Sarcoplasmic reticulum	Present as typical smooth endoplasmic reticulum, but uninvolved with Ca sequestration	Well developed; prominent terminal cisterns along I-A band interface	Less developed than skeletal; small, scattered terminal cisterns along Z line
Sarcolemma	Associated with dense bodies, intermediate filaments, and myofilament contraction	Invaginates to form T-tubules; associated with sarcoplasmic reticulum as triads	Invaginates to form T-tubules; associated with sarcoplasmic reticulum as dyads
Calcium binding and control	Calmodulin; by caveolae	Troponin C; by calsequestrin in terminal cisterns	Troponin C; by Ca from extracellular sources
Cell attachments	Forms basal lamina and gap junctions (nexi)	Forms basal lamina only	Forms basal lamina and intercalated disk (junctional complex)
Innervation	Autonomic	Somatic motor	Autonomic
Contraction	Involuntary: rhythmic	Voluntary: all (or none)	Involuntary: all (or none) in cell groups
Regeneration	Is able	Is able through satellite cell replication	Not able
Connective tissue associations	Endomysium	Endomysium, perimysia, epimysium	Endomysium

nective tissues of certain organs (prostate) or more often may form small bundles in the dermis.

SKELETAL MUSCLE

Skeletal muscle is composed of long bundles of parallel muscle fibers that individually can be long, up to 40 cm, but relatively narrow, 8 to 100 or more μm in diameter (see Figure 8-1). The skeletal muscle fiber contrasts in many ways when compared with the smooth muscle fiber (Table 8-1). Although the filament-ladened cytoplasm strongly reacts to eosin, longitudinal sections reveal distinct transverse striations throughout the body of each cell. This feature plus the presence of many nuclei within each muscle fiber, which are positioned peripherally next to the sarcolemma, provide excellent histologic characteristics that permit this tissue to be easily recognized

(Figure 8-7). Within each muscle fiber the myofilaments are arranged in cylinders that extend along the cell's entire length. The cylinders each measure between 1 and 2 μm in diameter and are called **myofibrils;** collectively the myofibrils give rise to the transverse striations when viewed longitudinally. The striations are due to the highly coordinated arrangement of actin and myosin myofilaments within the myofibrils, which, in turn, are aligned precisely so that individual striations appear as single entities (see Figure 8-7). Light microscopically, these striations have been designated as bands and a line. The **A band,** or anisotropic band, is characterized by both its staining reaction, being the most intensely stained band, and its birefrigency when viewed with polarized light. Within each A band is a central zone called the **H band,** which is less birefringent and stains lighter than the A band. Between the A bands there is another histologically, lighter region known as the **I**

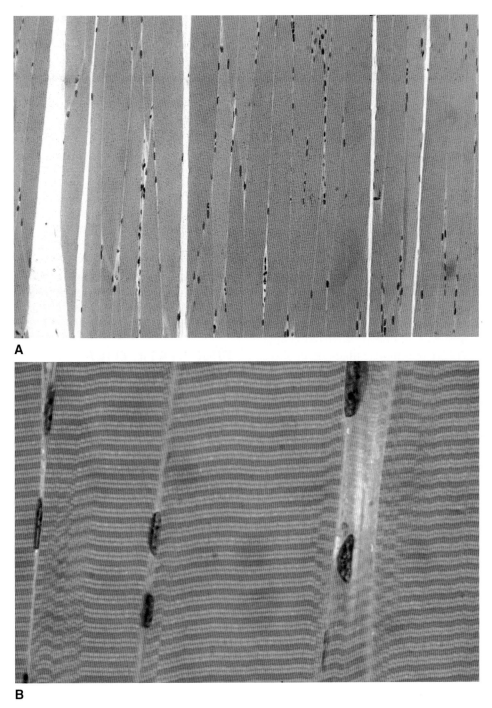

Figure 8-7. Light micrographs of skeletal muscle at **A,** low (×100) and **B,** high (×1000) magnification. The highly organized myofilaments form characteristic bands and lines, which are oriented horizontally in these micrographs, whereas the multiple nuclei are aligned vertically. (Plastic section, hematoxylin and eosin stain.)

TABLE 8-2   Fiber Types of Skeletal Muscle

TYPE	SUCCINIC DEHYDROGENASE LOCALIZATION	MITOCHONDRIA	FUNCTION
Red	Strong reaction	Numerous	Provides slow, enduring contraction; resistant to fatigue
White	Weak reaction	Comparatively few	Provides rapid contraction; easily fatigues
Intermediate	Intermediate reaction	Intermediate in number	Provides more rapid contraction than red and fatigues less easily than white

band, or isotropic band (nonbirefringent), which is bisected by a line, the Z **line,** or disk. The region from one Z line to the next is called the **sarcomere,** the smallest repeating unit within a myofibril.

Each muscle fiber is surrounded by a basal lamina and associated network of **reticular fibers** that collectively comprise the **endomysium.** The endomysium functions to hold adjacent muscle fibers together and is really the only component in skeletal muscle that is able to do this because there are no cell junctions between adjacent cells. It also provides an environment for capillaries and small fibrocyte-like cells (**satellite cells** [pericytes]) to reside. The satellite cell can be found occasionally within the skeletal cell's basal lamina. This cell is uninucleated and functions as a stem cell for new skeletal muscle fibers, especially in response to injury. Fully differentiated skeletal muscle fibers are incapable of further self-division, but can continue to increase substantially in their girth by adding new myofibrils peripherally. A group of parallel muscle fibers make up a single fascicle, and groups of fascicles, in turn, comprise individual muscles.

When observing individual muscles in cross section, individual skeletal muscle cells can differ markedly in diameter and color (histochemically) (Table 8-2). Based on cell width size and histochemical reaction to mitochondrial oxidative enzyme activity of **succinic dehydrogenase** reaction, muscle fibers can be divided into three categories: red, white, and intermediate fibers. **Red fibers** (type I) are the smallest in diameter and richest in oxidative enzyme activity, whereas **white fibers** (type II) are the largest in diameter and have fewer mitochondria and less oxidative enzyme activity. The red fibers are metabolically aerobic and referred to as slow-twitch (slow contracting) motor units, having a greater resistance to fatigue than white fibers. The white fibers, on the other hand, rely more on anaerobic respiration (glycolysis) and are called fast-twitch (fast contracting) motor units,

which generate greater muscle tension than red fibers, but fatigue more readily. **Intermediate fibers** do not easily fall into the red and white fiber categories, sharing instead characteristics of both.

FINE STRUCTURE

When viewed by electron microscopy, each sarcomere is composed of a highly organized arrangement of myofilaments in which the strands of actin are intercalated between the thicker myosin filaments (A bands) (Figure 8-8). In the region forming the H band, only myosin is found. The M line occurs within the center of this band, where adjacent myosin filaments are linked to one another by M-line filaments. The I bands are composed of actin filaments. As skeletal muscle contracts, the actin and myosin filaments slide over each other. As a result, the H band within the A band and the I bands on both sides of the A band become narrow (Figure 8-9). The Z line is actually the region where actin filaments of adjacent sarcomeres are interconnected. Beyond the resolution of the light microscope the myofilaments are held in position by assistance of three proteins: **α-actinin, titin,** and **nebulin.** The thin (actin) filaments are kept in place at the level of the Z line by the α-actinin. The Z line, which consists primarily of α-actinin, is then a proteinaceous sheet that transects the myofibril and allows the thin actin filaments to extend toward the centers of two adjacent sarcomeres. Each actin filament is further anchored by two long chains of nebulin that also wrap around the entire length of each thin filament and may be involved in their assembly and precise positioning. Titin, also anchored to the Z line, aids in the positioning of the myosin filaments and consists of a large, linear elastic protein that has a springlike base. Each myofibril is, in turn, held in register with adjacent myofibrils by the intermediate filaments, desmin and vimentin, that

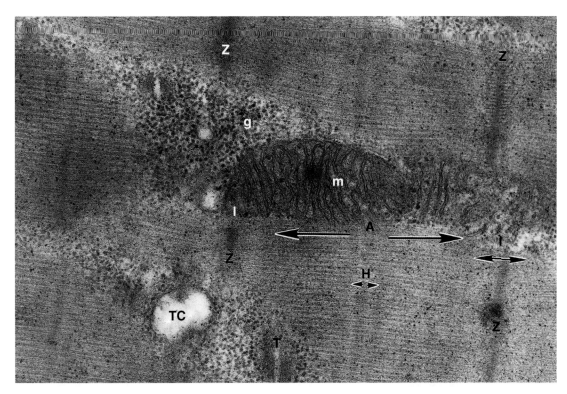

Figure 8-8. Transmission electron micrograph (×15,000) of canine skeletal muscle in longitudinal profile. The myofilaments, which are aggregated into myofibrils, are organized into A bands *(A with arrows)* and I bands *(I with arrows)*, with an additional H band *(H with arrows)* within the A band and a Z line within the I band. Each myofibril is separated from the other by mitochondria *(m)* and glycogen *(g)*. In addition, terminal cisternae *(TC)* of the sarcoplasmic reticulum and portions of a T-tubule *(T)* are evident.

interconnect neighboring myofibrils at the periphery of the Z lines.

MYOFILAMENT COMPOSITION AND MECHANISM OF CONTRACTION

As the thin actin filaments interact with the thick myosin filaments, they move or slide by each other, with the actin moving past the myosin toward the center of the sarcomere. This action results in the contracted state as shown in Figure 8-9. On a more molecular level, each actin filament consists of three components: **F-actin, troponin,** and **tropomyosin.** The F-actin provides the backbone of each thin filament with one end (plus end) attached to α-actinin of the Z line, and the other end projects to the middle of the sarcomere. The actin filament possesses two strands of F-actin that are helically coiled about one another (Figure 8-10). Each strand is composed of **G-actin** monomers, which are globular units that individually possess an active site for the binding of

myosin. These units are polymerized in a way that allows each molecule to have the same spatial orientation along the length of the strand, giving the actin filament many binding sites. The unidirectional assembly of G-actin units or molecules also gives the F-actin chains polarity with the plus end of each filament being attached to the Z line (by α-actinin). The active site of the G-actin unit will bind specifically to the head portion of myosin. The positioning of the active sites is instrumental for the myofilaments to slide by each other during contraction. During periods of resting and stretching, the sites are shifted out of alignment from the myosin head region. The tropomyosin component of the actin filament consists of thin molecules that form a narrow intertwining chain of comparatively short length within the grooves of the F-actin chains (Figure 8-11; see also Figure 8-10). This component and the thin filament's third component, troponin, play critical roles in the appropriate positioning of the G-actin active site. Troponin consists of a three-globular-polypeptide molecule that is attached to each tropomyosin polymer chain, the F-actin, and has a binding site for calcium as well.

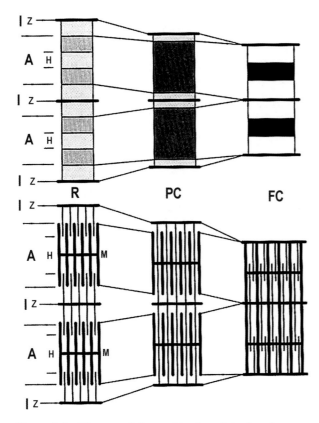

Figure 8-9. Diagram of the positioning of the bands during states of contraction and relaxation (R). *FC,* Full contraction; *PC,* partial contraction. *(Modified from Bergman RA, Afifi AK, Heidger PM Jr:* Histology, *Philadelphia, 1996, Saunders.)*

The thick myofilament consists of several hundred molecules of myosin, each being constructed of two heavy chains that wrap helically around one another and end in globular pieces that resemble golf clubs and are associated with two pairs of light chains (see Figure 8-11). The globular pieces are composed of **heavy meromyosin,** forming cross-bridges with the actin in the presence of calcium and ATP. The rest of the chain is made up of **light meromyosin.** The myosin molecules are arranged in a staggered manner as they form the thick filament, with the globular pieces protruding outwardly all along the filament's perimeter except in the center of the thick filament—the region of the H band—which lacks the globular pieces.

With the release of calcium into the myofibrils, calcium binds to that portion of troponin that has a strong affinity for calcium and, in effect, changes the conformation of the entire troponin molecule, which, in turn, results in the repositioning of tropomyosin and simultaneously reveals the myosin-binding sites along the actin filament (see Figure 8-11). By having the binding sites available, the myosin heads each with an ATP molecule now contact the actin. Through the hydrolysis of the ATP, the heads bend and bind temporarily and the actin causes the thin filament to move approximately 10 nm. By a number of repetitive interactions between the actin and myosin, the actin filaments are pulled toward the center of the sarcomere, which shortens considerably. At the end of contraction, the calcium is actively removed from the myofibrils, and the troponin and tropomyosin components of the actin filament become repositioned to form a complex that prevents the myosin cross-bridge from linking with the actin monomers.

In conjunction with the extensive amount of myofilaments within each fiber is an elaborate system of membranes called the **sarcoplasmic reticulum** (SR). The SR is essentially a smooth endoplasmic reticulum that extends throughout the sarcoplasm in an orderly fashion, closely associated with the myofilaments as it forms a canalicular network around each myofibril (Figure 8-12). The SR, in fact, contributes to the separation of the myofibrils within the skeletal muscle fiber, which can be visualized histologically when examining this tissue in cross section (Figure 8-13). This network has terminal cisternae at or near the end of each sarcomere (see Figure 8-12). As apposing cisternae of adjacent sarcomeres come into contact with each other, a tubular invagination of the cell membrane (sarcolemma) also comes into contact with the cisternae. This invagination is usually referred to as the **T-tubule** (transverse tubule). The two terminal cisternae of the SR and the T-tubule collectively form a **triad.** In mammals, triad complexes are typically positioned between the I and A bands. As a result, each sarcomere is in contact with two sets of triads. By comparison, in amphibia they are shared between adjacent sarcomeres as they occur along the Z lines.

The sarcolemma T-tubular system markedly increases the cell surface and its exposure to the extracellular environment. The presence of this finger-like network of tubules, which branch as necessary, permits a uniform contraction of the many sarcomeres within a single myofibril. In large muscle fibers the T-tubules have to extend at least the length of the radius of each cell. Contraction depends directly on the availability of intracellular calcium ions, which is regulated by the SR. By depolarizing the SR, the calcium ions, which are concentrated within the SR cisternae, are released into the myofilaments, causing a bridging action and subsequent sliding action to occur between actin and myosin at the expense of ATP. Depolarization of the SR is mediated through the surface-initiated depolarization of the sarcolemma. This latter depolarization

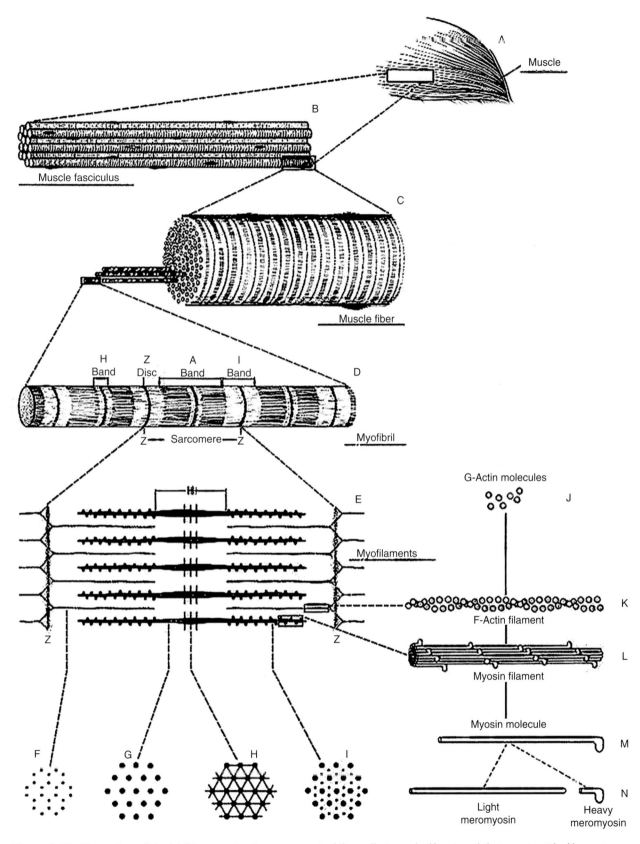

Figure 8-10. Illustration of the highly organized arrangement of the cells (muscle fibers) and their contractile filaments (actin and myosin) that is associated with skeletal muscle. *(From Fawcett DW: Bloom and Fawcett: a textbook of histology, ed 11, Philadelphia, 1986, Saunders.)*

Myofilaments

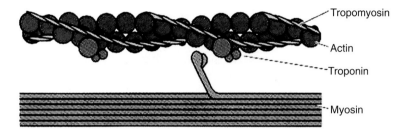

Tropomyosin

Actin

Troponin

Myosin

Figure 8-11. Illustration of the arrangement and interaction of actin and myosin. *(From Gartner LP, Hiatt JL:* Color textbook of histology, *Philadelphia, 1997, Saunders.)*

Myosin molecule

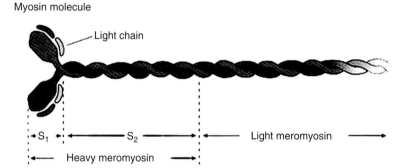

Light chain

S_1

S_2

Light meromyosin

Heavy meromyosin

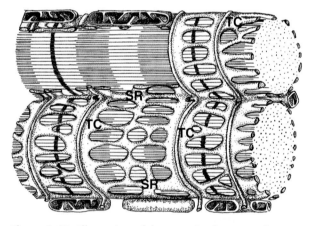

Figure 8-12. Illustration of the organized system of sarcoplasmic reticulum *(SR)* and adjacent mitochondria that envelops each myofibril within mammalian skeletal muscle. The terminal cisternae *(TC)* of the SR and transverse tubular invaginations (T-tubules) of the sarcolemma form two sets of triads along each sarcomere at the junctions where the A and I bands interact.

is triggered by the release of a neurotransmitter, **acetylcholine,** which is held within the **motor endplate** of myelinated motor nerve. Unlike smooth muscle, contraction of skeletal muscle (and striated in general for that matter) is uniform, rapid, and of comparatively short duration. Immediately after each

passage of depolarization, calcium is resequestered by the SR with further expenditure of ATP.

The source of ATP for both calcium sequestration and myofilamentous contraction originates from oxidative phosphorylation within the mitochondrion. As one might expect, the skeletal muscle fiber possesses many mitochondria, especially red muscle fibers. The mitochondria are housed along each myofibril next to the SR (see Figure 8-12). During episodes of extensive contractive activity, adenosine diphosphate (ADP) can be rephosphorylated by the glycolytic pathway, which concomitantly results in lactic acid accumulation, and by phosphocreatine kinase activity, which is able to transfer high-energy phosphate from creatine phosphate to ADP.

INNERVATION

Initiation of muscle fiber contraction comes from the activity of motor neurons that when excited release the acetylcholine that is stored within the numerous synaptic end bulbs at the terminations of their axons (see Chapter 9 for further description). These synaptic end bulbs comprise the motor endplates that contact the myocytes. Each physical contact made between the muscle fiber and the axonal ending is a **myoneural junction** (Figure 8-14). At the site of a myoneural junction, the synaptic end bulb lies

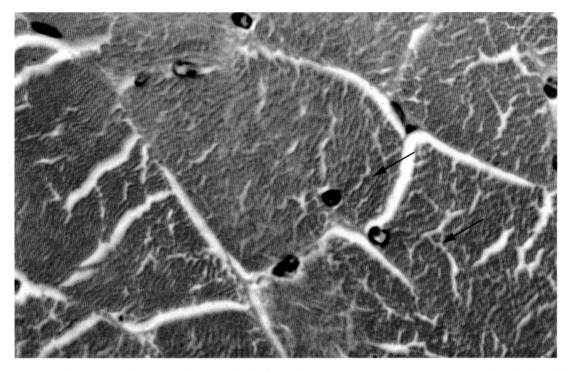

Figure 8-13. Light micrograph (×600) of bovine skeletal muscle in cross section. Arrows point to individual myofibrils.

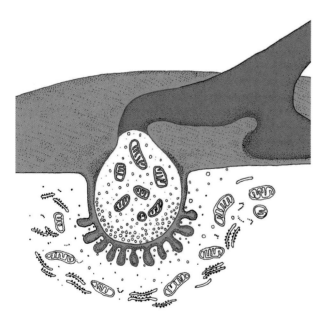

Figure 8-14. Illustration of the myoneural junction involved in the voluntary innervation of skeletal muscle.

within a depression called the **primary synaptic cleft,** and is bordered by junctional folds or infoldings of that portion of the muscle fiber. The infoldings as well as the primary synaptic cleft are lined by the **external lamina,** which appears to be an extension of the muscle cell's basal lamina. When the neurotransmitter is forcefully released from the axon at the primary synaptic cleft, it quickly diffuses across the synaptic gap and binds to receptors in the sarcolemma **(postsynaptic acetylcholine receptors).** The receptors, in fact, consist of ligand-gated channels that open when bound to an appropriate substance, such as acetylcholine. With the opening of the channels (i.e., ion influx), the sarcolemma becomes depolarized and an action potential or impulse is formed. The impulse moves rapidly throughout the cell by way of the T-tubular system. The presence of the enzyme, acetylcholinesterase, which is attached to the external lamina, breaks down acetylcholine into choline and acetate and prevents the released neurotransmitter from initiating further impulses.

CONNECTIVE TISSUE INVESTMENTS

Skeletal muscle is ensheathed by a layer of dense connective tissue known as the **epimysium** (Figure 8-15). From the epimysium thin septae of connective tissue penetrate inwardly, surrounding individual fascicles. These septae are called **perimysia** and are connected to a thin, delicate layer of connective tissue, the **endomysium,** which lines each muscle fiber and is similar to the basal lamina in epithelia.

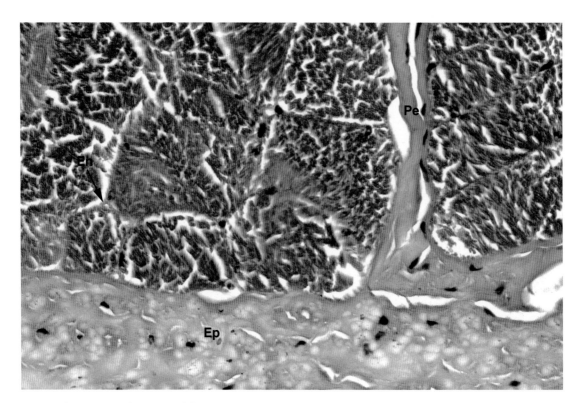

Figure 8-15. Light micrograph (×200) of the connective tissue components associated with bovine skeletal muscle consisting of the endomysium *(En)*, perimysia *(Pe)*, and epimysium *(Ep)*.

CARDIAC MUSCLE

Cardiac muscle resembles skeletal muscle in several ways. Both have multinucleated muscle that possess organized myofibrils, giving the tissue histologically a striated appearance. Both also have a well-developed SR and complementary T-tubule system. Nevertheless, cardiac muscle has sufficiently distinct morphologic characteristics that help distinguish the two tissues (see Table 8-1).

Individual cardiac muscle fibers have only a few nuclei, usually one or two centrally placed within the sarcoplasm (Figure 8-16). The muscle fibers are also shorter and frequently branched, binding to fibers in adjacent chains. The lengths of cardiac muscle fibers are mostly between 80 and 90 μm. They are essentially tubular in shape, having an averaged diameter of 15 μm. The most distinguishing characteristic is the presence of darkly stained transverse lines that intermittently cross chains of cells. These lines are **intercalated disks** and represent specialized cell-to-cell attachments or junctional complexes (see Figure 8-16).

INTERCALATED DISK

The intercalated disk is essentially a junctional complex that involves the entire face of the transverse cell surface in a highly undulated region consisting of only I band (actin myofilaments) material (Figure 8-17). The opacity of the disk is largely due to the presence of a specific junction that is similar to the macula adherens where I band actin filaments insert into dense material along the sarcolemma. Due to their similarity with desmosomes, but much more extensive, this cell junction is called the **fascia adherens** (see Figure 8-17). Also, scattered between these junctions are nexi or gap junctions that provide ionic channels between cells, and maculae adherentes (desmosomes) that further bind the cells together.

MYOFILAMENT ORGANIZATION AND OTHER ORGANELLES

Subcellularly, cardiac muscle cells can be distinguished from skeletal muscle cells by the presence of

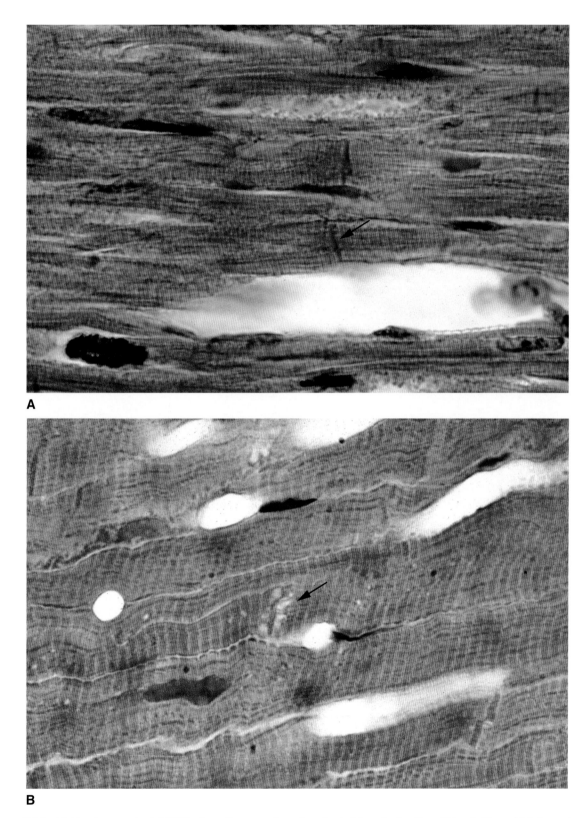

A

B

Figure 8-16. Light micrographs (×1000) of cardiac muscle cells oriented longitudinally within. **A,** The rabbit (hematoxylin and eosin stain) and **B,** the dog (plastic section, hematoxylin and eosin stain). Arrows point to intercalated disks.

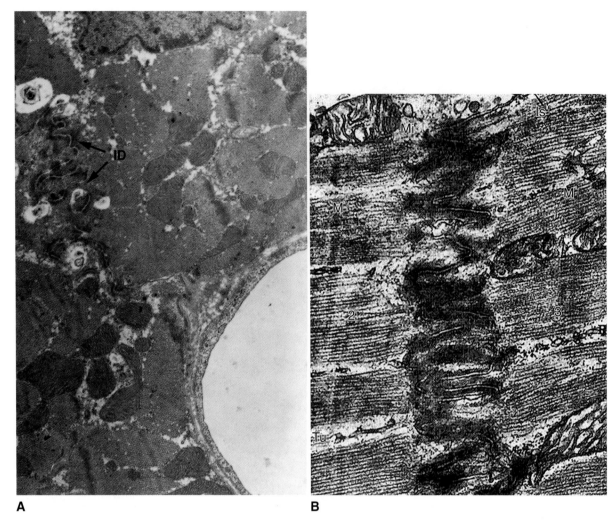

A   **B**

Figure 8-17. **A,** Transmission electron micrograph (×8000) of canine cardiac muscle with an intercalated disk *(ID)* linking adjacent cells. **B,** Close-up of an intercalated disk with fascia adherens. *2* and *3* denote adjacent cells; *Is,* intercellular space; *M,* M-line within the H band; *Mi,* mitochondrion; *Tu,* sarcoplasmic reticulum. *(From Gartner LP, Hiatt JL: Color textbook of histology, Philadelphia, 1997, Saunders.)*

numerous mitochondria that are packed in longitudinal rows (Figure 8-18). Nearly one third of the cytoplasmic volume is filled by this organelle (Figure 8-19). It is not unusual to find glycogen in these cells because it is used as a form of energy supply, along with triglycerides. The contractile apparatus is the same as that in skeletal muscle except that discrete myofibrillar units are not formed in cardiac tissue. Myofilaments are arranged discretely into A and I bands that form sarcomeres identical to those in skeletal muscle. Although sarcoplasmic reticulum is elaborate, the terminal cisternae, which are prominent in skeletal muscle fibers, consist of small dilatations that contact the T-tubules less frequently in cardiac muscle fibers. When the terminations of the SR occur along the T-tubule they are referred to as **diads,** or couplings (see Figure 8-18). Transverse tubules and associated

couplings are found to be aligned with the Z lines (reminiscent of the T-tubule system in amphibian skeletal muscle). The tubules are more than twice the diameter of that seen in skeletal muscle of the same animal and possess an **external lamina.** These differences may reflect a slower contraction rate seen in cardiac muscle when compared with skeletal muscle and the need to have calcium ions actively pumped into cardiac muscle fibers from the external environment.

Cardiac myocytes vary to some extent in size according to location within the heart. Cells within the atrium are generally slightly smaller than those that comprise the ventricles. The atrial muscle cells also form small membrane-bound granules that hold **atrial natriuretic peptides,** which can lower blood pressure by lowering water retention and relaxing vascular smooth muscle.

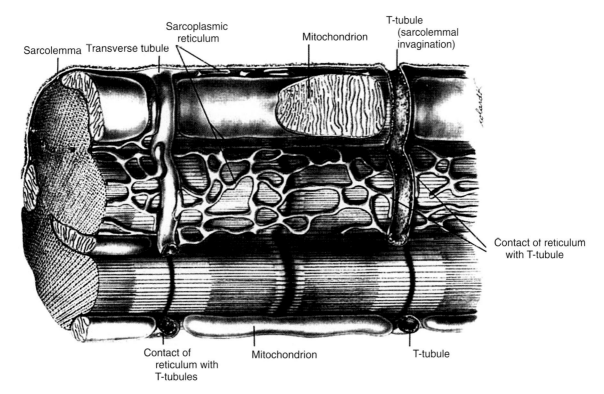

Sarcolemma   Transverse tubule   Sarcoplasmic reticulum   Mitochondrion   T-tubule (sarcolemmal invagination)

Contact of reticulum with T-tubule

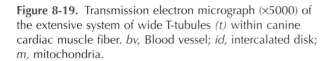

Contact of reticulum with T-tubules   Mitochondrion   T-tubule

Figure 8-18. Illustration of the lines of mitochondria (sarcosomes) lying next to the sarcoplasmic reticulum and intersected regularly by T-tubules. *(From Fawcett DW:* Bloom and Fawcett: a textbook of histology, *ed 11, Philadelphia, 1986, Saunders.)*

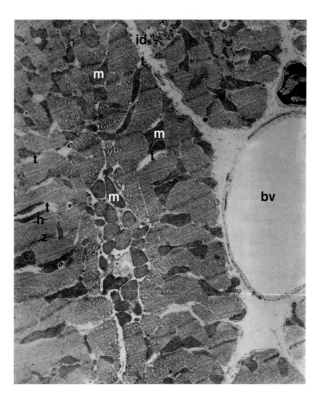

Figure 8-19. Transmission electron micrograph (×5000) of the extensive system of wide T-tubules *(t)* within canine cardiac muscle fiber. *bv,* Blood vessel; *id,* intercalated disk; *m,* mitochondria.

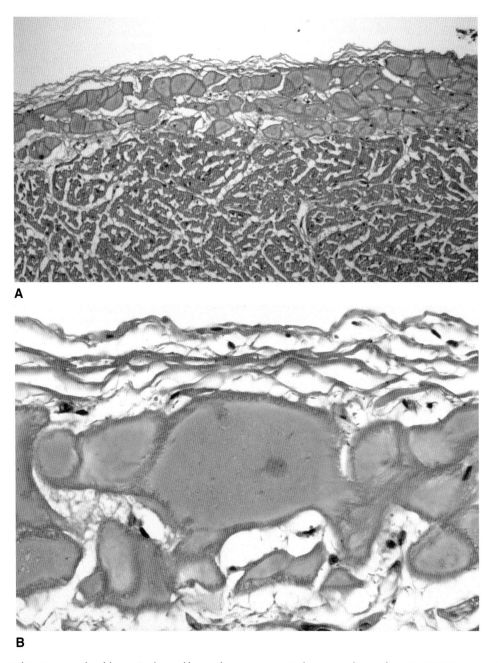

Figure 8-20. Light micrograph of large Purkinje fibers of a manatee. (**A,** hematoxylin and eosin [H&E] stain; ×200; **B,** H&E stain; ×1000.)

Also, within cardiac muscle lie enlarged cells, **Purkinje fibers** or **impulse conduction fibers,** which form the atrioventricular (AV) bundle that transmits impulses from the AV node to the ventricle of the heart (Figure 8-20). These cells are specialized muscle fibers modified for impulse conduction. Each cell contains few myofibrils and one or two central nuclei surrounded by large quantities of glycogen and are recognizable by the lightly stained cytoplasm and large size (Figure 8-21, A).

As in skeletal muscle, cardiac muscle fibers are externally lined by an endomysium. However, in this tissue a rich capillary network lines the cells. The capillary bed is responsible for providing the appropriate aerobic environment essential to maintain the high level of metabolic activity in this tissue (Figure 8-21, B).

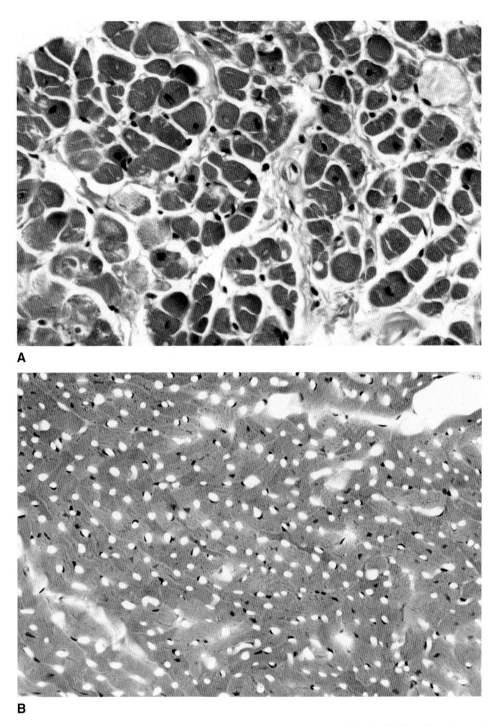

A

B

Figure 8-21. Light micrographs (×200) of cardiac muscle in cross section reveal the highly developed vascular bed associated with the cardiac muscle cells. (**A,** Rabbit, hematoxylin and eosin [H&E] stain; **B,** dog, perfused heart, plastic section, H&E stain.)

SUGGESTED READINGS

Andrews FM, Spurgeon TL: Histochemical staining characteristics of normal horse skeletal muscle, *Am J Vet Res* 47:1843, 1986.

Bergman RA, Afifi AK, Heidger PM Jr: *Histology,* Philadelphia, 1996, Saunders.

Burkholder TJ, Lieber RL: Sarcomere length operating range of vertebrate muscles during movement, *J Exp Biol* 204:1529, 2001.

Chadwick DJ, Goode JA editors: *Role of the sarcoplasmic reticulum in smooth muscle,* New York, 2002, Wiley.

Chen JC, Goldhammer DJ: Skeletal stem cells, *Reprod Biol Endocrinol* 13:101, 2003.

Dickinson PJ, LeCouteur RA: Muscle and nerve biopsy, *Vet Clin North Am Small Anim Pract* 32:63, 2002.

Fawcett DW: *Bloom and Fawcett: a textbook of histology,* ed 11, Philadelphia, 1986, Saunders.

Gartner LP, Hiatt JL: *Color textbook of histology,* Philadelphia, 1997, Saunders.

Gropp KE: *Morphology, morphometry, and development of skeletal muscle in muscle-type phosphofructokinase-deficient dogs,* PhD thesis, University of Florida, Gainesville, 1991.

Michael J, Xiang Z, Davenport G, et al: Isolation and characterization of canine satellite cells, *In Vitro Cell Dev Biol Anim* 38:467, 2002.

Severs NJ: Cardiac muscle cell interaction: from microanatomy to molecular make-up of the gap junction, *Histol Histopathol* 10:481, 1995.

Stolzenburg JU, Schwalenberg T, Dorschner W, Salomon FV, Jurina K, Neuhaus J: Is the male dog comparable to human? A histological study of the muscle systems of the lower urinary tract, *Anat Histol Embryol* 31:198, 2002.

Whitmore I, Notman JA: A quantitative investigation into some ultrastructural characteristics of guinea-pig oesophageal striated muscle, *J Anat* 153:233, 1987.

Nervous Tissue

KEY CHARACTERISTICS

- Highly cellular and vascularized
- Primary cell, neuron, is specialized for generation and transmission of electrical signal
- Subcellularly, highly differentiated with special terms associated for specific structures including neurolemma, neurotubule, neurofilament, axon, axon hillock, dendrite, Nissl body, perikaryon
- Separate population of support cells:
    Central nervous system glia: fibrous and protoplasmic astrocytes, oligodendrocytes, microglia, ependyma
        Peripheral nervous system glia: Schwann cell, amphicyte

Nervous tissue is basically an integrated communications network distributed throughout the entire body. The main component of this tissue is the **neuron,** which transmits impulses. In addition to neurons, **glial cells** (or **neuroglia**) provide support and protection to neurons.

Anatomically, nervous tissue is subdivided into two portions: the **central nervous system (CNS)**—the spinal cord and brain—and the **peripheral nervous system (PNS)**—**nerve fibers** and small aggregates of neurons, **ganglia.** Except for certain sensory epithelia and the associated ganglion cells of certain cranial nerves, the CNS and PNS are derived from a specialized region of ectoderm—the **neuroectoderm**—that lies along the dorsal midline of the embryo.

The function of the nervous system in its entirety is twofold. It detects, analyzes, and possibly uses and transmits all information generated by sensory stimuli including heat, light, mechanical, electrical, and chemical changes that occur externally **(exteroception)** and internally **(interoception).** And it organizes,

integrates, and coordinates different functions of the body as a whole, including motor, visceral, endocrine, and mental activities.

NEURON

Neurons, or nerve cells, are specialized cells that respond to changes in their environment through alterations of the electrical potential differences between the inner and outer surfaces of their cell membrane. An appropriate stimulus then modifies or changes the electrical potential within the cell (Figure 9-1). Modification of the electrical potential may occur only at the region that received the signal or may be spread throughout the entire cell by the membrane, eliciting a **nerve impulse** that is subsequently transmitted to other neurons and tissues (Figure 9-2). Specifically, a temporary change in the ion concentrations of sodium and potassium occurs at the level of the cell membrane. Normally there is an established difference in the concentrations of Na^+, K^+, and Cl^-

179

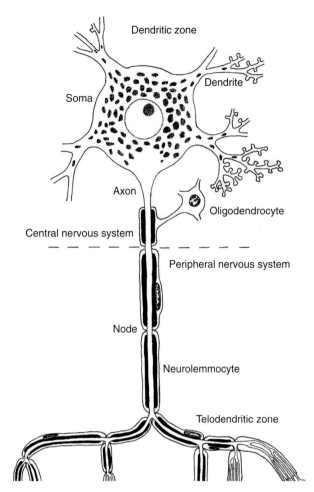

Figure 9-1. Illustration of a neuron with its specialized processes. Dendrites arise from the cell body (soma) to collectively form the dendritic zone, which is receptive to an appropriate stimulus. A newly formed nerve impulse flows from the dendritic zone to the cell's single axon, where it is transmitted to its branched endings that form the telodendritic zone.

inside and outside the cell, known as the **resting potential,** with Na⁺ and Cl⁻ considerably higher outside the cell and K⁺ higher inside. With an appropriate stimulus, such as a neurotransmitter, a short-lived leakage or exchange of Na⁺ to the inside and K⁺ to the outside occurs, resulting in an **action potential.** Initially the voltage-gated Na⁺ channels open at the site of stimulation, resulting in a quick buildup of this ion and **depolarization** of this region of the cell membrane. At this point, the Na⁺ channels close and the voltage-gated K⁺ channels open, causing K⁺ to leak extracellularly and in doing so restore the resting potential at which point the K⁺ channels subsequently close. The action potential generated is immediately spread along the neuron's excitable membrane.

In conjunction with the presence of an excitable membrane, neurons possess highly developed cellular processes **(dendrites)** that can be extremely long and have specialized contacts **(synapses).** As a specialization of the cell, dendrites expand the surface area of the neuron in a very cellular environment and as a result enhance the cell's capability to receive signals. The region of the neuron designed to perform this activity is the **dendritic zone** and can include the cell body (Figure 9-3; see also Figure 9-1). The dendritic zone accepts excitable input at discrete locations (the synapses) that consist of modified cellular contacts between the transmitting cell and the receiving cell. The transmitting cell delivers the excitable input (i.e., the nerve impulse) by a different group of processes that comprise the **telodendritic zone** (Figure 9-4; see also Figure 9-1). The telodendritic zone consists of the branched endings of the **axon,** which is the lone entity that transmits the impulse from the dendritic zone to the telodendritic zone. Neurons, then, are usually divided into three regions or parts: the dendritic zone, consisting of the perikaryon and its dendrites, the axon, and the axon's terminations, the telodendritic zone.

CELL BODY

The cell body is the **perikaryon,** or **soma,** and can range broadly in size from 3 to 120 μm in diameter. The nucleus is often large, particularly when compared with the entire perikaryon (Figure 9-5). It is also usually spherical and euchromatic. Prominent nucleoli (one or more) as well as satellite bodies, including Barr bodies, are often seen in these nuclei. The cytoplasm within the perikaryon is characterized by the presence of chromatophilic (basophilic) granular areas, the **Nissl bodies.** When examined by electron microscopy, Nissl bodies are found to be clusters of free ribosomes and rough endoplasmic reticulum (rER). The concentration of Nissl bodies varies with regard to the type of neuron and its present functional state, being numerous in the larger neurons (e.g., motor neuron). Besides Nissl bodies, the Golgi apparatus is normally well formed in the soma of neurons, lying adjacent to the nucleus. The Golgi apparatus is largely involved in the synthesis of neurochemical transmitters. The neurochemical transmitters are held in the secretory vesicles, which are transported within the axon to the telodendritic zone where they are released as synaptic vesicles. The cell body also contains mitochondria needed for the synthesis of the neurotransmitters and is fairly ladened with filaments, called **neurofilaments,** and microtubules **(neurotubules).** The cytoskeletal component of the cell body is especially prominent within the area known as the **axon**

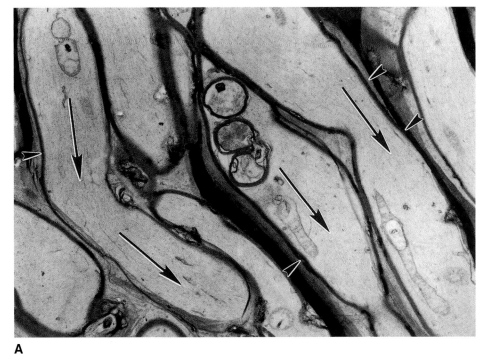

A

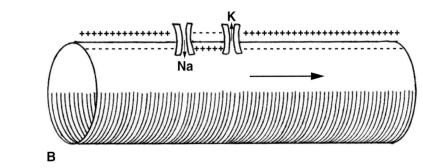

B

Figure 9-2. A, Layered transmission electron micrograph (×4000) of adjacent axons, each able to transmit nerve impulses *(arrows)* along their cell membranes that are individually insulated by myelin sheaths *(arrowheads).* **B,** Schematic diagram of a nerve impulse consisting of a propagated action potential whereby sodium *(Na)* temporarily enters the axon while potassium *(K)* is extruded.

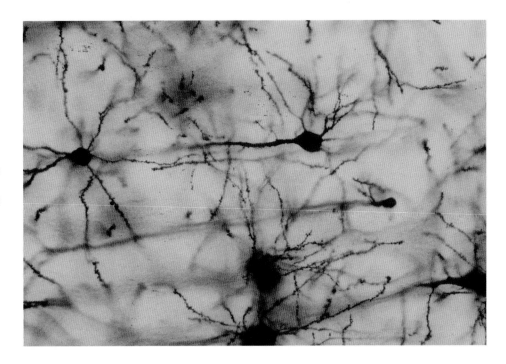

Figure 9-3. Light micrograph of silver-impregnated neurons with sparsely populated and evenly dispersed dendritic zones. (Rat brain, Golgi-Cox stain; ×400.)

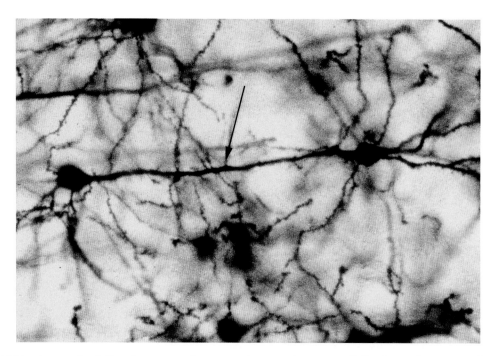

Figure 9-4. Light micrograph of silver-impregnated neurons. Arrow points to a radially directed axon. (Rat brain, Golgi-Cox stain; ×400.)

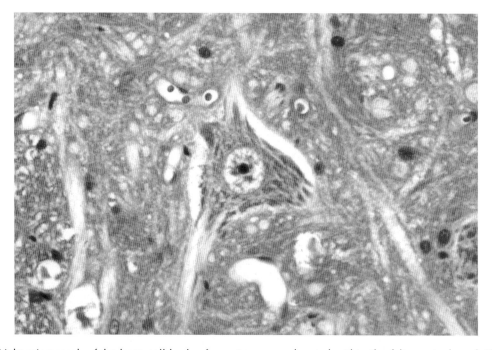

Figure 9-5. Light micrograph of the large cell body of a motor neuron located within the feline spinal cord. The cell body or soma houses a large euchromatic nucleus with prominent nucleoli and numerous basophilic Nissl bodies. (Hematoxylin and eosin stain; ×400.)

hillock, which leads to the cell's lone axon. Neurons that remain active and possess axons that extend great distances, 10 to 100 cm or more in length, such as motor neurons, form numerous Nissl bodies and a well-developed Golgi apparatus that make these cells among the largest in the body (see Figure 9-3). However, neurons that possess short axons, typically less than 1 mm long, can have little cytoplasm within each perikaryon that is often dominated in appearance by the nucleus, which may be heterochromatic (Figure 9-6).

DENDRITE

Dendrites consist of multiple elongated cellular processes specialized for receiving excitable stimuli. These processes can be numerous and highly branched, causing the receptive area of the cell to be increased greatly. In these instances, a single neuron is able to receive and integrate axon terminals from many neurons (see Figures 9-1 and 9-3). However, a neuron may have only a single dendrite with few branches and receive signals from a few neurons, or in some instances just one (Figure 9-7).

Cytologically, dendrites are nearly identical to the perikaryon, containing Nissl bodies, mitochondria, neurofilaments, and neurotubules. Outside of the nucleus and associated centrioles, the only organelle that is absent in this region is the Golgi apparatus. In smaller, branched dendrites most organelles are found with less regularity as occasional mitochondria; rough

endoplasmic reticulum (rER) and lysosomes are generally scattered throughout aggregates of neurotubules and neurofilaments. Dendrites usually possess numerous small projections called **dendritic spines** or **gemmules.** Rather than come to a fine point, the spines

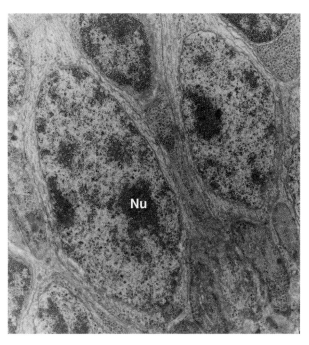

Figure 9-6. Transmission electron micrograph (×10,000) of the small cell bodies of bipolar cells within the inner retina of the pig. *Nu,* nucleolus.

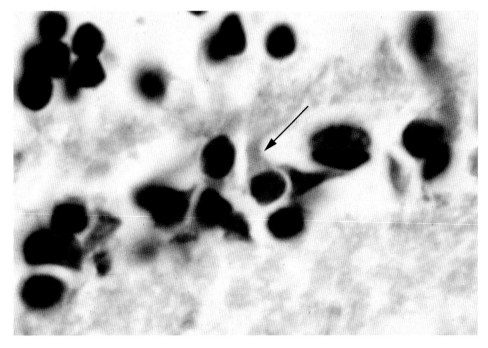

Figure 9-7. Light micrograph of the same neurons *(arrow)* seen in Figure 9-6. (Plastic section, toluidine blue stain; ×1000.)

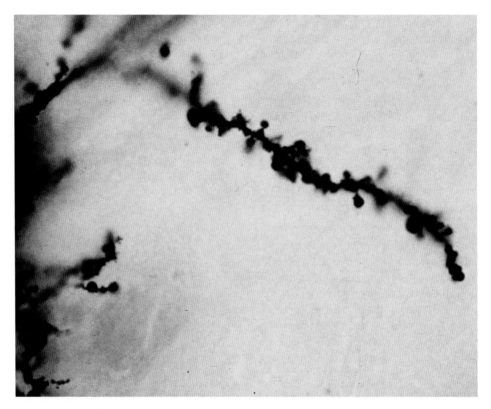

Figure 9-8. Light micrograph of silver-impregnated dendrite with numerous spines. (Rat brain, Golgi-Cox stain; ×1000.)

are pedicellate structures with expanded tips that offer specific sites for synaptic contact (Figure 9-8).

AXON

The axon is a cylindrical, long cellular process that varies in length and diameter according to the size and type of nerve cell. For the most part, cells with the longest and thickest axons have the largest soma. Some axons can attain lengths of 100 cm or more (e.g., motor neurons from the spinal cord). Each neuron possesses only one axon, and its axon arises from a pyramidal extension of the perikaryon—the **axon hillock.** The axon hillock lacks rER and free ribosomes and as a result can be distinguished cytologically from dendritic bases by the absence of Nissl bodies (Figure 9-9; see also Figure 9-6). Neurotubules and neurofilaments within the axon hillock are arranged in fascicles as they lead into the axon. The density of these cytoskeletal elements is sufficient enough to keep the other organelles free of this portion of the perikaryon's cytoplasm, but at the same time allow the secretory vesicles filled with a specific neurotransmitter to move from the cell body into the axon's cytoplasm. The axon, in general, has few organelles that are mostly mitochondria scattered throughout the neurotubules and neurofilaments (Figure 9-10). The cytoplasm within the axon is the **axoplasm,** and the cell membrane that surrounds the axoplasm is the **axolemma.** Cytoplasmic or axoplasmic streaming is extensive in axons, facilitated by the presence of the numerous neurotubules and neurofilaments. The streaming rapidly moves the secretory vesicles to be used in synaptic activity to the telodendritic zone and effectively causes mitochondria and axoplasmic fluid to move from the axon hillock to the synaptic ends and back again. This active streaming compensates greatly for the lack of protein synthesis and other metabolic activities that otherwise go on in the rest of the cell. **Axoplasmic flow** can be slow and fast, depending on what substances are being moved and how they are being moved. Slow axoplasmic flow involves the movement of filaments and cytosolic proteins at a rate of approximately 5 mm or less per day. Rapid or fast axoplasmic flow expends energy and involves the microtubule-linked transport of the secretory vesicles and mitochondria. The rate of rapid axoplasmic flow can occur up to 100 times faster (400 mm/day) than that of the slower form of streaming. Streaming proceeds both from the cell

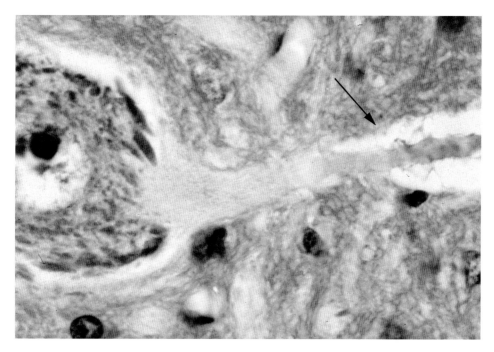

Figure 9-9. Light micrograph of the axon hillock of a motor neuron leading to the not-too-distantly myelinated axon *(arrow)*. (Hematoxylin and eosin stain; ×1000.)

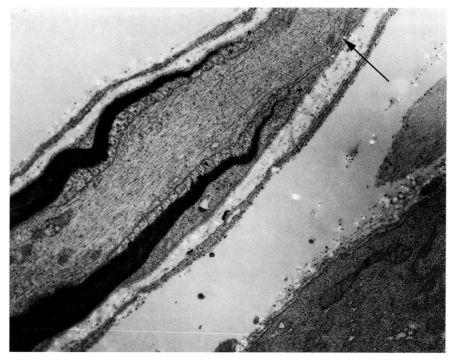

Figure 9-10. Transmission electron micrograph (×10,000) of the cytoskeletal-ladened axoplasm of a myelinated axon approaching a nodal *(arrow)* region (node of Ranvier).

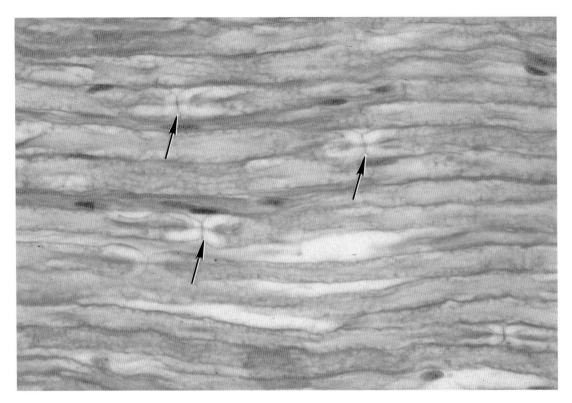

Figure 9-11. Light micrograph of a nerve bundle within the peripheral nervous system, characterized by the presence of nodes *(arrows)*. (Hematoxylin and eosin stain; ×400.)

body to the axonal ending **(anterograde transport)** and from the end of the axon to the soma **(retrograde transport).** In retrograde transport, the fast axoplasmic flow is about 200 mm/day or one half that of the fastest rate, which occurs anterogradely. Retrograde transport involves the movement of the subunits of the neurofilaments and microtubules as well as substances that will undergo degradation. It is important to keep in mind that in addition to cytoplasmic materials, intracellular pathogens, including viruses, such as the rabies virus or feline herpesvirus-1, can readily be spread from soma to nerve ending throughout portions of the body.

Axons may be enveloped by special sheaths provided by support cells. These sheaths help protect axons and aid in the conduction of the nerve impulse, with thicker sheaths providing faster axonal conduction. Axons that are ensheathed by single or multiple folds of a sheath cell are sometimes referred to as **nerve fibers.** Multiple ensheathment of an axon consists of cellular wrappings from a sheath cell that wind around an axon. This type of ensheathment is referred to as being **myelinated** (i.e., consisting of **myelin sheaths**) (see Figures 9-2 and 9-10). In the CNS, sheath cells are called **oligodendrocytes,** and in the PNS they are **neurolemmocytes** or **Schwann cells.** As the cellular

sheaths envelop the axon most of the cytoplasm within the sheaths is removed or "squeezed out," leaving only small, confluent portions of cytoplasm, known as **clefts (of Schmidt-Lantermann),** in what has become a whirl of tightly wrapped cell membrane. An axon in both the CNS and PNS is ensheathed by more that one oligodendrocyte and Schwann cell, respectively. The region where two adjacent myelin ensheathments (from two adjacent sheath cells) meet is the **node of Ranvier** (Figure 9-11; see also Figure 9-10). In the CNS the nodes of Ranvier are not encapsulated at all by neighboring myelin sheaths of oligodendrocytes. By comparison, in the PNS the nodes are covered by the loose interdigitations of neighboring Schwann cells (Figure 9-12).

Not all nerve fibers in the CNS and PNS are myelinated. In the PNS unmyelinated nerve fibers are seen mostly among smaller axons. These axons are enclosed singly or in clusters within a simple cleft of the Schwann cell. Nodes of Ranvier do not exist here because adjacent Schwann cells are laterally connected, forming a continuous sheath. In the CNS, unmyelinated axons, of which there are many, also can be unsheathed but still lined by glial tissue.

Axons typically branch before they end, a process sometimes referred to as terminal arborization. The

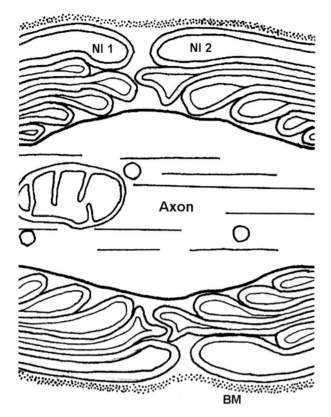

Figure 9-12. Illustration of a node between two neurolemmocytes (*N1₁* and *N1₂*) that insulate a portion of an axon within the peripheral nervous system (PNS). *BM,* Basement membrane.

result of this arborization is the formation of a **telo-dendritic zone** (see Figures 9-1 and 9-4). At the terminations of this zone, axons usually dilate into **boutons (boutons terminaux)** or **synaptic end bulbs** (Figure 9-13). **Preterminal bulbs (boutons en passage),** which consist of dilations along the axon, can occur as well.

SYNAPSES

Synapses are the contacts of axons with dendrites or the perikaryon. These are the regions where the nerve impulses are transmitted from one neuron (the presynaptic cell) to another (the postsynaptic cell). Postsynaptic cells can be nonneuronal, especially when located within the PNS, and frequently include glandular cells and muscle fibers. The synapse then is composed of the **terminal membrane** or **presynaptic membrane** at the preterminal or synaptic end bulb, a **synaptic gap** (synaptic cleft), and a **postsynaptic membrane** belonging to a dendrite or perikaryon of another neuron (Figure 9-14; see also Figure 9-13).

Numerous synaptic vesicles, approximately 40 to 65 nm in diameter, help identify synaptic end bulbs ultrastructurally. **Synaptic vesicles** hold materials **(neurotransmitters)** that are needed for transmitting a nerve impulse across the synaptic gap. The vesicles, which may be dark and granular or clear, can contain

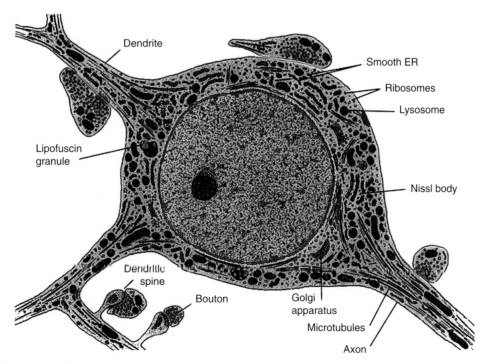

Figure 9-13. Illustration of an ultrastructural representation of a neuronal soma with direct and adjacent synaptic associations. *(Modified from Lentz TL: Cell fine structure: an atlas of drawings of whole-cell structure, Philadelphia, 1971, Saunders.)*

a wide variety of substances ranging from amino acids such as glycine and glutamate to peptides such as somatostatin and to monoamines, including catecholamines. The different populations of neurotransmitters occur separately with only one type of neurotransmitter formed within the neuron. As a result, neuronal terminals use acetylcholine as the neurotransmitter, catecholamines, or other types of signaling molecules. Many of the various neurotransmitters are synthesized at the level of the bulb and are collected and packaged within the vesicles that become clustered at the presynaptic membrane. Other neurotransmitters, including peptides, are assembled within the perikaryon's Golgi apparatus and are transported within the vesicles by rapid axoplasmic flow.

In addition to the numerous vesicles, the bulbs contain scattered elements of smooth ER, mitochondria, microtubules, and microfilaments. The synaptic vesicles are packed at the membrane site of their release. The presynaptic membrane contains dense material that becomes closely associated with those vesicles that lie next to the membrane and will release their contents at the moment that the nerve impulse arrives (see Figures 9-13 and 9-14). Behind these vesicles is a reserve of synaptic vesicles attached to actin filaments, facilitating the movement of these vesicles to the presynaptic membrane, along with a group of small proteins, including **synapsin-I** and **synapsin-II.** With the arrival of an action potential, the opening of voltage-gated channels occurs at the presynaptic membrane, allowing Ca^{++} to enter freely and enzymatically activate the phosphorylation of synapsin-I, which, in turn, mobilizes the vesicles closest to the membrane and permits them to merge with it and release their contents by exocytosis.

The released neurotransmitter now enters a narrow gap of approximately 20 to 30 nm wide. Extracellular protein within the gap facilitates the diffusion of the neurotransmitter to the postsynaptic membrane. Quickly the molecules of the neurotransmitter bind to a specific protein receptor attached to the postsynaptic membrane; this interaction results in the opening of ion channels and initiates a nerve impulse affecting that cell. Activity at the postsynaptic membrane ends when the neurotransmitter is sufficiently degraded. The degradation is performed by enzymes released by the stimulated cell at the site of the postsynaptic membrane. The degradative products are then taken in by the bulb, recycled, and resynthesized. When neurotransmitters act as inhibitors, hyperpolarization rather than depolarization of the postsynaptic membrane occurs. In those instances, the axonal bulbs are often positioned along the cell body, typically at the base of dendrites (i.e., **axosomatic synapses**), or along the axon of the neuron to be stimulated (i.e., **axoaxonic synapses**) and can thus function more effectively to block excitatory impulses (see Figure 9-13).

The postsynaptic membrane is similar in appearance to the presynaptic membrane in that the plasmalemma is thickened and opaque, containing the receptor protein that is responsible for the depolarized or hyperpolarized response. As in the presynaptic membrane, numerous filaments are associated with the postsynaptic membrane, but are much more visible than those seen presynaptically because of the lack of vesicles in the postsynaptic element (see Figures 9-7 and 9-14).

NEUROTRANSMITTERS

The driving force behind synaptic activity is provided by the neurotransmitter. Neurotransmitters consist of a variety of signaling molecules that act directly on receptor protein associated with ion channels. The response time involved in this process is usually short, less than 1 msec. Not all signaling molecules are directly involved with ion channels. Some act on G proteins or receptor kinases, which instead result in the activation of a second messenger. In these instances, the signaling molecules are called **neuromodulators** and the time associated with this process can be considerably longer, lasting up to several minutes.

Nearly 100 neurotransmitters and neuromodulators have been found. These signaling proteins can be divided into three groups: gases, small molecule transmitters, and neuropeptides. **Gases** represent the smallest and most recently discovered group, consisting of nitric oxide (NO) and carbon monoxide (CO), both of which have the potential to function as neuromodulators. The next smallest signaling proteins are the **small molecule transmitters,** which are subdivided into **amino acids,** which include gammaaminobutyric acid (GABA), glutamate, glycine, and aspartate; **acetylcholine;** and **biogenic amines,** which include catecholamines (epinephrine, norepinephrine, and dopamine) and serotonin. The third group consists of **neuropeptides,** many functioning as neuromodulators, and include opioids, gastrointestinal peptides, and various hormones.

NEURONAL SHAPE AND CLASSIFICATION

Neurons are classified according to the number and size of the processes extending from their cell bodies. The simplest category is the **unipolar** neuron, which possesses one cell process leading away from the perikaryon. Two branches may serve as an axon and

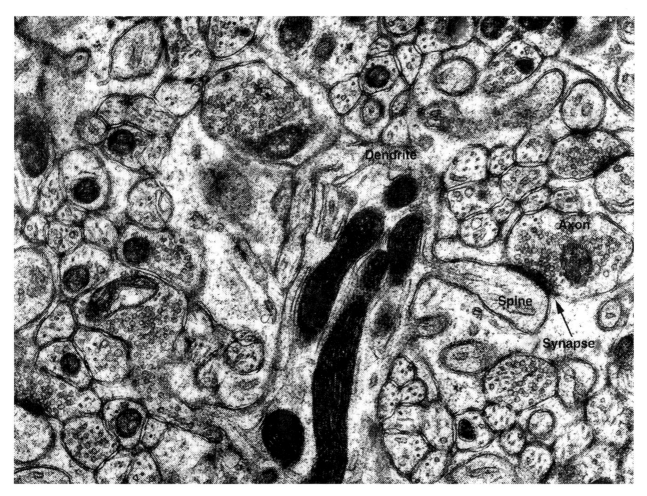

Figure 9-14. Transmission electron micrograph of a portion of the cerebellum with an extensive entanglement of glial processes and axons and dendrites, collectively called *neuropil.* Among the neuropil a dendritic spine forms a synapse (arrow) with an axonal ending (synaptic end bulb). Within the dendrite are several long mitochondria. *(From Fawcett DW: Bloom and Fawcett: a textbook of histology, ed 11, Philadelphia, 1986, Saunders.)*

dendrite or simply as an axon. True unipolar neurons are rare in vertebrates. Instead, a **pseudounipolar** neuron represents a modification of this category (Figure 9-15). The pseudounipolar neuron appears morphologically similar to the true unipolar neuron at maturity, but in fact originates embryologically as a neuron with two cell processes. During development, both processes move toward one side of the cell and fuse for a short distance from the perikaryon. Pseudounipolar neurons are found in dorsal root ganglia as well as some sensory ganglia of cranial nerves and amacrine cells in the retina. Neurons that possess two processes are referred to as **bipolar.** In these cells, an axon arises from one "pole" of the cell body, and a single dendrite arises from the opposite pole (see Figure 9-15). These cells are mostly associated with sensory apparatuses, being found in the retina and within vestibular and acoustic ganglia. The most common form of neuron is that which possesses several or more processes **(multipolar).** These neurons can

possess elaborate dendritic trees and may be grouped according to shapes of the dendritic patterns.

Neurons also may be classified on the basis of **direction of nerve impulse** as seen in the PNS, consisting of **afferent** neurons (toward the CNS) and **efferent** neurons (away from the CNS), and **type of function—sensory, motor,** and **integrative**—with sensory and motor being synonymous with afferent and efferent, respectively (Table 9-1).

NEUROGLIA

In addition to neurons a variety of support cells, or *neuroglia,* comprise much of the nervous tissue, and are found between neurons and along fiber tracts (Figure 9-16). Cells of this type provide physical as well as physiological support. Their functional roles, which have yet to be fully understood and appreciated, are

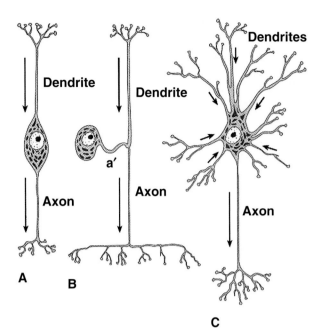

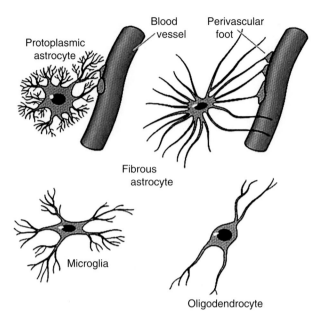

Figure 9-15. Diagram of the three basic morphological types of neurons that occur in domestic species. **A,** Bipolar neuron; **B,** pseudounipolar neuron (*[a'],* common process to the dendrite and axon); **C,** multipolar neuron. *(Modified from Bergman RA, Afifi AK, Heidger PM Jr: Histology, Philadelphia, 1996, Saunders.)*

Figure 9-16. Illustration of the types of neuroglia within the central nervous system (CNS). *(Modified from Gartner LP, Hiatt JL: Color textbook of histology, Philadelphia, 1997, Saunders.)*

TABLE 9-1	Classification of Neurons		
METHODS	**CATEGORY**	**PRINCIPAL CHARACTERISTIC**	**ADDITIONAL INFORMATION**
Shape	Unipolar	Single process associated with the soma	Domestic species do not possess unipolar neurons; pseudounipolar and bipolar neurons are most often associated with sensory innervation
	Pseudounipolar	Two processes combine for a short distance as one during development	
	Bipolar	Single axon and dendrite associated with the soma	
	Multipolar	Single axon and more than one dendrite associated with the soma	
Direction	Afferent	Directs signal (nerve impulse) toward CNS	Mostly sensory innervation
	Efferent	Directs signal away from CNS	Mostly motor innervation
Location	Central nervous system (CNS)	Present within the brain and spinal cord	Consisting of whole cells and soma with dendritic zone
	Peripheral nervous system (PNS)	Present outside the brain and spinal cord	Consisting of nerve fibers and localized ganglia (small clusters of neurons)
Type of functional innervation	Motor	Directs effector organs including muscle, glands, and other neurons	Synonymous with efferent
	Sensory	Responds to sensory stimuli, internally and externally	Synonymous with afferent
	Inter(neuron)/integrative	Interconnects and establishes network circuitry between motor neurons and sensory neurons	Number and complexity increase with evolution of mammals

TABLE 9-2   Key Characteristics of Neuroglia

CELL TYPES OF THE CENTRAL NERVOUS SYSTEM (CNS)	SHAPE	LOCATION	FUNCTION	OTHER FEATURES
Protoplasmic astrocyte	Numerous short, branched processes arranged in a stellate manner	Gray matter	Contributes to the blood-brain barrier; provides scaffolding for neuronal processes; maintains cation balance, especially K$^+$	Forms vascularly attached end feet; abundant cytoplasm and large, oval euchromatic nucleus
Fibrous astrocyte	Sparsely branched processes arranged in a stellate manner	White matter	Contributes to the blood-brain barrier; provides scaffolding for nerve fibers	Forms vascularly attached end feet; high concentration of intermediate (glial) filaments; smaller, oval, less euchromatic nucleus
Oligodendrocyte	Small round cell body with scattered thin processes	Gray and white matter	Myelinates axons in white matter and those present in gray matter; otherwise serves as perineuronal satellite cells without determined function	Myelinates small portions of more than one axon; possesses small, round partially heterochromatic nucleus
Microglia	Small oval cell body with fine spiny processes	Gray and white matter	Phagocytic/antigen-presenting capability	Well-developed lysosomal system; member of the mononuclear phagocyte population within the body
Ependyma	Cuboidal to columnar with sparsely ciliated apical surface	Line ventricles and central canal	Forms cerebrospinal fluid (CSF) within the ventricles and moves CSF within ventricles and central canal	Round to oval nucleus; possesses basal process that can provide further scaffolding, especially in the spinal cord
Cell Types of the Peripheral Nervous System				
Neurolemmocyte	Elongated and flattened; wrapped circularly around a portion of an axon	Within nerve bundles outside the CNS	Myelinates a portion (up to 1 mm) of an axon and ensheathes its smaller branches	Forms a basal lamina; elliptically shaped, partially heterochromatic nucleus located outside the myelin
Satellite cell	Small cuboidal	Nerve ganglion	Not determined	With other satellite cells envelops individual neurons; small, round partially heterochromatic nucleus

listed in Table 9-2. New studies have continued to redefine their association with neurons.

ASTROCYTES

Of the different cells that compose the neuroglia, the **astrocyte** is perhaps the largest, having many long processes that may be highly branched. As the name implies, this cell appears star shaped as the long processes surround a fairly small soma that is filled with a large, spherical nucleus. Although the function of the astrocyte is still being researched, it is thought to

provide scaffolding for the assemblage of neurons and their processes. Potassium ions within the small extracellular domain are pump regulated by these cells. Glutamate and α-aminobutyrate also are believed to be astrocyte regulated. Two types of astrocytes have been distinguished, both of which occur solely in the CNS. **Protoplasmic astrocytes** are found in gray matter, and have highly branched processes that contain granular and comparatively abundant cytoplasm. The nucleus in this cell type is centrally placed within the cell body, and when compared with other glial cells it is large and euchromatic (Figures 9-17 and

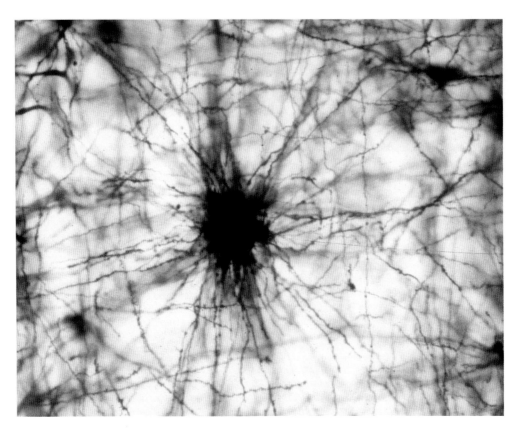

Figure 9-17. Light micrograph of silver-impregnated protoplasmic astrocyte with numerous radiating processes. (Cat brain, Golgi-Cox stain; ×200.)

9-18). These astrocytes mostly envelop the surface of neurons, synaptic areas, and blood vessels. When in contact with blood vessels, the ends of the processes expand to some degree and form vascular **end feet** or **pedicles** that may contribute to the blood-brain barrier (see Figure 9-16). **Fibrous astrocytes** by comparison occur in white matter; they have long slender, smooth, and relatively unbranched processes that are rich with thin filaments. The cytoplasm, which surrounds the centrally placed mostly euchromatic nucleus, possesses considerably fewer organelles than that of protoplasmic astrocytes (see Figures 9-16 and 9-18). End feet arise at the distal tips of those processes that contact blood vessels. Both types of astrocytes form a unique type of intermediate filament of **glial fibrillar acidic protein (GFAP).** Although GFAP is more concentrated in the fibrous astrocyte, it can quickly increase in amount in the protoplasmic astrocyte during an episode of injury.

Oligodendrocytes

The **oligodendrocyte** is a small cell type of neuroglia, possessing fewer, relatively short processes than found in astrocytes and a round, darkly stained nucleus (see Figure 9-16). This cell, which is found in both white and gray matter of the CNS, is cytoplasmically richer than the astrocyte, having numerous mitochondria, rER, and a prominent Golgi apparatus next to a small, round nucleus. In white matter, oligodendrocytes act as sheath cells that envelop and myelinate axons. Myelin consists of multiple wrappings of the oligodendrocyte's cell membrane, which function to insulate the axon so that the nerve impulse is able to travel great distances without a substantial loss of its action potential. A single oligodendrocyte is able to myelinate short regions of several or more adjacent axons (Figure 9-19). In gray matter, these cells are often positioned next to perikaryons, where they ensheathe their axons and partially line the perikaryon.

Microglia

Microglial cells—dense, elongated cells with numerous small, branching processes—are among the smallest cell types of the neuroglial element (see Figure 9-16). In the normal CNS, microglia are sparse and have a defense role, much like the macrophage in connective tissue. Many of the cells that have

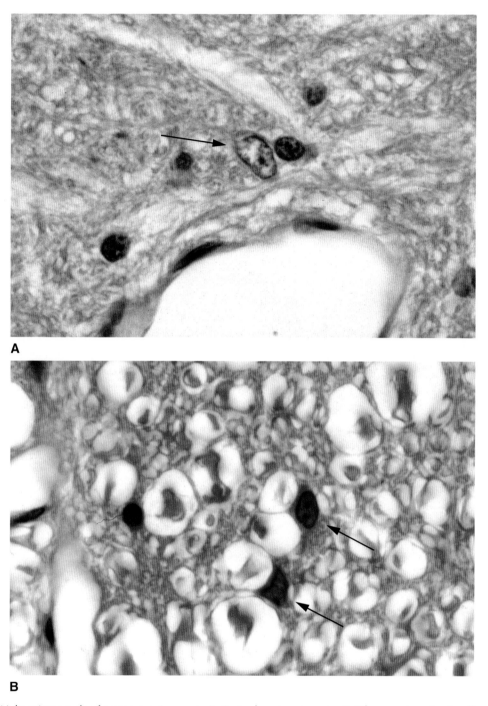

Figure 9-18. Light micrograph of astrocytes *(arrows)*. **A,** Protoplasmic astrocyte. **B,** Fibrous astrocyte. Smaller round nuclei belong to nearby oligodendrocytes. (Feline spinal cord, hematoxylin and eosin stain; ×1000.)

been described light microscopically have been demonstrated as oligodendrocytes or glioblasts (immature neuroglia) for the formation of new oligodendrocytes and astrocytes. Recently these cells have been proposed to be multipotential stem cells, having the capability of giving rise to neurons as well. However, some of the cells have been found to be derived from blood-borne monocytes and mesodermally derived from the bone marrow: these are true microglia. In response to an injury or infection, microglia (of the macrophage-monocyte system) become involved in phagocytic activity (Figure 9-20).

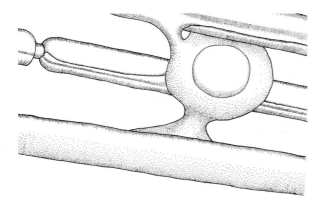

Figure 9-19. Illustration of an oligodendrocyte that is involved in the myelination of adjacent axons. As each sheath ends, it leaves the node exposed.

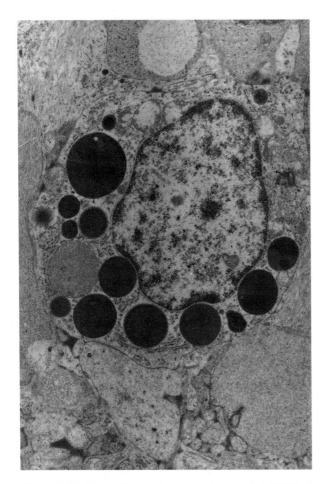

Figure 9-20. Transmission electron micrograph (×7000) of an active microglial cell in the dog.

Ependyma

Ependymal cells comprise those cells that line cavities in the CNS (i.e., the ventricles of the brain and the central canal of the spinal cord). These cells morphologically retain their neuroepithelial embryonic derivation and have an epithelial arrangement, forming ciliated simple cuboidal or columnar layers (Figure 9-21). Adjacent cells are closely joined by cell junctions that include nexi (gap junctions) and zonula adherens. In adults, cilia can be lost except for small, patchy regions. Although their apices line the cavities, their bases often extend into single long processes that travel from the center of the brain to peripheral connective tissue, especially in the young, developing individual. Although they shorten with maturation, these processes may nevertheless contribute further support to neuronal elements. Within the ventricles of the brain the ependyma becomes a modified special secretory epithelium that is cuboidal and lines the choroid plexi that form cerebrospinal fluid (CSF). These ependymal cells form tight junctions (zonula occludens) and in doing so maintain the blood-brain barrier as the capillaries are fenestrated in these plexi.

Neurolemmocytes

Neurolemmocytes are glia or **Schwann cells** of the PNS—the counterpart to oligodendrocytes of the CNS, because these cells are similarly involved in axonal ensheathment. Each cell forms a single, myelinated internodal segment (Figure 9-22). These cells, in effect, line up end-to-end for the length of the axon, and in an analogous manner resemble a long passenger train with its central corridor. It is important to note that the entire cell is involved in axonal

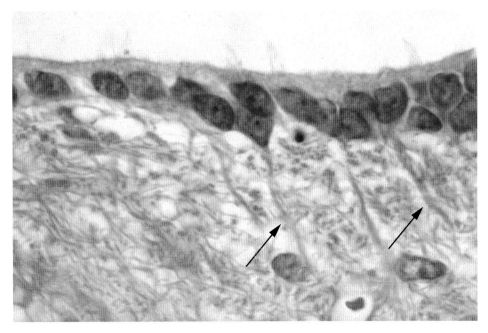

Figure 9-21. Light micrograph of ependymal cells lining the central canal of a feline spinal cord. Arrows point to the basal processes. (Hematoxylin and eosin stain; ×1000.)

ensheathment and that its innermost portion is able to coil around the axon repeatedly (up to 50 times). The cytoplasm within the multiple windings becomes "squeezed," or removed toward the outermost portion, leaving a small amount of cytoplasm along its inner cell membrane (Figure 9-23; see also Figure 9-10). As a result of the removal of the cytoplasm from the multiple windings, the wrappings of the cell membrane and residual cytoplasm become fused and are referred to as **myelin.** The fusion of the Schwann cell's plasmalemma forms **major dense lines** that consist of the cell membrane's inner leaflet and any associated cytoplasm, and **intraperiod lines,** consisting of the membrane's outer leaflet. It is thought that there is a very fine space within the intraperiod line, called the **intraperiod gap,** that may allow small molecules to reach the axon. This gap extends from the innermost wrapping of the neurolemmocyte's cell membrane **(the inner mesaxon),** and extends helically to the outermost wrapping **(the outer mesaxon).**

The inner and outer cytoplasmic portions of a neurolemmocyte are not entirely cut off from one another because of narrow cytoplasm connections or avenues that helically wind from one region to another, known as **clefts** or **incisures (of Schmidt-Lantermann).** These clefts, which can be seen by plastic-embedded specimens (Figure 9-24; see also Figure 9-22), function to keep the inner portion oxygenated and nourished.

In neurolemmocytes or Schwann cells that are long, up to 1 mm, and possess thick myelin, numerous clefts can be observed. The bulk of the cytoplasm and the nucleus of the neurolemmocyte, which is oval, are located within the outer portion (see Figure 9-24). In large neurolemmocytes (those that are long and have thick myelin), the nucleus protrudes to some extent into the myelin. At the end of each cell, a cleftlike avenue of cytoplasm is retained, interconnecting the inner and outer portions. The apposing ends of adjacent neurolemmocytes along the same axon, which are referred to as **nodes (nodes of Ranvier),** overlap to some extent and in doing so continue to ensheathe the axon in the absence of myelin (see Figures 9-10 and 9-12). This arrangement contrasts to that found in the CNS, which lacks any nodal ensheathment. Nodal and internodal regions along each axon within the PNS are further lined by a basal lamina that is made by each neurolemmocyte. With the approaching termination of each axon, the degree of myelination is reduced and eventually disappears. In these instances, the associated neurolemmocyte simply envelops the axon and its branches (Figure 9-25).

Before reaching the synaptic terminations of the axon, Na^+ ions can cross the axolemma only in a depolarized manner at the nodes of Ranvier, where Na^+ ion channels are clustered. However, because the

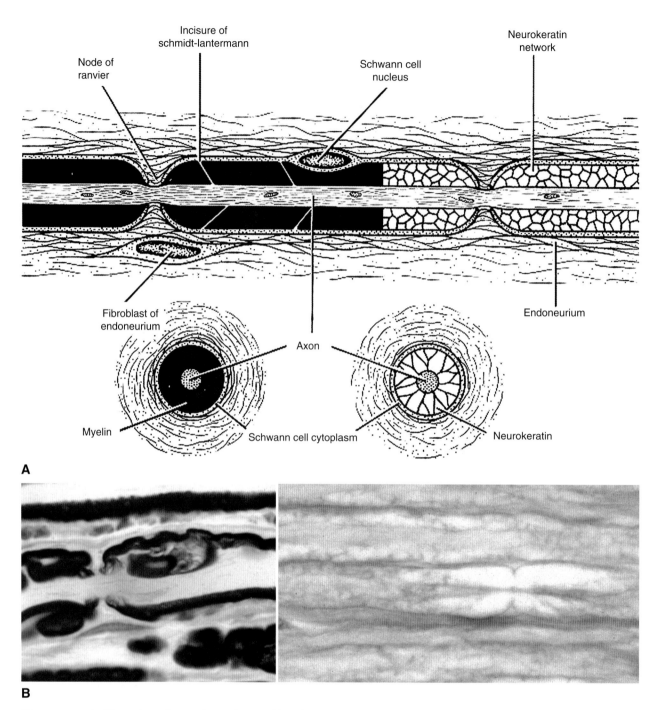

A

B

Figure 9-22. A, Illustration of a myelinated nerve fiber that represents the changes resulting from two different fixatives; the portion on the left has been preserved for electron microscopy, and the portion on the right has been preserved for traditional light microscopy with paraffin-embedded material. In traditionally prepared specimens of nerve fibers, much of the myelin's lipid component has been extracted, causing the structure to appear fragmented, and described years ago as consisting of neurokeratin. **B,** Light micrographs (×1000) of the illustration in **A.** The left side was embedded in plastic and stained with toluidine blue, whereas the right side was embedded in paraffin and stained with hematoxylin and eosin. (**A** *from Fawcett DW:* Bloom and Fawcett: a textbook of histology, *ed 11, Philadelphia, 1986, Saunders.*)

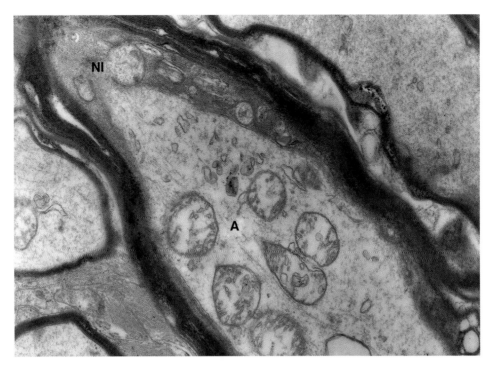

Figure 9-23. Transmission electron micrograph (×20,000) of a partially oblique view of a nerve fiber, revealing the innermost portion of the cytoplasm of the neurolemmocyte *(NI)* lying inside the myelin sheath and just outside the axolemma of the axon *(A)*.

nodes are covered by the end processes of two adjoining neurolemmocytes, outward movement of the Na⁺ ions is blocked. As a result excess Na⁺ ions continue to diffuse through the axoplasm to the next node and initiate depolarization at that point. In this way, the impulse is moved by a surging action potential that "jumps" from each node to the next, causing **saltatory conduction.** The rapidity of this process is enhanced by the amount of myelination. Thus the degree of myelination by the neurolemmocyte has a direct bearing on the velocity that a nerve impulse is conducted along a nerve fiber.

At the termination of the nerve fibers, the myelin sheath disappears and the axon is ensheathed solely by the cytoplasm and the cell membrane of the neurolemmocyte. At this point the voltage-gated ion channels are spread along the entire axolemma rather than clustered as before. Consequently, the nerve impulse moves along the axolemma at a slower rate in a process called **continuous conduction.**

Satellite Cell

Another glial component in the PNS is the **satellite cell,** or **amphicyte.** This cell occurs in nerve plexi and ganglia, such as the dorsal root ganglia, which

are sensory ganglia that contain the perikarya of pseudounipolar neurons. Satellite cells form an envelope around the individual neurons within a ganglion. The satellite cell is comparatively much smaller than the neuron and is usually cuboidal (Figure 9-26). These cells are covered by their basal lamina, which, in turn, is encapsulated by connective tissue. The satellite cell is believed to provide both structural and physiological support for each neuron in the PNS. The connective tissue lining these cells is contiguous with the **endoneurium,** a connective tissue that lines the axons and associated neurolemmocytes.

PERIPHERAL NERVOUS SYSTEM

Nervous tissue within the PNS consists of bundles of nerve fibers (nerves) that are myelinated except at their terminal arborizations. **Cranial nerves** originate from the brain (which lies within the cranium) and **spinal nerves** are found in the spinal cord. In addition to nerves, clusters of neurons and their cell bodies can be found at discrete locations among the body's different organ systems. These clusters are **ganglia** (ganglion, singular) and are further subdivided into **autonomic ganglia,** which assist in directing activities

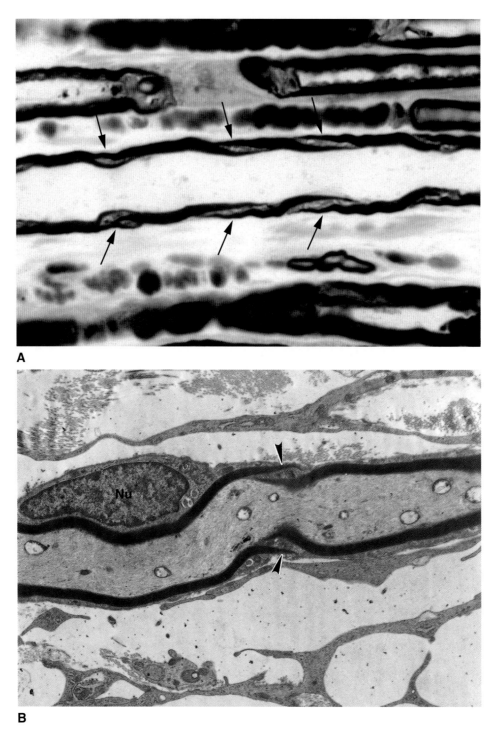

A

B

Figure 9-24. A, Light micrograph of multiple clefts *(arrows)* within the myelin sheath along an axon. (Plastic section, toluidine blue stain; ×400.) **B,** Transmission electron micrograph (×4000) of an encircling cleft *(arrowheads)* within the myelin sheath. *Nu,* Nucleus of the neurolemmocyte.

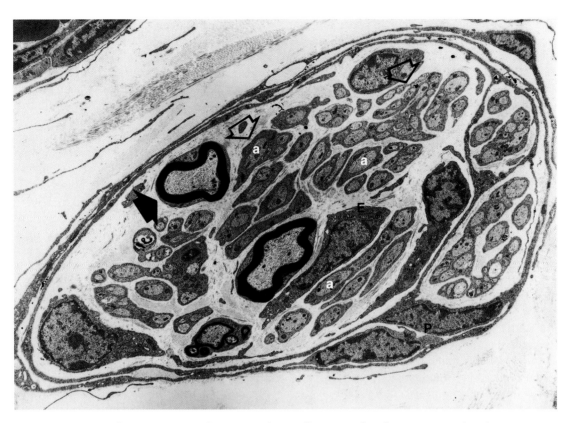

Figure 9-25. Transmission electron micrograph (×3000) of a small nerve within the canine peripheral nervous system (PNS), consisting of myelinated nerve fibers *(closed arrow)* and branched axons *(a)* that are ensheathed but not myelinated *(open arrow)*. The bundles of nerve fibers present are each separated by a perineurium *(P),* which in turn is lined externally by an epineurium. Each nerve fiber is lined by the endoneurium *(E).*

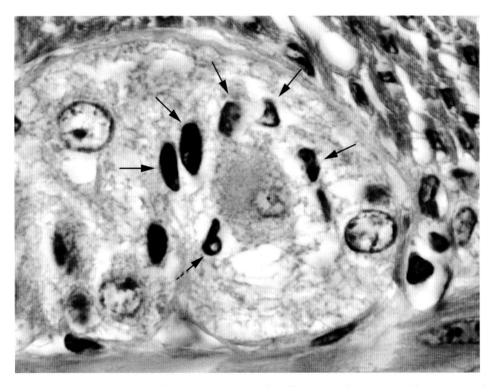

Figure 9-26. Light micrograph of satellite cells *(arrows)* surrounding the soma of a neuron within a nerve plexus within the small intestine of a dog. (Hematoxylin and eosin stain; ×1000.)

within the body associated with muscle under involuntary control (such as smooth and cardiac muscle) and glands; and **sensory ganglia,** which provide sensory innervation for both external and internal environments.

Autonomic ganglia are closely associated with neurons within the CNS that together with the neurons of the autonomic ganglia control the visceral portion of the body through their efferent or visceral motor innervation. The neurons with their cell bodies located within the CNS represent the first neurons of the autonomic chain. Their nerve fibers, **preganglionic fibers,** synapse with the neurons of the autonomic ganglia, which represent the second neurons of the autonomic chain. The second neurons (i.e., those of the autonomic ganglia) are multipolar with comparatively small amount of cytoplasm around the slightly displaced nuclei. Their axons, **postganglionic fibers,** are myelinated and terminate directly with smooth or cardiac muscle or specific glands.

Sensory ganglia are associated with both cranial and spinal nerves, being found within the cranial and dorsal spinal roots (dorsal root ganglia), and consisting of pseudounipolar neurons except for those associated with the sensory organs for smell (olfaction), vision, balance (vestibulation), and hearing (audition), which consist of bipolar neurons. The neurons are lined by neuroglia (satellite cells) that lie closely pressed to each neuron's soma, and a capsule of connective tissue (see Figure 9-26). The pseudounipolar neurons consist of exteroceptors and interoceptors, which possess specialized afferent processes that direct generated impulses from either external or internal stimulation to the CNS.

A nerve within the PNS that holds afferent fibers for interoception, exteroception, and proprioception also contains efferent nerve fibers. These latter fibers originate from somatic efferent neurons that function to innervate skeletal muscle cells. A somatic neuron and all of the muscle cells that it can potentially stimulate comprise a **motor unit.** Although muscle units can involve as many as 200 to 300 or more myocytes or even up to 1000 cells along the abdominal wall. They can have few units that are resistant to extensive activity or many units that are used mostly for intense contraction over a short duration. As one might suspect, the size of the motor neuron generally reflects the size of the motor unit in that smaller neurons innervate smaller units and larger neurons innervate larger units.

The innervation of the muscle cells by the neuron is performed by the synaptic activity of the **motor endplate,** which consists of several short axonal endings lying within pocket-like invaginations along a muscle fiber (see Figure 8-14). Each ending (synaptic end

bulb) forms a **myoneural junction** with the muscle fiber. The composition of this junction was previously described in Chapter 8. Acetylcholine is the neurotransmitter contained within the tens of thousands of synaptic vesicles that lie next to the presynaptic membrane of each terminal. Once released, the acetylcholine quickly binds to the many receptors along the primary and secondary clefts, causing ligand-gated ion channels to open and depolarization of the muscle fiber. The reaction caused by the neurotransmitter is short lived because of the presence of acetylcholinesterase within the secondary clefts, which almost instantaneously dissembles acetylcholine into acetate and choline. The choline within the synaptic cleft is then readily transported back to the axonal terminal and recycled by choline acetyltransferase so that a functional amount of the neurotransmitter is always present under normal circumstances.

CONNECTIVE TISSUE ASSOCIATED WITH THE PERIPHERAL NERVOUS SYSTEM

Within the PNS the nerve fibers are aggregated into bundles or fascicles that grossly appear white because of their myelination. As peripheral nerves, the fascicles are encapsulated by several layers of connective tissue elements that collectively form a fibrous protective sheath. The outermost layer consists of a dense fibrous coat, the **epineurium** (Figure 9-27). In peripheral nerves that contain more than a single fascicle, the epineurium occurs between adjacent nerve bundles as well. The thickness of the epineurium is most pronounced where the nerves emanate from the spinal cord.

Individual nerve bundles are enveloped by a sleeve of epithelioid-like cells that are joined to each other along their lateral borders by tight junctions. This cellular sleeve or sheath (the **perineurium**) can be comprised of more than one layer in larger fascicles, which becomes reduced to a single layer in smaller fascicles (see Figure 9-25). The cells form a basal lamina, and when more than one layer exists, small amounts of extracellular fibers coexist between the adjacent cellular layers. The perineurium provides a seal that preserves a microenvironment suited for maintaining nerve fibers and the conduction of their impulses. Internally the perineurium branches and lines a fine network of loose connective tissue that surrounds the neurolemmocytes or Schwann cells—the **endoneurium.** The loose connective tissue consists primarily of reticular fibers produced by the neurolemmocytes, fibroblasts and their collagen and elastin, capillaries, and occasional histiocytes and

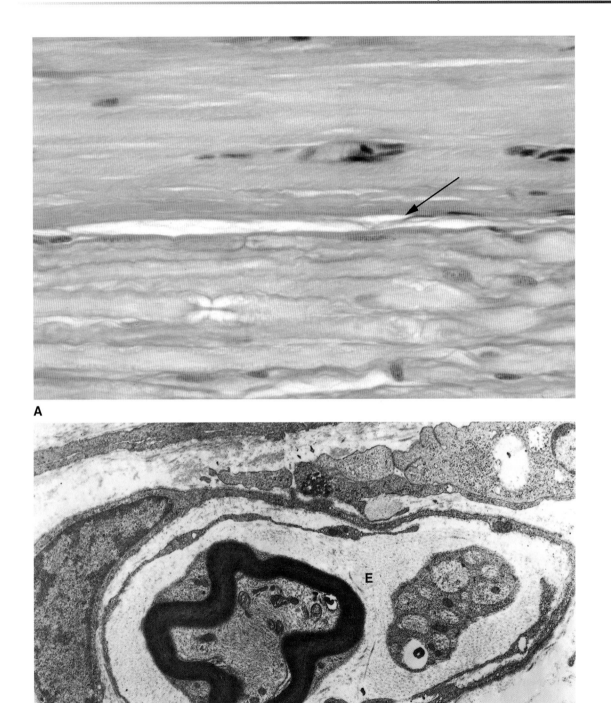

A

B

Figure 9-27. A, Light micrograph of a nerve bundle within the peripheral nervous system (PNS) sealed by the perineurium *(arrow)* and further protected by an outer connective tissue coat, the epineurium. (Hematoxylin and eosin stain; ×400.) **B,** Transmission electron micrograph (×6000) of individual nerve fibers in a dog that continue to be lined by the perineurium *(P)* and endoneurium *(E).*

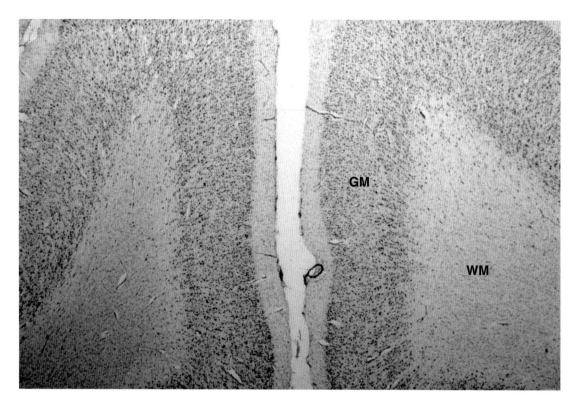

Figure 9-28. Light micrograph of the feline cerebrum with the gray matter *(GM)* located externally to the white matter *(WM)*. (Nissl [cresyl violet] stain; ×20.)

mast cells. The perineurial and endoneurial portions of the connective tissue investment of peripheral nerve are present up to the axonal endings (see Figure 9-27).

CENTRAL NERVOUS SYSTEM

The brain (the cerebellum, cerebrum, and brainstem) and the spinal cord make up the CNS, which is gross anatomically and histologically divided into two major components: gray matter and white matter. The gray versus white appearance is due to the amount of myelinated axons present. In **gray matter** the nervous tissue consists largely of the perikarya or soma of neurons, their dendrites, glia, blood vessels, and a small amount of nerve fibers that may be myelinated (Figure 9-28). The numerous cell branches associated with the different glia, dendrites, and axons are referred to as **neuropil** and can appear in the two-dimensional world of the histological slide as a confusing entanglement of processes (see Figure 9-14). Consequently, thick specimens (sections measuring from 50-200 μm in depth) combined with impregnation stains are often used to appreciate the full morphology of an entire cell, whether a neuron or one of

the neuroglia (Figure 9-29; see also Figures 9-3 and 9-17). The chief morphological characteristic of gray matter then is the presence of the neuronal cell bodies with the comparatively large, round nuclei surrounded by variable amounts of Nissl bodies (see Figure 9-5). In the brain, gray matter is located along the periphery, forming the cortex of the cerebrum and the cortex of the cerebellum (see Figure 9-28). In the spinal cord the gray matter is formed centrally, is H shaped, and surrounds the **central canal** (Figure 9-30). The gray matter, in turn, is surrounded by white matter.

White matter, in general, contrasts sharply from gray matter histologically in its absence of perikarya and in its prevalence of myelinated axons (see Figures 9-5, 9-9, 9-18, and 9-30). Although some unmyelinated nerve fibers may occur within white matter, the hallmark feature of this tissue is the presence of myelinated nerve fibers, which can be aggregated into bundles by neuroglia (fibrous astrocytes). These bundles consist of tracts that largely involve nerve fibers that originate and terminate in the same locations.

Within the brain there are loci of gray matter that are more or less surrounded by white matter and are referred to as **nuclei.** Each nucleus typically receives nerve impulses (input) from one or more tracts that

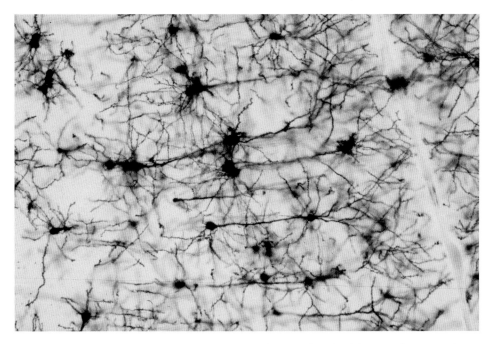

Figure 9-29. Light micrograph of silver-impregnated neurons and glia within the feline cerebrum. (Golgi-Cox stain; ×100.)

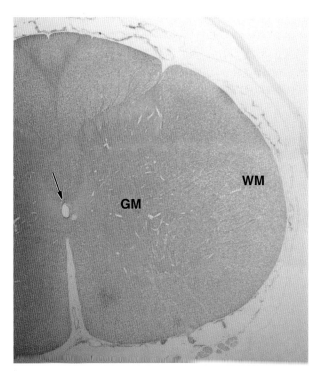

Figure 9-30. Light micrograph of a feline spinal cord, with the white matter *(WM)* located externally to the gray matter *(GM)*. Arrow points to the central canal. (Hematoxylin and eosin stain; ×20.)

come from other nuclei or areas of gray matter within the cortex of the cerebrum or the cerebellum. Likewise, each nucleus provides output and projects nerve impulses along one or more tracts to other centers of neurons. Within a nucleus is a population of small neurons—**interneurons**—that receive the input signal. These cells assist in selecting the appropriate output response. An example is the interneuron cell found in the **dorsal horns** (the upper or dorsal vertical bars of the H) of the spinal cord, which receives input from the sensory neurons (located in the dorsal root ganglion (see Figure 9-30). These cells then communicate with the large multipolar motor neurons located in the *ventral horns* (the lower vertical bars of the H) and form an integration network between the body's sensory and motoneurons. Interneurons in general comprise most of the total population of neurons within the CNS.

CEREBRAL CORTEX

Most of the neuronal cell bodies of the brain lie within the cerebral and cerebellar cortices. The **cerebral cortex** integrates sensory signals, initiates motor response, and is involved in learning and memory activities. It contains six distinguishable layers that form the periphery of the cerebral hemispheres. In domestic species the layers follow a highly undulating surface that consists of ridges **(gyri)** and grooves

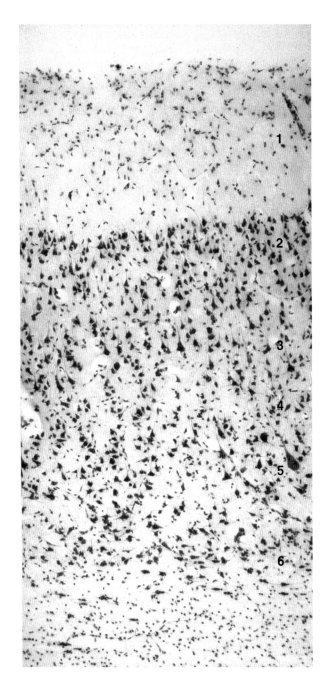

Figure 9-31. Light micrograph of the feline cerebrum and its six layers. *1.* Molecular layer, *2.* external granular layer, *3.* external pyramidal layer, *4.* internal granular layer, *5.* internal pyramidal layer, and *6.* multiform layer. (Nissl [cresyl violet] stain; ×200.)

matter to the cortical surface and measure up to several hundred micrometers in diameter. The principal neuron involved with the vertical integration is the pyramidal cell, which is designed in a way that directs its processes—dendrites and axon—from one layer to another.

Layer I—molecular layer is composed of nerve fibers that originate from other regions of the brain and are mostly oriented tangentially, running parallel with the cortical surface. It can be referred to as the plexiform layer because of the presence of extensive neuropil, which includes dendrites from pyramidal cells that lie farther in the cortex (layer III) and synapse with the incoming afferent fibers.

Layer II—external granular layer (or outer granular layer) contains small stellate interneurons (granule cells) and neuroglia.

Layer III—external pyramidal layer also contains neuroglia and small to large pyramidal neurons that become increasingly larger as they move toward the next inner layer (away from the surface). The neurons in this layer are distinctly pyramidal.

Layer IV—internal granular layer is a comparatively thin layer, consisting of smaller, more closely packed stellate neurons than seen in any other layer of the cortex. These neurons can receive sensory input, and in those areas of visual input—the visual cortex—this layer is quite prominent.

Layer V—internal pyramidal layer is composed of large pyramidal cells distantly arranged from one another, having the least cell density of the cerebral cortex. In motor areas of the cerebral cortex, these cells can be especially large. Their nerve fibers contribute to the white matter.

Layer VI—multiform layer (fusiform layer) possesses neuroglia and neurons that are spindle shaped but can vary a good deal in form and orientation.

CEREBELLAR CORTEX

As in the cerebrum, the gray matter of the cerebellum (the **cerebellar cortex**) forms the periphery of this portion of the brain. Neurons within this tissue are involved in directing activities associated with vestibulation (balance), skeletal coordination, and muscle tone. The cerebellar cortex receives input from proprioceptors associated with skeletal muscle and joints as well as spontaneously from cerebellar nuclei. The cerebellar cortex is divided histologically into three layers that vary little in appearance according to which area of the cerebellum is examined.

The outermost first layer is known as the **molecular layer** and consists of neuropil from dendrites of neurons located within the middle layer and axons of neurons located within the innermost layer. In

(sulci) (Figure 9-31; see also Figure 9-28). Although each layer lacks a well-delineated boundary to demarcate one from the other, they can be distinguished on the basis of prevalent cell type(s) and processes and to a lesser extent on cell densities. Each layer is interconnected with the others in a vertical manner, resulting in columns that extend from the underlying white

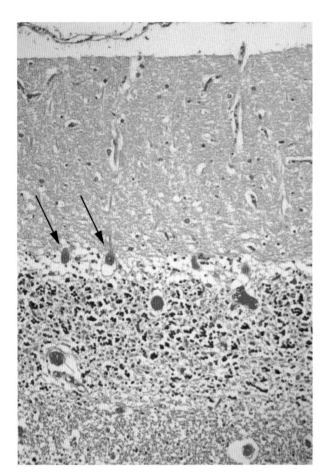

Figure 9-32. Light micrograph of the cerebellum of a manatee. Arrows point to the prominent piriform (Purkinje) cells along the outermost layer. (Hematoxylin and eosin stain; ×100.)

are two other populations of neurons to consider: the basket cell and the Golgi cell. The **basket cell** is an inhibitory neuron located within the innermost regions of the molecular layer next to the layer of piriform cells. Its axonal arborizations form a basket-like lining around the piriform soma, and its dendrites extend into the molecular layer. **Golgi cells** are stellate inhibitory interneurons that lie along the outermost region of the granular layer.

Within the granular layer of the cerebellar cortex are regions called **glomeruli**—synaptic complexes between axons entering the cerebellum, that is, input axons, and the dendrites of granule cells. The input axons form terminations called **mossy endings** (or mossy fibers) that synapse with dendritic branches of adjacent granule cells.

SPINAL CORD

The gray matter and white matter of the tubular-shaped spinal cord are localized in the reverse manner of that which composes the brain. The externally positioned white matter is organized into bundles of ascending and descending nerve fibers (Figure 9-33). Because most of the fibers extend along the longitudinal axis of the spinal cord, only a few are observed entering the white matter from the interior gray matter region. However, occasional bundles of nerve fibers can be found externally within the meningeal covering, either entering or exiting the spinal cord. Nerves exiting the spinal cord (efferent nerves) can be found ventrally, whereas those entering the spinal cord (afferent nerves) are seen dorsally.

When gray matter is viewed histologically in cross section, it appears as a misshapen H or perhaps, more accurately, a butterfly profile, with a **central canal** located in the middle connecting region, known as the **gray commissure** (see Figure 9-30). The ventral and dorsal prongs are the anterior and posterior horns, respectively. Within the horns, especially the anterior horns, the cell bodies of the neurons can be large, consisting of the motor neurons discussed earlier. Interneurons, including those associated with the somatic motor neurons, are largely located within the posterior (dorsal) horns. By comparison, visceral neurons are located predominantly between the ventral and dorsal horns in a more lateral position. These neurons are innervated by neurons of the dorsal root ganglion.

CONNECTIVE TISSUE OF THE CENTRAL NERVOUS SYSTEM

The connective tissue association with the nerve tissue comprising the CNS is considerably more for-

addition are scattered stellate neurons (Figure 9-32). The second or middle layer is thin and is made of a single layer of large neurons known as **piriform cells,** or **Purkinje cells,** which are flask shaped and have enormous dendritic trees that extend into the molecular layer. The axons of these cells are myelinated and project into and through the adjacent innermost third layer, the granular layer, and enter the white matter. In fact, these cells are the only neurons of cerebellar cortex that leave the CNS, acting as efferent neurons that provide inhibition and use GABA as the neurotransmitter. The granular layer (granule cell layer) is characterized by the presence of numerous small neurons **(granule cells),** whose axons are directed in the opposite direction of the piriform cells, projecting into the molecular layer and synapsing with extensive dendritic processes of piriform cells within the molecular layer. In addition to these two major populations of neurons that comprise most of the cerebellar cortex,

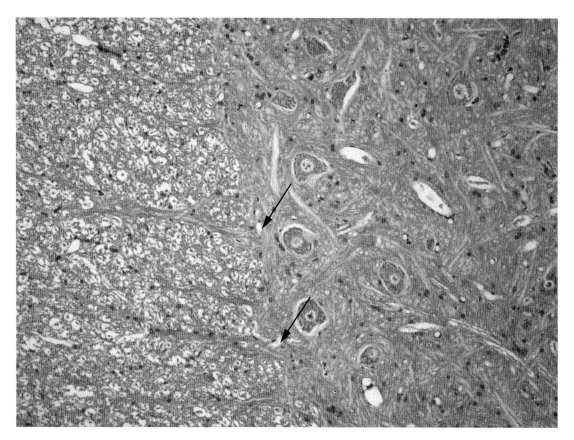

Figure 9-33. Light micrograph of nerve fibers *(arrows)* within gray matter moving from or to the surrounding white matter. (Hematoxylin and eosin stain; ×200.)

midable in providing protection and serving the aerobic demands for neurons than that found in the PNS. Externally, the CNS is lined by the skull and vertebral column, whereas internally it is enveloped by layers of connective tissue called the **meninges.** The meninges consists of three fibrous membranes that completely envelop the CNS: dura mater, arachnoid and pia mater. The **dura mater** (pachymeninx) is the outermost membrane and is composed of two layers: the **periosteal dura,** which is continuous with the periosteum of the inner surface of the cranial bones, and **meningeal dura,** which lies inside the periosteal dura and consists of a variably thick layer of dense connective tissue with fibroblasts. Both layers contain small blood vessels but are well developed in the periosteal dura. The meningeal dura is lined internally by a **border cell layer** composed of one or more layers of epithelial-like fibroblasts that interconnect with each other through gap junctions and desmosomes and are surrounded by a proteoglycan-rich extracellular matrix. Within the vertebral column the dura mater **(spinal dura)** is separated from the periosteum of vertebrae by an **epidural space,** which, in fact, is not a space, but consists of loose connective tissue, adipose, and a network of small veins. Within the cranial dura, sinuses drain the venous blood of the brain.

Internal to the dura mater is the **arachnoid,** which consists of two components: an external membrane of connective tissue that is in direct contact with the dura mater of the brain and a system of trabeculae extending from the membrane of the arachnoid to the pia mater (Figure 9-34). The dura and the arachnoid loosely interface but do not have solid connections with each other. As a result, there is a potential space (subdural space) for fluid such as blood to be held in this area upon injury. Occasionally, in the brain the arachnoid penetrates the dura mater, ending as small protrusions **(arachnoid villi)** into the venous sinuses of the dura mater. The space between the trabeculae comprises the **subarachnoid space,** which contains CSF and blood vessels that course along it sending branches into and away from the nervous tissue. The arachnoid tissues that extend into the venous sinuses of the dura (i.e., the arachnoid villi) are outflow apparatuses for the removal of CSF. When the internal pressure of the CSF within the arachnoid space exceeds the venous blood pressure, the villi dilate and open in a way that facilitates CSF removal from the brain. If the internal pressure within the subarachnoid space is less than that of the venous blood pressure, the villi collapse and prevent blood reflux into the spaces that carry CSF.

The **pia mater** lies immediately adjacent to the nervous tissue. This third portion of the meninges is a thin connective tissue membrane that extends along the irregular surface of the CNS and is able to penetrate it for some length as it lines entering and exiting blood vessels. The pia mater is composed of fine collagenous and elastic fibers and numerous small blood vessels along the external surface of the CNS, resting in contact with the glia beneath. This membrane also is covered by an epithelial-like fibroblastic layer of cells similar to those found in the arachnoid and not unlike that found in serous membranes in general.

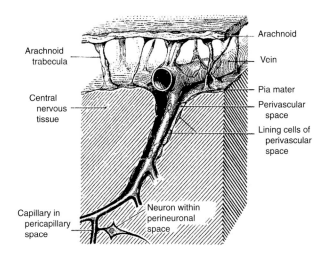

Figure 9-34. Illustration of a portion of the meninges associated with the cerebral cortex. *(Modified from Fawcett DW: Bloom and Fawcett: a textbook of histology, ed 11, Philadelphia, 1986, Saunders.)*

CEREBROSPINAL FLUID AND THE BLOOD-BRAIN BARRIER

The CNS is bathed in its own serum **(CSF)** that is suitable for its functional activities and provides a fluid cushion or shock absorber. CSF is a clear, watery material that electrolytically has a close resemblance to plasma, but contains considerably less protein. CSF is produced by discrete vascular beds known as **choroid plexi** within the ventricles of the brain, where it then continues to flow, eventually leaving through lateral apertures and entering the subarachnoid space and continuing to diffuse freely throughout the nervous tissue as well as be subsequently removed. It also enters the central canal of the spinal cord and bathes that portion of the CNS. The choroid plexi consist of ependymal cells arranged as a simple cuboidal epithelium that comes into direct contact with a capillary bed of the pia mater, which is lined by a fenestrated endothelium (Figure 9-35). The

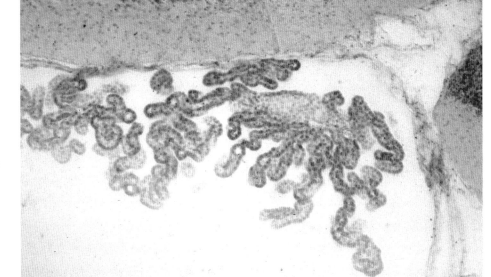

Figure 9-35. Light micrograph of the choroid plexus of a rat. (Nissl [cresyl violet] stain; ×100.)

choroid plexus epithelium passively secretes CSF by diffusion and actively pumps CSF by Na^+ secretion.

The **blood-brain barrier** maintains the differences between the composition of CSF and blood. This barrier is established by the presence of **continuous capillaries** that serve to nourish and oxygenate the neurons and their support cells within the nervous tissue. These vessels are lined by endothelial cells that form tight junctions (fasciae occludentes) and contribute greatly to the selective barrier. Vesicular movement of materials is performed by **receptor-mediated transport.** Different carrier proteins facilitate the movement of glucose, amino acids, and other molecules from blood into the nervous tissue. The end feet of the astrocytes, which form the **perivascular glia limitans,** also contribute to the blood-brain barrier through their selective absorption and subsequent movement of materials to and from adjacent neurons.

SUGGESTED READINGS

Bergman RA, Afifi AK, Heidger PM Jr: *Histology,* Philadelphia, 1996, Saunders.

Bray D, Gilbert D: Cytoskeletal elements in neurons, *Ann Rev Neurosci* 4:505, 1981.

Colombo JA, Fuchs E, Hartig W, et al: "Rodent-like" and "primate-like" types of astroglial architecture in the adult cerebral cortex of mammals: a comparative study, *Anat Embryol* 201:111, 2000.

Fawcett DW: *Bloom and Fawcett: a textbook of histology,* ed 11, Philadelphia, 1986, Saunders.

Gartner LP, Hiatt JL: *Color textbook of histology,* Philadelphia, 1997, Saunders.

Lentz TL: *Cell fine structure: an atlas of drawings of whole-cell structure,* Philadelphia, 1971, Saunders.

Martinelli C, Sartori P, Leda M, Pannese E: Age-related quantitative changes in mitochondria of satellite cell sheaths enveloping spinal ganglion neurons in the rabbit, *Brain Res Bull* 61:147, 2003.

Morest DK, Silver J: Precursors of neurons, neuroglia, and ependymal cells in the CNS: What are they? Where are they from? How do they get where they are going? *Glia* 43:6, 2003.

Onteniente B, Kimura H, Maeda T: Comparative study of the glial fibrillary acidic protein in vertebrates by PAP immunohistochemistry, *J Comp Neurol* 215:427, 1983.

Peters A, Palay SL, de F Webster H: *The fine structure of the nervous system: the neurons and supporting cells,* Philadelphia, 1976, Saunders.

Szalay F: Development of the equine brain motor system, *Neurobiology* 9:107, 2001.

Yokoyama A, Yang L, Itoh S, et al: Microglia, a potential source of neurons, astrocytes, and oligodendrocytes, *Glia* 45:96, 2004.

Circulatory System

KEY CHARACTERISTICS

- Designed to carry blood gases, nutrients, waste materials, cells of defense, lymph, and hormones throughout the body
- Consists of blood and lymphatic vascular systems:
   Blood vascular system is composed of an arrangement of heart-pumped vessels interconnected throughout the body with walls of incremental thickness and permeability:
   artery, arteriole, capillary, venule, and vein
   Lymphatic vascular system is composed of thin-walled, nonpumped vessels, restricted in range and interconnected with lymph and the blood vascular system
- Separate population of support cells:
   Pericyte

Among domestic animals the delivery and removal of nutrients, hormones, waste materials, and gases are essential or tantamount for the survival of any tissue within the body. The movement of these substances is provided by a network of conduits that collectively constitutes the circulatory system, subdivided into the **cardiovascular system,** which transports blood throughout the body by way of the **heart,** and the **lymphatic vascular system,** which carries excess extracellular tissue fluid that is watery and comparatively cell free and empties it into the cardiovascular system.

CARDIOVASCULAR SYSTEM

The movement of blood within the cardiovascular system is performed by the heart and its ability to push blood into two separate circuits: the **systemic circuit** (involved in the circulation of blood to all organs of the body) and the **pulmonary circuit** (circulates blood only to the lung). Both circuits are composed of a series of vessels that decrease in diameter as they move away from the heart.

BLOOD VESSELS

In the systemic circuit the **arteries** are vessels that direct blood to the different organs of the body; they branch a number of times and become smaller in luminal diameter with each branch. Eventually, arteries end in thin-walled vessels (**capillaries**) that possess narrow lumens and form various anastomosing arrangements known as **capillary beds** (Figure 10-1). The capillary and its bed offer the optimal environment for the exchange of nutrients, wastes, gases, and other substances to occur between blood and adjacent tissues. Capillaries and their beds empty into **veins** that progressively increase in diameter and become

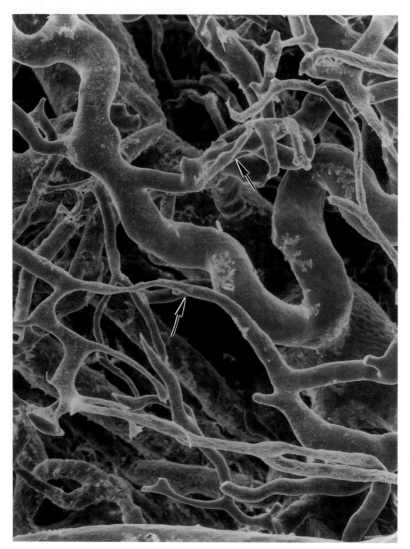

Figure 10-1. Scanning electron micrograph of a corrosion casting of an equine vascular bed. Arrows point to the smallest vessels, consisting of capillaries. (×210.)

fewer as they converge and course their way back to the heart.

Throughout the body, each type of blood vessel—artery, vein, and capillary—has its own distinguishing structural features. Overall, in a specific tissue, the artery is a high-pressure vessel that has a broader and more developed wall surrounding a smaller luminal diameter than that of a corresponding vein. Wall thicknesses of the different blood vessels also may vary according to their location with regard to a specific species. For example, the arteries of the iris within the eyes of pigs are unusually thick walled when compared with those of other domestic species and characteristic for that animal. Similar variations of blood vessel morphology occur in long-necked ungulates such as the giraffe and in deep-diving marine mammals.

Typically, each blood vessel is composed of two or three concentric layers or tunics (Figure 10-2). The innermost portion of the interior layer—the **tunica**

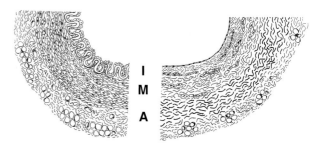

Figure 10-2. Diagram of a typical middle-sized artery (left) and vein (right) and their three layers as seen in cross section. *I,* Tunica intima; *M,* tunica media; *A,* tunica adventitia.

intima—is a cylinder of simple squamous epithelium that lines the vessel lumen. The cells of this epithelium (usually referred to as the endothelium) do not possess evenly shaped widths and lengths as in other simple squamous epithelia, but are more elongated in the direction of the vessel axis. The endothelium forms a basal lamina that is attached to a **subendothelial layer,** consisting of a variable amount of loose connective tissue and scattered smooth muscle fibers. Outside the subendothelial layer may be the **internal elastic lamina,** composed of a fenestrated sheet of elastin that can be prominent in muscular arteries.

Outside the internal elastic lamina, cells consisting primarily of smooth muscle fibers are concentrically arranged in layers and interspersed with elastic fibers and collagen (type III). This region is the **tunica media,** which is prominent in the large muscular arteries, and can have an **external elastic lamina** that is composed of a thinner, less prominent layer of elastic fibers found in the internal elastic lamina of the tunica intima. The tunica media is essentially associated with the artery and nearly disappears as the arteries become small and join the capillary.

The **tunica adventitia** or **tunica externa** forms the external-most layer of blood vessels, consisting of variable amounts of fibrocytes, collagen (type I), and elastic fibers that are largely oriented along the longitudinal axes of the vessels and merge seamlessly with adjacent connective tissues.

ARTERIES

Arteries are vessels that move blood from the heart to capillary beds, and possess the triple-layered walls previously described. Arteries specifically originate from the right and left ventricles as the **pulmonary trunk** and **aorta,** respectively. The pulmonary trunk and arteries derived from it are described in Chapter 11. Immediately from the aorta, the right and left coronary arteries arise, supplying the cardiac muscle tissue with an extensive labyrinth of blood vessels. As the aorta moves away from the heart, large arterial branches initially arise from its arch and form the right brachiocephalic, the left carotid and the left subclavian arteries that supply the anterior-most regions of the body. Posteriorly, the aorta continues to send off branches to the body wall and viscera and eventually bifurcates abdominally into the right and left common iliac arteries. Each of the major vessels originating from the aorta undergoes a series of branches that result in vessels that become progressively smaller. Along with changes in the size of the arteries, other morphological differences occur, allowing arteries to be characterized into three categories or types: elastic arteries, muscular arteries, and arterioles (Table 10-1).

Elastic Arteries

The largest arteries, including the aorta and its branches, are elastic arteries, also known as **conduct-** **ing arteries.** These vessels have extremely thick, three-layered walls (tunics) and possess abundant elastin to the point that they can appear yellow in their gross morphological appearance. Their innermost layer, the tunica intima, has a simple squamous endothelial lining; its cells' lengths typically measure two to three times greater than their widths and are oriented in the direction as the artery's axis (Figure 10-3). The endothelial cells are tightly attached (zonula occludens) and contain membrane-bound rodlike inclusions, **Weibel-Palade bodies,** that help facilitate the coagulation of platelets during blood clotting. The tunica intima, also, consists of the basal lamina of the endothelium and a thin, enveloping subendothelial area or layer of connective tissue, including fibroblasts; collagen, which is oriented for the most part longitudinally; occasional smooth muscle cells; and an outer mesh of elastic fibers (internal elastic lamina). The middle layer, the tunica media, is by far the most developed of the three tunics, possessing multiple layers or sleeves of concentrically arranged smooth muscle fibers, with each sleeve separated by and attached to a meshwork-like lamella of elastin fibers (see Figure 10-3). Although the tunica intima is able to receive its nourishment and oxygen by direct diffusion through the endothelial lining, the entire tunica media cannot be supported by direct diffusion and instead is supplied by the **vasa vasorum,** composed of small arteries that originate from the large artery and penetrate the densely packed smooth muscle-elastic fiber environment of the tunica media. The outermost region of the tunica media is made up of one last sheet of elastic fibers, the **external elastic lamina or membrane,** which is less developed than the other elastic lamellae and forms an interface with the tunica externa. The tunica externa of these large arteries is comparably thin, often less than half the thickness of the tunica media, and is composed mostly of loosely arranged collagen and elastic fibers, intermixed with fibrocytes, occasional histiocytes and elements of the vasa vasorum and nerve **(nervi vasorum).**

Muscular Arteries

As the elastic arteries branch and become smaller, including the less prominent arteries that extend from the aorta, the muscular arteries are formed. These arteries are characterized by the abundance of smooth muscle within their walls and comprise most of the named arteries found throughout the body. The tunica intima of muscular arteries has an endothelial lining and subtending basal lamina that are similar to those of elastic arteries. The adjacent subendothelial layer of muscular arteries, however, differs in that it is

TABLE 10-1	Characteristics of Different Types of Blood Vessels		
BLOOD VESSEL	TUNICA INTIMA	TUNICA MEDIA	TUNICA ADVENTITIA
Elastic artery (conducting artery) large arteries	Endothelium with Weibel-Palade bodies and basal lamina, and subendothelial layer lined incompletely by a thin internal elastic lamina	Numerous elastic membranes, each interspersed with smooth muscle and additional connective tissue, within outer portion; thin external elastic lamina including vasa vasorum	Thin adventitial tissue with vasa vasorum and nerve (bundles and fibers)
Muscular artery (distributing artery) medium to small arteries	Endothelium with Weibel-Palade bodies and basal lamina, and subendothelial layer lined by a thick internal elastic lamina	Few to many layers of smooth muscle with a single elastic membrane consisting of a thick external elastic lamina	Thin adventitial tissue with small vasa vasorum and nerve (bundles and fibers)
Arteriole (100 μm or less in diameter)	Endothelium with Weibel-Palade bodies and basal lamina, and thin subendothelial layer without an internal elastic lamina	One to two layers of smooth muscle	Thin adventitial tissue with nerve (fibers)
Metarteriole	Endothelium and basal lamina	Discontinuous smooth muscle forms precapillary sphincter	Thin loose connective tissue
Capillary	Same with pericytes	No smooth muscle	Same
Venule	Endothelium and basal lamina with pericytes	Thin connective tissue with oriented occasional circularly smooth muscle cells when enlarging to small vein	Thin loose connective tissue
Medium and small veins	Endothelium and basal lamina with valves in some, subendothelial connective tissue	Thin connective tissue with occasional circularly oriented smooth muscle cells	Thick adventitial tissue, forming bulk of the wall
Large vein	Endothelium and basal lamina with valves in some, subendothelial connective tissue with elastic membrane in some	Thin connective tissue with occasional circularly oriented smooth muscle cells	Thick adventitial tissue, forming bulk of the wall with bundles of longitudinally oriented smooth muscle cells

thicker (in large vessels) and contains a prominent internal elastic lamina (Figure 10-4). In these arteries all components of the tunica intima often appear undulated, especially in cross section. Much of the undulation is due to the contraction of the smooth muscle during fixation and processing of the blood vessel, which also results in a reduction of the luminal diameter and amount of blood contained within. In smaller arteries that become naturally reduced in size (by branching not fixation), the meshlike internal elastic lamina concomitantly thins, and occasional cell processes of the endothelium extend to the innermost smooth muscle cells of the tunica media and form gap junctions with them. The tunica media consists of smooth muscle that for the most part is circularly arranged as in elastic arteries. However, unlike the tunica media of elastic fibers, the muscle cells are enveloped by their own basal laminae and collagen (type III) with only a relatively small amount of elastic fibers. Elastic lamellae are essentially absent throughout most of the tunica media except along the outer-

most region, where an **external elastic lamina** is formed that is prominent in larger muscular arteries, consisting of several or more layers of thin, fenestrated sheets of elastic fibers (see Figure 10-4). The tunica adventitia of muscular arteries is much like that of elastic arteries, having loosely arranged collagen and elastic fibers, interspersed with fibrocytes, nerve fibers and their endings, and occasional histiocytes.

Arterioles

Arteries that are generally less than 0.1 mm in diameter are referred to as **arterioles.** The triwalled construction seen in elastic and muscular arteries is greatly reduced. The tunica intima continues to consist of an endothelial sheet that lines the lumen, its subtending basal lamina, a small amount of collagen and elastic fibers (i.e., the subendothelial layer) that disappears as the arterioles become confluent with capillaries, and an internal elastic lamina. The tunica media can contain up to several layers of

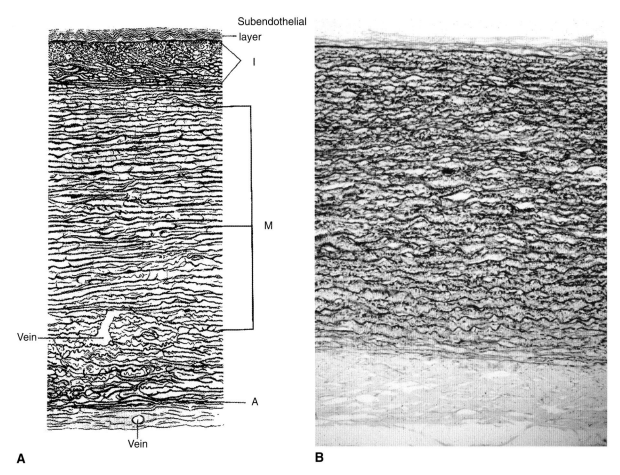

A
B

Figure 10-3. A, Diagram of an elastic artery in the longitudinal plane. *I,* tunica intima including subendothelial layer; *M,* tunica media; *A,* tunica adventitia. **B,** Light micrograph of the aorta. (Elastic [Verhoeff] stain; ×100.) *(A modified from Fawcett DW:* Bloom and Fawcett: a textbook of histology, *ed 11, Philadelphia, 1986, Saunders.)*

smooth muscle cells surrounded by their basal laminae and collagen and elastic fibers. In the smallest arterioles, the smooth muscle cells form a single layer, which is still concentrically arranged, and interfaces directly with the equally sparse tunica externa (Figure 10-5). The external elastic lamina that occurs in elastic and muscular arteries is not present in arterioles. As arterioles connect with capillaries, the smooth muscle can become separated into small bundles or simply become individually isolated. These vessels are **metarterioles,** and the muscle of these vessels can function as a precapillary sphincter that assists blood flow regulation. Metarterioles can also directly connect with small veins and bypass or shunt a capillary bed altogether (Figure 10-6).

CAPILLARIES

Capillaries are blood vessels designed for the exchange of a variety of substances between blood and adjacent tissues, including nutrients, wastes and gases.

The design is simple in construction—a single layer of squamous-shaped endothelial cells and their basal lamina with a very small amount of adventitial material and occasional undifferentiated, stemlike cells (pericytes). The luminal diameters of capillaries are typically small, allowing the flow of blood cells to move through them in single file (Figure 10-7). The diameters are not identical throughout the body, varying from tissue to tissue. They mostly range from 5 to 10 μm, but change very little within a specific tissue.

As in arterial vessels, the lengths of capillary endothelia (usually 25 μm and longer) travel in the same direction as the vessel and are two to three times greater than their widths. These cells can be extraordinarily thin. In the lung's alveoli, or air sacs, the capillaries' endothelia can be less than 0.2 μm thick, which is necessary for proper blood gas exchange (Figure 10-8). The curvature of the cells is more accentuated in these vessels than in arteries and veins due to the small luminal diameters, which

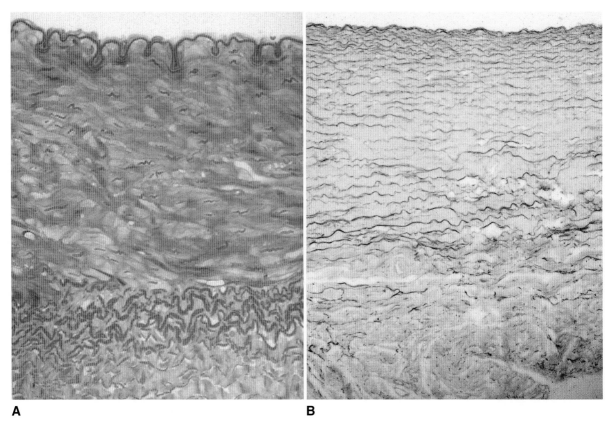

A   **B**

Figure 10-4. A, Light micrograph of a contracted muscular artery of the monkey in cross section. (Hematoxylin and eosin stain; ×100.) **B,** Light micrograph of a canine muscular artery in longitudinal section. (Elastic [Verhoeff] stain; ×100.)

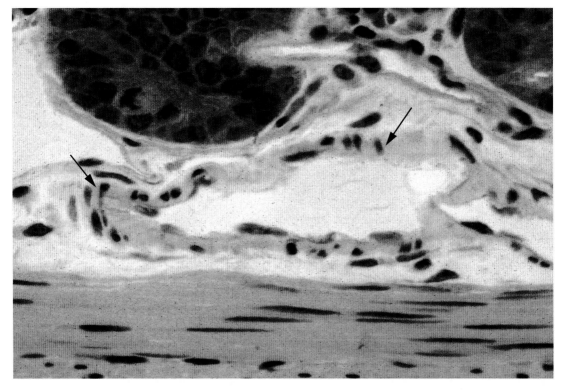

Figure 10-5. Light micrograph of an arteriole of the mouse mostly oriented in the longitudinal plane. Arrows point to the single layer of smooth muscle that encircles the endothelium of this blood vessel. (Plastic section, hematoxylin and eosin stain; ×400.)

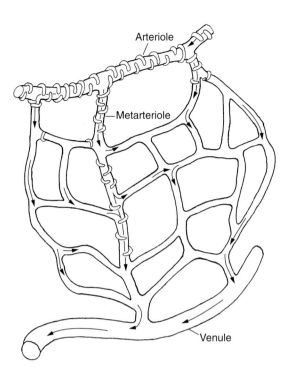

Figure 10-6. Diagram of a capillary bed and a metarteriole arising from an arteriole. Arrows point to the direction of blood flow.

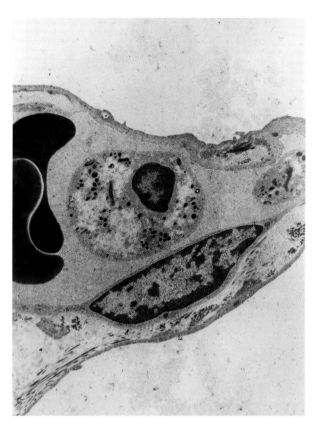

Figure 10-7. Transmission electron micrograph (×7000) of a capillary within the alveolus of a canine lung.

permits only the passage of single cells. The cell's cytoplasm tends to be sparsely populated with organelles, which consist of occasional mitochondria, rough endoplasmic reticulum (rER), polysomes, and a Golgi apparatus. Intermediate filaments, desmin or vimentin, coexist, but largely around the nucleus. The most numerous and readily observed feature is the presence of numerous small vesicles, specifically pinocytotic vesicles closely associated with the cell membrane (see Figure 10-7). Variations of endothelial morphology do occur and have resulted in the construction of several categories: continuous, fenestrated, porous, and sinusoidal.

Continuous Capillaries

Continuous capillaries are blood vessels not interrupted by any physical space such as a pore. The endothelial cells associated with these vessels are interconnected along their lateral sides by cell junctions that include tight junctions (zonula occludens) that, in turn, prevent any substances from circumventing this cellular lining. As a result any material that resides inside the lumen of this capillary must pass through the endothelium before entering the adjacent tissue and vice versa. In many continuous capillaries the exchange of materials is performed by a combina-

tion of endocytosis and exocytosis, a process known as **transcytosis,** and usually occurs from the luminal side toward adjacent tissue. As a result many pinocytotic vesicles are often within the cytoplasm of the endothelial cell (see Figure 10-8). Other transport systems, including the use of enzymes such as Na^+K^+ ATPase, may be present along the sides of these cells. The continuous capillary is common throughout the body and especially prevalent in nervous tissue. The undifferentiated perivascular cell **(pericyte)** is often associated with the continuous capillary. Pericytes share the basement membrane of the endothelium, and are encapsulated by it. Cell processes of pericytes can come into contact with the endothelium, forming gap junctions with the latter. Further angiogenesis (the formation of new blood vessels) can be contributed by cell division of pericytes. Pericytes also are able to be transformed into other mesodermally derived cells, including fibroblasts and smooth muscle.

Fenestrated Capillaries

Fenestrated capillaries do not form a continuous cellular lining around the lumen, but instead possess numerous round fenestrae, approximately 60 to 80 nm in diameter, that are spanned by a diaphragm-like

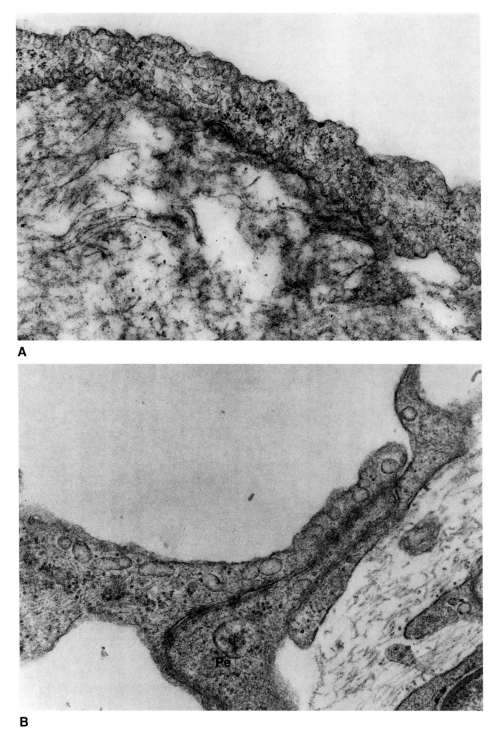

A

B

Figure 10-8. A, Transmission electron micrograph (×40,000) of pinocytotic vesicles within the cytoplasm of an endothelial cell lining a capillary. **B,** Transmission electron micrograph (×40,000) of adjoining endothelial cells and adjacent pericyte *(Pe)* lining a continuous capillary.

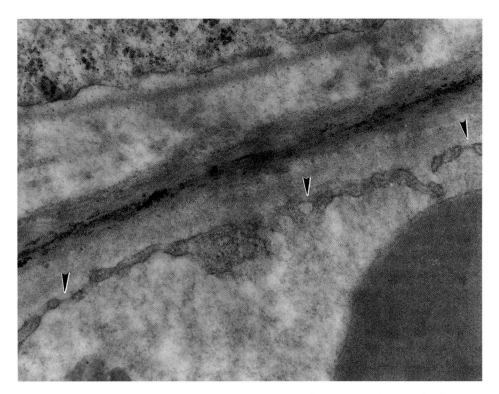

Figure 10-9. Transmission electron micrograph (×50,000) of a fenestrated capillary in the pig. The fenestrae *(arrowheads)* can be seen in profile as well as face-on.

structure that is thinner than the thickness of the cell membrane (Figure 10-9). The fenestrae are believed to facilitate the movement of molecular materials, which can be considerably large, into and out of the capillary lumen. Fenestrated capillary beds are associated with components of the endocrine system and the gastrointestinal tract. A form of the fenestrated capillary is the **porous capillary** in the kidney, specifically the region known as the *renal glomerulus*. In this instance, the pores lack diaphragms and much of the orderly arrangement that fenestrae often have.

Sinusoidal Capillaries

In certain regions in the body where blood becomes pooled and conforms to the shape that has been made available. Vessels within these regions are known as **sinusoids** or **sinusoidal capillaries** and occur within the liver, spleen, and other lymphoidal organs, bone marrow, and selected glands of the endocrine system. Sinusoids have often asymmetrical lumina and are porous, having variably sized diameters, some quite wide, and lacking the diaphragms that are characteristic of fenestrae. Blood flow varies greatly—from rapid in the choroidal sinusoids of the eye to slow to nearly nonexistent in the hematopoietic tissues.

VEINS

Unlike arteries, veins are characterized and categorized less on architectural construction and more on size. Consequently, they are traditionally described as small, medium, and large. This is not to say that veins lack the tunics found in arteries, because the three tunics—tunica intima, tunica media and tunica adventitia—do exist, but they are not usually as defined as those in arteries. In fact, the walls of veins are for the most part conspicuously thinner and less developed than those of the associated arteries within a specific portion of the body. However, because of the variety of mechanical conditions in different areas of the body that can influence venous structure, substantial variations of venous architecture can be found. For example, veins can possess **valves**—semilunar flaplike extensions of the tunica intima. This is especially true for veins that lie within the limbs of the body.

The smallest veins are **venules** and correspond to arterioles with regard to both location and function (see Figure 10-6, *inset*). Venules, in turn, empty into **medium-sized veins,** also known as **collecting veins,** and correspond functionally and by location to the muscular arteries. **Large veins** direct blood back to the

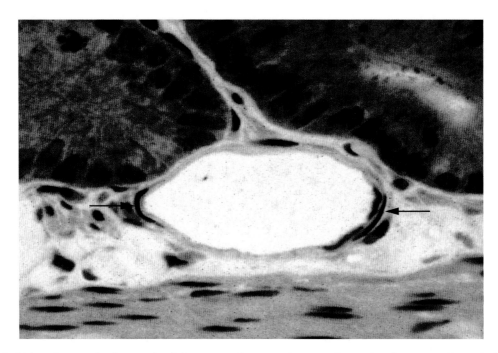

Figure 10-10. Light micrograph of a venule of the mouse. Arrows point to pericytes that lie next to the endothelium of this blood vessel. (Plastic section, hematoxylin and eosin stain; ×400.)

heart and from there to the lung. These veins, which include the jugular, renal, pulmonary, and portal veins and vena cava, correspond to the aorta and its principal branches (see Table 10-1).

Small Veins

Veins that are immediately associated with and drain capillaries are **postcapillary venules** and have the same construction as the adjoining capillaries, differing primarily in their luminal diameters, which range from 15 to 25 μm (Figures 10-10 and 10-11). Typically the endothelium can be vasoactively stimulated (by histamine and other similar agents) and is surrounded by a layer of pericytes and a small amount of connective tissue (tunica adventitia or externa). As the venules gradually increase in diameter, 30 μm and greater, they become enveloped by one or two incomplete layers of smooth muscle, constituting a tunica media, and an outer sheath of connective tissue, comprising the tunica externa. These vessels **(muscular venules)** eventually become larger and lead into small veins. The venules that arise from a continuous capillary bed are often more permeable in construction than the associated capillaries, especially regarding cell junctions, such as occluding and adhering junctions. Consequently, vasodilators, which are released during allergic reactions and inflammation, are effective in enhancing venule permeability, even more

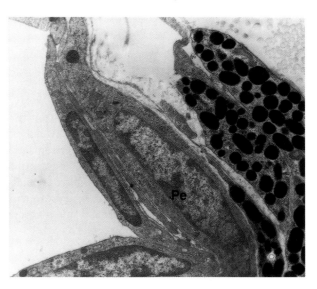

Figure 10-11. Transmission electron micrograph (×5000) of a venule in the iris of the pig. *Pe,* Pericyte.

than that in continuous capillaries, and result in the translocation of white blood cells and concomitant extravasation of plasma into adjacent tissues. The small veins are largely similar to the muscular venules, having increased diameter widths and closely spaced smooth muscle, which at this point forms a continuous layer (Figure 10-12).

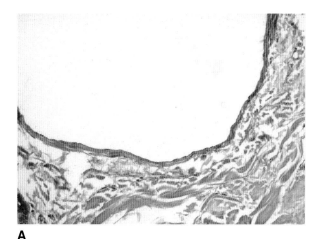

A

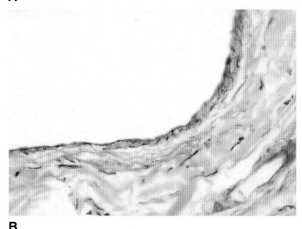

B

Figure 10-12. Light micrographs of a small vein. **A,** Hematoxylin and eosin stain; ×200. **B,** Elastic (Verhoeff) stain; ×400.

Medium Veins

As the small veins enlarge in diameter, they transform into medium veins with three well-developed tunics. Medium veins are typically less than 1 cm in diameter and drain most of the body into the large veins. The tunica intima, here, contains a small amount of subendothelial connective tissue, including elastic fibers, that forms a thin network around the endothelium rather than the lamina seen in arteries. In many medium veins, extensions of the tunica intima form valves, projecting on an angle into the lumen as a pair of bileaflets in the direction of blood flow. In this way, blood flow is further facilitated as it is directed to the heart, while at the same time the potential for the backflow of blood is blocked. The tunica media possesses smooth muscle loosely woven and circularly wound around the tunica intima. The tunica externa of medium veins is usually well defined, and thicker than the tunica media. Its elements—collagen, elastic

fiber meshwork, fibroblasts, and occasional small bundles of smooth muscle—are oriented along the longitudinal axis of each vein (see Figure 10-2). Although the amount of muscle within the outer two tunics is considerably less than that of corresponding arteries, there is fairly wide variation in this amount due to the different physical forces exerted, especially within the body's extremities.

Large Veins

Large veins comprise the major veins of the body, which, as mentioned, are those that return blood back to the heart. Their construction differs from medium veins in several ways. The tunica intima is more pronounced than that of medium veins, having a thicker subendothelial layer and an elastic fiber network (Figure 10-13). The tunica media differs from that of medium veins even more by being generally much less developed. In most instances, the tunica media is thin to nonexistent, having very little smooth muscle associated with it. However, the tunica externa of large veins is similar to that of medium veins—comparably thick and with its components, including smooth muscle, oriented longitudinally or spirally.

ARTERIOVENOUS SHUNTS

Although most arteries end by joining capillary beds, some deliver blood directly to the venous portion of the vascular system. In these instances, **arteriovenous anastomosis** occurs, resulting in shunts that bypass capillaries (see Figure 10-6). These shunts, which may occur within a capillary bed itself, influence substantially the blood flow of capillaries within a specific tissue, including portions of the reproductive tracts, gastrointestinal tract, and integument. When open, blood flow within these anastomoses can reduce blood flow within adjacent capillaries markedly. Conversely, when the shunts are closed, capillary blood flow increases. The proximal arterial segment **(metarteriole)** is structurally identical to the typical arteriole and equipped with smooth muscle that functions as a sphincter and in effect closes the shunt. Similarly, branches of the arterioles leading to the capillary bed possess their own sphincter, the **precapillary sphincter,** which when contracted reduces capillary blood flow (see Figure 10-6).

HEART

Blood flow within the cardiovascular system is provided by its single largest component, the heart. The heart with its powerful wall of muscle consists of four

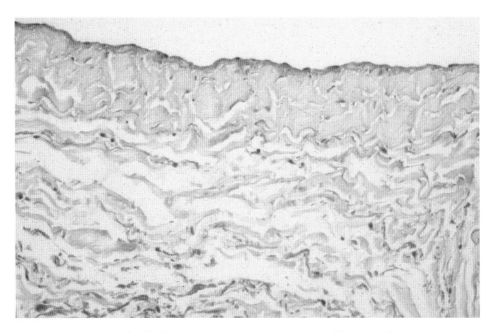

Figure 10-13. Light micrograph of a large vein (vena cava) in the dog. (Hematoxylin and eosin stain; ×200.)

chambers: two of which receive blood, the **atria,** and lead to two that discharge blood, the **ventricles.** Each atrium is separated from the respective ventricle by a valve that functions to prevent the backflow of blood (Figure 10-14). Venous blood from most of the body empties into the right atrium by way of the **superior** and **inferior cavae.** With the opening of the intervening valve **(right atrioventricular valve),** blood enters the right ventricle and is propelled to the lung by the right and left pulmonary arteries. With the return of oxygenated erythrocytes from the pulmonary veins, blood reenters the heart and goes into the left atrium. Upon the opening of the **left atrioventricular valve,** blood fills the left ventricle before being discharged back to the body via the aorta. The wall of the heart with its richly endowed muscle is composed of three layers: the **epicardium,** the **myocardium,** and the **endocardium.** In some ways, they are homologous to the three tunics of the blood vessel: the tunica externa, tunica media, and tunica intima, respectively.

EPICARDIUM

The outer lining of the heart is the **epicardium** and consists of an external serous layer or mesothelium—the **visceral layer of the pericardium**—and an inner fascia-like layer of connective tissue—the fibrous layer. The fibrous layer, which internally lies next to the mesothelium, externally attaches to the myocardium. This layer consists of a thin lining of loose connective tissue housing coronary vessels,

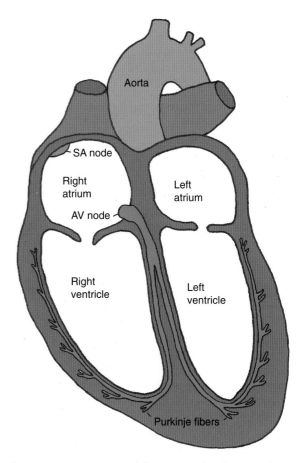

Figure 10-14. Diagram of the mammalian heart with its four chambers exposed along the coronal plane. *AV,* Atrioventricular; *SA,* sinoatrial.

nerves, and ganglia as well as adipose tissue. Where the major vessels exit the heart, the mesothelium continues along their outermost portion and then reflexes around the heart as the **parietal layer of the pericardium.** As a result, the heart lies in a thin cavity filled with serous fluid, which is lined by the mesothelia that form the visceral and parietal layers of the pericardium.

MYOCARDIUM

The **myocardium,** as the name implies, is the layer that contains the cardiac muscle and easily the thickest portion of the heart wall, being more developed along the ventricles than the atria. Although the vast majority of the myocytes are linked to each other in an end-to-end manner, forming spirally oriented, interwoven chains of cells around each chamber, some of these cells are modified to attach to the fibrous connective tissue element within this layer as well as along the borders of the epicardium and endocardium. Other muscle cells are modified to function in a nerve-like manner, providing impulse conduction, and even others function as endocrine cells.

Within the junction of the superior vena cava and the right atrium, there are specialized cardiac muscle cells that control the contraction of the entire heart (i.e., the heart rate) (see Figure 10-14). These cells are able to depolarize anywhere from 30 to 250 times per minute and comprise the **sinoatrial (SA) node**—the pacemaker of the heart. The generated impulse is spread through the atrial walls by internodal pathways, some ending at the atrioventricular node. These pathways consist of small branching modified muscle fibers that lack the typical intercalated disks and contain only sparse amounts of myofilaments. The **atrioventricular (AV) node** is positioned above the tricuspid valve within the septal wall. This node, which is composed of cells that are similar in morphology to those associated with the internodal pathways, gives rise to the **atrioventricular bundle.** The atrioventricular bundle transmits the impulse down the interventricular septum within the subendocardial connective tissue. The cells of this bundle have centrally placed nuclei, contain large amounts of glycogen that lie inside of scattered, peripherally placed myofibrils, and are interconnected end-to-end by intercalated discs. As the bundle branches, these cells **(Purkinje fibers)** (see Figure 8-20) eventually connect with the traditional muscle cells of the myocardium.

Even though the myocardium is not governed directly by the CNS, it does vary the rate of the heartbeat and its stroke volume. Through the stimulation of sympathetic innervation, which increases the rate, and parasympathetic innervation, which decreases the rate, the autonomic nervous system is able to regulate the activity of the heart.

The myocardium of both atria and ventricles is embraced by connective tissue in a way that forms a fibrous **cardiac skeleton,** to which some of the muscle cells are attached. The cardiac skeleton consists of: **fibrous rings** of interwoven collagen bundles that are located around the aorta and pulmonary arterial openings and those associated with the atrioventricular valves; the connective tissue that joins the fibrous rings, which is referred to as the **fibrous triangle;** and the fibrous bundles of collagen that form the membranous portion of the **interventricular septum.** Although the construction of the cardiac skeleton is similar among domestic species, the fibrous triangle varies considerably in its composition, ranging from dense irregular connective tissue in the cat and pig, fibrocartilage in the dog, and hyaline cartilage in the horse, to bone in the cow.

ENDOCARDIUM

The lining of the heart's cavities within the atria and ventricles is the **endocardium** and is similar in structure to the tunica intima of adjoining blood vessels. The innermost layer consists of the single-layered squamous endothelium that overlies inner and outer subendothelial layers (Figure 10-15). The **outer subendothelial layer** (subendocardial layer) contains loose connective tissue, including small blood vessels, nerves, and in localized areas impulse-conducting cells (Purkinje fibers). This layer, in turn, is connected to the **inner subendothelial layer,** which contains an elastic dense irregular connective tissue interwoven with smooth muscle cells. The cardiac valves can be considered a flaplike extension of the endocardium, having an abundant amount of collagen that merges with the fibrous rings and triangle.

LYMPHATIC VESSELS

In addition to the system of vessels that channel plasma and blood cells throughout the body, is the **lymphatic vascular system**—an adjoining network of vessels that functions to collect excess tissue fluid called **lymph** and contribute to the body's defense. Lymph is not circulated throughout the body in the way that blood is, but rather moves passively by diffusion from the interstitial spaces of adjacent tissues, usually loose connective tissue, into **lymphatic capillaries,** the smallest of the lymphatic vessels. From there, lymph is progressively emptied into larger vessels until it reaches **collecting ducts,** which drain the lymph into venous portion of the circulatory system.

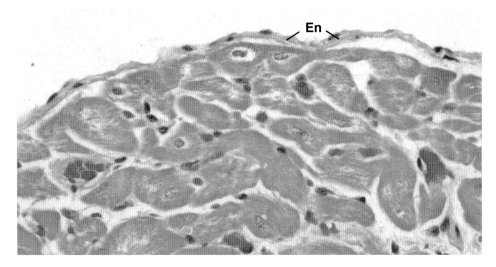

Figure 10-15. Light micrograph of the endocardium *(En)* of the pig. (Hematoxylin and eosin stain; ×400.)

LYMPHATIC CAPILLARIES

The smallest of the lymphatic vessels, the lymphatic capillaries are not open-ended as in blood capillaries, but end blindly in a loose connective tissue environment. These vessels vary in diameter, being often larger than that of blood capillaries, and are lined by endothelia that consist of a single-layered epithelium that either lacks a basal lamina or possesses an incompletely formed one. Tissue serum moves into the capillary lumen by passing through the cells or within spaces of variable sizes between adjacent endothelial cells because they do not possess tight junctions. Consequently, these vessels are freely permeable to protein and quite capable of removing protein-rich fluid. Overall, lymphatic capillaries can resemble blood capillaries, especially porous capillaries, but generally lack the more defined organization that blood capillary endothelia have. Adjacent endothelial cells can be attached to each other by desmosomes or simply overlay each other for a short distance. In the absence of a well-formed basal lamina, the base of each of these cells is connected to adjacent collagen and elastic fibers by their own filaments, **lymphatic anchoring filaments** that are organized in tufts and believed to participate in keeping the lumen open or patent (Figure 10-16).

SMALL AND MEDIUM LYMPHATIC VESSELS

Lymphatic capillaries lead into small lymphatic vessels (Figure 10-17) that, in turn, drain into medium-sized lymphatic vessels. Both small and

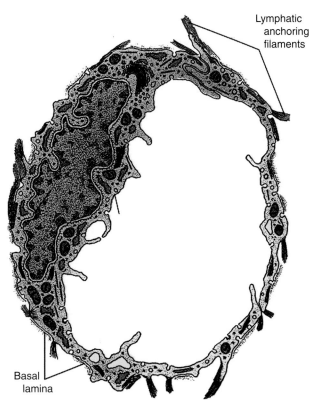

Lymphatic anchoring filaments

Basal lamina

Figure 10-16. Diagram taken from an ultrastructural representation of a lymphatic capillary. *(From Gartner LP, Hiatt JL: Color textbook of histology, Philadelphia, 1997, Saunders; modified from Lentz TL: Cell fine structure: an atlas of drawings of whole-cell structure, Philadelphia, 1971, Saunders.)*

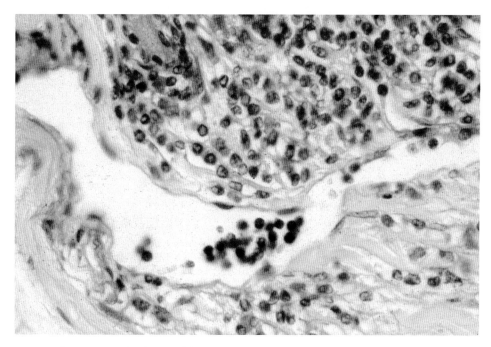

Figure 10-17. Light micrograph of a small lymphatic vessel in the dog. (Hematoxylin and eosin stain; ×400.)

medium lymphatic vessels possess valves that can be closely spaced. The endothelium of these vessels now forms continuous basal lamina. The region surrounding the endothelium resembles that found in veins, but is not as developed. As the lymphatic vessels increase in diameter, a subendothelium is present, consisting of a thin layer of connective tissue, surrounded by a variably developed layer of smooth muscle.

LARGE LYMPHATIC VESSELS AND DUCTS

The large lymphatic vessels and ducts resemble comparably sized veins to some degree, but generally have less-developed walls. Moreover, the construction of the wall is inconsistent; making it difficult to apply the tunic terminology used for blood vessels. A thin layer of elastic fibers may be found within the subendothelial region. A layer of smooth muscle outside the subendothelium varies in amount and is surrounded by collagen and elastin that likewise can vary in amount depending on the region of the body and species. The extracellular fibers merge imperceptibly with adjacent tissues.

SUGGESTED READINGS

Cliff WJ: *Blood vessels*, New York, 1976, Cambridge University Press.

Fawcett DW: *Bloom and Fawcett: a textbook of histology*, ed 11, Philadelphia, 1986, Saunders.

Gartner LP, Hiatt JL: *Color textbook of histology*, Philadelphia, 1997, Saunders.

Karlstrom K, Essen-Gustavsson B, Hoppeler H, et al: Capillary supply and fibre area in locomotor muscles of horse and steer—a comparison between histochemistry and electron microscopy, *Acta Anat* (Basel)145:395, 1992.

Kwak BR, Shah DC, Mach F: A starting point for structure function relationships in the canine pulmonary veins, *Cardiovasc Res* 55:703, 2002.

Lentz TL: Cell fine structure: *an atlas of drawings of whole-cell structure*, Philadelphia, 1971, Saunders.

Pauza DH, Skripka V, Pauziene N: Morphology of the intrinsic cardiac nervous system in the dog: a whole-mount study employing histochemical staining with acetylcholinesterase, *Cells Tissues Organs* 172:297, 2002.

Schmidt EE, MacDonald IC, Groom AC: Comparative aspects of splenic microcirculatory pathways in mammals: the region bordering the white pulp, *Scan Microsc* 7:613, 1993.

Schraufnagel DE, Pearse DB, Mitzner WA, Wagner EM: Three-dimensional structure of the bronchial microcirculation in sheep, *Anat Rec* 243:357, 1995.

Stone EA, Stewart GJ: Architecture and structure of canine veins with special references to confluences, *Anat Rec* 128:239, 1988.

Respiratory System

KEY CHARACTERISTICS

- Tubular system with conducting and respiratory portions
- Within conducting portion, specialized region for smell: olfactory region
- Within respiratory portion, highly areolar and vascularized
- Major cell: alveolar cell extremely thin and designed for gaseous exchange

The respiratory system functions to provide appropriate levels of oxygen to the different tissues throughout the body by means of the circulatory system and at the same time remove the potentially deleterious buildup of carbon dioxide from these same tissues. Respiration, from which this system's name is derived, consists of four events or steps: (1) ventilation, (2) external respiration, (3) gas transport, and (4) internal respiration. As the name suggests, **ventilation** is concerned with the movement of the air between the atmosphere and the lungs. **External respiration** involves the diffusion (and exchange) of the two gases at the level of the airway. Thus the first two, ventilation and external respiration, are associated with the respiratory system directly. Gas transport and internal respiration involve primarily the circulatory system. **Gas transport** is the process of moving oxygen and carbon dioxide to and from cells throughout the body, and **internal respiration** is the exchange of the two gases in the immediate region of a specific cell. Functionally and structurally, normal, healthy respiration then requires the close integration of both the respiratory and circulatory systems.

Components of the respiratory system include those that direct the passage of air into and out of the body (the **conducting portion**), and those that actually perform gaseous exchange (the **respiratory portion**) (Figure 11-1). The conducting portion is composed of a system of tubes that facilitate the movement of air as unobstructively as possible and at the same time makes the air suitable for gaseous exchange within the respiratory portion. As the conducting portion functions as a unit to deliver to and remove air from the respiratory portion, each of its components share structural similarities, including a suitable epithelial lining and surrounding support tissues, such as cartilage, smooth muscle, and strong contributions of elastic fibers. Table 11-1 outlines the essential tissues associated with each component or region of the conducting portion, and when looking at it one can easily see the shared similarities of their composition. The respiratory portion, by comparison, lacks most of the features found in the conducting portion and instead consists of tissues, principally simple squamous epithelia and scant loose connective tissue, that assist in the diffusion of substances, which in this case are the gases oxygen and carbon dioxide.

The conducting portion begins from its outermost structure, the nasal cavity, which is then followed consecutively by the nasopharynx; pharynx; larynx; trachea; primary, secondary, and tertiary bronchi; and bronchioles (see Figure 11-1).

TABLE 11-1 Structural Features of the Respiratory Tract in Domestic Mammals

REGION	SUPPORT	EPITHELIUM	CELL TYPES	GLANDS	SPECIAL FEATURES
		Conducting	*Extrapulmonary*		
Vestibular nasal cavity	Hyaline cartilage and dense connective tissue	Keratinized stratified squamous	Epidermal with melanocytes	Sweat and sebaceous	Presence of vibrissae
Respiratory nasal cavity	Hyaline cartilage, bone, and dense connective tissue	Ciliated pseudostratified columnar (respiratory)	Ciliated, brush, goblet, and basal	Mostly serous, branched tubuloacinar	Presence of erectile tissue (cavernous stratum)
Olfactory nasal cavity	Bone and dense connective tissue	Thick ciliated pseudostratified (olfactory)	Sustentacular, olfactory, and basal	Serous, branched tubuloacinar	Olfactory cells are bipolar neurons with receptive cilia from "vesicle"
Nasopharynx	Skeletal muscle and dense connective tissue	Respiratory	Ciliated, brush, goblet, and basal	Mucous, serous, and mixed branched tubuloacinar	Presence of diffuse and nodular lymphatic tissue; prominent elastic fibers
Larynx	Hyaline and elastic cartilage and dense connective tissue	Stratified squamous and respiratory	Basal, polyhedral and squamous; ciliated, brush, goblet, and basal	Mostly mucous, branched tubuloacinar	Presence of diffuse and nodular lymphatic tissue
Trachea and primary bronchi	C-rings of hyaline cartilage, smooth muscle and dense connective tissue	Respiratory	Ciliated, brush, goblet, basal, and neuroendocrine	Mucous and seromucous, branched tubuloacinar	Smooth muscle (trachealis) extends between ends of the C-ringed cartilage
		Conducting	*Intrapulmonary*		
Secondary and tertiary bronchi	Plates and islands of cartilage with smooth muscle helically oriented, and dense connective tissue	Respiratory	Ciliated, brush, goblet, basal, and neuroendocrine	Seromucous branched tubuloacinar	Crisscrossing ribbons of muscle further reinforced by helically patterned elastic fibers
Primary bronchioles	Smooth muscle helically oriented, and dense connective tissue	Simple columnar to simple cuboidal	Ciliated and nonciliated, Clara (bronchiolar exocrine), and neuroendocrin	None	Continued elastic fiber reinforcement
Terminal (tertiary) bronchioles (TB)	Smooth muscle and dense connective tissue with strong elastic fiber component	Simple cuboidal	Ciliated and nonciliated, Clara (bronchiolar exocrine), and neuroendocrine	None	Multiple (2-4) generations of TB in ruminants, pigs, horses, and rodents
		Respiratory			
Respiratory bronchioles (RB)	Smooth muscle bundles and dense connective tissue with strong elastic fiber component	Simple cuboidal and simple squamous	Ciliated and nonciliated, Clara (bronchiolar exocrine), and neuroendocrine, type I and type II alveolar	None	RB are not present in all species; most prevalent in carnivores with multiple (2-4) generations
Alveolar ducts	Smooth muscle bundles and dense to loose connective tissue with strong elastic fiber component	Simple squamous	Type I and type II alveolar and occasional macrophage (septal and alveolar)	None	Lack a true wall, completely lined by alveoli
Alveolar sacs	Loose connective tissue with strong elastic fiber component	Simple squamous	Type I and type II alveolar and occasional macrophage	None	Alveoli share common opening (atrium)
Alveoli	Loose connective tissue with strong elastic fiber component	Simple squamous	Type I and type II alveolar and occasional macrophage	None	Basic respiratory unit; interstitium between type I alveolar cell and vascular endothelium is extremely attenuated

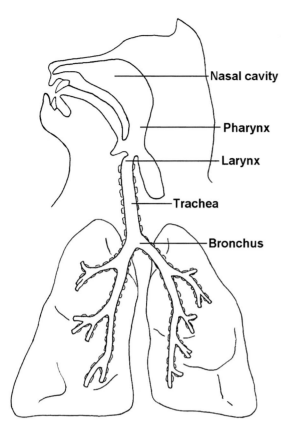

Figure 11-1. Diagram of the conducting portion of the airway in the cat. This portion of the airway system in domestic animals consists of the nasal cavity, pharynx, larynx, trachea, bronchi, and subsequent divisions leading to the respiratory portion.

The diagram labels, from top to bottom:
- Nasal cavity
- Pharynx
- Larynx
- Trachea
- Bronchus

NASAL CAVITY

The nasal cavity is made up of an external vestibule that extends into internal nasal fossae. The **vestibule** is the anterior portion of the nasal cavity and forms the true entrance into the respiratory system at the **nares,** or nostrils, of the nose. At its outermost region, the integument that lines the nares and extends into the vestibule for variable distances, depending upon the species, is referred to as **cutaneous region.** In most instances, the lining consists of a highly pigmented, thickened stratified squamous epithelium (Figure 11-2). As the epithelium continues within the nasal cavity, it gradually thins and becomes less keratinized and eventually is confluent with stratified cuboidal to columnar epithelia, both nonciliated. This region is the **transitional zone.** It is not unusual to see dermal papillae, especially in the dog, which provide a useful environment for cells of defense to temporarily reside. Vibrissae also can be encountered rostrally, as in the horse. The thick hairs, associated typically with numerous sebaceous glands, help filter out large particles that might otherwise be inhaled. Sweat glands also can be abundant in this region.

The remainder of the nasal cavity, the **nasal fossae,** is lined mostly by a ciliated pseudostratified columnar epithelium. The fossae lie within the **nasal septum,** two large chambers separated by a bony partition. Each fossa is responsible for conditioning the inspired air before entering the lungs. As mentioned, the conditioning or treatment of the air before it reaches the distal, respiratory portion of the respira-

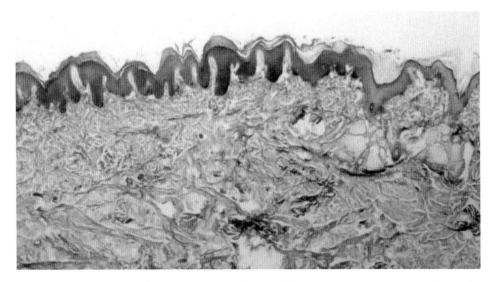

Figure 11-2. Light micrograph of the epidermal and dermal lining of the canine nares. (Hematoxylin and eosin stain; ×40.)

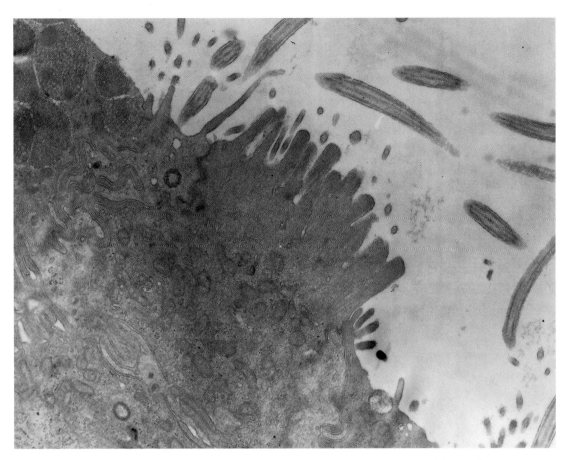

Figure 11-3. Transmission electron micrograph (×12,000) of a brush cell along the mucosal lining that forms respiratory epithelium of the upper canine airway.

tory system is one of the principal functions of the conducting portion. This treatment involves the cleansing, warming, and moistening of inspired air as it moves to the lungs. Specifically, as air flows through the nasal fossae, its mucosal lining ensnares particles such as dust, pollen, and fungal spores and some of the impure gases that might be contaminating the air. At the same time, this lining adds moisture to the air, which helps protect the cell lining within the respiratory portion from drying out. The warmth is contributed by the extensive vascular network that lies immediately beneath the mucosal lining.

The ciliated pseudostratified columnar epithelium **(respiratory epithelium)** found within the nasal cavities contains the usual three types of cells: basal, ciliated columnar (with and without microvilli), and secretory, as well as a fourth type, the **brush cell,** which is typically sparsely populated and possesses the hallmark thick and sometimes blunted microvilli (Figure 11-3). The secretory cells within the respiratory epithelium are typically goblet cells, but there are cells that form secretory materials more proteinaceous

and glycoproteinaceous than those found in goblet cells. Variations in the contents of the secretory cells may vary according to species and/or location within the nasal cavity. Caudally, the connective tissue subjacent to the mucosal lining of the nasal cavities increases its vascular bed and becomes the **cavernous stratum,** an erectile tissue (Figure 11-4). The cavernous stratum contributes to the warming of inspired air and houses serous or mixed nasal glands (simple branched, tubuloacinar) that discharge their contents into the nasal cavities, humidifying the air at the same time. Through neural stimulation of the blood vessels in this region, vascular constriction can occur, resulting in rhythmic or episodic mucosal congestion. Usually, the vascular activity alternates from one side or half of the nasal cavity to the other over a relatively short span of time (several hours or less).

OLFACTORY REGION

Within the dorsocaudal region of the nasal cavity is the **olfactory region** that lines the ethmoid and

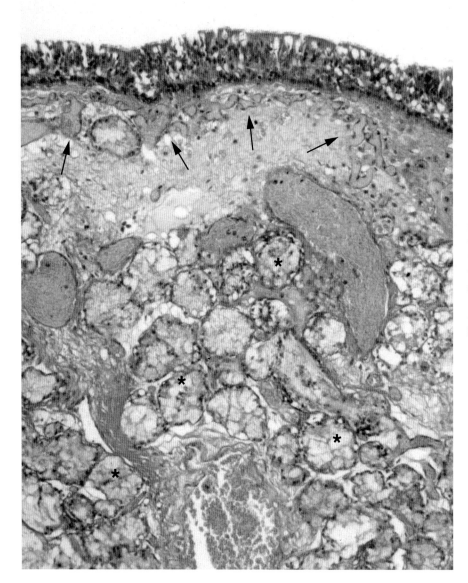

Figure 11-4. Light micrograph of the cavernous stratum in the manatee. Arrows point to the vascular bed, which is surrounded basally by numerous mixed nasal glands *(asterisks).* (Hematoxylin and eosin stain; ×100.)

nearby dorsal turbinates or conchae. The mucosa in this region consists of a very well-developed pseudo-stratified columnar epithelium that has up to a dozen or more layers of nuclei (Figure 11-5). This epithelium, which is responsible for smell or olfaction, is unique in its construction because it has three cell types: sustentacular, basal, and olfactory (neurosensory). Much of the volume of this epithelium is contributed by the **sustentacular cells,** whose columnar bodies are largest toward the airway and smallest toward the basal lamina that they help form (Figure 11-6). Their apical margins are striated, often with branched microvilli that internally lead to a well-

developed network of actin. The nuclei in these cells are positioned above the olfactory nuclei, located mostly in the apical third of their protoplasm (see Figure 11-6). The nuclei, which are broadly elliptically shaped and lightly stained, are surrounded by a yellow pigment, which may be a part of the mineralocorticoid receptor pathway that has been recently discovered in these cells. Mineralocorticoid hormones are able to regulate secretion and absorption in a wide variety of epithelial tissues and may play an important role in controlling olfactory secretion and/or sensory transduction. The sustentacular cells serve the olfactory cells that their cell bodies surround. They not

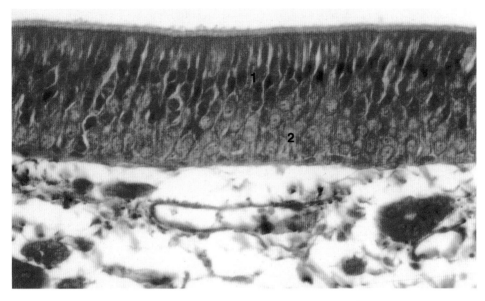

Figure 11-5. Light micrograph of the olfactory epithelium. Nuclei of the sustentacular cells are positioned apically *(1)*, and those of the neurosensory nerves *(2)* are located within the basal portion. (Hematoxylin and eosin stain; ×400.)

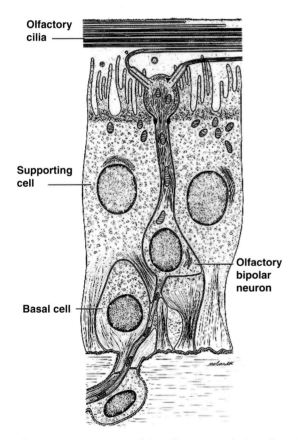

Olfactory cilia

Supporting cell

Olfactory bipolar neuron

Basal cell

Figure 11-6. Diagram of the olfactory epithelium based on transmission electron microscopy with foreshortened height. *(Modified from Fawcett DW: Bloom and Fawcett: a textbook of histology, ed 11, Philadelphia, 1986, Saunders.)*

only provide physical support for the neurosensory portion of this epithelium but also insulate the olfactory cells and facilitate its nutrition.

The **basal cells** consist of small pyramidal cells with round to oval, dark nuclei and occupy the lower one third of the epithelium (see Figures 11-5 and 11-6). As in all pseudostratified columnar epithelia, their apices do not reach the luminal surface. These cells have strong pleuripotential ability and can give rise to either sustentacular cells or olfactory cells, depending on the need. Both sustentacular and olfactory cells have a limited life span and are replaced on a regular basis. However, when the olfactory region suffers from a particular insult and an inordinate amount of sustentacular cells or olfactory cells is lost, the basal cells divide and produce an appropriate number of the missing population. With age, the ability to replicate olfactory cells may decrease more than with sustentacular cells, and as a result the ability to smell may become compromised.

The **olfactory cell,** the primary component of this epithelium, is a sensory-receptor bipolar neuron that responds to airborne chemicals (i.e., odorant substances) and thus provides the sense of smell. The receptive (dendritic) portion of the olfactory cell consists of the **olfactory vesicle,** a bulblike vesicle from which long, nonmotile cilia extend along the epithelial surface (see Figure 11-6). It is thought that an airborne odorant substance initially diffuses into the mucoserous layer that lines the olfactory epithelium and then binds with a long receptor protein associated with the ciliary membrane. Once enough odorant molecules have come into contact with the receptor molecule, adenylate cyclase becomes activated and a subsequent action potential arises (via the production of cyclic adenosine monophosphate [cAMP]). This action potential or nerve impulse is directed down the cell body to its axon, which then moves the signal to the olfactory bulb within the central nervous system. The receptor proteins can be likened to antibodies that are sensitive to specific antigens and thus have different sites for different odorant substances. It is possible that a single odorant substance may bind to several odor receptor sites on more than one neuron.

The connective tissue beneath the olfactory epithelium, the lamina propria, not only provides the proper environment for vascular support of the olfactory epithelium and the emigration of its nerve fibers but also houses the **olfactory glands.** Through their continuous secretions, these glands essentially refresh the epithelial surface and make sure that the same odorant molecule does not repeatedly elicit a protracted response. The olfactory glands are generally simple branched tubuloacinar in form and serous in their secretions.

VOMERONASAL ORGAN

Parallel with the base of the rostral nasal septum and located within its mucosal lining is a paired, tubular structure known as the **vomeronasal organ.** It is incompletely supported by hyaline cartilage, the **vomeronasal cartilage,** which encloses most of the organ except for the dorsolateral part. It is internally lined by an epithelial duct, the vomeronasal duct, which consists mostly of the respiratory epithelium (ciliated pseudostratified columnar epithelium), both rostrally and caudally except along the medial wall of the caudal part, which consists of a modified olfactory epithelium. The vomeronasal organ is connected to the oral cavity by the incisive duct (except in equine species, which lack any connection to the oral cavity). This structure functions to increase the sensitivity of chemoreception in domestic and wild species. Specifically, aerosol and liquid compounds of low volatility known as pheromones can be detected and influence hormonal and reproductive functions and sexual behavior of both genders. These compounds can be taken in via the incisive duct by licking, oral ingestion, or direct inhalation. The signals generated by the vomeronasal epithelium are sent to an accessory olfactory bulb, which acts in most species as the first neural integrative center for the vomeronasal sensory system.

Whereas the neurosensory epithelium is composed of sustentacular cells, basal cells, and olfactory cells, and has an olfactory epithelial appearance, there are some differences. This epithelium lacks both cilia, having microvilli in their place, and dendritic bulbs (except in dogs). The microvilli and their receptors are able to detect specific chemicals at remarkably low thresholds.

As in much of the olfactory region, the vomeronasal organ possesses the **vomeronasal glands,** which lie in the well-vascularized subjacent connective tissue (lamina propria submucosa). Their secretions, which can be either serous, mucous, or both, are deposited into the vomeronasal duct.

PARANASAL SINUSES

Extensive spaces within the ethmoid, frontal, maxillary, and sphenoid bones are adjacent to the nasal cavity and collectively constitute the **paranasal sinuses.** These spaces or sinuses freely open into the nasal cavity and are lined by a pseudostratified columnar epithelium with goblet cells, but there may be areas where the lining consists of either a simple squamous or cuboidal epithelium. In any case, the epithelium is supported by a thin lamina propria submucosa and together form the **mucoperiosteum** (because of the mucociliary apparatus associated with the epithelium) of the bone that supports these large spaces. In general, the glands are more sparsely populated in this region.

NASOPHARYNX

The **nasopharynx** is essentially the caudal continuation of the nasal cavity that lies dorsally to the soft palate and extends to the opening of the larynx (see Figure 11-1). The respiratory epithelium, present throughout much of this region of the conducting portion of the respiratory system, is replaced caudodorsally along the soft palate by a stratified squamous epithelium. The lamina propria submucosa is composed of loose connective tissue that contains mixed glands and lymph nodules (which can be abundant dorsally), forming the **pharyngeal tonsil.**

LARYNX

The distal-most region of the nasopharynx joins the **larynx,** the next component of the conducting portion, which along with the nasopharynx has an open tubular shape that typifies the airflow passageways in this system. The tubular shape, which can be asymmetrical, is maintained by skeletal muscle and rings of cartilage attached to one another and to the nearby trachea by ligaments. It is the muscle that controls the movement of the individual bodies of cartilage from one another that occurs during either the act of swallowing or vocalization. The cartilage is both hyaline and elastic in its composition. The elastic form occurs within the epiglottis, and the cuneiform and corniculate processes (or cartilages). The equine epiglottis, for example, is supported by a prominent wall of elastic cartilage intermixed with unilocular fat and mixed tubuloacinar glands (Figure 11-7). Two separate muscles are involved with the movement of the larynx: **extrinsic** and **intrinsic.** Those located extrinsically contract during swallowing and thus normally prevent liquids, saliva, and food from entering the airway. In most species, the epiglottis downfolds during swallowing. Specifically, the action known as **reflex apnea** is triggered by stimulation of receptors of the laryngeal nerve located within the epithelium. Intrinsically located muscle, on the other hand, contracts and relaxes during phonation as well as respiration (Figure 11-8).

As in the conducting portion before it, the respiratory epithelium lines most of the larynx with its pseudostratified columnar epithelium. Only the surfaces of the vocal folds or cords and epiglottis are composed of nonkeratinized stratified squamous epithelia (see Figure 11-8). Taste buds may occur within the epithelium lining the epiglottis, aryepiglottis, and arytenoids in most domestic species except the horse. These taste buds may work as chemosensory detectors to begin the reflex reaction that protects oral substances from entering the airway during drinking and swallowing. The lamina propria submucosa is composed of loose connective tissue, housing cells of defense, diffuse lymphatic tissue, scattered lymph nodules, and mixed glands, the last being absent in the vocal and vestibular folds. The lamina propria submucosa becomes dense irregular beneath those areas lined by the stratified squamous epithelium.

TRACHEA

At the end of the larynx the airway becomes the **trachea,** a flexible tube of varying length depending on the species, which extends and bifurcates into the primary bronchi within the thoracic cavity. The mucosal lining, once again, is composed of respiratory epithelium that is surrounded by a submucosa and a well-developed subtending adventitia with incomplete cartilaginous rings (Figure 11-9).

The mucosa is a tall ciliated pseudostratified columnar epithelium consisting of six cell types: basal cells, ciliated columnar cells, brush cells, goblet cells, Clara cells, and neuroendocrine cells. The **basal** and **ciliated columnar cells** easily constitute the majority of the total cell population. They are virtually identical to the basal cells and ciliated columnar cells described previously for the other portions of the conducting portion of the respiratory system, functioning to replace dying columnar, brush, and goblet cells and move mucus and entrapped particulates to the nasopharynx, respectively (Figure 11-10; see also Figure 3-12). The **goblet cells** also are numerous and continually produce secretory vesicles filled with mucigen, which when released into the lumen of the airway is hydrated and becomes **mucin,** a sticky substance that easily holds on to inspired foreign particles and eventually is removed by the ciliary action of the columnar cells (Figure 11-11; see also Figure 11-10). The nucleus of the goblet cell is often crescent shaped and located basally within the cell at the same level of the basal cell (see Figures 4-2 and 4-3). The rough endoplasmic reticulum (rER), ribosomes, and Golgi apparatus surround the nucleus.

The brush cells, Clara cells, and neuroendocrine cells constitute only a small amount (10% or less) of the total cell population. The **brush cells** are narrow columnar cells with microvilli and can be species

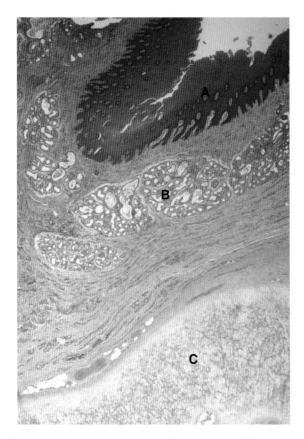

Figure 11-7. Light micrograph of an equine epiglottis consisting of *(A)*, a stratified squamous epithelium, *(B)*, with subtending glands, and *(C)*, elastic cartilage. (Hematoxylin and eosin stain; ×40.)

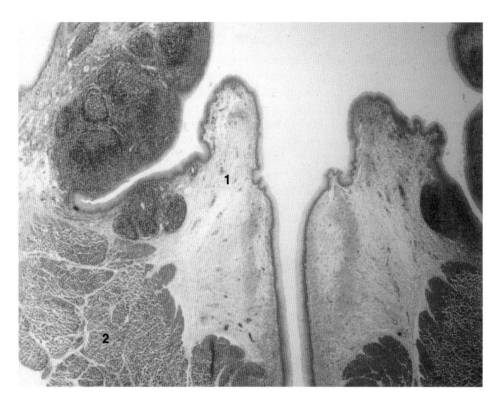

Figure 11-8. Light micrograph of the cranial portion of the vocal fold *(1)* and intrinsic skeletal muscle *(2)* of the larynx. (Hematoxylin and eosin stain; ×40.)

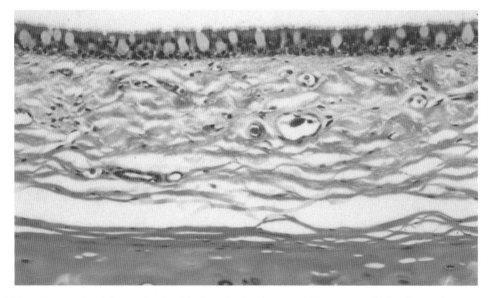

Figure 11-9. Light micrograph of the tracheal epithelium in the dog overlying scattered blood vessels, an occasional mixed branched gland, and hyaline cartilage. (Hematoxylin and eosin stain; ×200.)

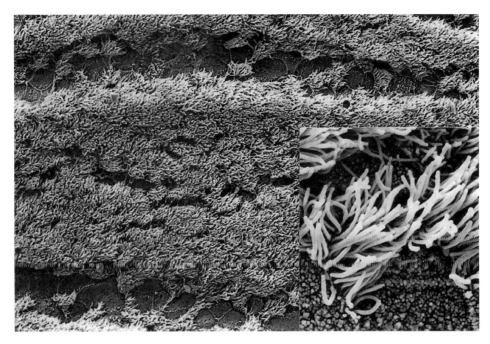

Figure 11-10. Scanning electron micrographs of a ferret trachea taken at ×1000 and ×5000 *(inset)* magnifications, respectively. The heavily ciliated epithelium is separated by furrows of nonciliated cells that run longitudinally within the airway.

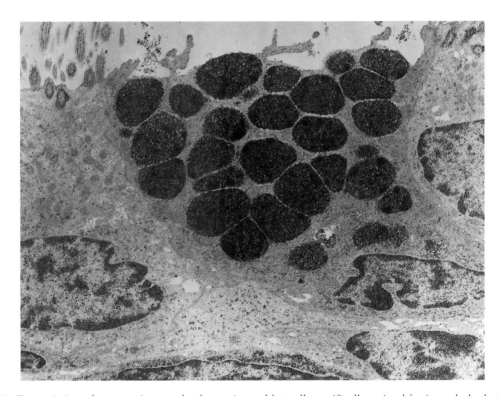

Figure 11-11. Transmission electron micrograph of a canine goblet cell specifically stained for its carbohydrate-laden mucin. (Silver methenamine stain; ×8000.)

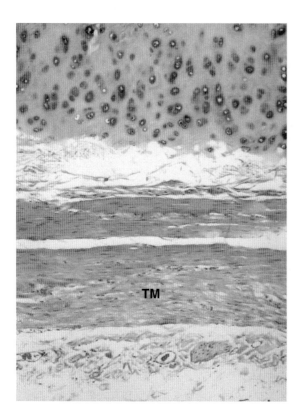

Figure 11-12. Light micrograph of tracheal cartilage in the dog along with the trachealis muscle *(TM)*. (Hematoxylin and eosin stain; ×200.)

variable in height, lacking any cilia. Although their function remains unknown, they have been associated with endings of the trigeminal nerve (CN V) and may play a sensory role. It has also been suggested that they are goblet cells void of their secretory vesicles, having just released most if not all of their mucigen. These cells, which can be easily distinguished when viewed from the perspective of the lumen, can form "tracks" because they are aligned along the same longitudinal axis of the trachea.

The **Clara cells** are rare in most mammalian trachea, more often found within the bronchial tree. Like brush cells, these cells also are columnar and have less populated apical microvilli than columnar cells. They differ especially in that they appear to be secretory and contribute to the airway fluid as they form granules filled with protein and glycoprotein that lie apically within the cytoplasm.

The **neuroendocrine cells** are more pyramidal than columnar and brush cells and produce granules that lie basally within the cytoplasm and appear to be released into the adjacent lamina propria.

The lamina propria of the trachea is generally composed of loose connective tissue that surrounds and houses sentinel cells of defense, simple mucous and mixed tracheal glands that empty into the lumen,

and associated nervous and vascular elements. Even though the epithelial cells contribute to the fluid lining its apices, the tracheal glands provide most of the secreted fluid. At the base of ducts of these glands and along the outer portion of the lamina propria are an increased number of elastic fibers that can form a layer or lamina adjacent to the submucosa. The **submucosa** is composed mostly of irregular dense connective tissue with interspersing glands, blood vessels, and lymphatics. Its outermost boundary is enveloped by the **adventitia,** which consists of dense connective tissue and intervening incomplete rings or C-shaped pieces of hyaline cartilage. Each "ring" of cartilage is incomplete dorsally; its free ends are filled or bridged by smooth muscle, the **trachealis muscle** (Figure 11-12). The outermost regions of the adventitia anchor the trachea to adjoining connective tissue structures of the neck, including those of the esophagus.

BRONCHIAL TREE

At the end of the trachea the first division of the airway occurs, resulting in the right and left extrapulmonary primary bronchi. This bifurcation subsequently arborizes and gives rise to the bronchial trees that form the basis of the right and left lungs within the thoracic cavity. Each **bronchial tree** consists of an extrapulmonary primary bronchus and the sequential intrapulmonary orders of airways that are connected, including intrapulmonary bronchi, bronchioles, terminal bronchioles, and respiratory bronchioles (Figure 11-13). These intrapulmonary divisions eventually give rise to the area of gaseous exchange, the aveolar ducts and sacs, which collectively constitute the parenchyma. The bronchial trees, in turn, are enveloped by a layer of connective tissue and epithelium collectively known as the **visceral pleura.**

BRONCHI

The **primary bronchi** are anatomically constructed in the same manner as the trachea, but smaller in diameter (Figure 11-14). Each bronchus is equipped with its own nervous, vascular, and lymphatic "trunk" lines that concomitantly branch with each division of the airways. In general, as the conducting airways subdivide, becoming progressively smaller in diameter, the respiratory epithelium becomes shorter with fewer goblet cells, and the amount of glands and connective tissue including cartilage becomes less. Only the elastic and smooth muscle tissues increase with regard to the thickness of the wall of the airway, and the Clara cells within the

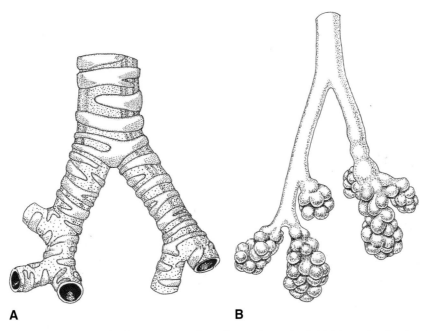

Figure 11-13. **A,** Diagram of the bronchial tree starting from the trachea. The initial branches begin with the two extrapulmonary bronchi. Upon entering the lung, they branch, forming intrapulmonary bronchi, all possessing supportive cartilaginous plates. **B,** Diagram of the terminal bronchioles that either form respiratory bronchioles *(on the right)* or end directly into alveolar ducts *(on the left).*

Figure 11-14. Illustration of a portion of bronchi and associated vasculature within a pulmonary lobule. *(Modified from Fawcett DW: Bloom and Fawcett: a textbook of histology, ed 11, Philadelphia, 1986, Saunders.)*

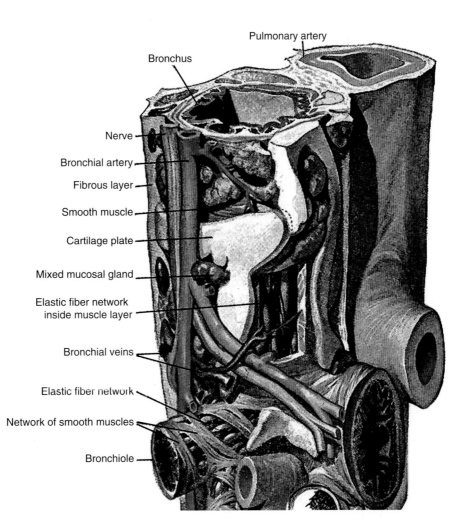

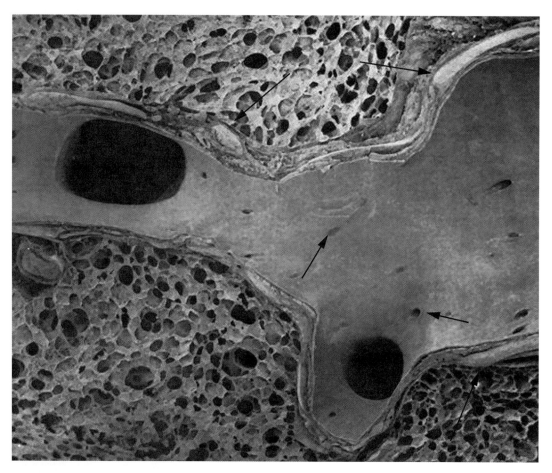

Figure 11-15. Scanning electron micrograph (×40) of branching segmented bronchi. Large arrows point to the cartilage plates and small arrows point to some of the many ducts of glands located along the conducting airways.

respiratory epithelium become more numerous. Each primary bronchus divides one or more times to give rise to the **intrapulmonary bronchi,** which can be considered secondary and tertiary bronchi (see Figure 11-13). This intrapulmonary bronchus also can be referred to as the **lobar bronchus** because it leads to an individual lobe of the lung, entering the lung at its hilum (see Figures 11-1 and 11-13). Lobar bronchi subsequently divide into two branches that, in turn, divide into two more branches. This pattern of division in which one structure separates into two is known as dichotomous branching, which is the principal branching pattern in the lung. The bronchi derived from the lobar bronchi provide the airways for the portions of the lung referred to as **bronchopulmonary segments** or **segmental bronchi** (Figure 11-15). Each of the successive branches or generations of bronchi has decreasingly smaller airways but possesses a greater surface area than the preceding generation. Within these smaller generations of intrapulmonary bronchi, the hyaline cartilage becomes not only smaller

but also irregular in its placement or organization. With the loss of the C-ring configuration, the airways lack a flattened region and have become entirely round. Smooth muscle is the major component of the submucosa, consisting of two apposing layers. Simple mixed glands are still present but have decreased in size and density (Figure 11-16). The connective tissue of the adventitia is now more loosely constructed, containing variable amounts of elastic fibers that can extend and connect with the elastic fibers from the adventitia of other portions of the bronchial tree. Nervous tissue can be found as nerve plexi within the submucosa and adventitia and as nerve endings within the respiratory epithelium.

BRONCHIOLES

The last branching of the intrapulmonary bronchi results in the formation of the **bronchioles,** which usually branch and form several generations before

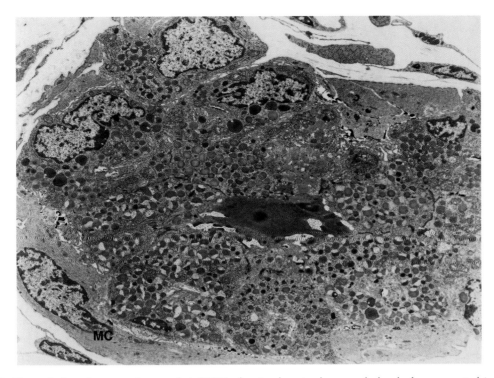

Figure 11-16. Transmission electron micrograph (×5000) of a simple mixed mucosal gland of a segmented (secondary) bronchus in a canine lung. *MC,* Myoepithelial cell.

ending as terminal bronchioles (see Figure 11-13). The first generation of bronchioles, the primary bronchiole, forms the airway for a pulmonary lobule. Bronchioles arise after 10 or so generations of dichotomous branching have occurred within the lung. With the continued decrease in the height of the respiratory epithelium, the cells have become more cuboidal, especially in the smaller bronchioles, but still well ciliated. Goblet cells tend to be sparse and basal cells are absent altogether, making the epithelium either a simple columnar or simple cuboidal one. **Clara cells,** also known as **bronchiolar exocrine cells,** are more frequently encountered in the epithelial lining of these airways (Figure 11-17). The Clara cell can absorb and secrete because it contains glycoproteinaceous secretory granules that when released line and protect the bronchiolar epithelium. This cell also has the ability to degrade some inhaled toxic substances. And the Clara cell has the stem cell capability to divide and reform the bronchiolar epithelium as needed.

The lamina propria of bronchioles consists of glandless loose connective tissue subtended by smooth muscle (see Figure 11-17). The smooth muscle is still layered in an apposing manner but is less developed than in the bronchi. The adventitia lacks cartilage altogether, but still possesses an extensive network of elastic fibers around the smooth muscle layers and

outer portion of the lamina propria. As air is inspired and the lung becomes inflated, the elastic fibers and smooth muscle are able to exert an evenly distributed opposing force and thus maintain the integrity or patency of the bronchiolar shape.

The bronchioles branch into several smaller **terminal bronchioles** that form the last component of the conducting portion of the respiratory system (Figure 11-18). In these bronchioles the epithelium is generally simple cuboidal, and Clara cells can be numerous, especially in carnivores, in which it is the predominant cell type.

RESPIRATORY BRONCHIOLES

Each terminal bronchiole undergoes a final subdivision to form respiratory bronchioles. In terms of its structure, the **respiratory bronchiole** can be thought of as a continuation of a terminal bronchiole that occasionally is interrupted by thin-walled outpocketings called **alveoli** (Figure 11-19; see also Figure 11-18). The alveolus is that portion of the respiratory system involved in gas exchange and for that reason represents the parenchymatous unit of the lung. Thus the respiratory bronchiole along with the alveolar ducts, alveolar sacs, and alveoli comprise the respiratory portion of the respiratory system. Because respira-

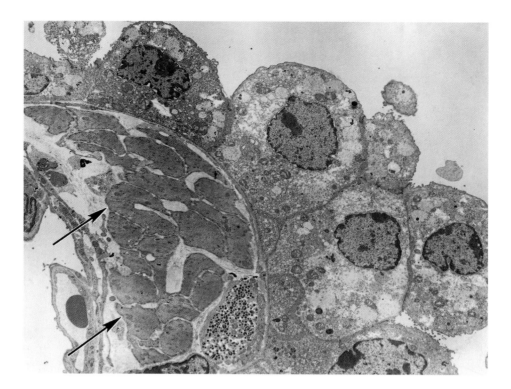

Figure 11-17. Transmission electron micrograph (×5000) of Clara cells (bronchiolar exocrine cells) lining a portion of a bronchiole. Arrows point to smooth muscle cells lying beneath the epithelium.

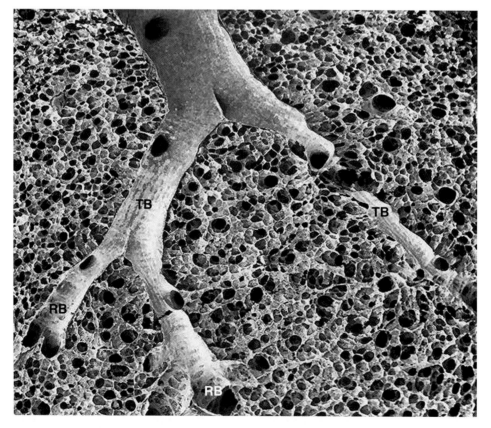

Figure 11-18. Scanning electron micrograph (×30) of a terminal bronchiole *(TB)* that branches into respiratory bronchioles *(RB)* within a pulmonary lobule of a ferret.

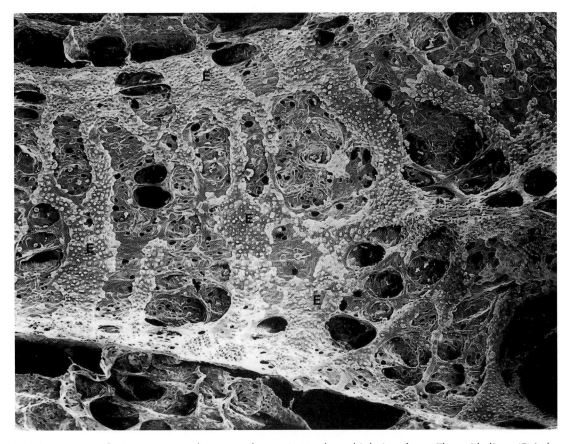

Figure 11-19. Scanning electron micrograph (×200) of a respiratory bronchiole in a ferret. The epithelium *(E)* is frequently interrupted by numerous outpocketings of alveoli and alveolar sacs.

tory bronchiole possesses alveoli along its longitudinal axis, the structural composition of the epithelium, lamina propria, and submucosa become markedly altered wherever the alveoli occur, causing the epithelium to become transformed from simple cuboidal to simple squamous and the submucosa and its smooth muscle to move around each outpocketing. The length and overall amount of respiratory bronchioles vary among domestic species, being much more prominent among carnivores than herbivores and among mammals can be absent altogether in small rodents and humans (see Table 11-1).

ALVEOLAR DUCTS AND ALVEOLAR SACS

Respiratory bronchioles branch or simply end in **alveolar ducts,** which are structures in which the airways continue in their linear manner, but are lined only by alveoli, having no bronchiolar epithelium and subtending smooth muscle (Figures 11-20 and 11-21). There may be areas along the alveolar duct, especially

at its end, where a small cluster of alveoli (two or more) form a blind outpocketing known as an **alveolar sac** (see Figures 11-19 through 11-21). The alveoli of each sac share the same common space that the airway has emptied into: the **atrium.**

ALVEOLI

The functional units of the respiratory system are **alveoli** and occur as small outpocketings of the respiratory bronchiole, alveolar duct, and alveolar sac (see Figures 11-19 through 11-21). As the basic unit for gaseous exchange, the alveolus is a semiglobar air space lined by a squamous respiratory epithelium and closely associated capillary network (Figure 11-22). Consequently, the main cell type of this tissue is the **squamous alveolar epithelial cell,** also known as the **type I alveolar cell** or **type I pneumocyte.** Whereas the nucleus appears flattened, the rest of the cell is exceedingly squamous and, of course, thin when viewed in cross section. In fact, the cytoplasm of the

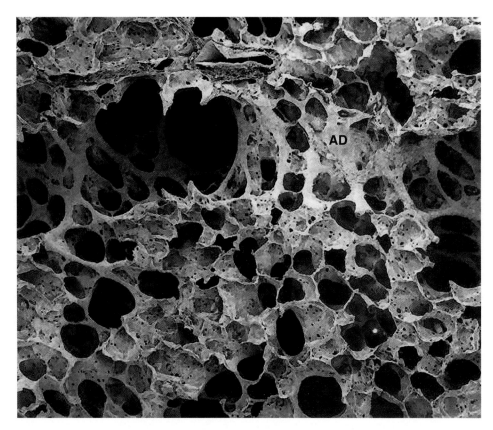

Figure 11-20. Scanning electron micrograph (×100) of an alveolar duct *(AD)* in the ferret.

type I cell can become attenuated to a thickness of less than 200 nm and not be seen histologically because it's at the margin of resolution of the light microscope (see Figure 11-22). The few organelles that help comprise the cytoplasm of the type I alveolar cell include mitochondria, rER, and polysomes, and are located in the vicinity of the nucleus. Endocytotic vesicles, also present, are more diffusely distributed throughout the cytoplasm. Adjacent squamous cells form tight junctions (zonulae occludentes), preventing serum leakage into alveolar lumina. The type I alveolar cell occupies more than 95% of the surface area of each alveolus and is intimately associated with the underlying well-vascularized connective tissue.

Another native cell of the respiratory epithelium is the **type II alveolar cell,** or **type II pneumocyte,** which is distinctly morphologically different from the type I cell, being more or less cuboidal (Figure 11-23). The apical portion of the cell distinctly projects in a domelike fashion into alveolar lumen. When considering the entire lung, this cell is actually more numerous than the type I. The type II alveolar cell contains a round centrally placed nucleus, both smooth and rER, a well-developed Golgi apparatus, mitochondria, and secretory vesicles. Scattered short microvilli project along the cell's apical/luminal surface. The

type II alveolar cells are most abundant at the septal portion of the alveolus, where one alveolus abuts another and together share the adjoining septum (see Figure 11-21). For that reason they are also referred to as **septal cells.** Among the secretory vesicles are **lamellar bodies** that form the most characteristic feature of this cell type. Lamellar bodies contain layers of membrane-bound material that is high in phospholipid content and when secreted functions as the **pulmonary surfactant.** During respiration, alveoli

Figure 11-21. A, Diagram of a respiratory unit of the lung, which includes the respiratory bronchiole, alveolar ducts *(AD)*, alveolar sacs *(AS)*, and alveoli. The area where alveolar ducts end and alveolar sacs begin is recognized as an atrium. **B,** Transmission electron micrograph (×3000) of the thickened adluminal end that lines the alveolar duct indicated as *1* in the diagram. *MC,* Mast cell; *SM,* smooth muscle. **C,** Transmission electron micrograph (×3000) of the thickened adluminal end that lines the atrium indicated as *2* in the diagram. *(A modified from Fawcett DW:* Bloom and Fawcett: a textbook of histology, *ed 11, Philadelphia, 1986, Saunders.)*

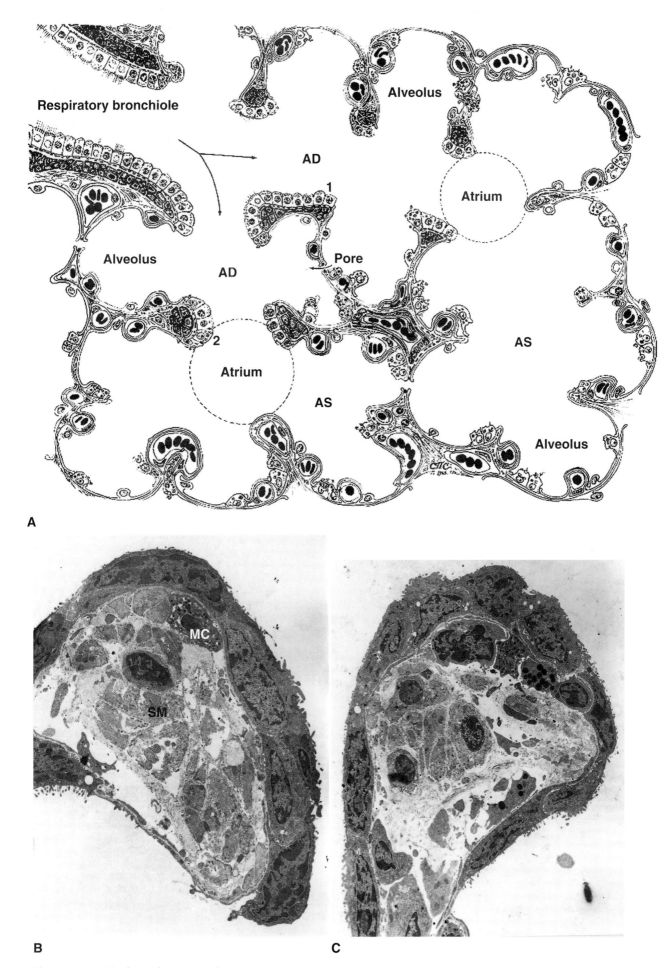

Respiratory bronchiole

Alveolus

AD

1

Pore

AD

Alveolus

2

Atrium

AS

Atrium

AS

Alveolus

MC

SM

A

B

C

Figure 11-21. For legend see opposite page

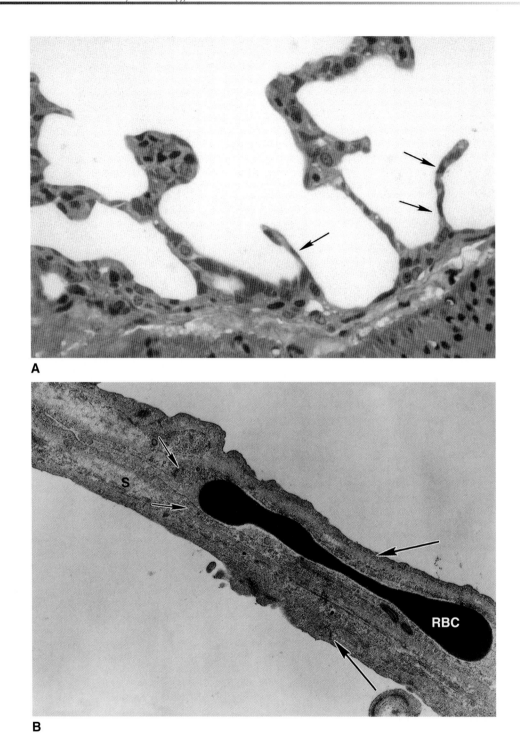

A

B

Figure 11-22. A, Light micrograph of rat alveoli lined by type I alveolar cells *(arrows).* (Plastic section, hematoxylin and eosin stain; ×1,000.) **B,** Transmission electron micrograph (×25,000) of the extremely thin cytoplasm of the type I alveolar cells *(large arrows)* that line equally thin stroma *(S)* and an endothelial cell of an adjacent capillary *(small arrows)* in the dog. *RBC,* Red blood cell.

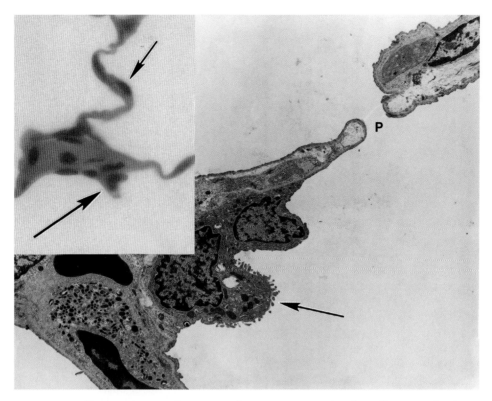

Figure 11-23. Transmission electron micrograph (×7000) of a type II canine alveolar cell *(arrow)* that lies in the septa of adjacent alveoli. *P,* pore. Inset is a light micrograph of an alveolar septum in the cow. Large arrow points to a type II alveolar cell and small arrow points to nearby type I cell. (Hematoxylin and eosin stain; ×400.)

change shape and there is the potential for alveolar collapse. The presence of a surfactant creates a gas-liquid interface that is largely hydrophobic and reduces surface tension. As a result, alveoli of different sizes are able to work and coexist in equilibrium. In short, it minimizes the work of breathing and the possibility of alveolar collapse. In addition to the phospholipids the lamellar bodies also release surfactant proteins that become lodged within an aqueous coat between the external film of phospholipids and the cell membranes of the type I alveolar cell. This external assemblage of the phospholipids and proteins along the respiratory epithelium is known as **tubular myelin.** Recently it has been suggested that in addition to controlling fluid balance and surface tension, the surfactant produced by the type II alveolar cell may play a role in host defense.

Although type I and II alveolar cells are the predominant cell types found within the alveoli, cells of defense can be encountered, especially macrophages and mast cells. Pulmonary macrophages arrive in this region as blood-borne monocytes that migrate into the pulmonary interstitium and are sometimes referred to as **septal macrophages.** They generally move between type I alveolar cells and enter the luminal airway where they become **alveolar macrophages** (Figure 11-24). Alveolar macrophages engulf fine particles, such as bacteria and dust that has reached the air sacs. These cells, which enter the pulmonary air lumina by the tens of millions each day, also remove some of the surfactant, which is constantly replaced. Most of the macrophages move proximally within the airways toward the trachea and then pharynx where they are eliminated by swallowing or expectoration.

As in bronchi and bronchioles, **mast cells** are encountered within the alveoli, but normally are much fewer than the alveolar macrophage (Figure 11-25; see also Figure 11-21). They lie interstitially between an adjacent capillary and the epithelium, particularly at the junction of three alveoli. These cells can be activated by a wide variety of agents, including allergens, and contribute to difficulties in respiration, such as in asthma. In domestic cats and other members of the cat family (Felidae), asthma can occur within the small airways, resulting in multifocal areas of alveolar wall fibrosis.

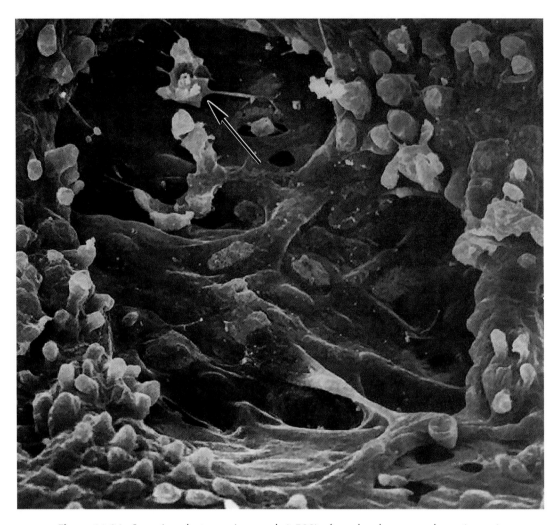

Figure 11-24. Scanning electron micrograph (×500) of an alveolar macrophage *(arrow).*

INTERALVEOLAR SEPTUM

A major portion of any alveolus within the lung is connected to adjacent alveoli. The area where two adjacent alveoli are joined forms the **interalveolar septum** (see Figures 11-22 and 11-23). Interalveolar septa may be very thin, consisting of a flattened capillary lined on both sides by type I alveolar cells. Small openings, **alveolar pores,** occasionally interrupt the septum and allow the air spaces of the two alveoli to be shared. In the regions where three alveoli are interconnected are usually other connective tissue elements besides the blood vessel. Two of these elements, the macrophage (septal macrophage) and the mast cell, have been mentioned. Fibrocytes and components of the extracellular matrix also are present in varying amounts. Collagen (type I and III) and elastic fibers form a network instrumental to the parenchymal micromechanics within the lung (see Figure 11-25). The greatest density of collagen and elastic fibers occurs within 10 to 20 μm of an alveolar duct. The amount and degree of penetration of the fibers, especially elastic fibers, into alveolar septae vary from species to species but are most likely greater in lungs with larger alveoli. Age can also influence the structure of the interalveolar septum. In older individuals, increases in thickness of the alveolar wall and septum and associated elastic fibers can occur. These changes would appear to offset increases in the overall alveolar size that occur concomitantly.

The thinnest portions of the interalveolar septae, which possess capillaries, are involved in gaseous exchange and are known as the **blood-gas barriers.** Although any increase in the thickness of this barrier has the potential to impede gaseous exchange, its presence is necessary in order to prevent the leakage of any plasma or serum into the air space of the alveolus. The blood-gas barrier is composed of the thickness of the capillary endothelium and its basal lamina, the thickness of any intervening connective tissue, the thickness of the alveolar type I cell and its basal lamina, which may be shared with that of the capillary endothelium, and the overlying surfactant (see Figure 11-22).

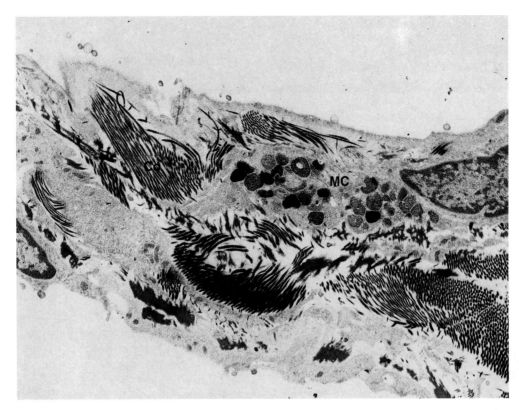

Figure 11-25. Transmission electron micrograph of a mast cell *(MC)* within the stroma near the junction of several alveoli. Collagen *(Co)* within the stroma can vary considerably in thickness. (Barium permanganate stain; ×8000.)

Actual gas exchange occurs primarily at the site of the red blood cell within the capillary. Oxygen, which has diffused through the blood-gas barrier, is taken up by available hemoglobin within the erythrocyte, resulting in **oxyhemoglobin.** Concomitantly, carbon dioxide (CO_2) is released, which like O_2 moves by passive diffusion through the different elements of the blood-gas barrier and enters the luminal air space of the alveolus. Specifically, CO_2 is diffused throughout the cytosol of the erythrocyte and is held at a different location within the hemoglobin molecule, **carbaminohemoglobin.** Carbon dioxide within its cytosol may be converted temporarily into carbonic acid (H_2CO_3) by the enzyme, carbonic anhydrase. The H_2CO_3 readily dissociates into bicarbonate and hydrogen ions (HCO_3^- and H^+). The bicarbonate ion may leave the cytosol and diffuse into the plasma with a concomitant influx of Cl^-. This exchange (chloride for bicarbonate) is the **chloride shift** and can occur in either direction. Plasma bicarbonate ions, in turn, will eventually reenter the erythrocyte (with the chloride shift), reassociate with hydrogen ions to form carbonic acid, and then be broken down into CO_2 and H_2O by the carbonic anhydrase. The diffusion of each gas is driven by the partial pressure within the alveolar air space and the lumen of the alveolar capillary.

PLEURA

As in many organs of the body, each lung is located in its own cavity, the thoracic cavity, and lined by a serous membrane called the **pleura.** The pleura consists of variably developed dense, irregular connective tissue covered by a simple squamous to simple cuboidal epithelium **(mesothelium).** In large domestic species such as the horse, the connective tissue component is thick when compared with that of the dog and cat. The portion that forms the external lining of each lung is the **visceral** or **pulmonary pleura,** which reflexes at the hilum and pulmonary ligament onto the **parietal pleura,** which is attached to the walls of the thoracic cavity. The connective tissue of the visceral pleura intermixes with that of the external-most alveoli and their septae and houses the nerves and blood vessels associated with bronchioles, alveolar ducts, sacs, and so forth in this region. Lymph vessels also occur here, forming a superficial system that drains into larger vessels that empty into bronchopulmonary lymph nodes at the hilar region of each lung. The visceral and parietal pleura are separated by the **pleural cavity,** which holds a small amount of serous fluid and provides a frictionless environment for the lungs to push against during internal respiration. The mesothelial cells can possess bushlike long microvilli that along with hyaluronans-laden lubricants minimize the effort of breathing.

During inhalation each lung expands and causes the visceral pleura to push against the pleural cavity and parietal pleura. Inhalation itself is a catabolic process, requiring contraction of the diaphragm and intercostal and other various accessory respiratory muscles. As the result of their contraction, the volume of the thoracic cavities grows, which, in turn, causes a change in the pressure within the pleural cavities. The differential between the pressure of the pleural cavities and that of the atmosphere becomes the driving force for the intake of air. As air continues to be inhaled and individual alveoli expand, each lung expands, stretching and pushing the entire visceral pleura against the pleural cavity. When the same muscles that contracted now relax, the pressure within the pleura cavities returns to its previous level, and the elastic fibers within the entire system (including the pleura) help force the respired air out of the lungs.

The proximal and distal airways of the pulmonary system are innervated by sympathetic and parasympathetic elements of the nervous system. The parasympathetic nerve fibers, which are supplied by the vagus nerve, innervate the bronchial smooth muscle, causing them to contract, resulting in bronchoconstriction. The sympathetic nerve fibers are supplied by the thoracic sympathetic chain ganglia (middle cervical and cervicothoracic ganglia). They innervate the smooth muscles of the bronchi but cause their relaxation and resultant bronchodilation. These nerves also innervate the smooth muscle associated with the arteries and veins within the pulmonary tract.

RESPIRATORY VASCULATURE

Blood for each lung is primarily provided by the pulmonary arteries. These arteries are large and elastic, and they originate from the pulmonary trunk arising from the right ventricle of the heart. As the right ventricle contracts, deoxygenated blood is pumped to the lungs by the right and left pulmonary arteries. Upon entering the lung, branches of the pulmonary arteries accompany the primary bronchi and follow down the bronchial tree, branching to the level of the respiratory bronchioles (see Figure 11-4). From there they divide and form a capillary network for the air sacks, where gaseous exchange occurs. Subsequently, the oxygenated blood is returned by pulmonary veins in a reversed, ascending, treelike manner to the heart's left atrium.

AVIAN SYSTEM

Whereas the respiratory system in birds is comparable with that in mammals, its anatomy is different, especially regarding the lung, which is overall not as elaborate or developed but small and compact, and does not change volume during respiration. The system consists of the nasal cavity, larynx, syrinx, 4 orders of conducting airways (versus up to 15 orders in mammals), and a compact spongy parenchyma.

The nasal cavity is similar to the mammalian nasal cavity, having mostly a respiratory lining with the vestibular region containing a stratified squamous epithelium and the dorsocaudal portion containing the olfactory epithelium. The respiratory epithelium contains intraepithelial glands consisting of clusters of mucus-secreting cells arranged in simple acini. The connecting larynx has similarities to the mammalian structure; however, unlike mammals, the avian larynx lacks vocal cords and has little ability to create usable sounds. The adjoining trachea is constructed along the same lines as mammalian trachea, including the presence of the cartilaginous tracheal rings. Tracheal rings in birds, however, completely encircle the trachea as opposed to mammalian tracheal rings, which are incomplete. The smooth muscle that lines mammalian trachea is absent in birds. The intraepithelial glands associated with the avian respiratory epithelium are especially well developed in the trachea.

At the junction of the trachea and extrapulmonary primary bronchi is a diverticulum called the **syrinx.** The syrinx provides a bird's ability to vocalize. Although its construction varies from one species to another and undoubtedly contributes to the enormous range of avian phonations, the syrinx is basically an inverted Y-shaped structure with a **median vocal fold** in the syringeal lumen where the syrinx bifurcates. This fold and two **lateral vocal folds** (lateral tympanic membranes) are used for phonation and are lined by thinly layered stratified squamous epithelia. Through the contraction and relaxation of ventral and dorsal skeletal muscles associated with the syrinx, a bird is able to finely control the syringeal airways, regulate the timing of phonation, and determine the frequency of sound.

The avian lung occupies considerably less area in the thoracic cavity than the mammalian lung and as mentioned does not change in size during inhalation and exhalation. However, each lung is continuous with air sacs, which do change in volume during breathing. The primary bronchi are referred to as **mesobronchi** upon entering the lungs. Each mesobronchus has lateral branches that form the **secondary bronchi** (Figure 11-26). The secondary bronchi empty either into air sacs or tertiary bronchi (Figure 11-27). The **tertiary bronchi (parabronchi),** which interconnect secondary bronchi, give rise to many **atria,** also known as small **air vesicles,** that extend radially from the tertiary bronchi (Figure 11-28). The atria give rise to **air capillaries**—continuous loops of fine airways where the gas exchange occurs. The epithelial lining of the air capillaries include type I and type II cells, both of which are similar to those seen in mammalian lungs. Likewise, the epithelium of the mesobronchi is similar to that lining the primary bronchi and trachea

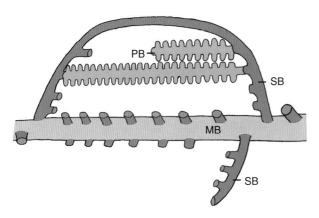

Figure 11-26. Diagram of the bronchial branching pattern in the avian lung. *MB,* Mesobronchus; *SB,* secondary bronchi; *PB,* parabronchi (tertiary bronchi).

in mammals. Initially, walls of the extrapulmonary bronchi also are similar to mammalian tracheal and bronchial walls because they include hyaline cartilage and smooth muscle. The cartilaginous rings, however, become replaced by plaques of cartilage and disappear in the initial portion of the mesobronchi. Except for the absence of the goblet cells, the respiratory epithelium of the secondary bronchi is similar to that of the mesobronchus. There is still a lamina muscularis mucosae but less confluent and more multidirectional than in the primary bronchi. Both secondary and tertiary bronchi become interrupted by atria. At the site where atria arise, the epithelium becomes transformed into a simple cuboidal and simple squamous epithelium.

The caudal end of each mesobronchus empties into an air sac (abdominal air sac), which, like other air sacs connected to secondary bronchi, are lined by simple cuboidal to simple squamous epithelia. Like mammals, avian ventilation is governed by abdominal muscle activity. This activity directly influences the size and volume of the air sacs, resulting in the movement of air through the air pathways, including the air capillaries.

Overall, regardless of anatomical differences between birds and mammals, the respiratory tissues of both groups of animals possess comparable mechanical behavior. Still, birds of active flight have efficient methods for gas exchange not found in mammals. The

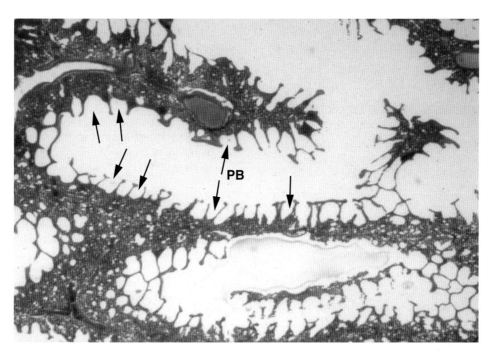

Figure 11-27. Light micrograph of the tertiary bronchi (parabronchi) *(PB)* and atria *(arrows)* of an avian lung. (Hematoxylin and eosin stain; ×20.)

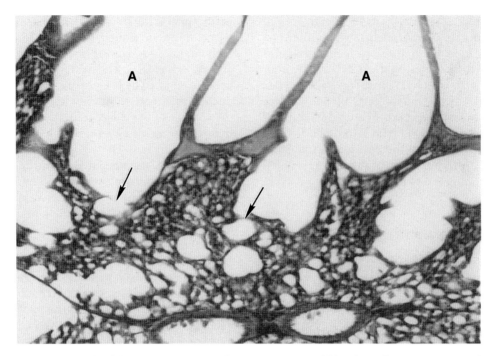

Figure 11-28. Light micrograph of the atria *(A)*, air capillaries *(arrows)*, and blood capillaries in an avian lung. (Hematoxylin and eosin stain; ×100.)

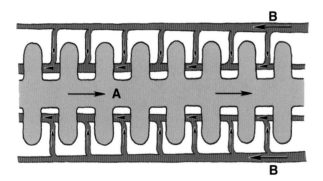

Figure 11-29. The orientation of the gas exchange in the avian lung provides a countercurrent relationship between the air *(A)* and blood *(B)* capillaries.

interaction of airflow in the parabronchial lumen with incoming blood at the level of the exchange tissue is crosscurrent as the directions of flow between the gas exchange media occur perpendicularly to each other. Concomitantly, the interaction between the air capillary and blood capillary occurs in a countercurrent way as blood flows to the parabronchial lumen while air flows in the opposite direction, toward the periphery (Figure 11-29).

SUGGESTED READINGS

Barnas GM, Hempleman SC, Harinath P, Baptiste JW: Respiratory system mechanical behavior in the chicken, *Respir Physiol* 84:145, 1991.

Fawcett DW: *Bloom and Fawcett: a textbook of histology,* ed 11, Philadelphia, 1986, Saunders.

Hlastala MP, Robertson HT, editors: *Complexity in structure and function of the lung,* New York, 1998, Dekker.

Hyde DM, Samuelson DA, Blakeney WH, Kosh PC: A correlated scanning and transmission electron microscopic study of the ferret lung, *Scan Electron Microsc* III:891, 1979.

Kwak BR, Shah DC, Mach F: A starting point for structure function relationships in the canine pulmonary veins, *Cardiovasc Res* 55:703, 2002.

Maina JN: What it takes to fly: the structural and functional respiratory refinements in birds and bats, *J Exp Biol* 203:3045, 2000.

Maina JN: Some recent advances on the study and understanding of the functional design of the avian lung: morphological and morphometric perspectives, *Biol Rev Camb Philos Soc* 77:97, 2002.

McLaughlin RF, Tyler WS, Canada RO: A study of the subgross pulmonary anatomy in various mammals, *Am J Anat* 108:149, 1961.

Nettum JA: Combined bronchoalveolar-vascular casting of the canine lung, *Scan Microsc* 10:1173, 1996.

Nowell JA, Tyler WS: Scanning electron microscopy of the surface morphology of mammalian lungs, *Am Rev Resp Dis* 103:313, 1971.

Pirie M, Pirie HM, Cranston S, Wright NG: An ultrastructural study of the equine lower respiratory tract, *Equine Vet J* 22:338, 1990.

Schraufnagel DE, Pearse DB, Mitzner WA, Wagner EM: Three-dimensional structure of the bronchial microcirculation in sheep, *Anat Rec* 243:357, 1995.

Wang NS: Anatomy and physiology of the pleural space, *Clin Chest Med* 6:3, 1985.

Immune System

KEY CHARACTERISTICS

- Highly cellular, within the framework of areolar connective tissue with reticular fibers, either encapsulated fully, partially or not; cells diffusely aggregated or clustered in nodules (follicles) with or without germinal centers
- Major cells: lymphocytes B and T with subpopulations, plasma cell, antigen-presenting cells, and macrophages provide protective response known as immunity

The body is constantly faced with the prospect of being invaded and damaged by a variety of foreign agents, living and nonliving. The immune system incorporates all the components within the body, enlisting tissues and organs and their specific cells that directly protect against such invasions. Cells that offer this protection normally have the ability to discern **self-**substances (the body's own molecules) from **nonself** substances (foreign, or not from a part of the body), and destroy or inactivate the latter. This cellular ability is **immunocompetence,** and the protective response provided by immunocompetent cells is **immunity.** Immunocompetent cells consist of antigen-presenting cells, lymphocytes, and plasma cells. Antigen-presenting cells and lymphocytes are able to start the immune process in response to the presence of nonself substances **(antigens).** Their exposure to antigens initially results in the formation of **cytokines**—proteins that can be exogenously released to signal or inform other cells of the present antigenic interaction. In addition, the immunocompetent cells (lymphocytes) exposed to foreign or nonself substances may either form specific proteins called **antibodies** that can bind directly to the presenting antigens or induce other cells to destroy or kill the foreign substance if it should be an invading organism or an abnormally altered preexisting cell. The recruit-ment of other cells to eradicate nonself substances is **cell-mediated immunity,** and the production of antibodies to incapacitate nonself substances is traditionally referred to as **humoral immunity.** The antibodies produced by domestic animals consist of five classes or isotypes: immunoglobulin M (IgM), immunoglobulin A (IgA), immunoglobulin G (IgG), immunoglobulin D (IgD), and immunoglobulin E (IgE), each able to perform specific duties.

In mammals the antigen-presenting cells and lymphocytes are derived from bone marrow. Lymphocytes differ from antigen-presenting cells in that they not only have self-/nonself recognition capability but also **memory, specificity,** and **diversity.** In terms of their development and functional roles, lymphocytes can be separated into two cell types: **B lymphocytes** and **T lymphocytes.** B lymphocytes are not only formed in the bone marrow but develop their immunocompetence there as well. T lymphocytes, however, must first migrate from the marrow to the thymus before developing their immunocompetence. Bone marrow and the thymus are then the **primary lymphoid organs** of the immune (lymphoid) system (Table 12-1). Once immunocompetent, T and B lymphocytes can move to other portions of the immune system, making up the **secondary lymphoid organs**—the spleen, lymph nodes, and diffuse lymphoid tissue—the lattermost

TABLE 12-1 Histological Features of Lymphoid Organs in Domestic Mammals

ORGAN	STROMA	PARENCHYMATOUS ORGANIZATION	VASCULAR ASSOCIATIONS	FUNCTIONS	SPECIAL FEATURES AND SPECIES VARIATIONS
Thymus	Encapsulated by thin, dense, irregular connective tissue with incomplete septa (trabeculae); the cortex and medulla are supported by the epithelial reticulum	Separated into cortex and medulla; cortex consists of many T cells and resident macrophages lined by the epithelial reticulum, which forms blood-thymus barrier; medulla has less-populated T cells among a larger epithelial reticulum	Lacks afferent and efferent lymph vessels; arterial supply is at the corticomedullary junction via stromal septa; tight cortical capillaries drain into medullary venules	Early in development, center for T cell production; naive T cells become immunocompetent in cortex	Epithelial reticular cells of the medulla form whorled thymic corpuscles
Lymph node	Encapsulated by thin, dense, irregular connective tissue with incomplete septa (trabeculae); reticular fibers and stellate reticular cells support the parenchyma within the cortex, paracortex, and medulla	Separated into cortex, paracortex, and medulla; cortex consists of lymphatic nodules (B cell germinal centers) and diffuse lymphoid tissue; paracortex has many T cells; medulla has lymph sinuses and cords of lymphocytes, plasma cells and macrophages	Presence of afferent and efferent lymph vessels; afferent lymph vessels enter along entire capsule; blood vessels and efferent lymph vessels are connected to a hilum	Filters lymph by removing foreign substances including invading microorganisms; provides B and T cell production	Lymph sinuses contain stellate cells for slowing forward movement of lymphocytes; trabeculae are highly developed in the ox; cortex is located centrally and medulla peripherally in the pig
Spleen	Encapsulated by thin, dense, irregular connective tissue along with smooth muscle; trabeculae can be entirely smooth muscle; reticular fibers and stellate reticular cells support the white pulp and splenic cords of the red pulp	Separated into white and red pulp; white pulp consists of periarterial lymphatic sheaths (PALS) with nodules; cells include B and T cells, plasma cells, macrophages, and antigen-presenting dendritic cells; red pulp consists of network of venous sinusoids (sinuses) and cords of lymphocytes, plasma cells, and macrophages	Lacks afferent lymph vessels; blood vessels and efferent lymph vessels are connected to a hilum; arterioles from the white pulp lead to capillaries in the red pulp, which can be sheathed and open or closed	Fetally, a site for hematopoiesis; continues to provide B and T cell production; immunologically filters blood, removes and breaks down old blood, and recycles iron; acts as a blood reservoir	Red pulp is well developed in domestic species, especially so in the dog and horse, allowing extensive red blood cell storage to occur in these animals
Diffuse lymphatic tissues: gut-associated lymphatic tissue (GALT), bronchus-associated lymphatic tissue (BALT)	Nonencapsulated to partially encapsulated (tonsils of the caudal oral cavity and pharynx); stroma of nodules consist of modified branching reticular cells	Consist of nodules: rounded aggregates of mostly B cells surrounded by T cells and antigen-presenting cells (follicular dendritic cells); and diffuse tissues: unorganized concentration of lymphocytes with scattered plasma cells and macrophages	Presence of afferent and efferent lymph and blood vessels; in tonsils, afferent lymph vessels are absent	Immunologically filter lymph; provide B and T cell production; a primary center for B cell formation in the lymphatic nodules of the developing ileum of ruminants	Among the GALT aggregates of lymphatic nodules form Peyer's patch, especially in the ileum

lacking a connective tissue sheath or fascia and instead is unencapsulated, whereas the other components are encapsulated (see Table 12-1).

CELLS OF THE IMMUNE SYSTEM

B LYMPHOCYTE

The B lymphocyte, or **B cell,** is formed and becomes immunocompetent in the bone marrow of mammals and the diverticulum of cloaca called the bursa of Fabricius (thus the designation B) in birds. Morphologically, B cells are typical of lymphocytes in general: they are small and round, with a prominent heterochromatic nucleus surrounded by a small rim of cytoplasm (see Figure 7-18). Without the assistance of determining the presence of **antigen receptors** that are specific for B cells, this cell type cannot be distinguished from the T lymphocyte or **T cell** based on its histological appearance. The antigen receptors, also known as **immunoglobulins** or antibodies, are molecules exposed to the cell surface along its plasma membrane, and function to recognize the presence of a foreign substance. Antigen receptors of B cells are constructed in a way that will allow them to capture or bind the antigen (Figure 12-1). Each antigen has

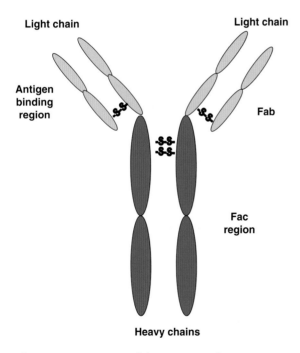

Figure 12-1. Diagram of the structure of a prototype antibody molecule, immunoglobulin G (IgG), consisting of the two pairs of two different proteins—light chains and heavy chains—with the light chains binding epitopes and the heavy chains binding receptors (Fc receptors) on the surface of various cells.

specific sites or regions called **epitopes** (antigenic determinant) that are a part of its structure and can potentially react with the antigen receptors. Typically, epitopes are a small handful of amino acids (six or fewer) and/or sugar moieties. Small antigens have only a single epitope, whereas larger ones, such as microbial organisms, have a variety of antigenic sites.

As B cells become immunocompetent, each lymphocyte produces tens of thousands of immunoglobulins that insert into the cell membrane, projecting outwardly along its surface—**surface immunoglobulins (SIGS).** Before each B cell is exposed to an antigen for the first time, it is in a **naïve** or virgin state. When a naïve or virgin B cell comes into contact with an antigen, a chain of events is initiated that results in its activation and subsequent proliferation. Newly formed cells can become either **plasma cells** (actively produce more antibodies specific for that antigen) or **memory cells** (develop a higher affinity for the antigens than their predecessors, but remain uninvolved in the immune response that had spawned them). The memory cells are able to exist for long periods (up to years) and can result in faster, more powerful responses to reexposure of the same antigen. Because of the continued production of antibodies by the plasma cells that was initiated by the B cells, a **humorally mediated immune response** is generated.

The immunoglobulins or antibodies formed by B cells change with the progression of the antigenic exposure and immune response. Naïve B cells produce the IgM antibody, the first isotype of immunoglobulin to be generated in the primary immune response. The IgM class takes on a pentameric form as the heavy chains or Fc regions are bound to one another by J-protein links. This large antibody is designed to activate the complement system and is short lived. On subsequent exposure, the B cells, which are now plasma cells, undergo a process known as *class switching* and produce other classes of antibodies, including IgA, IgE, and IgG with IgG, and IgA, comprising the largest amount of immunoglobulin found in the blood. These antibodies, especially IgG, appear to bind and combat antigens more effectively. In most instances, foreign substances will not induce a humoral immune response until T cell intermediaries have become involved. Still, there are antigens—**thymic-independent antigens**—that will generate a humoral immune response without T cell involvement, but in these instances B memory cells are not formed and as a result only IgM is released.

T LYMPHOCYTE

Like the B cell, the T lymphocyte, or **T cell,** is created in bone marrow, but unlike the B cell, the T cell must first migrate to another region—the thymus—before it can become immunocompetent. The T cell morphology is identical to that previously described for the B cell. The principal difference between the two lymphoid cell types is in antigen receptors that each type possesses. As mentioned, the B cell receptors consist of antibodies that have excellent binding properties. T cell receptors, however, do not consist of antibodies per se, but do have similar properties. **T cell receptors** extend outwardly along the cell membrane of T cells in much the same way as do B cell receptors. Most important, they function as antigen receptors, being able to recognize antigens and bind with their epitopes. However, they have only a single antigen-binding site as opposed to the two binding sites associated with the B cell receptors (see Figure 12-1). Intracellularly, the membrane-bound component of the T cell receptor interacts with other, separate membrane-bound proteins, including CD3, CD8, and CD 28, each of which forms a complex and helps facilitate the receptor-epitope binding and resultant signal transduction of a specific subtype of T cell (Figure 12-2).

The T cell becomes activated only when the T cell receptor is able to perceive an epitope of an antigen that is attached first to the cell membrane of another cell. The antigen, in fact, is bound to the other cell by a specific glycoprotein known as a **major histocompatibility complex (MHC) molecule,** which can be divided into two classes: MHC-I molecules and MHC-II molecules. Whereas most cells of the body contain the class-I MHC molecule, certain cells known as antigen-presenting cells contain both classes of molecules within their cell membranes. Even if a T cell receptor is able to bind to an epitope of an antigen, activation of the T cell will not proceed unless an accompanying MHC molecule is recognized as well (see Figure 12-2).

Like B cells, T cells can be divided into subtypes: T memory cells, T helper cells (1 and 2), cytotoxic T cells, and T suppressor cells. The **T memory cell** is similar to the B memory cell, and is made as a member of a clone after an initial exposure to a specific foreign material that has an immunological memory for it. Activated T cells can produce and release different cytokines that direct the activities of other lymphoid cells. These T cells are called **T helper cells** and consist of two types: T helper cell 1 (T_H1) and T helper cell 2 (T_H2). T_H1 creates cytokines that regulate cellularly mediated immune responses, whereas T_H2 creates cytokines that regulate humorally mediated immune responses (see Figure 12-2). **Cytotoxic T cells** have the ability to attach to target cells, such as cells transformed by viruses, and subsequently kill them. And **T suppressor cells** are able to inhibit the

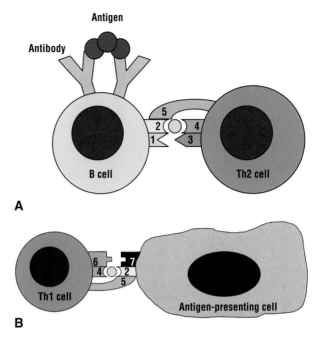

Figure 12-2. Schematic diagram of the interaction between **A,** lymphocytes and **B,** lymphocyte and antigen-presenting cell. In **A,** the interaction between the B cell and the Th(helper)2 cell by the class II MHC-epitope complex *(2),* the T cell receptor *(4)* and CD4 molecules *(5)* along with CD40 *(1)* and CD40 receptor *(3)* results in thymic-dependent, antigen-induced B memory and plasma cell formation. In **B,** the Th(helper)1 cell similarly binds to an antigen-presenting cell by the class II MHC-epitope complex with the T cell receptor and CD4 molecules. In this event the antigen-presenting cell subsequently expresses B7 molecules *(7)* that bind the CD28 *(6)* to the Th(helper)1 cell, which then results in the release of interleukin 2 (IL-2). *(After Gartner LP, Hiatt JL: Color textbook of histology, Philadelphia, 1997, Saunders.)*

activities of other T and B cells and, in effect, reduce or repress the immune response.

ANTIGEN-PRESENTING CELLS

Cells of the monocyte-derived lineage, including macrophages, Kupffer cells, Langerhans cells, dendritic cells, and others throughout the body make up the **antigen-presenting cells** of the immune system. These and the lymphoid cells, B cells and epithelial reticular cells of the thymus, are able to phagocytize and process antigens so as to become "antigenic" when presented to effector cells by attaching MHC-II molecules to the epitopes (see Figure 12-2). In a manner similar to T helper cells, antigen-presenting cells also form cytokines that signal and activate target cells (T cells and macrophages) that then can effectively attack the foreign substance.

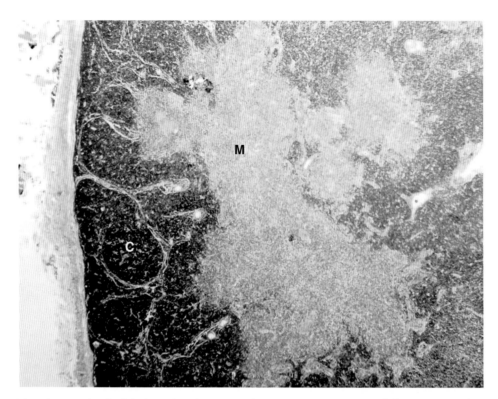

Figure 12-3. Light micrograph of a lobule within the canine thymus. *C,* Cortex; *M,* medulla. (Hematoxylin and eosin stain; ×20.)

In addition to these cells is another population of lymphocytes that comprises the **natural killer cells.** Similar to the cytotoxic T cell, this cell type is able to recognize various tumor- and virally affected cells as foreign and subsequently eradicate them, but without the need or use of the MHC molecule. For that reason, natural killer cells are not required to go to the thymus for immunocompetence. These cells—able to recognize their Fc region—prefer to attack cells coated with antibodies, but they also can destroy cells that are not Fc region presenting. In these antibody-independent instances, the natural killer cells are able to recognize receptors on specific tumor cells or those virally transformed.

THYMUS

The thymus is a bilobed, lymphoepithelial organ located in the cranial mediastinum. During embryonic development it originates along with the parathyroids from the third and possibly fourth pharyngeal pouches. Because the thymus initially was an epithelial structure, a well-formed vascular bed infiltrates the thymic parenchyma, resulting in the formation of the epithelial reticulum. In conjunction with the development of the vasculature, loosely arranged connective tissue

elements form a capsule that covers each lobe and penetrate the parenchyma as incomplete septa, creating lobules that are not entirely separated from each other, but are attached to a central lobe. With maturation, the connective tissue of the capsule becomes dense irregular. The epithelial reticulum consists of stellate cells that remain connected to one another by desmosomes as they are associated with perivascular spaces. Other epithelial cells line the internal periphery of each lobule. Undeveloped lymphocytes (lymphoblasts) originating from the bone marrow invade the epithelial reticulum. Each lobule consists of a central medulla and surrounding cortex (Figure 12-3).

CORTEX

The cortex is composed of lymphocytes and the epithelial reticulum (Figure 12-4). T lymphocytes **(thymocytes),** which have left the bone marrow in an immunologically incompetent state, have migrated and invaded the cortex. At this point they have further divided and been directed to become immunocompetent deep within the cortex. Because of the extensive population of these cells, the cortex of each lobule appears as the darkest region (see Figure 12-3).

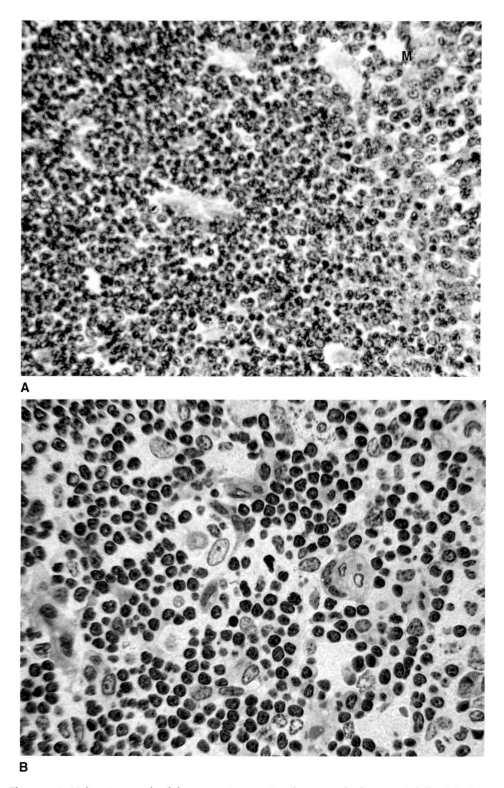

A

B

Figure 12-4. Thymus. **A,** Light micrograph of the cortex in a canine thymus and adjacent medulla *(M)*. (Hematoxylin and eosin [H&E] stain; ×100.) **B,** Light micrograph of the cortex from a plastic section of the thymus of a monkey. (H&E stain; ×400.)

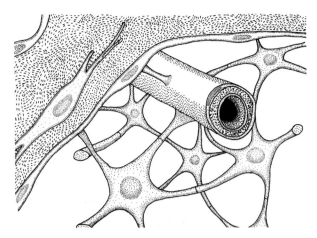

Figure 12-5. Illustration of the epithelial reticular cells within the cortex of the thymus showing the sealed environment of their labyrinth spaces for housing thymocytes (T cells).

Cells of the epithelial reticulum (epithelioreticular cells) can be solely stellate and with their desmosomal attachments to one another form a supportive network called the **cytoreticulum** within the cortex (Figure 12-5). These cells contain numerous intermediate filaments reminiscent of astrocytes of the central nervous system. Other epithelial reticular cells form a continuous lining that separates the cortex from the stromal elements, including septa and associated blood vessels, and creates a tight seal through their occluding junctions while concomitantly extending to the nearby stellate cells (see Figure 12-5). Similar cells isolate the cortex from the medulla. In this way the epithelial reticulum is able to isolate the cortex and the developing thymocytes contained within from potentially incidental antigenic substances as well as present self-antigens to these thymocytes. If the T cell receptors of these developing thymocytes recognize self-proteins or they cannot recognize the self-antigens presented to them by the epithelial reticular cells, these cells are killed before migrating to the medulla. As a result only a small number of the thymocytes leave the cortex.

In addition to the thymocytes and the epithelial reticular cells is a population of resident macrophages. The macrophages are responsible for the removal for the vast number of thymocytes that are killed and appear in greatest number at the boundary of the cortex and the medulla in most species.

MEDULLA

The appearance of the medulla contrasts strongly with that of the cortex in that there are far fewer lym-
phocytes in this region of the thymus, and a portion of the epithelial reticular cells is larger and has more epithelial morphology than those seen in the cortex (Figure 12-6). Overall, the pleomorphic epithelial reticular cells vary in shape. Some can be larger and more rounded than others, whereas some remain stellate. Moreover, some of the epithelial reticular cells form the medulla's most distinctive structures, the thymic corpuscles. Each corpuscle consists of a concentric array of squamous epithelial reticular cells that remain fastened to each other by desmosomes, holding keratohyalin granules and considerable amount of cytoplasmic filaments (Figure 12-7). In some instances, the centers of these whorled-arranged cells degenerate into cornifications or possibly become calcified.

Thymocytes in the medulla are small for the most part, and located within areas of the supportive network formed by epithelial reticular cells in a comparable manner to that seen in the cortex. These lymphocytes, however, tend to be more irregularly shaped than their cortical counterparts.

In the avian thymus, the medulla may contain a variety of unusual structures including myoid cells consisting of skeletal muscle, cystlike bodies with a brush-bordered epithelium, vacuolated epithelial reticular cells with microvilli, and mucus-bearing cells.

INVOLUTION OF THE THYMUS

The thymus is most active in the young, developing animal. With age, the thymus holds fewer lymphocytes than before, with a concomitant rise in both the number of adipocytes and size of the cytoreticulum. This process is referred to as the *involution* of this organ, a form of age-related atrophy, and is generally believed to occur among domestic species. The rate of involution, however, may vary considerably among animals. In sheep, the reduction of the composition of the peripheral T cell pool that is expected to transpire with age occurs very little in adults, and naïve T cells enter the peripheral T cell pool at about the same rate throughout much of their life. However, involution may be accentuated or accelerated by changes in diet, such as nutritional deficiencies, agents associated with infectious disease including bacterial endotoxin, and hormones involving the reproductive system and adrenal glands.

LYMPH NODES

Throughout the network of lymph vessels is a series of **lymph nodes** that filter lymph, including the

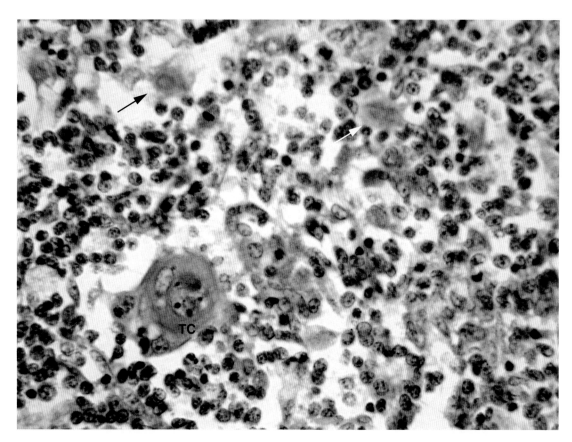

Figure 12-6. Light micrograph of the medulla in the canine thymus. Because the thymocytes are more sparsely populated, the stellate form of the reticular epithelial cells *(arrows)* is readily seen. *TC,* Thymic corpuscle. (Hematoxylin and eosin stain; ×200.)

removal of invading microorganisms and various other foreign materials. Each lymph node is oval and encapsulated, having both afferent and efferent lymph vessels. The latter, along with blood vessels, are located at a **hilum (hilus),** consisting of a small depression (Figure 12-8). Afferent lymph vessels, however, penetrate the rest of the capsule surface. These vessels possess valves, ensuring that only lymph will enter the node at these points. Likewise, the efferent lymph vessels have valves, ensuring in these instances that the filtered lymph will not be remixed with that still being processed in the node (see Figure 12-8). The lymph and blood vessels are housed in a stroma that forms an enveloping capsule of thin, dense irregular connective tissue (Figure 12-9) that broadens at the hilum and follows vessels as trabeculae into the parenchyma. From the trabeculae, an elaborate network of widely spaced reticular fibers (collagen type III) establishes the structural design for the cortical and medullary regions of the node (see Figure 12-9).

The parenchyma of lymph nodes consists of lymphocytes (both B and T), antigen-presenting cells,

and macrophages. Because the antigens are directed to a nearby node, the lymphoid cells respond immunologically. Macrophages actively engulf and digest the various microorganisms that enter the node. Collectively, these cells are found in three regions of the lymph node: the cortex, the paracortex, and the medulla. One should keep in mind that the relative number and organization of the cells within each node of an individual animal are influenced directly by the local response that these cells may be expressing toward varying amounts of antigens that are present within the range of the afferent lymph vessels that flow to a particular node. For that reason some lymph nodes may appear to be weakly developed under normal conditions. Others, such as those associated with the digestive system, can be considerably more active because of the frequent exposure of foreign material.

CORTEX

Along the periphery of each lymph node, concentrations of connective tissue extend inwardly as tra-

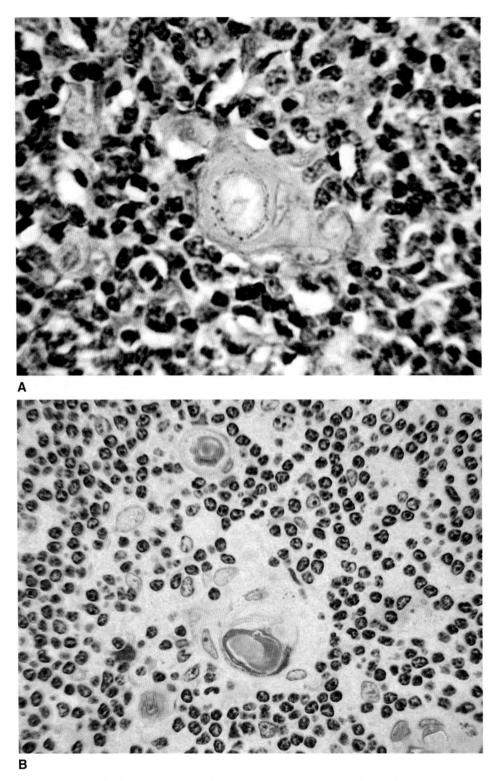

A

B

Figure 12-7. A, Light micrograph of a thymic corpuscle in a young pig. (Hematoxylin and eosin stain; ×400.) **B,** Light micrograph of an adult thymic corpuscle with concentric array of epithelial reticular cells. (Plastic section, hematoxylin and eosin stain; ×400.)

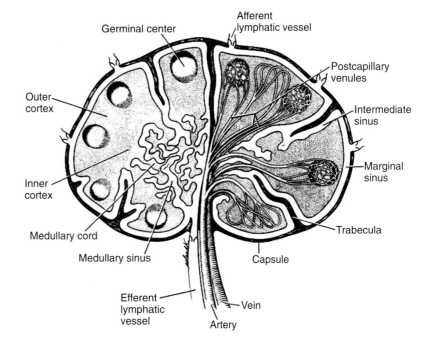

Figure 12-8. Diagram of a lymph node. The left side illustrates the system of lymphatic sinuses that originate beneath the capsule from afferent vessels and drain centrally into the medulla, then empty into the efferent vessel that exits the node at the hilum. The right side illustrates the vascular tree within the lymph node. *(Modified from Fawcett DW:* Bloom and Fawcett: a textbook of histology, *ed 11, Philadelphia, 1986, Saunders.)*

beculae from the capsule to form open-ended compartments that interface centrally with the medulla (see Figure 12-8). Concomitantly, each trabecula is lined by a sinus that arises from a subcapsular (marginal) sinus, which, in turn, is fed by afferent lymph vessels. From each trabecula small reticular fibers form a lacy network of structural support for the lymphoid cells to coexist (see Figure 12-9). The cortical parenchyma is usually arranged into spherically shaped **lymphatic (lymphoid) nodules** and **diffuse lymphoid tissue** (see Figure 12-9; Figure 12-10). Lymphatic nodules can be described as being **primary** and **secondary.** Primary lymphatic nodules are intensely stained areas that consist of B lymphocytes that have either entered the lymph node or are leaving it. Often the center of a primary nodule appears more lightly stained as a result of the plasma cells being formed as well as B lymphocytes and are now referred to as secondary nodules. These areas (also called **germinal centers**), develop when the node has been challenged antigenically. The lightly stained centers or light regions are lined externally by caps of small lymphocytes that are directed toward incoming lymph.

PARACORTEX

At the inner portion of the cortex is a region between the cortex and the medulla that is populated mostly by T lymphocytes. This region, the **paracortex,** merges the cortex with the medulla without obvious borders (see Figures 12-8 and 12-9). As B lymphocytes move toward the outer cortex, T cells remain in this

region, resulting in a **thymus-dependent zone.** When antigen-presenting cells arrive in the paracortex, the epitope MHC-II complexes are presented to the T helper cells and divide if activated.

MEDULLA

In most domestic species, the innermost portion of the lymph node, that lying near the hilum, is the **medulla**—loosely populated lymph sinuses interspersed with clusters of lymphocytes, plasma cells, and macrophages called **medullary cords** that become prominent in active nodes (Figure 12-11). The medullary cords are enriched with reticular fibers as well as reticular cells and are sites where lymphocytes have left the cortex to enter the medullary sinuses.

LYMPH SINUSES

Much of each lymph node consists of a system of sinuses that originate along the inside margin of the capsule, receiving the contents of afferent lymph vessels emptying into the node. These sinuses, the subcapsular sinuses, comprise a bowl-shaped cavity that flow along the perimeter of each trabecula, going toward the labyrinth of sinuses within the medulla (see Figure 12-8). The sinuses possess a meshwork of luminal stellate cells that function in part to slow the movement of newly entered material, allowing macrophages and lymphoid cells to react in a timely manner (Figure 12-12).

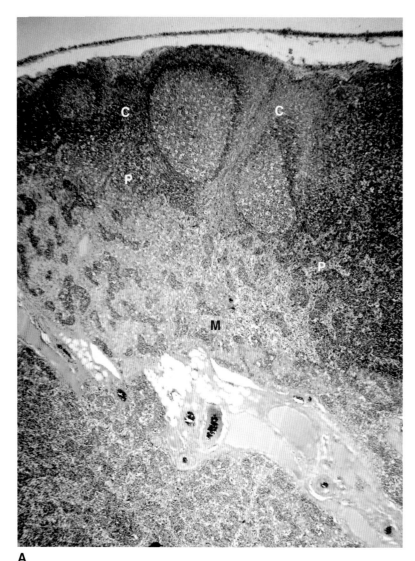

A

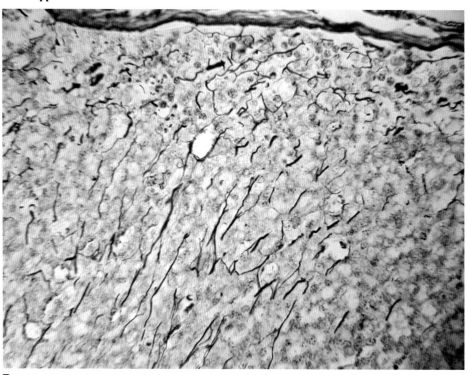

B

Figure 12-9. Lymph node. **A,** Light micrograph of the canine lymph node. *C,* Cortex; *M,* medulla; *P,* paracortex. (Hematoxylin and eosin stain; ×20.) **B,** Light micrograph of the reticular fibers within the cortex. (Silver stain; ×200.)

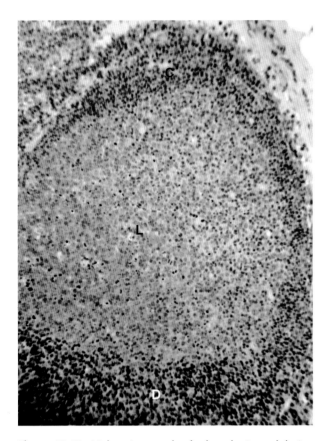

Figure 12-10. Light micrograph of a lymphatic nodule in the cortex of the canine lymph node. *C,* Cap; *L,* light region; *D,* dark region. (Hematoxylin and eosin stain; ×200.)

SPECIES VARIATIONS

The development and the relationship of the cortex and the medulla vary among domestic animals. In some species such as the ox, the cortex is well compartmentalized and clearly delimited by extensive trabeculae. In general, larger lymph nodes possess more developed trabeculae. In contrast with other animals, the pig has a differently constructed lymph node, with a medullary region that lies next to the capsule, surrounding a central cortex. In this animal the afferent vessels travel deeply by way of the trabeculae to the lymphatic nodules, where lymph filters outwardly toward the sinuses of the peripheral medulla. The centralization of efferent vessels is less evident in the pig, often making it difficult to recognize a defined hilum.

SPLEEN

Within the lymphatic system the **spleen** is the largest component, functioning in several capacities. In addition to serving as an area for T and B cell proliferation and antibody (Ab) formation of blood-borne antigens, it acts as a filter for blood by removing and breaking down old erythrocytes as well as recycling their iron. Moreover, the spleen in domestic species has the ability to add to the erythrocyte and granulocyte populations and can be a reservoir for red blood cells during periods of unusual demand.

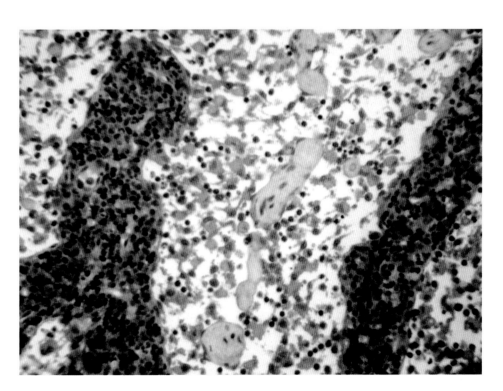

Figure 12-11. Light micrograph of the medulla of the canine lymph node. (Hematoxylin and eosin stain; ×200.)

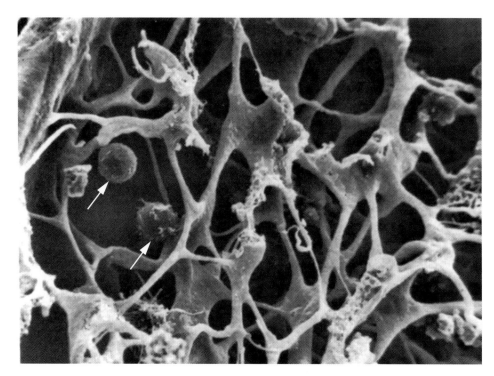

Figure 12-12. Scanning electron micrograph of a sinus within a canine lymph node containing numerous stellate cells. Arrows point to probable lymphocytes. *(Modified from Fawcett DW:* Bloom and Fawcett: a textbook of histology, *ed 11, Philadelphia, 1986, Saunders.)*

Like lymph nodes the spleen is covered by a capsule of dense irregular connective tissue oriented circumferentially. Unlike lymph nodes, there are no afferent lymph vessels that lead to the capsule. Collagenous cords or trabeculae extend radially from the capsule into the body of the spleen, separating the parenchyma into compartments. In many instances, smooth muscle may comprise much, if not most, of the capsule and trabeculae, helping facilitate the removal of blood from this organ (Figure 12-13). Within the spleen, the often highly congested parenchyma is lined by numerous reticular fibers.

Most of the capsular surface of the spleen is convex, converging into a recessed area, the **hilum (hilus).** At the hilum, the capsule broadens as arteries ingress and veins and lymph vessels egress. Branches of the arteries first enter the trabeculae **(trabecular arteries)** before eventually moving into the parenchyma. When leaving the trabeculae, the arteries are lined by a loosely arranged adventitia that holds a sheath of lymphocytes referred to as the **periarterial lymphatic sheath (PALS)** (Figures 12-14 and 12-15). Centrally located within these sheaths, these arteries are called **central arteries.** As these arteries enter nodules, they can be referred to as **nodular arteries.** At the end of each artery, the vessel, which is now reduced to arteriolar size, has entered the portion of the nodule

known as the red pulp (referred to as the pulp arteriole). The lymphatic sheath is absent around this vessel, which will soon branch into short capillaries that run approximately parallel to one another (see Figure 12-15). These capillaries can contain areas called **sheathed capillaries,** where its endothelial cells become tall and the surrounding regions have sheaths of a different kind. These sheaths consist of thickened walls of reticular fibers and reticular cells interspersed with red blood cells and macrophages (Figure 12-16; see also Figure 12-15). The areas of the capillary sheaths can vary in size—prominent in the cat and pig, but less so in the dog, horse, and ruminants. The shape of the sheathed capillary is commonly elliptical but can be spherical as well. In addition, before the termination of the nodular artery, small branches lead to capillary beds without reticular sheaths. These capillary beds and the sheathed capillaries empty into the venous outflow component, consisting primarily of **venous sinusoids,** of the spleen (see Figure 12-15). It may be that some of the capillaries empty directly into the venous sinusoids **(closed circulation),** whereas others end near the sinusoids **(open circulation).** In the latter instance, the blood of these vessels moves first into the extracellular matrix of the red pulp before entering the sinuses. It is not understood at this time whether domestic species possess both open and closed

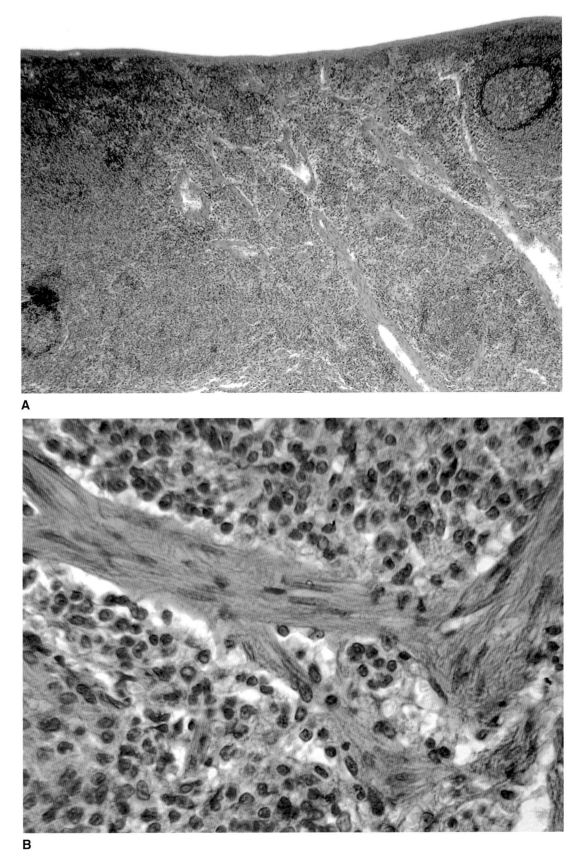

Figure 12-13. Light micrograph of a spleen of a cat with smooth muscle within the trabeculae, **A,** and capsule, **B.** (**A,** Hematoxylin and eosin [H&E] stain; ×25; **B,** H&E; ×250.)

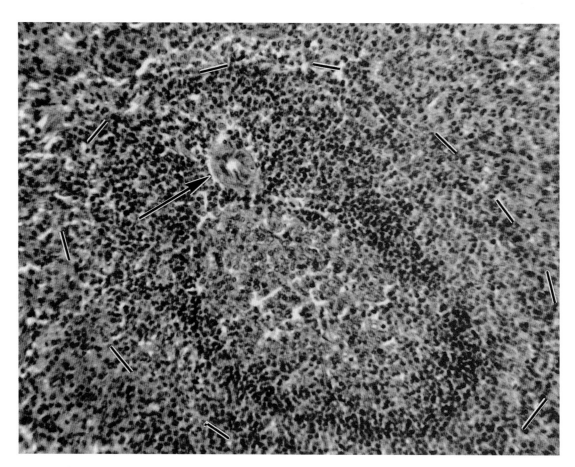

Figure 12-14. Light micrograph of a periarterial lymphatic sheath (PALS) outlined by the broken line in the feline spleen. A lymphatic nodule is positioned centrally of the PALS. Arrow points to the central artery, which here is pushed off to one side. (Hematoxylin and eosin stain; ×100.)

circulation or just one or the other. For some time the canine spleen had been thought to be open, but recently has been determined to be closed. In any case, the venous sinusoids empty into trabecular veins that coalesce into the splenic vein, which in turns flows into the portal vein.

Unlike the thymus and the lymph node, the parenchyma of the spleen is not readily subdivided into a cortex and a medulla. Instead, the architecture of the parenchyma follows closely that of the vasculature and as a result is composed of two regions or areas called pulps, the **white pulp** and the **red pulp,** that intertwine with one another and can be seen both grossly and histologically (Figure 12-17; see also Figure 12-15).

White Pulp

The central arteries leaving the trabeculae and the surrounding sheaths of lymphocytes, the PALS, comprise most of the white pulp (see Figures 12-14 and 12-15). Within the PALS may exist lymphoid nodules

that house numerous B cells and possess germinal centers, indicating antigenic activity. The construction of the periarterial lymphoid sheaths is comparable with that seen in paracortical regions of lymph nodes with the loosely knit arrangement of reticular fibers and associated reticular cells. T cells are predominantly located in proximity to the artery within the PALS. As the white pulp interfaces with the red pulp, the reticular cells, which become flattened at this point, and the reticular fibers are oriented circumferentially. Plasma cells and macrophages are more numerous here than in the rest of the white pulp, where they tend to be few. When the spleen is exposed to blood-borne antigens, the white pulp becomes filled with lymphocytes (many are large) as well as lymphoblasts and immature plasma cells. Lymphoid nodules become more apparent with well-defined germinal centers, including caps of small lymphocytes that are oriented toward the red pulp. These nodules can attain substantial size, occurring as localized expansions of the PALS, often displacing the central artery. In addition to these components are also lymph

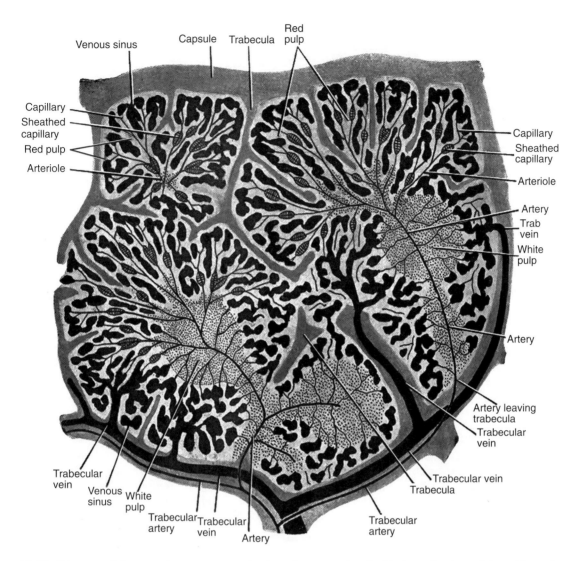

Figure 12-15. Diagram of the vascular arrangement in the spleen associated with the red pulp and the white pulp. *(Modified from Maximow AA, Bloom WA:* Textbook of histology, *ed 2, Philadelphia, 1934, Saunders.)*

vessels that originate in the white pulp and exit this region by way of the trabeculae, eventually joining and leaving the spleen at the hilum.

Red Pulp

Surrounding the white pulp is the **red pulp,** composed of a well-developed network of venous sinusoids with intervening cellular partitions known as **splenic cords,** plus continuations of the central arteries as pulp arterioles and their capillaries. The red pulp derives its name from the extensive vasculature in this part of the spleen seen grossly when compared with the gray pallor of the white pulp. The splenic cords contain numerous erythrocytes, lymphocytes, plasma cells, macrophages, and granulocytes intertwined and enveloped by stellate

reticular cells and their collagen type III fibers (Figure 12-18). Damaged red blood cells are engulfed and broken down by the large population of macrophages. This part of the spleen is involved in the degradation of hemoglobin and the recycling of iron.

The venous sinusoids or sinuses are lined by an unusually shaped endothelium consisting of cells that are fusiform shaped and widely spaced, oriented along the longitudinal axis of each sinus (Figure 12-19). When viewed light microscopically, the shape of the endothelial cells can appear cuboidal, with their nuclei positioned next to the vessel lumen. The elongated spaces between adjacent endothelial cells allow cells of the splenic cord to move into the sinuses (see Figures 12-18 and 12-19). Macrophages may also extend their processes through these spaces

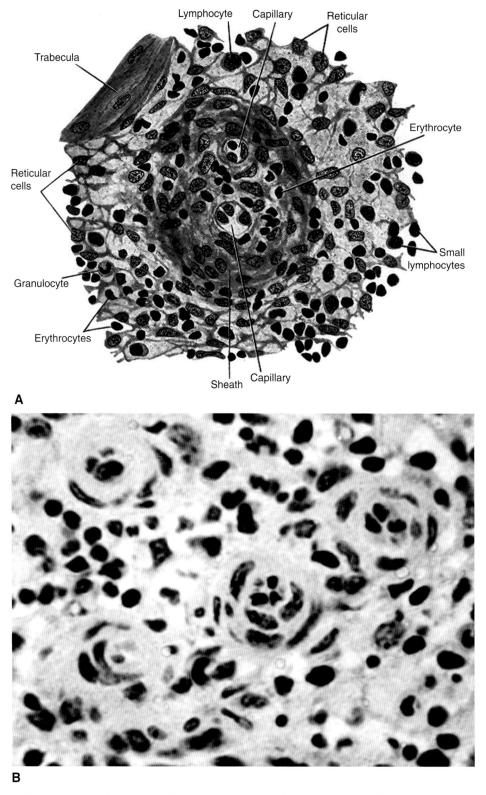

Figure 12-16. A, Illustration of a sheathed capillary in the dog. **B,** Light micrograph of closely located sheathed capillaries in the red pulp of a monkey. (Plastic section, hematoxylin and eosin stain: ×400.) *(**A** modified from Maximow AA, Bloom WA: Textbook of histology, ed 2, Philadelphia, 1934, Saunders.)*

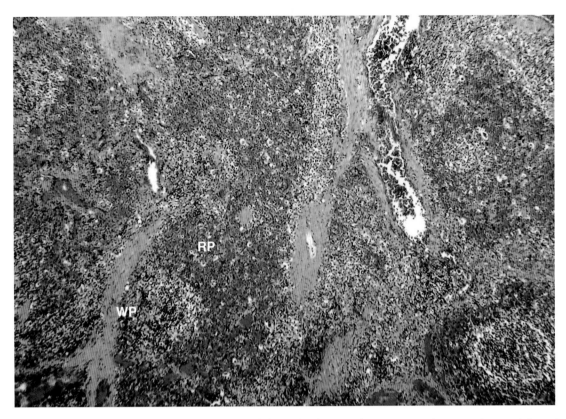

Figure 12-17. Light micrograph of white pulp *(WP)* and the red pulp *(RP)* that comprise the parenchyma of the spleen in the manatee. (Hematoxylin and eosin stain; ×20.)

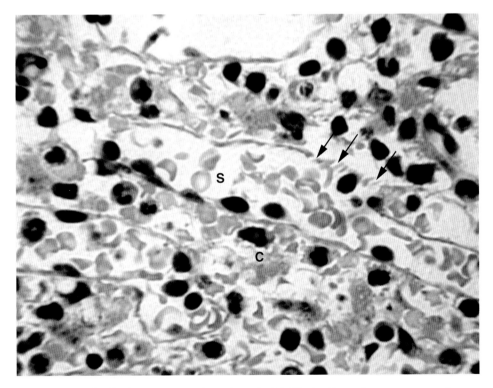

Figure 12-18. Light micrograph of splenic sinuses *(S)* and cords *(C)* filled with erythrocytes, macrophages, and a variety of leucocytes. Arrows point to the elongated spaces between endothelial cells. (Hematoxylin and eosin stain; ×400.)

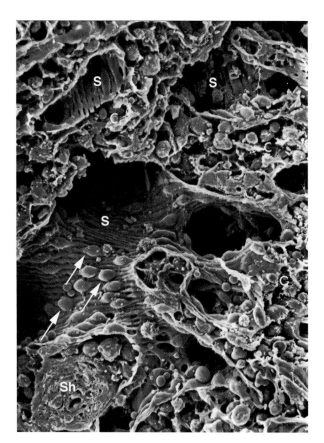

Figure 12-19. Scanning electron micrograph of splenic sinuses *(S)* and cords *(C)*. *Sh,* Sheathed capillary. Arrows point to the nuclei of the endothelial lining of the sinuses that protrude into its lumen. *(Modified from Leeson and Leeson TS, Leeson CR, Paparo AA:* Text/atlas of histology, *Philadelphia, 1988, Saunders).*

and in doing so monitor blood moving through each sinus.

In general, the red pulp of the spleen in domestic species is well developed, but by comparison, the white pulp appears much less developed. Nevertheless, the amount of white pulp varies, and is more prominent in the dog and horse than in the cat and ruminants. In the dog, as well as in the rat and human, an open-ended perimarginal cavernous sinus plexus occurs between the boundary of the white and red pulps. It is believed that in species with this plexus, about 90% of splenic inflow has the potential to exit by this route, bypassing the filtration beds of the red pulp. As noted, the size, shape, and prevalence of the sheathed capillaries vary substantially among domestic animals.

DIFFUSE LYMPHATIC TISSUES

Within the immune system is a collection of diffuse lymphatic tissues that consist of concentrated areas of lymphocytes, including lymph nodules (follicles). In contrast with the thymus, lymph nodes, and spleen, these tissues are nonencapsulated and associated with the mucosal portion of the gastrointestinal, urinary, and respiratory tracts (**mucosa-associated lymphatic tissue [MALT]).** When associated with the alimentary canal, they are usually referred to as **gut-associated lymphatic tissue (GALT),** and when associated with the respiratory tract, they are called **bronchus-associated lymphatic tissue (BALT).**

Lymph nodules are composed of circumscribed assemblies of lymphocytes packed tightly together and principally populated in B cells. Antigen-presenting cells and T cells typically surround the nodules in a loosely arranged manner. There is often a light staining area within a nodule, which represents a **germinal center** for lymphocyte proliferation. The proliferating cells, lymphoblasts, are responsible for the light stain reaction, because these cells are large when compared with the other lymphocytes, having fairly abundant cytoplasm and larger and less heterochromatic nuclei than the other cells (Figure 12-20). Generally, the mucosa-associated lymphatic tissues occur separately, and are isolated from one another. However, along specific areas of the gastrointestinal tract, especially the ileum of the small intestine, nodules can form clusters, sometimes referred to as *Peyer's patches.* Where the simple columnar epithelium usually lines that region, the lymph nodules are lined by flattened or squamous-like cells called M (microfold) cells. These cells are able to collect and transfer antigenic material of particle size to the nodule. Comparable nodules comprising BALT develop in the larger airways of the respiratory tract; they are located adjacent to the respiratory epithelium of the bronchi and proximal bronchioles. As in GALT, BALT is lined by M cells instead of the pseudostratified columnar epithelium.

Lymph nodules located within the caudal oral cavity and pharynx are clustered and partially encapsulated. These structures are called *tonsils* and specifically referred to by location. The palatine tonsils are located bilaterally at the junction of the oral cavity and pharynx. These tonsils are lined by a stratified squamous epithelium that can be smooth in carnivores or deeply invaginated in small ruminants and the horse (Figure 12-21). The lingual tonsils are found along the dorsal surface of the caudal portion of the tongue and like the palatine tonsils are covered by a stratified squamous epithelium. The pharyngeal tonsil is located along the roof of the nasopharynx and lined by a pseudostratified columnar epithelium. Diffuse lymphatic tissue generally lies next to the epithelia of each of these different tonsils. Much of the parenchyma is composed of lymph nodules, some having

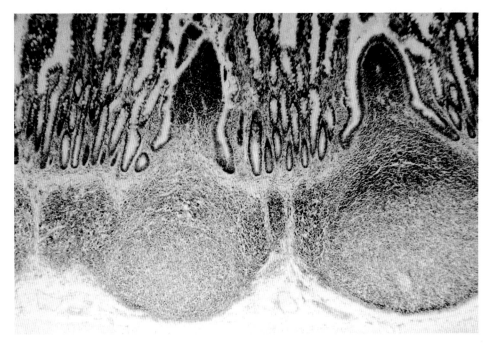

Figure 12-20. Light micrograph of a cluster of lymphatic nodules (Peyer's patch) in the ileum of a cat. (Hematoxylin and eosin stain; ×30.)

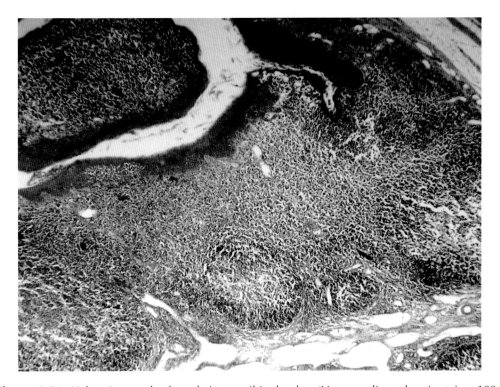

Figure 12-21. Light micrograph of a palatine tonsil in the dog. (Hematoxylin and eosin stain; ×100.)

germinal centers. The deep portion of each tonsil is separated from the adjacent tissue to some extent by a fibrous capsule that can be well developed in the palatine and pharyngeal tonsils.

AVIAN CLOACAL BURSA

In birds the **cloacal bursa (bursa of Fabricius)** is a lymphoid organ that is the thymus counterpart for B cells. It is believed that the bursa is a primary lymphatic organ for B cell differentiation. The precursors of the lymphoid cells originate elsewhere, quite possibly the spleen. The bursa, which is located dorsally in the cloaca, possesses a lymphoepithelial parenchyma comparable with that of the thymus. During embryonic development, lymphoid progenitor cells move into the developing bursa with subsequent formation of nodules (follicles). Concomitantly, epithelial buds extend inwardly to produce the reticuloepithelial cells that form the stroma of the medullary and cortical portions of this organ. During early development of the bursa, the formation of the tripeptide called *bursin*, which is a B cell–differentiation hormone, is essential for the normal development and subsequent activity of the pineal gland.

SUGGESTED READINGS

Alexandre-Pires G, Pais D, Esperanca Pina JA: Intermediary spleen microvasculature in *Canis familiaris*—morphological evidences of a closed and open type, *Anat Histol Embryol* 32:263, 2003.

Binns RM: Organisation of the lymphoreticular system and lymphocyte markers in the pig, *Vet Immunol Immunopathol* 3:95, 1982.

Binns RM, Pabst R: Lymphoid tissue structure and lymphocyte trafficking in the pig, *Vet Immunol Immunopathol* 43:79, 1994.

Cunningham CP, Kimpton WG, Holder JE, Cahill RN: Thymic export in aged sheep: a continuous role for the thymus throughout pre- and postnatal life, *Eur J Immunol* 31:802, 2001.

Fawcett DW: *Bloom and Fawcett: a textbook of histology,* ed 11, Philadelphia, 1986, Saunders.

Fournel C, Magnol JP, Marchal T, et al: An original perifollicular zone cell in the canine reactive lymph node: a morphological, phenotypical and aetological study, *J Comp Pathol* 113:217, 1995.

Gartner LP, Hiatt JL: *Color textbook of histology,* Philadelphia, 1997, Saunders.

Griebel PJ, Kugelberg B, Ferrari G: Two distinct pathways of B-cell development in Peyer's patches, *Dev Immunol* 4:263, 1996.

Li L, Hsu HC, Grizzle WE, et al: Cellular mechanism of thymic involution, *Scand J Immunol* 57:410, 2003.

Ploemen JP, Ravesloot WT, van Esch E: The incidence of thymic B lymphoid follicles in healthy beagle dogs, *Toxicol Pathol* 31:214, 2003.

Landsverk T, Halleraker M, Aleksandersen M, et al: The intestinal habitat for organized lymphoid tissues in ruminants: comparative aspects of structure, function and development, *Vet Immunol Immunopathol* 28:1, 1991.

Leeson TS, Leeson CR, Paparo AA: Text/atlas of histology, Philadelphia, 1988, Saunders.

Maximow AA, Bloom WA: *Textbook of histology,* ed 2, Philadelphia, 1934, Saunders.

Reynolds JD: Peyer's patches and the early development of B lymphocytes. *Curr Top Microbiol Immunol* 135:43, 1987.

Schmidt EE, MacDonald IC, Groom AC: Comparative aspects of splenic microcirculatory pathways in mammals: the region bordering the white pulp, *Scanning Microsc* 7:613, 1993.

Snook T: A comparative study of the vascular arrangements in the mammalian spleens, *Am J Anat* 87:31, 1950.

Sompayrac L: *How the immune system works,* Malden, Mass, 2003, Blackwell Science.

Suzuki T, Furusato M, Shimizu S, Hataba Y: Stereoscopic scanning electron microscopy of the red pulp of dog spleen with special reference to the terminal structure of the cordal capillaries, *Cell Tissue Res* 182:441, 1977.

Integument

KEY CHARACTERISTICS

- Highly cellular external lining; epidermis, covering dense connective tissue; dermis, which protects and houses glands; blood vessels; nerve endings
- Major cells of the epidermis: keratinocyte, Langerhans cell, melanocyte, Merkel cell
- Major cells of the dermis: fibrocyte, adipocyte, mast cell, histiocyte
- Modified appendages include hairs, claws, hoofs, horns

The external lining of the body consists of skin and its varied specializations, which among domestic species includes claws, hoofs, pads, and horns. The integument is actually the largest of all organs; it has a large surface area, especially in large ungulates, that can be several meters square or more, and considerably thick. Skin functions to protect the body against exposure to the external environment and continual changes occurring within the outside world while concomitantly interacting with the body's internal environment and its possible physiologic fluctuations. In addition, the skin contributes to external sensory awareness, thermoregulation, immunologic defense, and wound healing.

Skin is composed of two portions: the epidermis and the dermis. The **epidermis** consists of a stratified squamous epithelium that is usually cornified or keratinized. Inside and beneath the epidermis is a layer of connective tissue called the **dermis.** The development of both portions varies considerably from species to species, depending on protective needs of the animal against desiccation and abrasion (Figure 13-1).

In addition to the epidermis and dermis is another structure associated with skin—**hypodermis,** which lies internally to the dermis (see Figure 13-1). The hypodermis, also referred to as **subcutaneous tissue,** can be rich in adipose tissue and loose connective tissue, which serves to anchor the skin to adjacent structures, such as skeletal muscle, and forms the superficial fascia of gross anatomy.

EPIDERMIS

A keratinized stratified squamous epithelium, the epidermis is a seal that prevents the body from rapidly dehydrating. In its absence, extensive evaporation from the underlying tissues occurs. Whereas the epidermis is an absolute necessity for terrestrial animals, this external portion of the skin is also impermeable to water and thus is an essential feature for aquatic species. The epidermis is composed of two cell populations: **keratinocytes** (those that solely constitute the epithelium) and **nonkeratinocytes** (those cells that have migrated into the keratinized stratified squamous epithelium, including melanocytes, macrophages, and lymphocytes).

KERATINOCYTES

Keratinized stratified squamous epithelium consists of five discrete regions or strata (see Figure 3-15). The

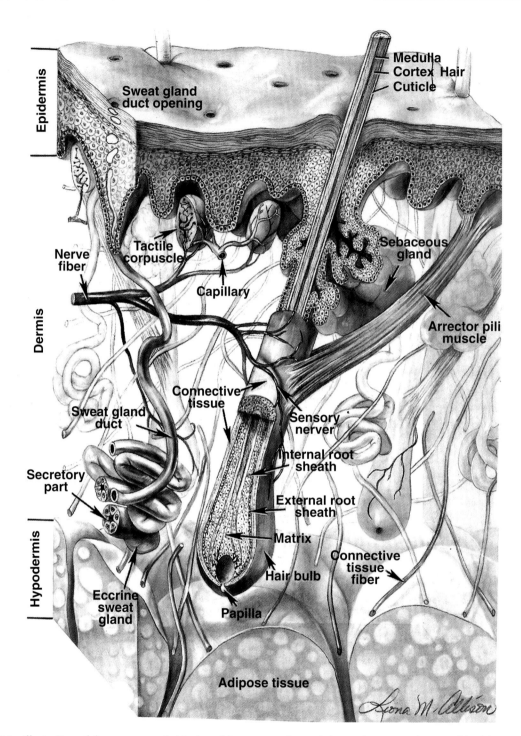

Figure 13-1. Illustration of the structure of skin found in many regions of domestic mammals. *(Modified from Leeson CR, Leeson TS, Paparo AA: Atlas of histology, ed 2, Philadelphia, 1985, Saunders.)*

first and innermost region is the **basal layer,** or **stratum basale,** which produces continuously (mostly at night) new cells to the epidermis as well as anchors the epidermis to the dermis through the basal lamina that it creates and the hemidesmosomes attached to it (Figure 13-2). The basal layer comprises a single layer of stem cells that can be columnar to cuboidal and mitose sporadically with one of the resultant cells contributed to the remaining strata of the epidermis. These cells become involved in tonofilament production early, with some of the tonofilaments being associated with the hemidesmosomes that attach the base of the epidermis to the dermis (see Figure 13-2). The tonofilaments made not only are associated with the numerous

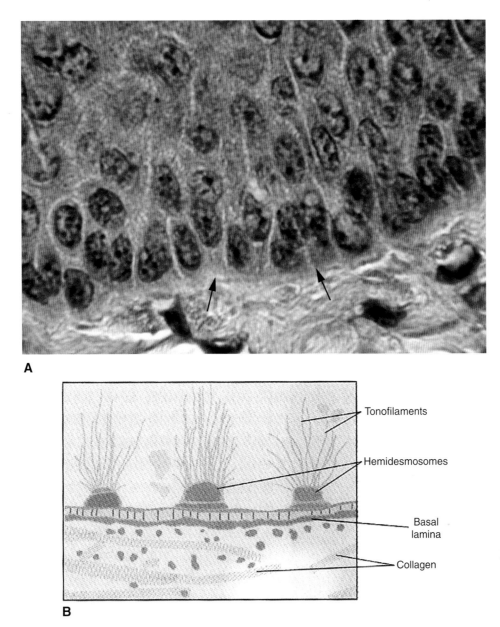

A

B

Figure 13-2. A, Light micrograph (×400) of the basal portion of the porcine epidermis and its attachment to the dermis by the basement membrane *(arrows).* **B,** Diagram of the anchoring structures, hemidesmosomes, that firmly secure the basal cells to the underlying extracellular matrix. *(From Bergman RA, Afifi AK, Heidger PM Jr:* Histology, *Philadelphia, 1996, Saunders.)*

desmosomes that form the primary attachment structure from one cell to another within the epidermis, but also form prekeratin bodies or plaques that mature into keratin in the cells of the other strata.

The keratinocytes derived from the basal or germinating layer form the **stratum spinosum,** which is one to three cell layers thick in hairy skin and often four or five cell layers thick in hairless (glabrous) skin, but can be prominent in regions where the skin thickens such as the nares of the nose or the pads of feet (Figure 13-3). The spiny cellular processes that extend

to every adjacent cell provide the principal morphological feature of this region of the epidermis. Each process ends as a desmosome, making this region of the skin highly resistant to the mechanical effects of stretching and pressing. The intercellular spaces between these processes may provide conduits for substances to be secreted eventually by the keratinocytes as they approach full development. Small membrane-bound **lamellar granules (Odland bodies)** become apparent in the oldest, outermost layers of this stratum (Figure 13-4). These granules appear round to

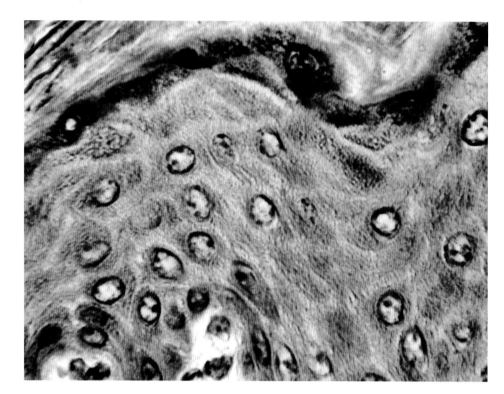

Figure 13-3. Light micrograph of the stratum spinosum in the epidermis of a pig. (Hematoxylin and eosin stain; ×4000.)

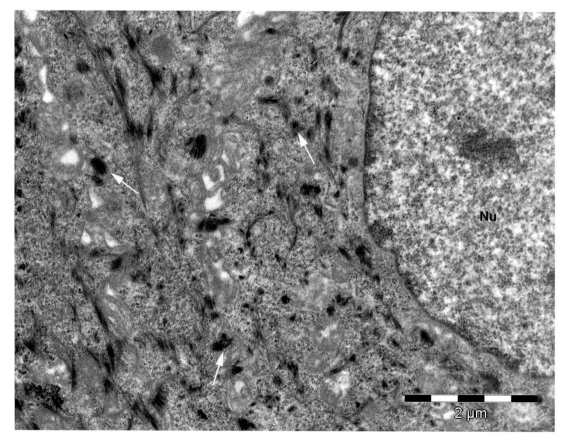

Figure 13-4. Transmission electron micrograph (×20,000) of the stratum spinosum in the epidermis of a pig. Arrows point to small lamellar granules forming within the cytoplasm of the older keratinocytes. *Nu,* Nucleus.

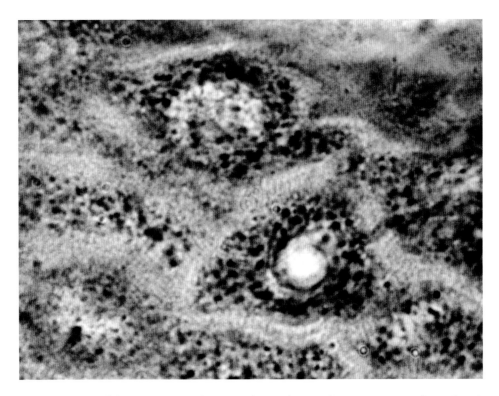

Figure 13-5. Light micrograph of the stratum granulosum in the epidermis of a pig. (Hematoxylin and eosin stain; ×400.)

branched tubular and most likely are derived from the Golgi apparatus.

With increased amounts of the lamellar granules, the spiny keratinocytes become transformed into granular cells and thus result in the formation of the third region of the epidermis, the **stratum granulosum.** The stratum granulosum is characterized by the presence of the granule-bearing keratinocytes that react basophically with stains such as hematoxylin (Figure 13-5). The granules are referred to as **keratohyalin granules,** which eventually fill much of the cytoplasm (Figure 13-6). The granules consist of profilaggrin, which is the precursor for **filaggrin.** Filaggrin is the protein responsible for keratin filament aggregation in the process of cornification. In addition, the lamellar granules continue to form within the cytoplasm. Histologically, the nuclei become difficult to distinguish because of the abundance of these granules, which contain lipid components as well as hydrolytic enzymes and other proteins. The lipid and enzyme portions are extruded or released into the intercellular spaces, becoming filled with ceramides, cholesterols, and fatty acids. As a result, the intercellular lipid mixture creates a watertight seal. This stratum is usually two or three cells thick, but can be as thin as a single cell layer or many layers in thickened skin. The oldest cells of the stratum granulosum undergo a necrobiotic process that involves the degeneration of

the nucleus and all associated metabolic apparatuses by the release and subsequent digestion of lysosomal enzymes. The combination of this event, the packaging of the granules and release of lipids, which undoubtedly facilitates the cell's death, culminates in the final keratinization process. Each keratinocyte, which has become squamous in form, is now organelleless and filled with keratin and its aggregated forms, keratohyalin. These cells are still lined by cell membranes coated by a lipid-rich matrix. Cells undergoing this final process comprise the **stratum lucidum** and can only be observed histologically in thickened skin where they appear as clear cells with a relatively homogeneous protoplasm (Figure 13-7).

When the keratinization process has been completed, the cells have joined other cells that had undergone the process before them to form the **stratum corneum,** the outermost region of the epidermis. The keratin filaments within each cell are oriented parallel to the surface of the skin. Keratinocytes of the stratum corneum tend to be chromophobic and cytologically homogeneous when treated with the traditional stains such as hematoxylin and eosin (see Figure 13-7). Within its innermost layers, the adjacent apposing (front and back) cells are tightly compressed against one another and, along with the numerous desmosomes and intercellular deposits, create a tight seal. Among the outermost cells (those immediately

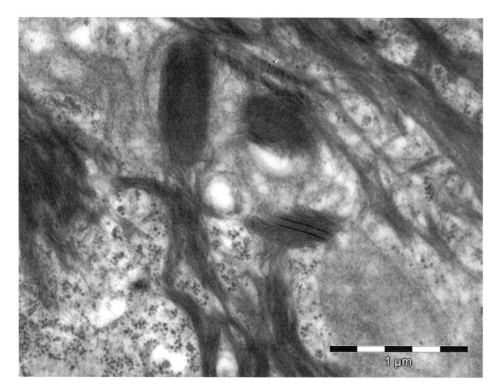

Figure 13-6. Transmission electron micrograph (×40,000) of forming keratohyalin granules in a keratinocyte within the stratum granulosum of the porcine epidermis.

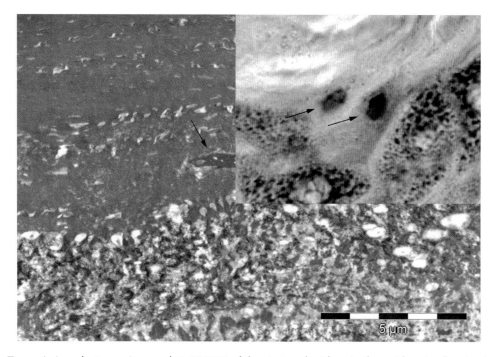

Figure 13-7. Transmission electron micrograph (×20,000) of the stratum lucidum in the epidermis of a pig. *Inset:* Light micrograph (×400) of the stratum lucidum. (Hematoxylin and eosin stain.) Arrows point to the fading nuclei within the cells of this ephemeral layer.

adjacent to the environment), the seal is weakened as fewer desmosomes and less-intercellular deposits are apparent. With casual abrasion these cells can be removed, a process known as **desquamation,** which is usually continuous, but can vary in rate. This superficial layer(s) of cells that are being normally removed is sometimes referred to as the **stratum disjunctum.**

NONKERATINOCYTES

Whereas the epidermis consists mostly of keratinocytes in the form of a keratinized stratified squamous epithelium, other cells reside within this portion of the skin that have migrated from the adjacent dermis or from the central nervous system (CNS) and developed with the surface ectoderm to form the epidermis. The cells that originate from connective tissue provide defense and protection for the integument, which consists of melanocytes and Langerhans cells.

Melanocyte

The **melanocyte,** a melanin-forming cell, is more closely associated with the integument than with any other system in the body. Although this cell type is found in the dermis, it is especially involved with the epidermis, located within the basal layer or lying immediately inside it (Figure 13-8). Typically these melanocytes possess a number of armlike processes that extend into the stratum spinosum. In active melanocytes, developing melanosomes move into

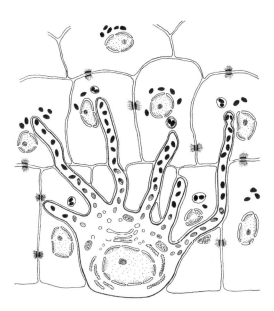

Figure 13-8. Diagram of a melanocyte along the basal layer of the epidermis with its finger-like processes that protrude into adjacent cells and insert melanin granules through tips that pinch off.

each process. Each process is able to push into either a basal cell or a young, developing keratinocyte of the stratum spinosum and give up its distal-most part, which includes mature melanosomes. Eventually, the cell membranes of both the melanocyte fragmented process and the keratinocyte's phagosome break down and allow the melanosomes to be moved freely within the cytoplasm of the keratinocytes and become positioned in a lid- or caplike manner over the nucleus (Figure 13-9). In this way the stem cells of the stratified squamous epithelium are protected against effects of too much light, particularly its ultraviolet components. The possible devastating and mutagenic effects of ultraviolet (UV) light on replicating deoxyribonucleic acid (DNA) are minimized. However, breeds of domestic species that are lightly pigmented or partially albinotic are highly susceptible to damaging effects of the sun.

Melanocyte shape and size can vary according to the density of their population. In areas of the body where they are relatively few, such as inside the limbs, their processes can be long and dendritic, and the cell bodies polygonal. By comparison, in areas of high population densities, as in the epidermal lining of canine nares, the processes are short and the cell bodies are round (see Figure 13-8).

Melanosome development occurs in four steps, beginning initially as a basic structural unit consisting of tyrosinase and a protein matrix that has been generated by the Golgi apparatus (Figure 13-10). The units become more structured during the second stage and an ordered pattern within the melanosome takes form. In stage III melanosomes, melanin biosynthesis occurs within the ordered pattern. As melanogenesis proceeds, the entire unit is filled and matures into a uniformly dense body that is generally referred to as a **melanin granule.** This type of development occurs in the form of melanin known as **eumelanin,** which is the most common occurring form, existing in most domestic and wildlife species including birds, reptiles, and amphibia. However, another form of melanin (**phaeomelanin**) is responsible for the reddish brown to yellow coloring of skin, hair, and feathers of different species and breeds of mammals and birds, including the junglefowl, Jersey buff turkey, llamas, horses, sheep, dogs, cats, and so on. In the formation of this melanin, the ordered pattern found in second and third stages of eumelanin development is absent. Instead, the units begin as small round structures that become opaque early in development and gradually increase in size, with new melanin added peripherally to the melansome until its full size is attained (see Figure 13-10). The melanin granules finally constructed are characteristically round, whereas those made of eumelanin are often oval. In both forms of

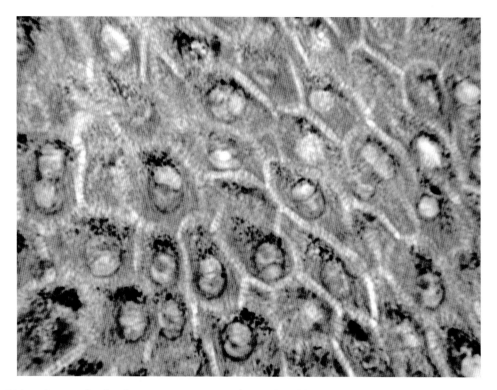

Figure 13-9. Light micrograph of melanin "caps" covering the nuclei of keratinocytes in the stratum spinosum of canine skin. (Hematoxylin and eosin stain; ×400.)

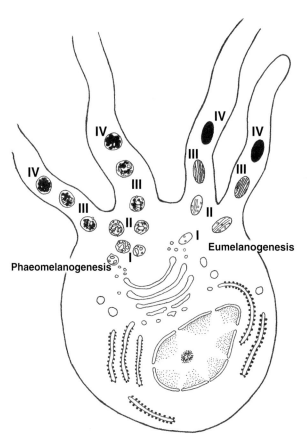

Figure 13-10. Diagram of the two forms of melanogenesis that can occur in the melanocyte: phaeomelanogenesis *(left)* and eumelanogenesis *(right)* form melanin granules in four stages. In the first stage, both types of melanin formation begin with vesiculoglobular bodies. In eumelanosomes, this process becomes coordinated with the formation of lamellae (stages II and III), whereas in phaeomelanosomes, the vesiculoglobular bodies are added peripherally in a more random manner. With rare exception the two forms of melanogenesis do not occur in the same cell.

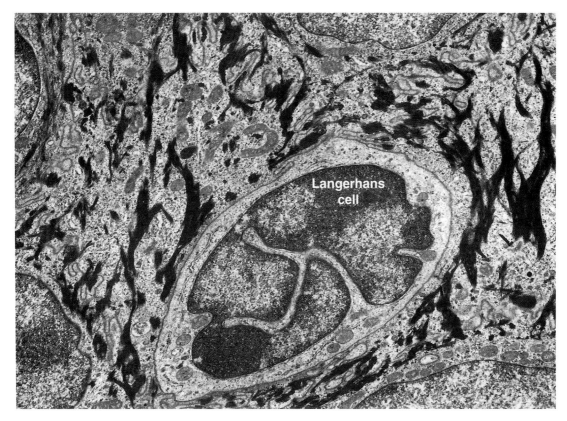

Figure 13-11. Transmission electron micrograph of a Langerhans cell, its polymorphous nucleus embraced by keratinocytes within the outer stratum spinosum. *(From Fawcett DW:* Bloom and Fawcett: A textbook of histology, *ed 11, Philadelphia, 1986, Saunders.)*

melanin, tyrosine is transformed by tyrosinase into **DOPA** (3,4-dihydroxyphenylalanine), which is then converted into dopaquinone and finally into melanin.

Even though there may be considerable variation in the density of melanocytes from one species to another, differently colored breeds of the species can have identical densities. In these instances, the difference in the coloration is due to the melanogenic activity of these cells. Melanogenic activity is generally controlled by genetic expression, which can result in myriad color patterns of the integument seen throughout the animal kingdom. Of course, melanization is strongly influenced by light, but it also is affected by the endocrine system in a variety of ways, especially by the release of melanin-stimulating hormone secreted by the pituitary. And remember that melanin has the capability to bind a variety of substances including drugs and metals. The length of time that this binding occurs may vary from substance to substance, and the effects of a drug may last considerably longer in darkly pigmented individuals and be toxic in highly pigmented regions of the body such as the uveal portion of the eye.

Langerhans Cell

Another nonkeratinocyte within the epidermis is the **Langerhans cell,** which typically resides in the stratum spinosum (Figure 13-11). It also can be found in the dermis and stratified squamous epithelia of the digestive and reproductive tracts. Like the melanocyte, the Langerhans cell has dendritic-like processes that extend in different directions. Although once believed to be of neural crest origin, they are now known to be formed (or at least their precursors formed) in the bone marrow, where they then migrate via the circulatory system to the epidermis and other portions of the body.

Langerhans cells have antibodies (Fc) and complement (C3) receptors attached to their cell membranes that sensitize and allow them to react to foreign substances as **antigen-presenting cells.** The recognized foreign substance is ingested by this cell and processed for lymphoid interaction. As the processing is performed, the cell migrates to a nearby lymph node and presents to the T lymphocytes epitopes of the processed foreign substance (see Figure 12-2).

Besides a dendritic appearance, the Langerhans cell has a well-developed lysosomal system and a pale, often indented nucleus. These features and their origin cause them to be placed in the mononuclear phagocyte system. In certain species, human beings and rats, the Langerhans cell possesses small granules **(Birbeck, or vermiform granules)** that are beyond the resolution of the light microscope. However, their presence in domestic species has yet to be found. The general morphology of the Langerhans cell, the absence of tonofilaments and elements of keratinization, in general, and their position within the epidermis are characteristics that can be used for their identification.

Merkel Cell

A third nonkeratinocyte that resides in the epidermis is the **Merkel cell.** This cell type lies within the basal cell layer and is specialized for sensory transduction (Figure 13-12). The Merkel cell tends to be oval to elliptical, its length running parallel to the surface of the epidermis. The cytoplasm tends to be clear when examined histologically. Unlike the melanocyte and the Langerhans cell, the Merkel cell is firmly attached to neighboring basal cells of the epidermis by desmosomes. The nucleus, which can be polymorphous or deeply indented, is surrounded by dense-cored granules also present in the cell's processes, which extend toward the stratum spinosum. The function of these granules, which can be viewed only ultrastructurally, is unknown. Each Merkel cell is believed to be in communication with an afferent, unmyelinated nerve ending. The nerve ending and the Merkel cell form a **Merkel cell-neurite complex** referred to also as the **tactile hair disk.** It is believed that this complex or disk functions as a receptor for touch because it is a slow-adapting mechanoreceptor.

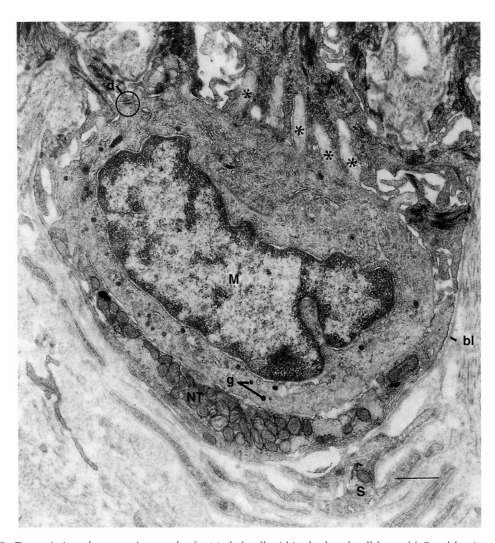

Figure 13-12. Transmission electron micrograph of a Merkel cell within the basal cell layer. *bl,* Basal lamina; *d,* desmosome; *g,* granule; *M,* Merkel cell; *NT,* nerve terminal; *S,* stromal cell of adjacent dermis; *asterisks,* spiny processes. *(From Gartner LP, Hiatt JL: Color textbook of histology, Philadelphia, 1997, Saunders.)*

DERMIS

The connective tissue that the epidermis contacts is the **dermis,** or **corium,** which consists of dense irregular connective tissue. In animals with glabrous to less hairy skin such as in the pig, the dermis can usually be separated into an outermost portion—the **papillary layer,** composed of a loose web of extracellular fibers, fibrocytes, cells of defense, and small vessels that form capillary loops and nerves—and an innermost portion—the **reticular layer,** which is much more compact and less cellular than the papillary layer (Figure 13-13). As in the epidermis, the dermis is thickest in those regions that routinely receive the most abrasion. In these regions the reticular layer is especially developed. In most domestic species, the skin is well populated with hair and there is a general absence of dermal papillae. In these instances, the terms **superficial** and **deep dermis** are used.

The dermis and epidermis are connected to each other by the **basement membrane.** The epidermis-dermis basement membrane is contributed by the basal cells of the epidermis and their ability to form a **basal lamina** and attach the base of their cells to the basal lamina by hemidesmosomes. Melanocytes and Merkel cells located within the basal cell layer also are partially attached to the basal lamina by hemidesmosomes. The hemidesmosomes become linked to the basal lamina by **anchoring filaments** that pass from the cell membrane and become embedded within the portion known as the **lamina densa** of the basal lamina (see Figures 3-26 and 13-2). Within the area of the anchoring filaments **(lamina lucida)** are also several glycoproteins, including fibronectin and laminin, that contribute to the adhesion of the base of the basal cells to the basal lamina. The lamina densa, however, is composed primarily of collagen type IV. Internally, the basal lamina is connected to nearby reticular fibers (collagen type III) by **anchoring fibrils** that consist of collagen type VII. This latter portion is known as the **reticular lamina** and is produced in varying amounts by the fibrocytes of the papillary layer.

PAPILLARY LAYER

As the superficial-most layer of the dermis, the papillary layer is critically important to the welfare of the epidermis. It is this portion that houses the

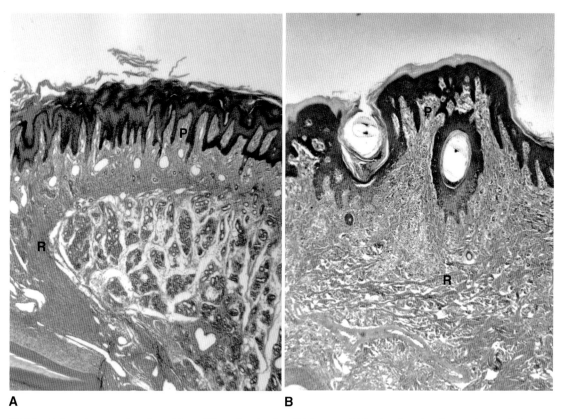

A   **B**

Figure 13-13. Light micrographs of papillary *(P)* and reticular *(R)* layers within the dermis of a canine pad, **A,** and a porcine back, **B.** (Hematoxylin and eosin stain; ×20.)

branching nerve endings and vascular capillary network that serve to link and nourish the keratinocytes and nonkeratinocytes of the epidermis and any modified structures associated with skin in this area. In areas of the body where the skin is thickened, the papillary layer may interdigitate with the epidermis, resulting in the formation of dermal papillae, which appears sawtoothed in shape and creates an interface between the dermis and epidermis for strong attachment (see Figure 13-13). The surface area of the basal lamina becomes markedly expanded, which provides a suitable way for increased numbers of hemidesmosomal attachments to occur. Each dermal papilla possesses a capillary bed or loop that not only nutritionally supports the epidermis but also assists in regulating body temperature. In keeping with the loose connective-tissue environment, sentinel cells of defense such as lymphocytes, histiocytes (macrophages), and mast cells randomly reside here.

RETICULAR LAYER

The reticular layer is characterized principally by the size and density of the extracellular fibers, which are larger and more compact than those comprising the papillary layer (see Figure 13-13). The irregular appearance of the collagen and elastic fibers is perhaps more pronounced in this region than in any portion of any other organ of the body. Animals with thick skins have very well-developed reticular layers, consisting mostly of collagen type I and proteoglycans that are dominant in dermatan sulfate. The elastic fibers are broad in this layer as opposed to those in the papillary layer, which are considerably smaller in diameter (Figure 13-14). The elastic fibers can continue to thicken and possibly harden with exposure to sunlight, a condition referred to as **elastosis.**

Although fewer cells of defense are normally seen in the reticular layer, they can be found as well as occasional melanophores, including melanocytes. The fibrocyte is the predominant cell type and is usually seen in fairly low densities except in areas where recent repair has been performed. Adipocytes also can be observed in this region in scattered clusters, especially where the reticular layer comes into contact with adjacent tissues, such as bone or skeletal muscle. It is at this point where the reticular layer of the dermis ends and a looser connective tissue, the **hypodermis** or **subcutaneous tissue (subcutis),** begins, being the outer fascia of an adjacent skeletal muscle or bone (Figure 13-15). In fact, the fat cells in this area can be numerous and result in the formation of the **panniculus adiposus.** This tissue contributes to body contour in addition to fat storage and heat insulation.

The glands and hair follicles of skin lie mostly within the deep or reticular layer. Their presence and number vary according to the location of the skin. In conjunction with each hair follicle is one or more small bundles of smooth muscle called the **arrector pili,** which has one end attached to the side of a follicle and the other end attached near the epidermis within the superficial dermis (Figure 13-16; see also Figure 13-1). When these bundles contract, the hairs, which are usually positioned at low angles, become erect and stand on end. The muscle fibers, which are innervated autonomically, will contract in low temperatures causing the raised hairs to trap air within the coat, which acts to insulate the body further. There can be other small bundles of smooth muscle within the dermis that occur mostly deep within the reticular layer of the dermis and have no association with hair follicles. These are found at specific sites of the body, including the penis, scrotum, and teats.

Nervous elements also can be found within the reticular layer. In addition to nerve bundles containing afferent and efferent nerve processes that course their way through the dense connective tissue elements to and from the papillary layer and epidermis, sensory receptors may be encountered. These receptors are encapsulated mechanoreceptors that function to detect (and respond) to vibration and are known as **lamellar corpuscles (pacinian corpuscles)** (Figure 13-17).

GLANDS OF THE SKIN

Skin glands consist of two types: sweat glands and sebaceous glands. Each type originates from the ectoderm and remains connected to the epidermis by a single duct. Because of this characteristic, both of these glands represent simple, exocrine glands found ubiquitously among the integument of domestic species.

SWEAT GLAND

The **sweat gland** consists of a **simple coiled tubular adenomere** that is associated with the skin throughout the body but can be modified and concentrated at selected regions (these latter glands are listed and briefly described in Table 13-1). The common sweat gland produces a clear, watery (99% water) secretion, sweat that contains salts, primarily the cations sodium and potassium, and perhaps a small amount of protein. With the release of sweat onto the surface of the epidermis and its subsequent evaporation, heat near and at the surface is dissipated, which provides a cooling effect for the body. Water loss

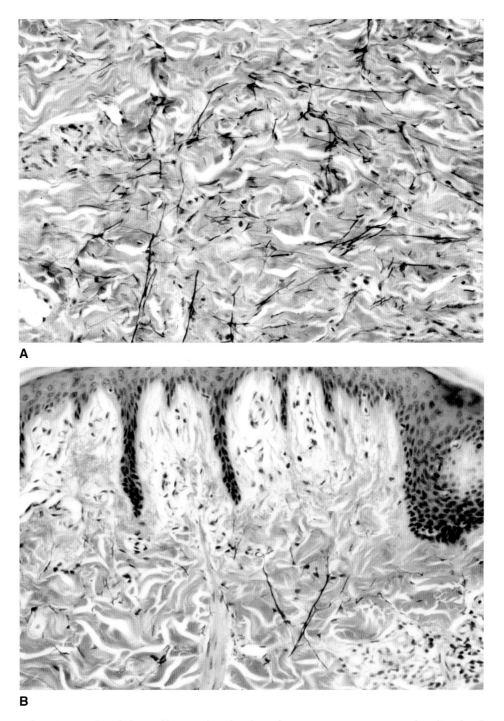

A

B

Figure 13-14. Light micrographs of elastic fibers within the skin of a pig, **A,** most pronounced within the deep portion of the reticular layer and **B,** much less developed in the papillary portion. (Elastin stain; ×200.)

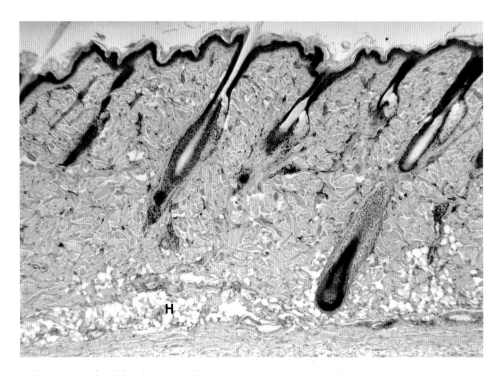

Figure 13-15. Light micrograph of the dermis and its innermost association with the adipose-laden hypodermis *(H).* (Hematoxylin and eosin stain; ×40.)

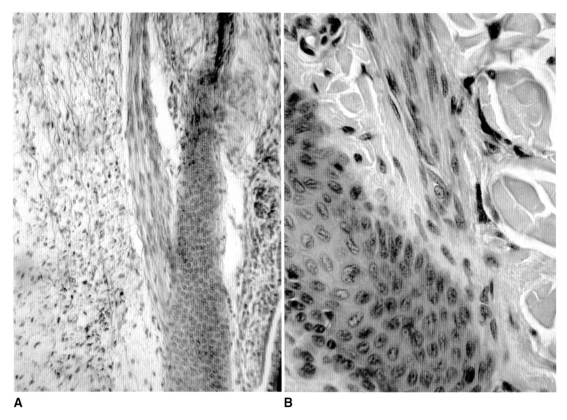

A   B

Figure 13-16. Light micrographs of attachment of the arrector pili muscle to the side of a canine hair follicle. (Hematoxylin and eosin stain; **A,** ×100; **B,** ×250.)

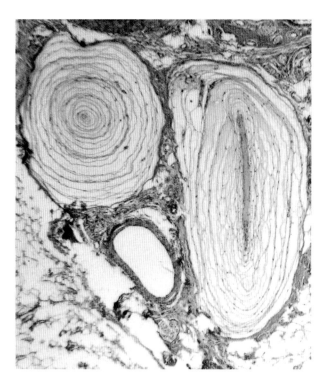

Figure 13-17. Light micrograph of lamellar bodies seen in cross section *(left)* and longitudinally *(right)* within the reticular layer. (Hematoxylin and eosin stain; ×40.)

hairless skin or within the distal-most portion of a hair follicle as described previously. Internally, the duct extends through the papillary layer of the dermis and much of its reticular layer before continuously joining the secretory unit (Figure 13-18). The duct can be more or less straight or become serpentine before it reaches the level of the secretory unit, at which point it may coil at variable lengths, depending on the species, the age of the individual, and perhaps even the gender (see Figure 13-18). The duct consists of a bilayered epithelium with cuboidal layers (Figure 13-19). The cells of the apical or luminal layer can be either similar in appearance to those of the basal layer or slightly smaller with regard to the amount of the cytoplasm and nucleus. At the point where the duct joins the adenomere, the apical layer becomes confluent with the layer of secretory cells that line the lumen. Concomitantly, the basal layer of the duct disappears and is replaced by a layer of **myoepithelial** cells that appear fibroblast-like and are oriented in the same plane as the axis of the lumen (Figure 13-20). The myoepithelial cells are, in fact, contractile cells with smooth muscle actin. When these cells are activated, the secretions held within the lumen of the adenomere become more quickly propelled to the surface.

The morphology of the secretory cells can differ according to the species and to their cells' activity, being most polarized and at their greatest height during active production of sweat. Thus the secretory cells can range in their morphology from low cuboidal to columnar. Active secretion can be apparent as apical portions of these cells extend into the lumen. In ruminants and pigs the lumens of the secretory units can be wide, making these glands more saccular in shape than tubular (see Figure 4-11). The normal activity of the sweat glands located throughout most of the integument is species variable, active in horses quiescent in dogs and cats. In dogs and cats, active sweat glands can be found in their footpads (see Figure 13-13). These glands are not apocrine, but instead eccrine or merocrine. The ducts of these simple tubular secretory units empty directly onto the epidermal surface rather than into the hair follicle as in the case of the rest of the integument. Similar eccrine sweat glands can be found in the planum rostrale and medial surface of the carpus in pigs, the planum nasolabiale of large ruminants, the planum nasale of small ruminants and the frog of ungulates in general.

through sweat gland secretion can range from a couple of hundred milliliters to several liters each day, depending on the size of the animal, ambient temperature, and amount of exercise during that period.

The sweat glands of most domestic species are believed to be of the **apocrine type,** in which a portion of the secretory cell, being residual cytoplasm, is contributed along with the secretory material. The ducts empty into adjacent hair follicles superficial to the sebaceous glands associated with the follicles. Verification of apocrine release has been made, but it is not known how extensive apocrine secretion occurs among mammals. Eccrine (or merocrine) secretion, which involves the release of only secretory material, is predominantly found in primate sweat glands, although apocrine glands are associated with axillary, perianal, and pubic regions in these species. Although the extent of the eccrine type among nonprimate mammals has not been determined, they do exist and are discussed later.

Although the sweat gland is the classic example of the simple coiled tubular gland, there is considerable variation in its morphology among animals, especially in terms of the degree of being coiled, the shape of the secretory end piece or adenomere, and the size or length and depth of the gland. The secretory duct empties at the surface of the epidermis in glabrous or

SEBACEOUS GLANDS

The **sebaceous gland** is a **simple, branched alveolar** gland that secretes an oily material—**sebum**—in a manner that requires the entire cell to be contributed,

TABLE 13-1	Glands of Mammalian Skin			
TYPE	SHAPE	LOCATION	SECRETION: MODE/PRODUCT	FUNCTION
Sebaceous	Simple, branched acinar	Throughout the body, closely associated with hair follicles	Holocrine; sebum: accumulation of fatty acids (i.e., oily lipid rich)	Lubricates hair and epidermis, contributes to antimicrobial protection, lowers evaporation and water loss
Tarsal: *specialized sebaceous*	Numerous acini emptying into one duct	Eyelids	Holocrine; oily layer of the preocular tear film	Provides an outer surfactant coat for tears, which lowers dehydration of the tear film and reduces tear overflow onto the face
Supracaudal: *specialized sebaceous*	Multiple, branched acinar associated with one hair follicle	Dorsally positioned near base of tail in dogs and cats	Holocrine; sebum: accumulation of fatty acids	Lubricates hair and epidermis, contributes to antimicrobial protection, lowers evaporation and water loss
Circumanal: *modified sebaceous*	Branched acinar and cords of hepatoid (hepatocyte-like) cells; and possibly simple, coiled, tubular in the dog	Subcutaneously, circumferentially around the anus	Holocrine and merocrine (and apocrine in the dog); sebum and possibly hormone-related substance(s)	Lubricates area and possible antimicrobial protection; other functions remain unknown; in the dog the apocrine sweat glands associated with the circumanal gland may provide chemoattractant (pheromone) activity; has clinical relevance in the dog as a principal site of tumor formation
Sweat	Simple, coiled tubular or saccular	Throughout the body, closely associated with hair follicles except in localized regions (carnivore footpad, frog, porcine carpus)	Apocrine (duct empties superficially into hair follicle) eccrine (merocrine), duct leads directly to skin surface; watery with some proteolytic enzymes, electrolytes (salts), and albuminoid substances	Cools body temperature as well as excretory; in carnivores, apocrine sweat glands are least active among domestic species and along with the goat may be involved in pheromone activity
Anal sacs: *modified sweat* (and *sebaceous*)	Simple, coiled saccular in the dog; and simple, branched acinar in the cat	Along the anocutaneous junction	Apocrine in domestic carnivores and holocrine as well in the cat and nondomestic carnivores; often dark and oily with a variety of substances, including amines, lipids, lysosomal enzymes, glycoproteins	Used as a marking fluid among carnivores and possibly involved with canine social recognition; the secretions along with adjacent excrement support extensive microbiota that may contribute to the function of this gland; in dogs excrement may occlude the duct
Carpal: *modified sweat*	Compound, coiled tubuloalveolar with large collector canals	Along the medial surface of the carpus in the pig	Eccrine (merocrine); watery with salts and glycosidic residues	Found only in the pig, wild and domestic; secretions are odorous and may be used as a marking fluid

a process referred to as **holocrine secretion.** Consequently, the lumen of each sebaceous gland is filled with cells; the oldest cells are pushed toward the duct (Figure 13-21; see also Figure 4-12). Newly formed cells that enter the lumen of each adenomere have round nuclei and an eosinophilic cytoplasm that contains the rough endoplasmic reticulum, mitochondria, and other metabolic machinery needed to assemble and collect triglycerides and cholesterol into lipid droplets or locules. The cells that give rise to the sebum-producing cells and are thus the secretory cells of this holocrine gland are small and cuboidal to squamous shaped. Once the sebum-producing cell is formed, it quickly grows in size and resembles a multilocular adipocyte except that the sebum-producing cell has lost all connections to the basal lamina and its nucleus is centrally positioned (Figure 13-22; see also Figures 4-12 and 13-21). As each cell is continu-

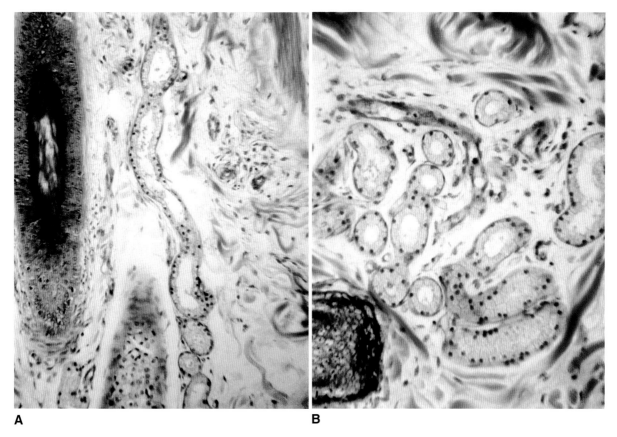

A   **B**

Figure 13-18. A, Light micrograph of a distal portion of an equine sweat gland that extends alongside a hair follicle. (Hematoxylin and eosin [H&E] stain; ×25.) **B,** Light micrograph of the end of the secretory portion of an equine apocrine sweat gland. (H&E stain; ×100.)

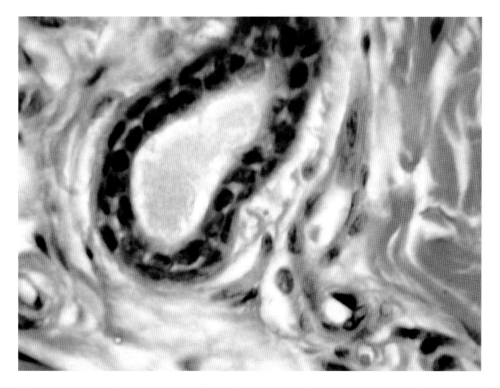

Figure 13-19. Light micrograph of a cross section of the duct portion of a porcine sweat gland. (Hematoxylin and eosin stain: ×400.)

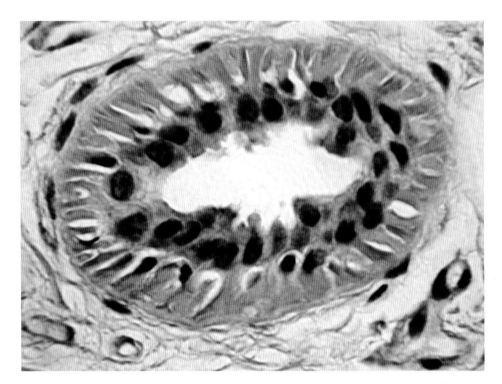

Figure 13-20. Light micrograph of a cross section of the secretory portion of a porcine sweat gland; the outer layer of myoepithelial cells appears contracted. (Hematoxylin and eosin stain; ×400.)

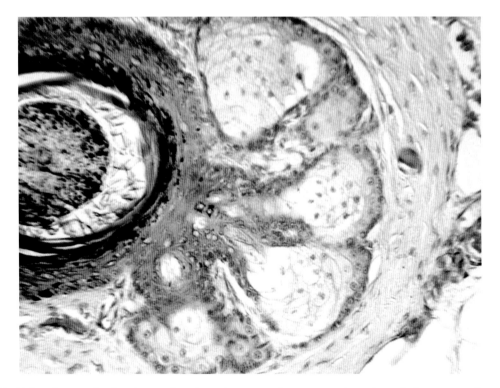

Figure 13-21. Light micrograph of a cluster of canine sebaceous adenomeres oriented nearly in cross section, lying next to a hair follicle. (Hematoxylin and eosin stain; ×100.)

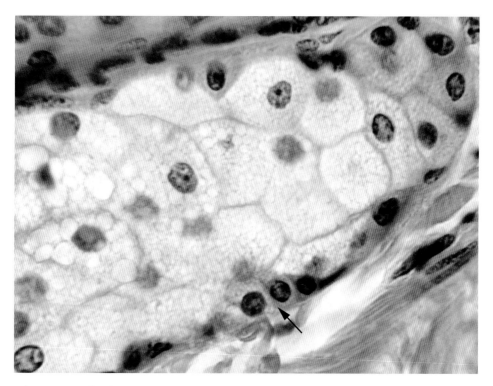

Figure 13-22. Light micrograph of a canine sebaceous gland. Arrow points to newly forming secretory cells. (Hematoxylin and eosin stain; ×250.)

ally pushed away from its origin, the organelles begin to break down and the nucleus becomes pyknotic.

For the most part, sebaceous glands are closely associated with hair follicles; they are appendages of hair follicles that discharge their content into their ducts and adjacent hair follicle, which together form the **pilosebaceous canal.** Often, the size of the sebaceous gland is inversely proportional to the size of the hair with which it is associated.

Each secretory unit is more flask shaped or pear shaped than it is round (see Figures 4-12 and 13-21). In some animals such as the horse, the secretory units are saccular or even broadly tubular (Figure 13-23).

In glabrous regions of the integument, sebaceous glands can still exist, such as the anus of most species and teat regions of the horse. In other glabrous regions including the footpads, claws, hoofs, and horns, sebaceous glands are absent. The sebaceous gland functions to lubricate the epidermis and hair and thus helps maintain their texture and flexibility. It also facilitates antimicrobial protection by providing a physical barrier at the opening of the follicles, inhibiting bacterial and fungal invasion. Sebum also contains antimicrobial agents, including fatty acids such as linoleic acid, the iron-binding protein transferrin, and immunoglobulin G (IgG) and IgA. Sebaceous gland activity is largely under the influence of the endocrine system—stimulated by androgens and testosterone while suppressed by corticosteroids.

Although sebaceous glands are found throughout the integument, their distribution and amount of development vary among domestic species, including the presence of specialized types of sebaceous glands (see Table 13-1). One of these specialized types is the **circumanal gland** that occurs in the dog. The circumanal glands are modified sebaceous glands that consist of a parenchyma of hepatocyte-like cells called **hepatoid cells** that lie deep within the dermis and are joined superficially by traditional-appearing sebaceous cells. Although it is speculated that they may be involved in hormonal activity, their function has yet to be determined.

Another specialized form is the **tarsal gland** (Meibomian gland) associated with the eyelids of domestic animals. The tarsal gland consists of multiple sebaceous glands that join a central duct and secrete an oily layer onto the tear film that covers the anterior portion of the eye (Figure 13-24; see also Figure 20-24).

HAIRS

One of the modifications of the epidermis is hair, a highly keratinized, rodlike structure that emerges

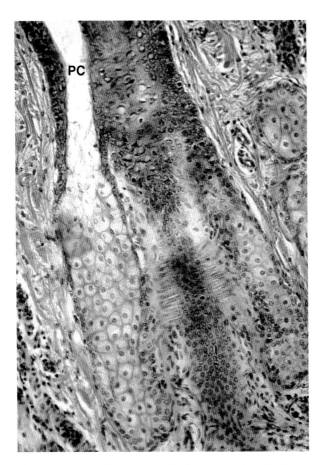

Figure 13-23. Light micrograph of a secretory end of an equine sebaceous gland that empties into a shared duct connected to the pilosebaceous canal *(PC)*. (Hematoxylin and eosin stain; ×100.)

from the epidermis. Mammals are characterized, in part, by the presence of hair, which in domestic species covers most of the body. The relatively few areas that are hairless or **glabrous** include the muco-cutaneous junctions of the body, footpads, hoofs, glans penis and teats of various species. Hair combined with sebum coating forms a water-resistant coat and helps insulate the body against cold temperatures as well as providing physical protection.

A variety of hairs are associated with different areas of the body. Regarding those that are a part of the general integument there are two basic types: the primary hair and the secondary hair. The **primary hair** is easily the larger of the two types in terms of its diameter and length and is usually deeply seated in the dermis. Sebaceous glands, sweat glands, and the arrector pili muscle are directly affiliated with this hair. The **secondary hair,** also referred to as *underhair,* is more superficially placed in the dermis than the primary hair and lacks associations with sweat glands and arrector pili muscle.

HAIR FOLLICLES

Hairs are formed by **hair follicles** that consist of invaginations of the epidermis that have invaded the dermis and even the hypodermis. Rather than be positioned at a 90-degree angle to the surface, the hair follicle is usually oriented more on a slant, which enhances its ability to provide thermal insulation and water resistance. At the base of the hair follicle is the **hair root** and an adjacent **dermal papilla** (hair papilla), which protrudes into the root (Figure 13-25).

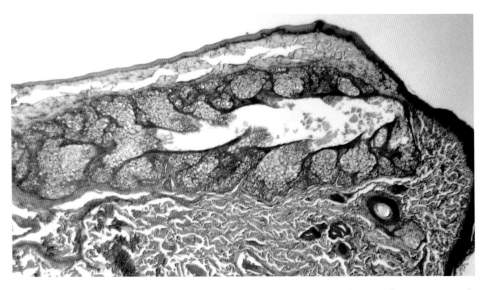

Figure 13-24. Light micrograph of a specialized sebaceous gland—the tarsal gland—in a dog. (Hematoxylin and eosin stain; ×25.)

The hair root and the dermal papilla can be collectively referred to as the **hair bulb.** The dermal papilla possesses a small plexus of blood vessels (capillaries) that feeds the root. The innermost portion of the root next to the papilla is the **hair matrix,** densely packed cells that undergo proliferation and are responsible for hair growth. The cells of the hair matrix are a specialized form of the basal layer of the epidermis. The cells derived from this portion of the hair root differ from those of the typical epidermis in that the composition of the keratin formed is different. Rather than create keratin that has a keratohyalin phase and produce lipid materials that will be later released as done by keratinocytes, the matrix cells form a keratin without keratohyalin but is high in sulfur content and immersed in little lipid. The resulting keratinized cells are considerably harder and more resistant to mechanical stress than the mature keratinized cells of the epidermis.

The cells within the central portion of the hair matrix form the **medulla**—the core of the hair that is composed of large, somewhat cuboidal cells that become less compact when further removed from the root (see Figure 13-25). Only primary hairs possess a medulla. Cells that envelop the medulla and thus are slightly peripheral to the center of the matrix give rise to the **cortex** of the hair. These cells become keratinized in the manner described above, forming a "hard" keratin. Outside the cortex of the hair, a single line of cells within the peripheral matrix becomes the **cuticle** of the hair, which consists of flat keratinized cells that overlap one another and form the outer boundary of the hair when exposed to air.

Melanocytes reside in the hair root next to the dermal papilla (Figure 13-26). In terms of their density, they can be especially concentrated in this region of the integument and are responsible for an animal's coat color. Melanocytes high in phaeomelanin content will give rise to tan, yellow, red, and red-brown fur, whereas those high in eumelanin content yield dark brown to black coats. Hair without any pigment appears white.

The peripheral portion of the hair bulb at the level of the matrix is lined by a **root sheath,** which is

Figure 13-25. A, Diagram of a hair follicle.   *Continued*

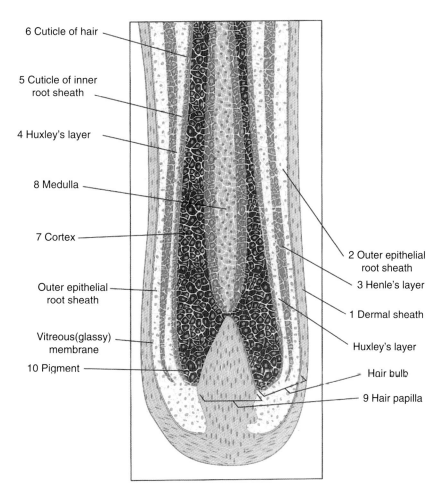

6 Cuticle of hair

5 Cuticle of inner root sheath

4 Huxley's layer

8 Medulla

7 Cortex

Outer epithelial root sheath

Vitreous(glassy) membrane

10 Pigment

2 Outer epithelial root sheath

3 Henle's layer

1 Dermal sheath

Huxley's layer

Hair bulb

9 Hair papilla

A

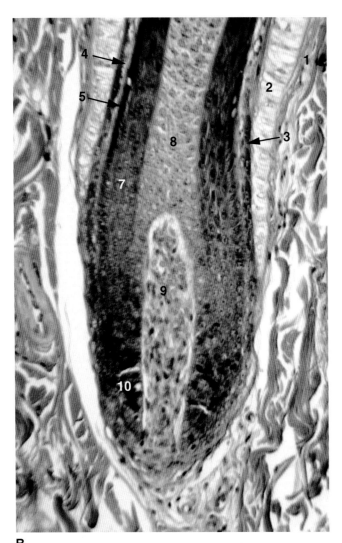

Figure 13-25, cont'd B, Light micrograph of a canine hair follicle. (Hematoxylin and eosin stain; ×30.) *(From Bergman RA, Afifi AK, Heidger PM Jr:* Histology, *Philadelphia, 1996, Saunders.)*

B

divided into internal and external portions. The **external root sheath** initially consists of a single layer of cells along the base of the hair bulb, but increases within a short distance to several layers in the direction of the surface (see Figure 13-25). Outside of the external root sheath is its basal lamina, which is called the **glassy membrane,** and is confluent with the epidermal basal lumina as the external root sheath becomes confluent with the epidermis. Inside the external root sheath and outside the matrix is an **internal root sheath** made up of three components: **Henle's layer** or **pale epithelial layer,** which is a single, external layer of cuboidal cells that lies against the innermost portion of the external sheath; **Huxley's layer,** or **granular epithelial layer,** which can consist of one or two layers of flattened cells that contain trichohyalin granules; and the **cuticle of the internal root sheath,** composed of scalelike cells that overlap one another and form the external lining of

the hair. All portions that comprise the hair within a follicle are referred to as the **hair root,** and the portion that extends above the epidermis is the **hair shaft.**

TYPES OF HAIR FOLLICLES

Hair follicles, like hairs of the integument can be divided into two basic types: simple follicles and compound follicles. **Simple follicles,** also known as *single follicles,* have one emerging hair shaft. In contrast, **compound follicles** have more than one hair shaft arising from a single opening (Figure 13-27). In compound follicles, the follicles are tightly clustered together and as a result share the same opening as well as auxiliary glands. It is not unusual to have a primary hair surrounded and reinforced by secondary hairs in this manner. Simple hair follicles can be fairly evenly distributed or clustered, depending on the species and

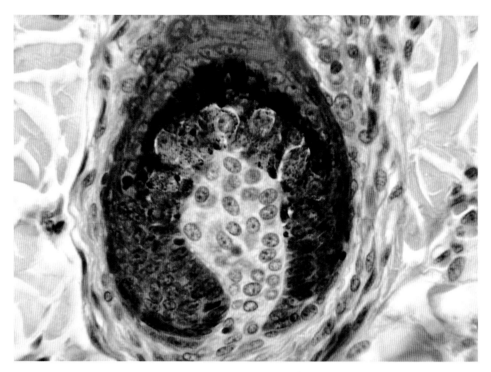

Figure 13-26. Light micrograph of a row of melanocytes within the cortex surrounding the dermal papilla. (Hematoxylin and eosin stain; ×250).

the location of the follicle along the body. Variations also are seen among animals with compound follicles regarding the number of primary and secondary hairs associated with each follicle.

In addition to the common follicles just discussed are specialized forms that give rise to modified hairs for tactile sensory reception. These hairs are known as **tactile hairs, sinus hairs,** or **vibrissae,** which are most commonly found within the nasal sinuses and peri-orally along the snouts of domestic mammals. Vibrissae have a very wide diameter and can be long. Their origin and composition are essentially identical to primary hairs in single follicles. The construction of the connective tissue adjacent to the follicle, however, is considerably different. The major distinguishing feature is the presence of a well-formed dermal sheath that contains a vascular sinus lying within its inner and outer layers. The sinus itself can be divided by differences in its morphology into upper and lower portions. The upper portion possesses an uninterrupted annular vascular sinus (without trabeculae), whereas the lower portion contains a network of connective-tissue trabeculae surrounded by blood within its cavernous chamber. Within the inner layer of the dermal sheath, the external root sheath of the follicle is lined by a thickened basement membrane (glassy membrane). In cats and dogs, the inner layer

of the dermal sheath within the region of the annular (nontrabecular) sinus is thickened into a sinus pad. A variety of innervations are associated with vibrissae, including free nerve endings and Merkel-cell tactile-hair disks.

HAIR CYCLE

All keratinized structures are replaced over various spans of time. The replacement of the cornified layers of the epidermis is a continual process. Although new layers are made to replace the old ones, it is done in a rhythmic manner. Mitotic divisions within the stratum basale occur generally at night. Hair is also replaced on a regular basis, but over a longer period. It usually takes 3 months to more than a year to grow to its normal length, depending, of course, on the length of the coat for a particular animal. The replacement of hair can occur steadily throughout the year or seasonally and can be influenced by external temperature; length of daytime; hormonal changes involving adrenal, thyroid, and reproductive glands; and nutrition. Among domestic species, a dense pelage forms in the fall, replacing the sparse coat formed previously during the spring. The increased production of the numerous fine hairs assists in trapping warm air and providing a more effective insulator.

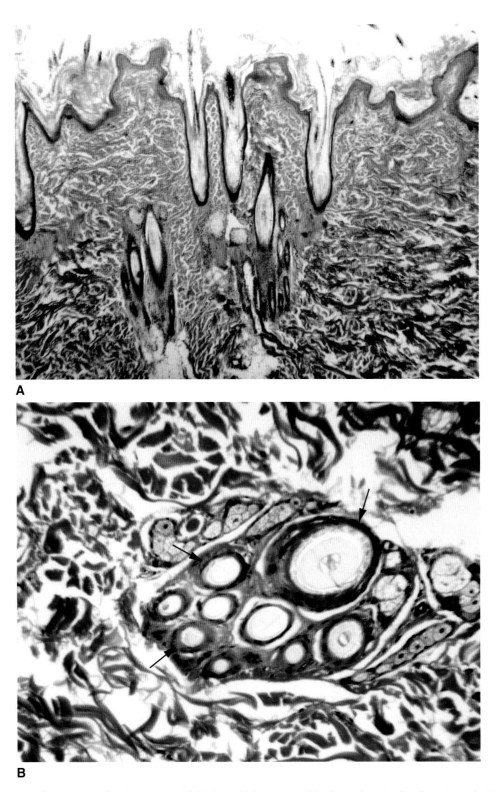

A

B

Figure 13-27. **A,** Light micrograph of compound follicles within canine skin that is longitudinally oriented. (Hematoxylin and eosin [H&E] stain; ×20.) **B,** Light micrograph of compound follicles in cross section with clusters of secondary hairs *(left arrows)* surrounding a primary hair *(right arrow).* (H&E stain; ×100.)

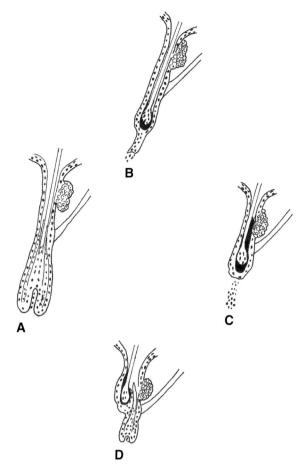

Figure 13-28. Diagram of the hair cycle: *(a)*, anagen, *(b)*, catagen, *(c)*, telogen, *(d)*, renewed anagen.

Hair formation and replacement occurs in a three-phase process. Initially, a hair bulb undergoes a phase of active cell division called the **anagen phase,** and develops a hair to its full length over a fairly long time as mentioned (Figure 13-28). At the end of the growing phase, the mitotic and keratinizing activities of the hair bulb disappear and the hair enters the **catagen phase.** The entire hair bulb becomes cornified and at the same time the base of the follicle moves toward the level of the sebaceous glands. During this regression of the hair follicle a new (secondary) germ layer and dermal papilla form beneath the older follicle. At this point, the hair and its follicle remain unchanged or dormant and are in the **telogen phase.** The hair may stay in the telogen or resting phase for some time. Eventually, the secondary germ layer becomes active and is transformed into a new hair bulb undergoing an early anagen phase. The new hair formed then pushes the old hair out of the follicle, causing it to be shed. As the new anagen phase proceeds, the hair follicle returns to its original depth within the dermis.

CLAWS

The claws of domestic carnivores are extensively developed portions of the epidermis and dermis that extend from the distal phalanges (Figure 13-29). The distal phalanx forms the **ungual process,** which has a clawlike morphology and is covered by the dermis, which is broadest dorsally. The overlying epidermis forms a very prominent and hard cornified stratum along the dorsal ridge (Figure 13-30). This part of the stratum corneum is called the **wall** or **wall epidermis** (claw plate) and becomes markedly attenuated at the **ungual crest.** A fold of skin, the claw fold, covers the dorsal base of the wall and is comparable to the periople of the hoof. The ventral portion of the epidermis lining the claw is called the **sole** and is composed of less compact or "softer" keratin than the wall keratin.

EQUINE HOOF

Like the claw, the hoof formed in horses is composed largely of cornified epidermal tissue. However, the cornified arrangement here is considerably more developed in its architecture, area and thickness (Figure 13-31). As before, the distal phalanges are lined by the dermis (the **laminar corium**), and together form a semiconical shape that is greatest in its height and width along the region of the toe (the medial axis) and tapers on both sides toward the heel. Fine layers of the superficial-most portion of the dermis interdigitate with infoldings of the epidermis, referred to as the **stratum lamellatum (stratum internum)** (Figure 13-32). These dermal layers, which project externally at right angles to the lamina corium, comprise the **primary laminar corium.** The stratum lamellatum is also called the **laminar epidermis,** which further interdigitates with the adjacent dermis, primary laminar corium, the latter forming the **secondary laminar corium** (see Figures 13-31 and 13-32). As a result, the surface area connecting the dermis and the epidermis in the equine hoof is enormous. The primary and secondary laminae of the corium are innervated and considered as the **sensitive laminae.** Innermost layers of the epidermis, which comprise the **secondary laminar epidermis,** are possibly innervated as well and may be included within the sensitive laminae. In contrast, the **primary laminar epidermis,** which consists of cornified epithelial cells, lacks nerve endings and comprises the **insensitive laminae.**

The epidermis comprises the **wall** of the hoof, which can be divided into three regions: the stratum externum, the stratum medium, and the stratum inter-

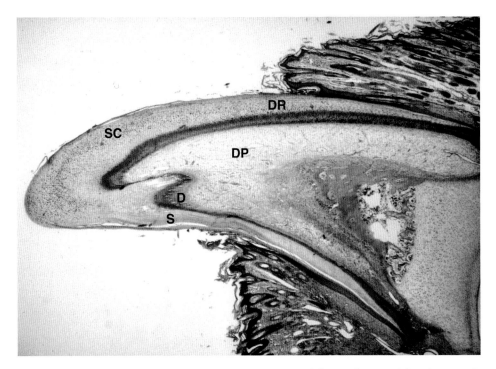

Figure 13-29. Light micrograph of a canine claw. *SC,* Stratum corneum of the epidermis of the claw; *D,* dermis of the claw; *DP,* distal phalanx; *DR,* dorsal ridge; *S,* sole. (Hematoxylin and eosin stain; ×2.)

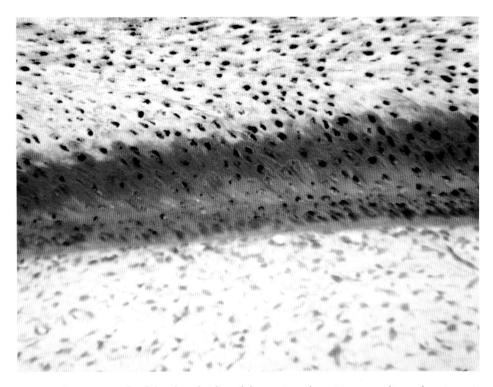

Figure 13-30. Light micrograph of the dorsal ridge of the canine claw. (Hematoxylin and eosin stain; ×100.)

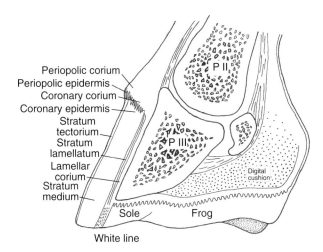

Periopolic corium
Periopolic epidermis
Coronary corium
Coronary epidermis
Stratum tectorium
Stratum lamellatum
Lamellar corium
Stratum medium
Sole   Frog
White line

P II
P III
Digital cushion

Figure 13-31. Diagram of an equine hoof as viewed longitudinally.

num. The **stratum internum** consists of the laminar epidermis that interdigitates with the dermal laminae as previously described. The cells produced by the stratum internum are interfaced with the **stratum medium** on one hand and the laminar corium on the other and thus help connect the wall tightly to the corium along its entire surface. Keratinocytes produced by the laminar epidermis (stratum lamellatum) are moved or pushed outwardly to join the stratum medium. The stratum medium is hard cornified material that originates from the **coronary epidermis** and **coronary corium** (papillary corium), which together form the coronary band and is located along the proximal-most border of the hoof's wall (Figure 13-33; see also Figure 13-31). At this point numerous hairlike papillae extend distally and form hard keratinized tubules, known as **tubular horn,** which appear round in cross section (Figure 13-34; see also Figure 13-32). Each tubule is constructed by keratinocytes that are cylindrically wrapped, resulting in an outer cortex and an inner medullary region where the cells are more loosely arranged as in the medulla of a hair. The cortex, which can be subdivided further into zones (see Figure 13-34), is surrounded, in turn, by hard keratinized tissue referred to as the **intertubular horn.** The tubular and intertubular horns comprise the stratum medium, by far the largest of the three strata, and become prominent in its overall thickness distally toward the front of the toe. As a result, the strength and support afforded by the wall are provided mostly by this stratum. The keratinocytes that are newly formed by the coronary epidermis for both tubular and intertubular horn are pushed in a downward direction, joining those arising from the stratum internum. The

rate of production and movement of the new keratinocytes in the two strata is comparable.

The outermost portion of the wall of the hoof consists of the **stratum externum (stratum tectorium),** which is much thinner than the stratum medium. The stratum externum originates from the **perioplic epidermis** (the epidermis of the periople), which lies proximal and external to the coronary epidermis and coronary corium and is bordered internally by the **perioplic corium** (the corium of the periople) (see Figures 13-31 and 13-33). This epidermis forms an outer shiny cover for the wall and is made of tubular and intertubular horn, like the stratum medium, but is much softer, differing in the content of cytokeratins. The corium of the periople interfaces proximally with the dermis of the skin that lies above the hoof and distally with the corium of the coronary band, and is papillated like the coronary corium. As in the coronary corium and stratum medium, these papillae facilitate the downward formation of the epidermis.

At the base of the hoof the third phalanx is lined by the dermis called the **sole corium,** which, in turn, is covered externally by the **sole epidermis.** The sole corium is a well-developed irregular dense connective tissue able to absorb considerable physical pressure exerted on it. Both the sole corium and the sole epidermis reflex caudally from the lamellar corium and the stratum lamellatum, respectively, at the distal tip of the third phalanx (see Figure 13-31). At the junction of the stratum lamellatum and the sole epidermis, the laminar epidermis of the former becomes directed toward the bottom of the hoof, and as a result, joins and interdigitates with the tubular and intertubular horn that is formed by the sole epidermis. The cornified epidermis arising from the laminar epidermis has a different level of compactness and hardness as well as pigmentation, which collectively results in the **white line (white zone).** The white line enables the wall of the hoof to be distinguished visually from the sole. Within the sole numerous papillae extend from the corium into the epidermis in a manner similar to that seen at the coronary band and results in the production of the tubular and intertubular horn, which along with the distal end of the wall form the hard baseplate of the hoof known as the ground border of the wall.

The ground border of the hoof can be divided into toe, quarter, and heel regions (see Figure 13-31). At the heel, the cranial reflection of the wall on each side forms the **bars.** Within the bars and caudal to the toe and quarter, is a wedge-shaped area of the ground surface of the hoof called the **frog.** The dermis or corium of the frog possesses adipose and along with its fibroelastic tissue thickens into a wedge-shaped structure that helps to absorb impact forces involved in

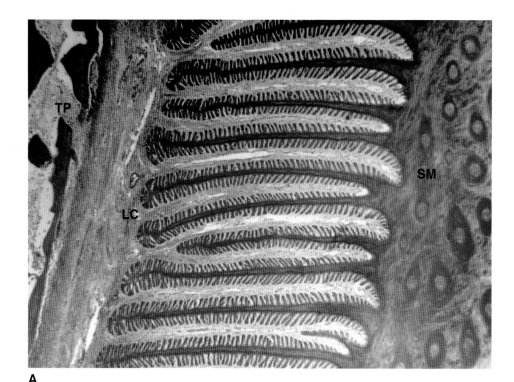

A

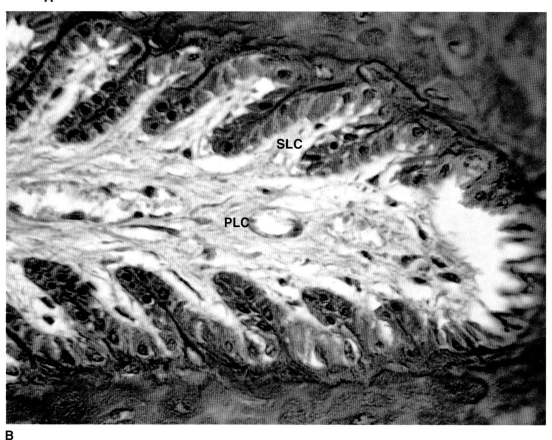

B

Figure 13-32. A, Light micrograph of the stratum lamellatum in the equine hoof. *LC,* laminar corium; *SM,* stratum medium; *TP,* third phalanx. **B,** Light micrograph of the outer portion of the equine hoof's stratum lamellatum. *PLC,* Primary laminar corium; *SLC,* secondary laminar corium. (Hematoxylin and eosin stain; **A,** ×25; **B,** ×250.)

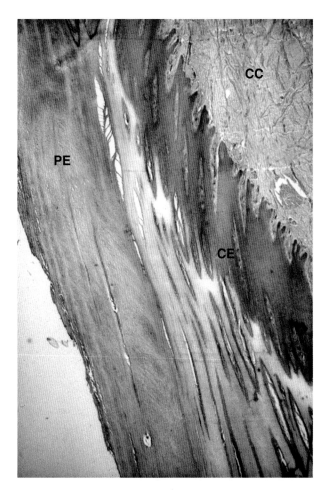

Figure 13-33. Light micrograph of the equine coronary band. *PE,* Perioplic epidermis; *CC,* coronary corium; *CE,* coronary epidermis. (Hematoxylin and eosin stain; ×2.5.)

walking and running. This portion of the hoof also includes the presence of branched and merocrine sweat glands. These glands are concentrated along the central ridge of the frog. The dermis forms smaller papillae than seen in adjacent sole, and the epidermis of the frog forms a softer cornified horn than that found in the nearby sole and wall. The water content for the frog is approximately 50% as compared with 25% and 33% for the wall and sole, respectively. Collectively, the ground border of the wall, the bars, the frog, and the white line are the portions of the hoof that contact the ground and bear the weight of the animal.

NONEQUINE HOOF

In domestic animals with cloven hoofs, such as ruminants and pigs, the digital organ is histologically very similar to the equine hoof. Overall, the construction of the wall and sole and adjacent corium is

nearly identical. Secondary laminae within stratum internum or stratum lamellatum do not occur in the nonequine hoof. Also, instead of a frog is a well-developed **bulb** lined by a thin, soft horn.

CHESTNUT AND ERGOT

In the horse, thickened skin, which lacks hair and glands, lines the supracarpel and tarsal chestnuts as well as the ergot at the flexion of the fetlocks. These areas possess a well-developed epidermis of tubular and intertubular horns associated with long dermal papillae reminiscent of that occurring along the coronary of the hoof (Figure 13-35).

HORNS

Among ruminants, outgrowths of the frontal bone known as **os cornua** form the foundation for the integumentary appendage called the **horn.** Each frontal process, or os cornua, possesses a papillated corium bordered externally by a hard cornified epidermis. The construction of the hard keratinized tissue is similar to the stratum medium of the hoof, consisting of tubular and intertubular horns. Each hard cornification is covered by a thin lining of soft keratin—the **epikeras**—made by the epidermis at the base of the horn. The epikeras is comparable to the stratum externum of the hoof and is continually shed and replaced.

AVIAN INTEGUMENT

The basic structure of avian integument is essentially the same as that of mammals. Nevertheless, a number of variations must be considered. The epidermis is generally much thinner than that seen in mammals, especially when associated with feathered skin. It consists of a keratinized stratified squamous epithelium that has a stratum basale; a stratum spinosum called the **stratum intermedium;** a **stratum transitivum,** which is the counterpart to the **stratum granulosum** but lacks the keratohyalin granules; and a stratum corneum (Figure 13-36). The keratinocytes can be called **sebokeratocytes,** because of their ability to produce a lipid emulsion in addition to keratin proteins. This emulsion fills the intercellular spaces and forms a surface lipid layer, which is high in neutral lipids and may act as a defense barrier.

The dermis, however, can be developed in birds, and along with the hypodermis can be subdivided into a number of layers or strata including a superficial layer the **stratum superficiale,** followed by a dense

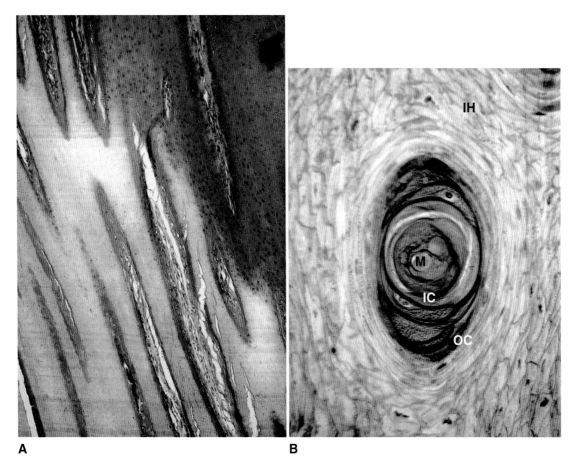

A   **B**

Figure 13-34. A, Light micrograph of the elongated papillary extensions of the coronary corium. (Hematoxylin and eosin [H&E] stain; ×40.) **B,** Light micrograph of one of the papillary extensions seen in **A,** but here in cross section, forming tubular horn. *IC,* Inner cortex; *OC,* outer cortex; *IH,* intertubular horn; *M,* medulla. (H&E stain; ×250.)

layer of **stratum compactum,** and then a loose one, the **stratum laxum,** which together comprise the deep **stratum profundum** (Figure 13-37). The stratum profundum is lined internally by a lamina elastica. The inner portion of the stratum profundum, the stratum laxum, can house large blood vessels, smooth muscle, adipose tissue, and feather follicles.

The one feature found in mammalian skin that is not seen in avian skin is glands. The sweat gland and the sebaceous gland that are associated with the epidermis and hair follicle of mammals are conspicuously absent (see Figure 13-37). In their place is a single, large sebaceous-like preen gland—the **uropygial gland.** Its holocrine secretion results in the production of an oily substance that has a sebaceous gland–like function and is especially well developed in aquatic birds, providing a waterproofing mechanism. The uropygial gland typically has two lobes and lies dorsally and caudally (near the base of the tail) and is spread along the feather-coated body by preening. The amount and content of the oily secretion are

governed in part by hormonal activity, particularly androgens.

From dermal-based follicles, feathers are hair-like epidermal specializations that usually extend far beyond the surface of the epidermis. Like hairs, the feathers and their follicles are positioned at an angle within the dermis, largely to control heat load by radiation. Because each follicle has a bundle of skeletal muscle attached to it, the normal resting position of each feather can be altered according to changes in the heat load as well as by other factors such as mating and defense. The feather follicle resembles a hair follicle, but forms a proximal umbilicus that leads to a distal umbilicus and then gives rise to the quill (see Figure 13-37). Above the epidermis, partitions called barbs branch away from the quill, and from the barbs barbules arise. Feather coloring, which can be extraordinary, results from the deposition of different pigments. Carotenoids provide much of the coloration. For example, xanthophylls give rise to brilliant plumages rich in bright yellows, oranges, and

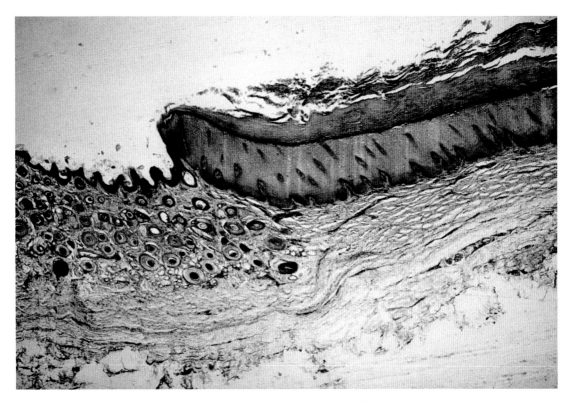

Figure 13-35. Light micrograph of the equine chestnut and its distinctively thickened epidermis provides a sharp contrast with adjacent hair-filled skin. (Hematoxylin and eosin stain; ×20.)

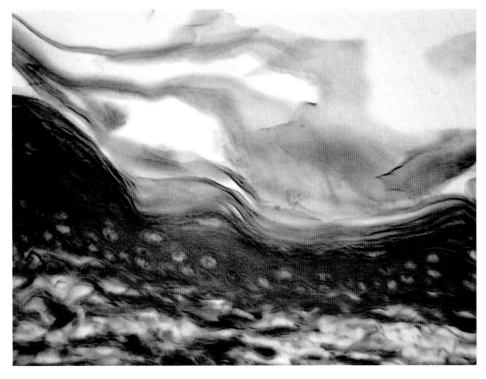

Figure 13-36. Light micrograph of the avian epidermis. (Hematoxylin and eosin stain; ×250.)

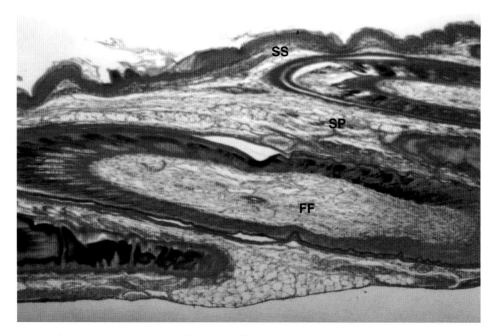

Figure 13-37. Light micrograph of avian skin with feather follicles *(FF)* within the stratum profundum *(SP)* of the dermis. *SS,* Stratum superficiale. (Hematoxylin and eosin stain; ×20.)

reds. Seasonal plumage change is usually due to simple chemical change in the carotenoids. However, changes in both color and the condition of feathers can be the result of environmental factors including nutrition, toxin exposure, and so on.

SUGGESTED READINGS

Abalain JH, Amet Y, Lecaque D, et al: Ultrastructural changes in the uropygial gland of the Japanese quail, *Coturnix coturnix,* after testosterone treatment. Comparison with the sebaceous gland of the male rat, *Cell Tissue Res* 246:373, 1986.

Atoji J, Yanamoto Y, Suzuki Y: Apocrine sweat glands in the circumanal glands of the dog, *Anat Rec* 252:403, 1998.

Aumuller G, Wilhelm B, Seitz J: Apocrine secretion—fact or artifact? *Anat Anz* 181:437, 1999.

Bergman RA, Afifi AK, Heidger PM Jr: *Histology,* Philadelphia, 1996, Saunders.

Fawcett DW: *Bloom and Fawcett: A textbook of histology,* ed 11, Philadelphia, 1986, Saunders.

Gartner LP, Hiatt JL: *Color textbook of histology,* Philadelphia, 1997, Saunders.

Leeson CR, Leeson TS, Paparo AA: *Atlas of histology,* ed 2, Philadelphia, 1985, Saunders.

Menon GK, Brown BE, Elias PM: Avian epidermal differentiation: role of lipids in permeability barrier formation, *Tissue Cell* 18:71, 1986.

Mishra PC, Leach DH: Electron microscopic study of the veins of the dermal lamellae of the equine hoof wall, *Equine Vet J* 15:14, 1983.

Ongpipattanakul B, Francoeur ML, Potts RO: Polymorphism in stratum corneum lipids, *Biochim Biophys Acta* 1190:115, 1994.

Pedini V, Socco P, Dall'Aglio C, Gargiulo AM: Detection of glycosidic residues in carpal glands of wild and domestic pig revealed by basic and lectin histochemistry, *Ann Anat* 181:269, 1999.

Prota G: *Melanins and melanogenesis,* San Diego, 1992, Academic Press.

Slominiski A, Pawelek J: Animals under the sun: effects of ultraviolet radiation on mammalian skin, *Clin Dermatol* 16:503, 1998.

Spearman RIC: *Comparative biology of skin,* London, 1977, Academic Press.

Stump JE: Anatomy of the normal equine foot, including microscopic features of the laminar region, *J Am Vet Med Assoc* 151:1588, 1967.

Wattle O: Cytokeratins of the equine hoof wall, chestnut and skin: bio- and immunohistochemistry, *Equine Vet J Suppl* 26:66, 1998.

Webb AJ, Calhoun ML: The microscopic anatomy of the skin of mongrel dogs, *Am J Vet Res* 15:274, 1954.

Digestive System I: Oral Cavity and Alimentary Canal

KEY CHARACTERISTICS

- Continuous tract, tubular and composed of four tunics: tunica mucosa, tunica submucosa, tunica muscularis, and tunica serosa
- Enhanced luminal (mucosal) modifications for digestion and absorption include plicae, papillae, and villi
- Major cells: ameloblast, odontoblast, chief cell, parietal cell, absorptive cell (enterocyte), goblet cell, enteroendocrine cell, acidophilic granule cell

Throughout the animal kingdom, the digestive system consists of sequentially connecting tubular organs that along with their glands function to ingest, break down, and absorb food substances and eliminate those portions that cannot be digested. Although among domestic mammals the types of organs and their sequence are largely the same, structural variations for each organ are often encountered. These variations are due to the different types of materials used as food sources. Among domestic species, plant eaters (herbivores) possess morphological features to facilitate the breakdown of cellulose-based substances and are not present in meat-eating or carnivorous species. Conversely, carnivores have structures that enhance the ingestion, breakdown, and absorption of meat. Some of the distinctions between the digestive tracts of herbivores and carnivores can be seen throughout the chapter, including Table 14-1, which lists mucosal characteristics of domestic mammals.

As mentioned, the digestive system is mostly tubular shaped with a repeatable histological pattern throughout, consisting of four major coats known as **tunics** (Figure 14-1). The innermost tunic forms a continuous lining for the entire length of the alimentary canal and is referred to as the **tunica mucosa,** also called the *mucosal lining* or *mucous membrane.* The tunica mucosa is composed of a variably developed epithelium that lines the lumen of the digestive tract and is usually covered along its apex by a film of a mucus-rich substance, including cellular detritus, mucin, and serous secretions. The epithelium, in turn, is attached to connective tissue called the **lamina propria,** which is usually loose and may be subtended by a small layer of smooth muscle, the **lamina muscularis.** Mucosal glands may be housed in the lamina propria. Glands may also be associated with the **tunica submucosa,** which lies immediately adjacent to the mucosa. This tunic consists of connective tissue that is more compact than that of the lamina propria and generally contains the largest blood vessels needed to serve that particular portion of the digestive system. In areas along the alimentary canal where the lamina muscularis does not exist, the lamina propria of the tunica mucosa may be difficult to distinguish from the tunica submucosa. In these instances, this area is the **propria-submucosa.** A third tunic—the **tunica muscularis**—consists of considerable amounts of smooth or skeletal muscle surrounding the tunica submucosa. When the muscle involved is smooth, it generally is organized into two layers, with the innermost layer oriented circumferentially (circularly) and the outermost layer oriented along the longitudinal axis of the

TABLE 14-1   Key Morphological Characteristics of the Gastrointestinal Tract of Domestic Species

ORGAN	EPITHELIUM AND ITS CELL TYPES	LAMINA PROPRIA AND ASSOCIATED GLANDS: MUCOSAL AND SUBMUCOSAL	CELLS OF GLANDS	MUSCLE: LAMINA MUSCULARIS MUCOSAE AND TUNICA MUSCULARIS	SPECIES VARIATIONS
Esophagus	Stratified squamous	Lymph nodules and scattered lymphatic tissue (pig); branched tubuloalveolar glands within submucosa of cranial portion in most domestic species and entire length in dogs	Mucous cells	Lamina muscularis is thin, longitudinal (absent in dogs); tunica muscularis: inner circular and outer longitudinal, skeletal cranially and smooth caudally; inner circular thickens and forms cardiac sphincter muscle at opening of the stomach	Keratinized in ruminants and less extent in horses; in horses and cats skeletal muscle of tunica muscularis extends caudally and in dogs and ruminants is entirely skeletal

Nonruminant Stomach Regions

ORGAN	EPITHELIUM AND ITS CELL TYPES	LAMINA PROPRIA AND ASSOCIATED GLANDS: MUCOSAL AND SUBMUCOSAL	CELLS OF GLANDS	MUSCLE: LAMINA MUSCULARIS MUCOSAE AND TUNICA MUSCULARIS	SPECIES VARIATIONS
Nonglandular	Stratified squamous	Nonglandular		Tunica muscularis: smooth muscle, inner longitudinal; outer circular; and outermost oblique	Nonexistent in carnivores, small in pigs, well developed in horses
Cardiac	Simple columnar with lamina propria forming gastric folds; gastric lining cell	Mucosal branched tubular coiled glands	Mucous cells, endocrine cells	Lamina muscularis is thickened, 2-3 layers; tunica muscularis: smooth muscle, inner helical/longitudinal; outer/middle circular, being most developed; and outermost oblique	Chief cells can be found in pigs and parietal cells in dogs; especially well developed in pigs and little developed in carnivores and horses
Fundic	Simple columnar with lamina propria forming gastric folds; gastric lining cell	Branched tubular coiled glands (longer than cardiac glands and subdivided into isthmus, neck, body and base)	Mucous (neck) cells, chief cells, parietal cells, endocrine cells	Similar to the cardiac region	In dogs this region consists of a light zone with a thinner mucosa and a dark zone with a thicker mucosa; next to the pyloric region
Pyloric	Simple columnar with lamina propria forming gastric folds; gastric lining cell	Deep gastric pits with short mucosal unbranched to branched tubular coiled glands	Mucous cells, endocrine cells	Similar to the cardiac region; middle circular broadens into pyloric sphincter	

Ruminant Stomach Regions

ORGAN	EPITHELIUM AND ITS CELL TYPES	LAMINA PROPRIA AND ASSOCIATED GLANDS: MUCOSAL AND SUBMUCOSAL	CELLS OF GLANDS	MUSCLE: LAMINA MUSCULARIS MUCOSAE AND TUNICA MUSCULARIS	SPECIES VARIATIONS
Rumen	Keratinized stratified squamous	Nonglandular with conical to tongue-shaped papillae with well vascularized connective tissue; lamina propria-submucosa		Lamina muscularis is absent; tunica muscularis: smooth muscle, inner circular; outer longitudinal	
Reticulum	Keratinized stratified squamous	Nonglandular with honeycombed reticular crests with smaller secondary crests and papillae extending from crests and between them		Lamina muscularis is present within apical portion of larger crests; tunica muscularis similar to the rumen	

TABLE 14-1 Key Morphological Characteristics of the Gastrointestinal Tract of Domestic Species—cont'd

ORGAN	EPITHELIUM AND ITS CELL TYPES	LAMINA PROPRIA AND ASSOCIATED GLANDS: MUCOSAL AND SUBMUCOSAL	CELLS OF GLANDS	MUSCLE: LAMINA MUSCULARIS MUCOSAE AND TUNICA MUSCULARIS	SPECIES VARIATIONS
Omasum	Keratinized stratified squamous	Nonglandular with laminae of different sizes (orders), primary being the largest; each lamina possess papillae		Lamina muscularis is well developed and extends into laminae; inner circular smooth muscle extends along with lamina muscularis into largest laminae	
Abosmasum	Simple columnar with lamina propria forming gastric folds; gastric lining cell	Branched tubular coiled glands	Mucous (neck) cells, chief cells, parietal cells, endocrine cells	Similar to the cardiac region	
Small Intestine					
Duodenum	Simple columnar with lamina propria forming villi; enterocytes, goblet cells, endocrine cells	Lymph nodules (Peyer's patches) and scattered gut-associated lymphatic tissue (GALT); simple branched and unbranched tubular glands (crypts); submucosal simple branched, tubuloacinar glands	Columnar lining cells, endocrine cells, goblet cells, acidophilic granule cells (Paneth)	Lamina muscularis is bilayered with strands of smooth muscle extending into the villi; tunica muscularis: smooth muscle, inner circular; outer longitudinal with myenteric plexus between	Submucosal glands are mucous in dogs and ruminants, seromucous in cats, and serous in horses and pigs; tunica muscularis is thickest in horses
Jejunum	Similar to duodenum; villi are thinner, smaller, and less dense than duodenum	GALT more developed and crypts less developed than duodenum	Similar to the duodenum	Similar to the duodenum	
Ileum	Similar to jejunum	GALT most developed	Similar to the duodenum	Similar to the duodenum	Lymph nodules most numerous in horses and largest in cattle
Large Intestine					
Cecum	Simple columnar	GALT is well developed throughout and concentrated at one end or the other; simple unbranched tubular glands	Goblet cells	Tunica muscularis: smooth muscle, inner circular; outer longitudinal with myenteric plexus between	GALT localized around ileal ostium in dogs, pigs, and ruminants and next to the colon in cats and horses; in horses and pigs outer longitudinal layer of tunica muscularis has flat muscle bands with elastic fibers: taeni ceci
Colon	Simple columnar	GALT is present throughout; simple unbranched tubular glands	Goblet cells	Similar to the cecum	In horses and pigs outer longitudinal layer continues to form flat muscle bands with elastic fibers: taeni coli
Rectum	Simple columnar	Similar to the colon	Goblet cells	Similar to the cecum but more developed	

alimentary canal. The fourth and outermost coat is the tunica serosa/tunica adventitia, which is composed of loose to dense connective tissue and forms an outer fascia for the different elements of the digestive system. In areas where this fascia is in contact with a serous cavity, such as the peritoneal cavity, the connective tissue is lined by a mesothelium and the fascial coat is known as the **tunica serosa.** However, in those areas where this portion of the alimentary canal directly abuts another structure and its outer covering, this tunic is called the **tunica adventitia.**

ORAL CAVITY

The entrance to the alimentary canal of the digestive system is the oral cavity and its opening, which forms a junction between the integument and the digestive tract. Among mammals, this junction forms the upper and lower lips, which extends as a cutaneous mucous membrane into the initial portion of the alimentary canal. The cavity itself is typically asymmetrically shaped and composed of the narrow vestibule, which lies between the lips and cheeks and the teeth and gingivae, and the relatively expansive buccal cavity, which extends internally between the oropharynx and the arches of the teeth. The functions of the oral cavity, which are many, consist of taking in and breaking down food both mechanically and chemically. Other functions include food lubrication, taste, bodily defense against foe, cellular defense against infection, and contribution to vocalization.

LIPS AND CHEEKS

In concert with the articulation of the mandible and maxilla, the upper and lower **lips** may part or remain sealed in controlling the entrance to the oral

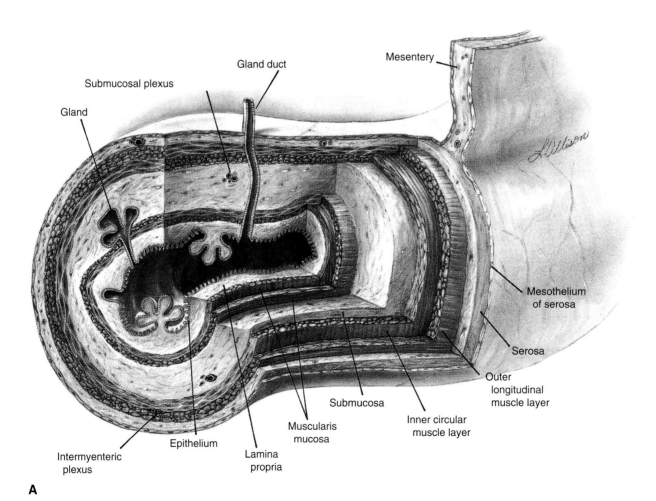

A

Figure 14-1. A, Illustration of the general organization of the gastrointestinal tract of a mammal. Light micrographs of four different portions of the tract in domestic species, each with varied development of the mucosal *(M)*, submucosal *(S)*, and muscular tunics *(T)*.

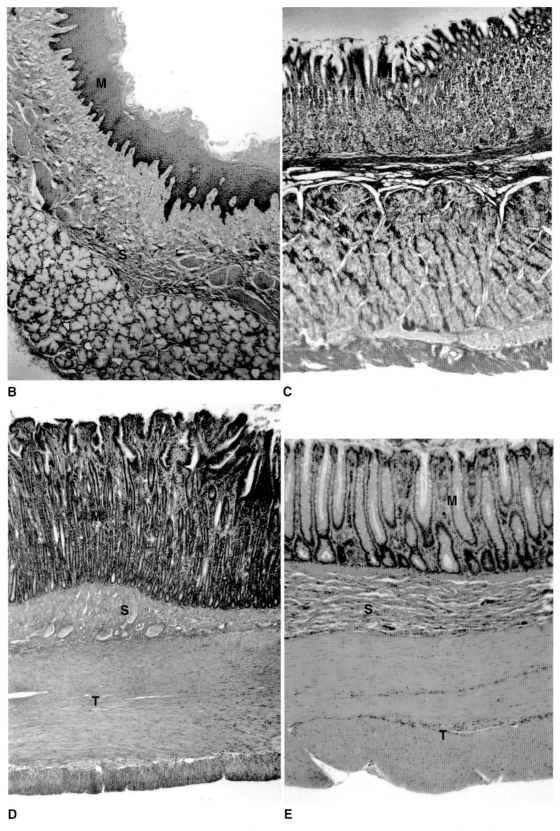

Figure 14-1, cont'd B, Esophagus. **C,** Stomach. **D,** Small intestine. **E,** Large intestine. (Hematoxylin and eosin stain; ×20.) *(A modified from Leeson CR, Leeson TS, Paparo AA:* Atlas of histology, *ed 2, Philadelphia, 1985, Saunders.)*

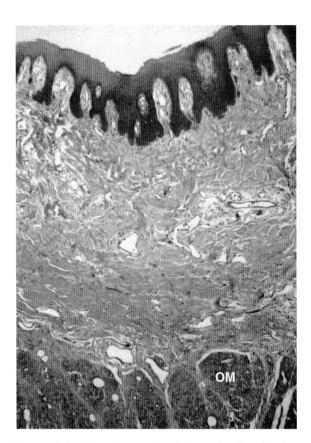

Figure 14-2. Light micrograph of the canine lip with the orbicularis muscle *(OM)*. (Hematoxylin and eosin stain; ×20.)

cavity. As a flexible "door" to the digestive tract, the lips and the cheeks contribute to food mastication and the phonetics of vocalization. Each lip has a core of skeletal muscle, the **orbicularis oris muscle,** that provides the extensive mobility associated with these structures (Figure 14-2). Externally, the lip is lined by a thin epidermis and typical dermis with hair follicles, sebaceous glands, and sweat glands. At the orifice where the upper and lower lips contact one another, hair and glands are absent, forming the **mucocutaneous junction** that typically has a thickened stratified squamous epithelium, forms the lamina epithelialis, and can be well keratinized or cornified in herbivorous animals (Figure 14-3). There can be a notable interdigitation between the epithelium and the lamina propria, which is well vascularized but may lack pigment, causing this area to appear pink; otherwise this region can be heavily melanized. The dermis becomes the lamina propria and submucosa without any obvious morphological difference. The internal portion of each lip forms the **mucous aspect,** which can contain serous or seromucous glands known as the **labial glands,** a form of salivary gland.

The external portion of the cheeks is much like that of the lips, consisting of skin that overlies the **buccinator muscle,** a well-developed layer of skeletal muscle. Internally, the buccinator muscle is lined by the mucosa, which may be keratinized among domestic species as previously described for the lips. The lamina propria of ruminants is elevated, forming **buccal papillae,** conical projections that contribute to the mastication of fibrous food. The submucosa houses compound tubuloalveolar glands called the **buccal glands,** minor salivary glands that can produce mucous or serous secretions or both.

TEETH

Like bone, teeth are heavily mineralized structures consisting of enamel, dentin, and cementum (Figure 14-4). Of the three components, **enamel** is the hardest and most durable, consisting of 96% to 99% calcium hydroxyapatite arranged in large crystals that are thinly coated with an organic matrix. The enamel is located along the external surface of the tooth known as the **crown,** which is exposed to the oral cavity. The enamel crystals can be very organized in their architecture, being variously arranged in rows of slender rods that extend longitudinally from the innermost region of the enamel, next to the dentin, to the oral cavity (Figure 14-5). In the pig, the rods closest to the dentin, the initial enamel layer, are straight, but become wavy in the inner enamel layer and form a staggered pattern in the outer enamel layer. These layers of enamel rods are produced by the **ameloblast,** which initially synthesizes and secretes **enamilin** and **amelogenin,** both keratin-like glycoproteins transported from the Golgi apparatus to the apical surface within secretory granules (see Figure 14-5). As the enamel of a tooth continues to be made, the ameloblasts gradually recede. Highly mineralized and solidly designed, the enamel of a tooth is able to withstand enormous pressure.

Internal to the enamel is another highly mineralized component of the tooth known as the **dentin.** Dentin is more elastic than enamel; it is composed of 60% to 70% calcium hydroxyapatite and 30% to 40% bound water and organic materials, including collagen, proteoglycans, and glycoproteins. Much of the tooth is composed of dentin, most of which lies beneath the gingiva (see Figure 14-4). This material is produced by columnar-shaped cells called **odontoblasts,** which are located along its inner margin next to the periphery of the pulp (Figure 14-6). The apex of each odontoblast form **odontoblastic processes,** long cytoplasmic processes that extend from the base

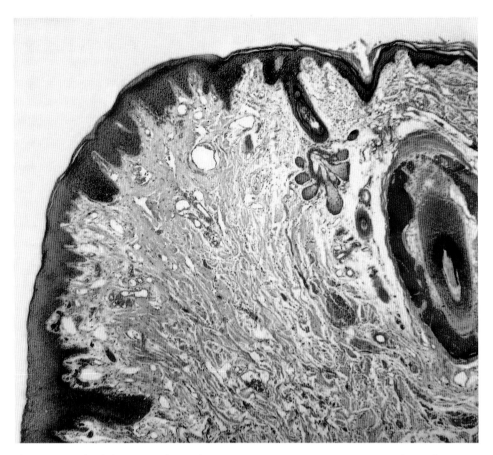

Figure 14-3. Light micrograph of the canine lip at the mucocutaneous junction. (Hematoxylin and eosin stain; ×20.)

of the dentin to the dentinoenamel junction in the area of the crown and to the dentinocemental junction below the crown (see Figure 14-4). The odontoblastic processes lie within tunnel-like spaces surrounded by peritubular dentin. Intertubular dentin lies between the peritubular dentin; this dentin is more mineralized than the peritubular type. Collagen (type I), proteoglycans, and glycoproteins, which have yet to be mineralized, are between the odontoblastic processes and the peritubular dentin. This portion represents **predentin** and is reminiscent of prebone or osteoid material associated with osteoblasts. Unlike ameloblasts, odontoblasts remain active during the longevity of a tooth, secreting predentin and mineralizing it, but usually at a reduced rate once the tooth has erupted.

Where the tooth has remained below the level of the gingival (i.e., the root of the tooth), the dentin is lined externally by the third mineralized component, the **cementum.** Cementum is the least mineralized of the mineralized portion of the tooth, composed of roughly 50% calcium hydroxyapatite with the remainder consisting of collagen (type I), proteoglycans, and

glycoproteins. The cells involved in the formation of cementum are **cementoblasts,** and are osteoblastic in form and function. In fact, cementum as a whole can be thought of as a bony structure. Much of the cementum is cellular, possessing osteocyte-like cells called **cementocytes** that lie in lacunae within the cementum. Each cell interconnects with adjacent ones by slender cytoplasmic processes that lie within canaliculi that can extend to the vascular peridental ligament. When cementocytes are present, this portion can be referred to as the **cellular cementum.** However, there is a portion that lacks cementocytes, the **acellular cementum,** which covers the upper region of the root.

Each adult tooth is attached to a surrounding bony socket known as the **alveolus** (see Figure 14-4). The attachment is provided by densely packed collagen fibers that form the **periodontal ligament.** The portion of the tooth that lies within the alveolus is the **root,** and the region of the tooth between the alveolus and the crown is the **cervix.** Although most of the tooth is mineralized, a central area—the **pulp**—consists of a loose connective tissue, including a well-developed

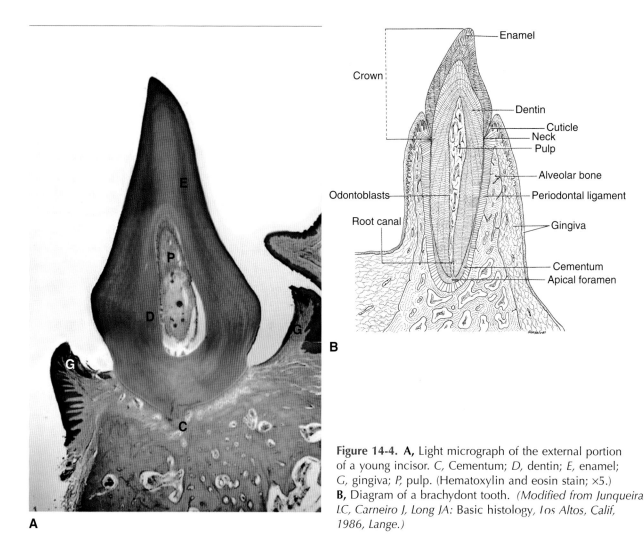

A

B

Figure 14-4. A, Light micrograph of the external portion of a young incisor. *C,* Cementum; *D,* dentin; *E,* enamel; *G,* gingiva; *P,* pulp. (Hematoxylin and eosin stain; ×5.) **B,** Diagram of a brachydont tooth. *(Modified from Junqueira LC, Carneiro J, Long JA: Basic histology, los Altos, Calif, 1986, Lange.)*

vascular bed and nerve supply. At the base of the tooth (i.e., the tip of the root) a small channel, the **root canal,** interconnects the pulp to the peridental ligament by way of the **apical foramen,** a small orifice. It is through this foramen that blood and lymphatic vessels and nerves enter the pulp.

The pulp is lined peripherally by a single layer of odontoblasts that collectively form the pulp's outermost zone, the **odontoblastic zone** (see Figure 14-6). At the base of the odontoblasts is a relatively narrow **cell free zone** that covers the innermost zone of the pulp, the **cell rich zone,** which is the largest of the three zones; it is composed of nerve, lymphatic, and vascular elements as well as fibroblasts and mesenchymal cells and associated extracellular fibers and proteoglycans. Because the odontoblasts remain active, adding new dentin internally throughout the life of an individual, the cavity occupied by the pulp is gradually diminished in size.

TYPES OF TEETH

Among domestic mammals are two types of teeth: brachydont and hypsodont. The morphological description given above applies to **brachydont** teeth or dentition, in which the crown is covered by enamel and visible above the gingiva. These teeth generally are short, ceasing to elongate or expand after they have erupted. The longevity of the ameloblast that forms the crown of the brachydont tooth is short lived and restricted to only the developmental stage of this type of tooth (see Figures 14-4 and 14-5). Members of the Carnivora and Primates possess only teeth of this construction. Pigs also have brachydont teeth except for canine teeth, which are of the hypsodont type. Ruminants have only incisor teeth that are brachydont.

The second type of tooth, the **hypsodont,** is able to continue to grow during the life of the individual,

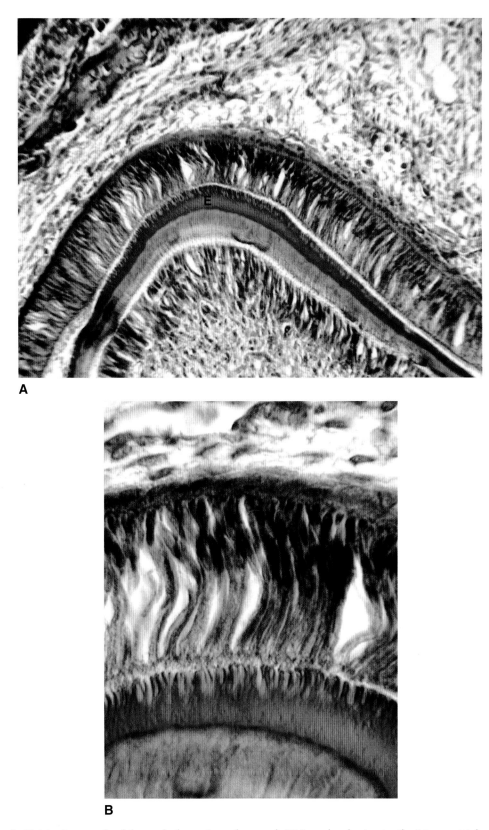

Figure 14-5. A, Light micrograph of the early formation of enamel *(E)* in a developing tooth. (Masson trichrome stain; ×100.) **B,** Light micrograph of the ameloblasts involved in the enamel formation. (Masson trichrome stain; ×400.)

Continued

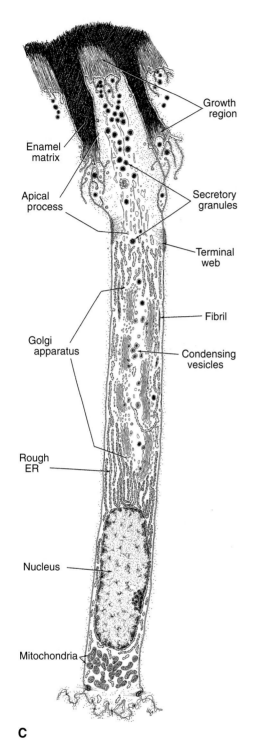

Growth region

Enamel matrix

Apical process

Secretory granules

Terminal web

Fibril

Golgi apparatus

Condensing vesicles

Rough ER

Nucleus

Mitochondria

C

Figure 14-5, cont'd C, Diagram of ameloblast taken from an ultrastructural observation. *ER,* Endoplasmic reticulum. *(Revised from Fawcett DW:* Bloom and Fawcett: a textbook of histology, *ed 11, Philadelphia, 1986, Saunders.)*

rather than cease in its development shortly after erupting through the gingiva. These teeth are characteristically long, especially in the instance of the porcine canine-tooth, which, for example, become tusks in boars. The morphology and organization of the mineralized components of hypsodont dentition are different than that of brachydont dentition. The cementum, which only occurs below the gingiva in brachydont teeth, forms a continuous outer lining of hypsodont teeth that extends above the gingiva as well as below (Figure 14-7). The cementum is internally lined by enamel, an arrangement not found in brachydont teeth (see Figure 14-4). The enamel, in fact, is formed along most of the length of a hypsodont tooth, ending near the tip of the root. Dentin forms the innermost mineralized component, lying next to the enamel, but not coming into contact with the cementum either above or below the gingiva (see Figure 14-7). Another morphological difference between the two types of teeth is the occurrence of **infundibula,** which consist of invaginations of both cementum and enamel at the tooth's surface as it becomes contoured during development as seen in molars (see Figure 14-7). Infundibula possess enamel plicae, which enhance the process of grinding, by providing greater resistance to the forces of physical compression. The hypsodont teeth then never form true enamel crowns as in brachydont teeth.

ODONTOGENESIS

During embryogenesis, the oral ectoderm proliferates and invaginates in a horseshoe-shaped manner into the subjacent mesenchyme, forming the **dental lamina** (Figure 14-8). From the dental lamina individual thickenings of epithelial cells arise, being primordia of developing teeth known as **enamel organs.** Each enamel organ initially becomes cup shaped and faces away from the oral cavity. The concavity of the cup becomes filled with ectomesenchymal cells, forming the **dental papilla.** The cells lining the internal surface of the cup are the **inner enamel epithelium** and those forming an external cover are the **outer enamel epithelium.** Both epithelia initially appear simple squamous in shape. Also epithelial cells are lodged between the inner and outer epithelia. These cells make up a middle layer and are called the **stellate reticulum** because they begin to acquire a mesenchymal-like morphology, forming cellular processes that attach to one another. The inner epithelium eventually becomes transformed into active, columnar-shaped secretory-like cells known as *ameloblasts,* which produce enamel (see Figure 14-5). Cells within the dental papilla differentiate into odontoblasts and begin to form the dentin (see Figure

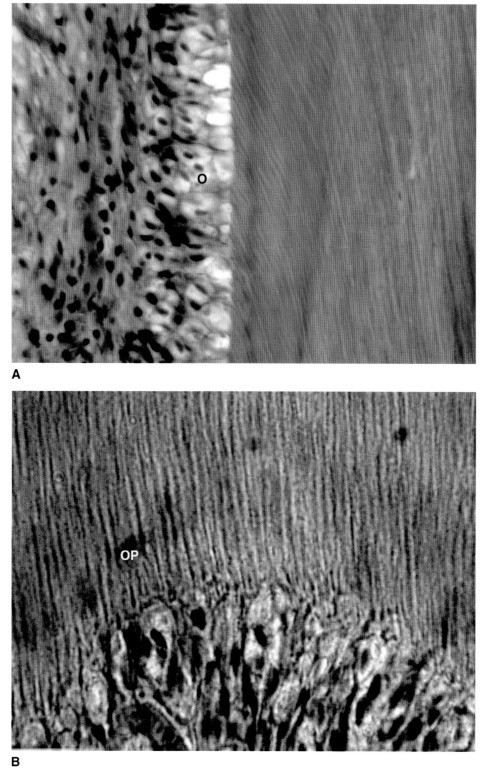

A

B

Figure 14-6. **A,** Light micrograph of odontoblasts *(O)* forming dentin in a nearly mature tooth. (Hematoxylin and eosin stain; ×200.) **B,** Light micrograph of the odontoblastic processes *(OP)* extending from the odontoblasts; the processes are involved in dentin production. (Hematoxylin and eosin stain; ×500.)

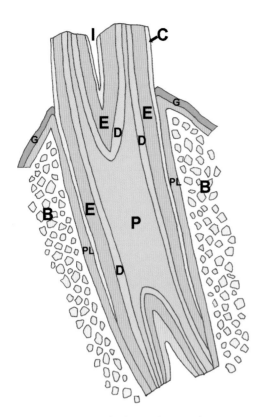

Figure 14-7. Diagram of a hypsodont tooth. *B,* Bone; *D,* dentin; *E,* enamel; *G,* gingival; *I,* infundibulum; *P,* pulp; *PL,* periodontal ligament.

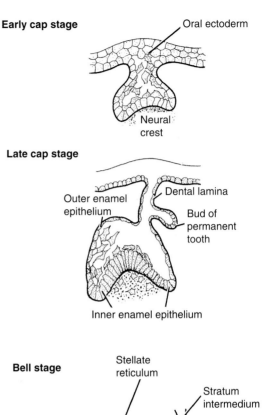

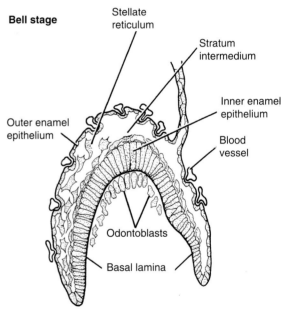

Figure 14-8. Schematic illustration of the development of a brachydont tooth. *(Revised from Warshawsky H: The teeth. In Weiss L, editor:* Histology: cell and tissue biology, *ed 5, New York, 1983, Elsevier Biomedical.)*

14-8). As the young ameloblasts and odontoblasts form the earliest mineralized portion of the developing tooth, the first enamel and dentin secreted become the **dentinoenamel junction** (see Figure 14-5). This junction begins at the apex of the crown of a brachydont tooth and progressively extends along the sides of the crown to the neck of the tooth. With the production of more dentin, odontoblasts are forced to move farther into what was the dental papilla or developing pulp.

At the junction of the inner and outer enamel epithelium, cells begin a downward growth into the developing adjacent connective tissue. These cells form the **epithelial sheath of Hertwig** and are responsible for the formation of the root. The epithelial cells become odontoblastic and the connective tissue that they ensheathe becomes the dental pulp. The odontoblasts create the dentin of the root and are continuous with those producing coronal dentin. This entire process, including the development of the enamel organ, occurs within a thickening capsule of connective tissue that represents the **dental sac.** At the point that the crown and its enamel coat have developed fully, the crown becomes exposed to the oral cavity as it ruptures through the dental sac. Along the root, the

dental sac collapses onto its sides and becomes concomitantly transformed into a lining of cementoblasts.

GINGIVA

The root of each tooth is lined by the **gingiva,** a dense, irregular connective tissue and an overlying stratified squamous epithelium (see Figure 14-4). Before this epithelium joins or becomes attached to

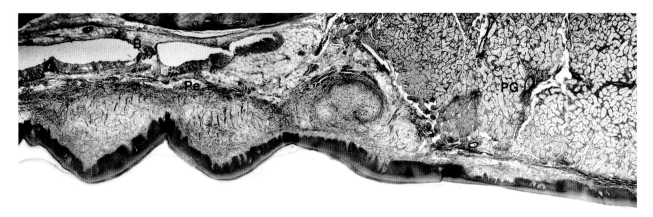

Figure 14-9. Light micrograph of the hard palate of a rabbit with rugae consisting of a ridged or dentated mucosa and stratified squamous epithelium. *PG,* palatine gland; *Pe,* periosteum; *B,* bone. (Hematoxylin and eosin stain; ×15.)

each tooth, it reflexes by several millimeters away from the oral cavity toward the root apex of the tooth, forming a gingival sulcus. In a collar-like manner, the epithelium is firmly attached to each tooth's enamel surface by hemidesmosomes and is referred to as the **junctional epithelium.**

PALATE

The oral cavity is separated from the nasal cavity of the respiratory system by the **hard palate,** a bony shelf that is fixed in placed and covered by a layer of irregular dense connective tissue, which, in turn, is lined by a keratinized stratified squamous epithelium. This mucosa, which is especially developed in ruminant species, is transversely ridged. The ridges are referred to as **rugae,** and the connective tissue here as well as within the rest of the papillary layer is directly fused with the submucosa (i.e., a propria-submucosa) and intermixes with the periosteal lining of the subtending bones (Figure 14-9). Posteriorly, the **palatine glands,** consisting of branched mucus and seromucous glands, are housed in this portion of the hard palate.

The soft palate by comparison possesses a core of skeletal muscle instead of bone that is covered ventrally by a nonkeratinized stratified squamous epithelium along the oropharyngeal surface. Its nasopharyngeal surface is caudally lined also by the stratified squamous epithelium and rostrally by a pseudostratified columnar epithelium. The adjacent irregular dense connective tissue is also continuous between the lamina propria and the submucosa, lacking a lamina muscularis. As in the hard palate, branched mucus and seromucous palatine glands are located within the propria-submucosa.

TONGUE

Arising cranially from the floor of the oral cavity and extending rostrally, the **tongue** is a large, usually flattened mass of intertwined skeletal muscle lined by a mucosal membrane with sensory awareness for gustation and touch. As a result, this structure is able to taste, acquire, and pull food into the oral cavity and subsequently help break it apart in concert with the teeth. In horses, a cord of hyaline cartilage and fibroelastic tissue, the **dorsal lingual cartilage,** lies mid-dorsally within skeletal muscle and provides additional support to the tongue. Among domestic species the epithelium of the mucosa is dorsally thick and keratinized stratified squamous (Figure 14-10). In contrast, the epithelium located ventrally is typically thin and nonkeratinized (Figure 14-11). In addition to having a thick mucosa, the dorsal portion of the tongue is highly papillated. The **lingual papillae** contribute to either prehension and mastication or gustation. Those papillae that provide the former functions are principally mechanical in their activity and serve to facilitate the movement of liquid and solid food materials into the oral cavity and toward the esophagus. These papillae possess one of several shapes: filiform, conical, or lenticular.

Filiform papillae, as the name implies, are narrow and filament-like. These papillae are usually the most numerous and help the tongue capture and bring ingesta into the oral cavity (Figure 14-12). This activity is partially contributed by the direction that the papillae are positioned, pointed to the pharynx. In addition to mucosal keratinization, each papilla has a vascular core that provides further support. In cats these papillae are especially well developed, having

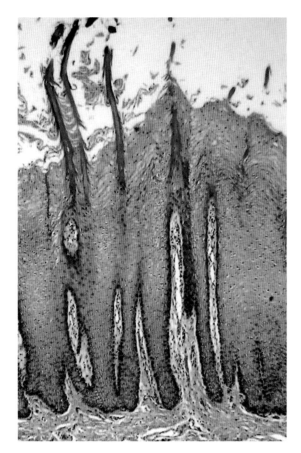

Figure 14-10. Light micrograph of the dorsal surface of the tongue of a horse with filiform papillae. (Hematoxylin and eosin stain; ×40.)

two caudally directed apices, one larger and more pointed than the other (see Figure 14-12). Canine filiform papillae are also well developed, although smaller and less pointed and keratinized than those of the cat. By comparison, filiform papillae in the horse are reduced in size, and composed of slender, caudally curved extensions of the mucosa (Figure 14-13; see also Figure 14-10).

In addition to the filiform papillae are conical and lenticular forms. **Conical papillae** are located along the root of the tongue in carnivores and pigs. They are generally less keratinized and larger than their filiform counterparts. In cats they contribute to the drinking of milk and water and transportation of food mass toward the pharynx. In pigs these papillae have lymphatic tissue within their connective tissue cores and resultantly can be called **tonsillar papillae;** they collectively form the **lingual tonsil. Lenticular papillae** are, as the name implies, lens shaped or flattened spherical, keratinized projections along the dorsal portion of the posterior or caudal third of the tongue. In the bovine tongue, this region is referred to as the **torsus linguae,** and has a mucosa that is especially well developed, with long connective tissue papillae intercalated by deep epithelial invaginations and intermittent lenticular papillae.

Lingual papillae involved in gustation include fungiform, circumvallate, and foliate types. **Fungiform papillae** are large mushroom-like bodies that extend

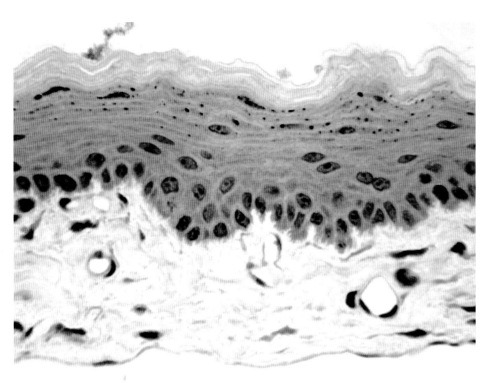

Figure 14-11. Light micrograph of the ventral surface of a cat's tongue, which lacks papillae. (Hematoxylin and eosin stain; ×20.)

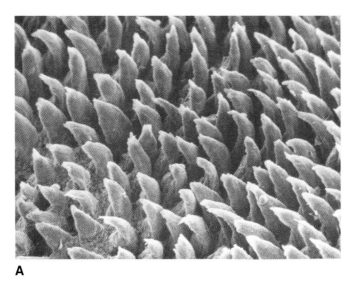

A

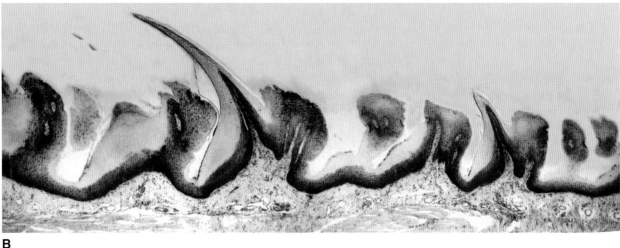

B

Figure 14-12. A, Scanning electron micrograph of a rabbit tongue with filiform papillae. **B,** Light micrograph of the dorsal surface of the tongue of a cat with filiform papillae. (Hematoxylin and eosin stain; ×10.) *(From Fawcett DW:* Bloom and Fawcett: a textbook of histology, *ed 11, Philadelphia, 1986, Saunders.)*

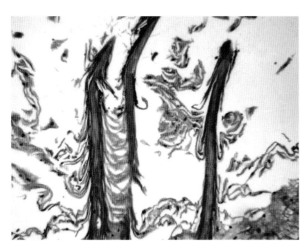

Figure 14-13. Light micrograph of the dorsal surface of the tongue of a horse with filiform papillae. (Hematoxylin and eosin stain; ×100.)

beyond the level of the apices of surrounding filiform papillae. The connective tissue of each of these papillae forms a stalk, containing appropriate capillary beds beneath a nonkeratinized mucosal epithelium. Among secondary papillae that occur dorsally along each dome of these structures, taste buds can be found, especially among the tongues of carnivores.

Circumvallate, or **vallate, papillae** are another type of lingual papilla associated with taste. These papillae are both fewest and largest encountered on the tongues of domestic species. Although they may have a domelike morphology, the circumvallate papillae lie within a sulcus that is lined by the mucosal epithelium (Figure 14-14). Along the sides of the sulcus, including its base, serous secretions are emitted by the ducts of serous gustatory glands. As in fungiform papillae, secondary papillae of the epithelium

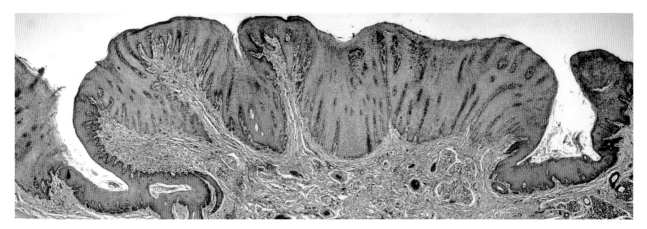

Figure 14-14. Light micrograph of the dorsal surface of the tongue of a horse with a vallate papilla. (Hematoxylin and eosin stain; ×4.)

and adjacent connective tissue can be seen in the circumvallate papillae. However, the taste buds are not located dorsally within the circumvallate papillae, but instead along their side or lateral margin.

A third form of lingual papillae for gustation are the **foliate papillae.** This leaflike type is arranged in parallel folds located posterolaterally along the dorsoventral margin of the tongue. Taste buds, when present, are positioned on each side of a foliate papilla. In cats taste buds partially develop within foliate papillae, but are rudimentary and without sensory function. In ruminants, taste buds are absent altogether in the foliate papillae.

TASTE BUDS

Gustation, or taste, is provided by the sensory apparatus known as the **taste bud.** Taste buds are oval intraepithelial organs that consist of clusters of spindle-shaped cells extending the length of the organ from its base against the basement membrane to a small opening, the **taste pore** (Figures 14-15 and 14-16). The spindle-shaped cells have been subdivided into three types: dark cells (type I), light cells (type II), and intermediate cells (type III). At this time, it is unclear whether all three types are involved in chemoreception, or only one or two. The dark and light cells possess microvilli at their tips, which were once referred to as taste hairs. In addition to the spindle-shaped cells is a fourth type, the basal cell, believed to be a stem cell that gives rise to the others (see Figure 14-16). Each taste bud contains an arborized nerve ending that terminates on the sensory cells. The sensory cells are able to distinguish the sensations: sweet, sour, bitter, and salty. Although each taste bud may have the capability to sense the different tastes, it is believed that different regions of the

tongue vary in their sensitivities to the four tastes. In the dog the taste buds located toward the front of the tongue are more sensitive to salt, whereas those located posteriorly are more sensitive to sweet substances.

SALIVARY GLANDS

As food is brought into the oral cavity, it is acted upon immediately by the secretions of the salivary glands. Salivary glands can be divided into two broad categories: those that are major, which include the parotid glands, the mandibular glands, and the sublingual glands; and those that are minor, including the buccal glands, labial glands, and palatine glands. Additional minor glands may be present that are specific for certain domestic species, such as the molar gland in the cat or the zygomatic gland in carnivores. The secretions of the salivary glands are mostly serous in composition, containing various enzymes that begin the digestive process, leaving most of this activity to occur in the stomach and intestines. Mucous secretions are also contributed by salivary glands, making these glands mixed with regard to their secretory product (see Table 4-1 and Figure 4-6). As the salivary glands function to moisten and lubricate ingested substances, these substances begin to break apart and dissolve, revealing more readily sweet, sour, bitter, and salty qualities that can be detected by the taste buds as described earlier.

Histologically, salivary glands consist of tubular, alveolar, and tubuloalveolar arrays of serous and mucus-secreting end pieces. Each of these shapes can be found in the same gland (Figure 14-17). The distinction between major and minor salivary glands is based on size; the major glands have numerous lobules and microlobules. The minor glands are compound glands as well, but generally less crowded with fewer

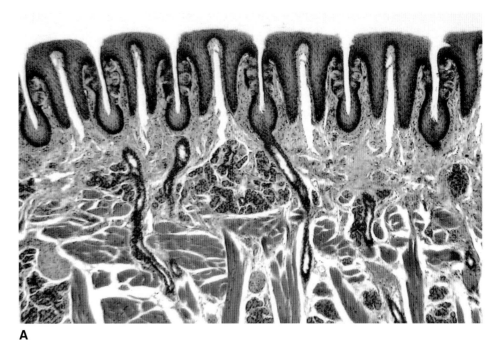

A

Figure 14-15. A, Light micrograph of the dorsal surface of the tongue of a rabbit with foliate papillae. (Hematoxylin and eosin [H&E] stain; ×20.) **B,** Close-up of the foliate papillae with taste buds. (H&E stain; ×600.)

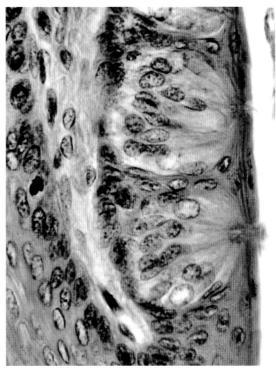

B

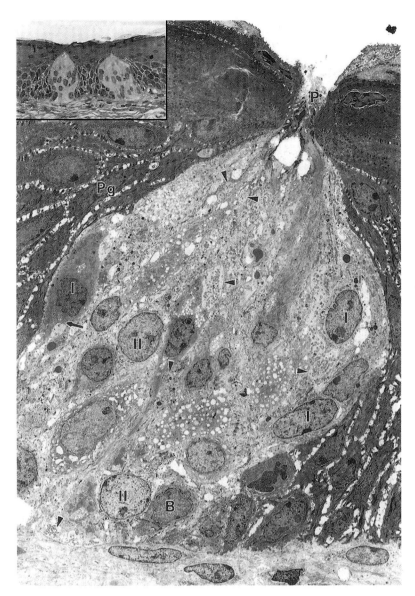

Figure 14-16. Transmission electron micrograph (×2600) of a taste bud from the sheep. *B,* Basal cell; *P,* taste pore; *Pg,* perigemmal cell; *arrowheads,* nerve fibers; *I,* type I cell; *II,* type II cell. *(From Gartner LP, Hiatt JL:* Color textbook of histology, *Philadelphia, 1997, Saunders.)*

lobules and microlobules. Further information about salivary glands is provided in Chapter 15.

ALIMENTARY CANAL

PHARYNX

The oral cavity leads into the **pharynx,** which is the beginning of the **alimentary canal.** Not only is the pharynx connected to the oral cavity by the **oropharynx,** it also opens into the nasal cavity by the **nasopharynx** and the larynx by the **laryngopharynx** (see Figure 11-1). The tunica mucosa consists mostly of a stratified squamous epithelium that may be keratinized, and a lamina propria that mixes directly with the adjacent submucosa and is sometimes referred to

as **propria-submucosa.** Along the nasopharynx, the epithelial lining is transformed into a pseudostratified columnar type. The tunica muscularis is entirely skeletal and lined externally by adventitia of varying development as it comes into contact with nearby structures.

ESOPHAGUS

The **esophagus** is a muscular channel that transports liquid and solid food that may have been previously masticated within the oral cavity by the laryngopharynx to the stomach. In carnivores, the junction between the esophagus and the laryngopharynx contains an internal circular fold, the **pharyngoesophageal lumen.** The length of the esophagus can

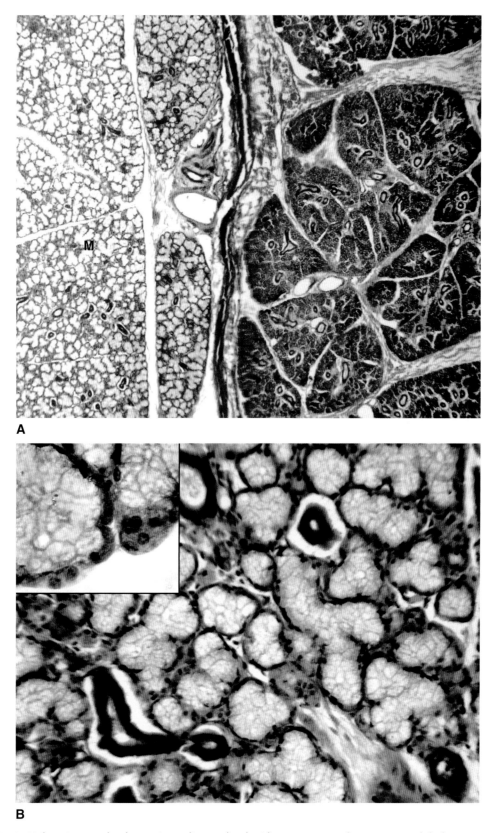

Figure 14-17. A, Light micrograph of a canine salivary gland with serous *(S)* and mucous *(M)* lobules. (Hematoxylin and eosin [H&E] stain; ×15.) **B,** Light micrograph of the secretory end pieces in the mucous portion of the salivary gland. (H&E stain; ×200.) **Inset,** close-up of serous-secreting cells, demilunes, that lie adjacent to mucous-secreting cells in a canine salivary gland. (Hematoxylin and eosin stain; ×500.)

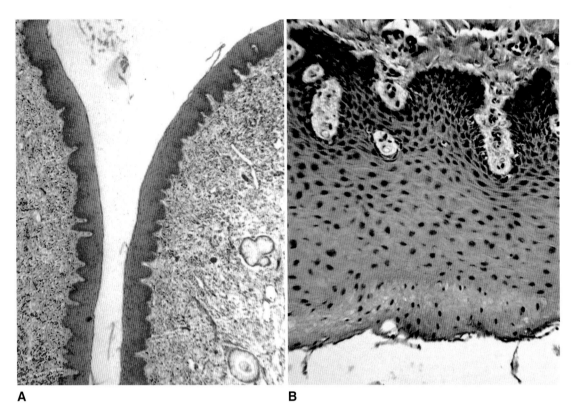

A   **B**

Figure 14-18. A, Light micrograph of the mucosal lining of a canine esophagus. (Hematoxylin and eosin [H&E] stain; ×25.) **B,** Light micrograph of the thickened stratified squamous epithelium along the esophagus of a pig. (H&E stain; ×125.)

vary sharply between species, especially herbivores. Each of the tunics is designed to be able to change markedly in its diameter so that ingested materials can be transported to the stomach without difficulty. This is especially true in the instance of carnivores in which the size of the bolus can be considerable.

The mucosa of the esophagus generally contains all three layers: the lamina epithelialis, which is stratified squamous; lamina propria; and lamina muscularis. Of the three, the epithelium is easily the most prominent, nearly 0.5 mm thick in the dog and greater than that in domestic herbivores. In carnivores and some herbivores such as pigs, the prominent epithelium is nonkeratinized (Figure 14-18). However, ruminant species and to a lesser extent horses possess keratinized epithelia. The connective tissue beneath the epithelium that forms the lamina propria consists of numerous tightly interwoven collagen and elastic fibers of relatively small size, which, in turn, is lined by a thin layer of smooth muscle that forms the lamina muscularis (Figure 14-19). The lamina muscularis consists of longitudinally oriented small bundles of smooth muscle that become confluent caudally. In the dog, this component of the mucosa is absent. At the pharyngoesophageal junction, coordinated activities of skeletal and smooth muscle allow food to move into

the esophagus, passing through a **pharyngoesophageal sphincter** (upper esophageal sphincter).

The submucosa houses the seromucous glands of the esophagus, the **esophageal glands proper,** among an extracellular matrix that differs little from the lamina propria. The esophageal glands may be present throughout the length of the esophagus as in the dog or restricted in location, such as in the pig, where they are found cranially. The glands can appear largely mucous, having serous-secreting cells restricted to demilunes that line the mucus cells (Figure 14-20). In addition to the glands, the major supporting vessels (i.e., arteries, veins, and lymph vessels) and nerves of the esophagus are located in the submucosa.

The tunica muscularis is composed of two layers: an inner circular bundle and an outer longitudinal one. In many species, the two layers cranially consist of skeletal muscle that caudally is replaced by smooth muscle. In the porcine esophagus both types of muscle occur within the middle third or so of its length (Figure 14-21). By comparison, in the horse and the cat the transition area where skeletal muscle is replaced by smooth is located toward the caudal end of the esophagus. In dogs and ruminants the skeletal muscle is never replaced by smooth muscle. In the regions where smooth muscle exists, parasympathetic

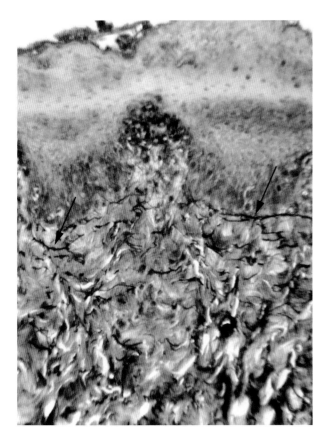

Figure 14-19. Light micrograph of the connective tissue of the mucosal-submucosal portion of the porcine esophagus. Arrows point to the elastic fibers that occur extensively in this area. (Elastin [Verhoeff] stain; ×100.)

nerve plexi, **Auerbach's myenteric plexi,** lie intermittently between the two layers. In each species as the tunica muscularis approaches the opening to the stomach, the inner circular layer broadens into the **cardiac sphincter muscle** (lower esophageal sphincter).

The outermost portion of the esophagus is lined by a tunica serosa for much of its length, especially the thoracic portion, where it is lined by the mediastinal pleura. Cranially, the tunica muscularis of the esophagus is covered by adventitia. In some domestic animals, the caudal or abdominal portion also has a serosal lining—the visceral peritoneum—as in cats, dogs, and horses. In others, including ruminants, the junction of the esophagus and the stomach is very close to the diaphragm and the abdominal portion lacks a serosa.

STOMACH

As a portion of the alimentary canal, the **stomach** is its widest or most dilated segment, allowing for a considerable volume of food substances to be held while being broken down to digestible components by gastric juice and peristalsis for further absorption, particularly within the intestines. The gastric juice is a viscous, acidic substance called **chyme,** rich in enzymes and hydrochloric acid. The four tunics previously described in the esophagus occur in the stomach, each contributing to the digestive roles that this organ plays. The tunics of the stomach vary quite

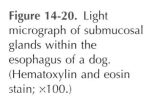

Figure 14-20. Light micrograph of submucosal glands within the esophagus of a dog. (Hematoxylin and eosin stain; ×100.)

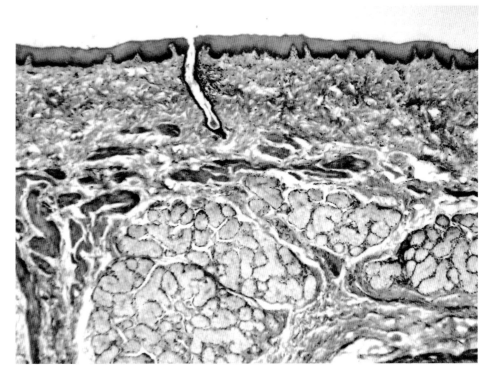

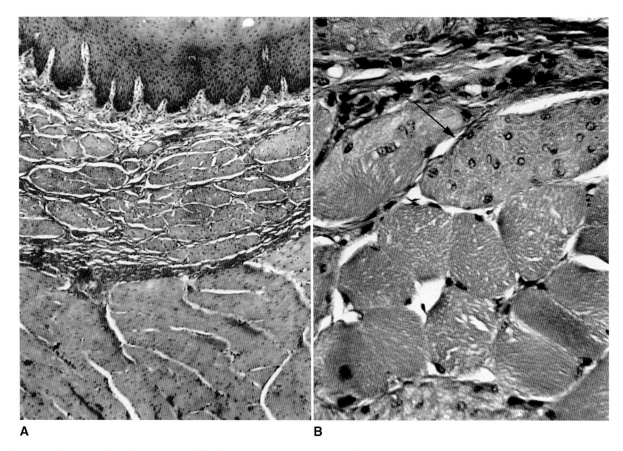

A   B

Figure 14-21. A, Light micrograph (×25) of the tunica muscularis within the esophagus of a pig. **B,** Within the caudal half, the skeletal muscle fibers are replaced by smooth muscle *(arrow)*. (Hematoxylin and eosin stain; ×250.)

a bit in their development, not only between species but also within different areas of the stomach.

The mucosa can be either entirely glandular as in carnivores or partially glandular as in herbivores. The epithelial lining in glandular mucosae lines **gastric folds,** which are numerous and prominent in height of stomachs that have emptied (Figure 14-22). As food is ingested these folds become flattened. Small infoldings or pits, **gastric pits,** are confluent with subtending glands, the **gastric glands.** Although the glandular mucosa has this arrangement of folds, pits, and glands, this tunic is histologically diverse with regard to the types of glands that are present and consequently is divided into three regions: **cardiac, fundic,** and **pyloric** (Figure 14-23).

Cardiac Gland Region

In stomachs entirely lined by glandular mucosae, the cardiac region is a narrow zone at the gastroesophageal junction. The only exception among domestic animals can be found in the pig, which has a considerably large cardiac region, comprising nearly half of the stomach's internal surface (see Figure 14-23). In most species

within this region, the stratified squamous epithelium that has continuously lined the esophagus is transformed into a columnar epithelium. At the base of the gastric pits, which are short compared with other regions of the stomach's mucosa, are branched, tubular, and coiled glands **(cardiac glands)** that release mucus-rich secretions, which then pass into the necks of each gland before entering the pit (Figure 14-24). Most of the secretory cells are mucus producing and cuboidal, especially toward the neck, but can become more columnar appearing toward the base of the gland.

Fundic Gland Region

This region of the gastric mucosa is generally more developed than the cardiac gland region, occupying between one quarter (pig) to half (carnivores) of the mucosal portion of the stomach (see Figure 14-23). The glands in this region, which are called the **proper gastric glands,** are numerous and crowded, reducing considerably the volume of connective tissue within the lamina propria. The glands are similar to that of the cardiac region in that they are tubular and

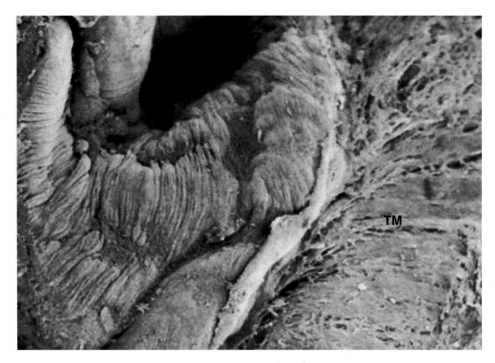

Figure 14-22. Scanning electron micrograph (×5) of the stomach (pyloric region) of a dog reveals the presence of the gastric folds and well-developed muscular tunic *(TM)*.

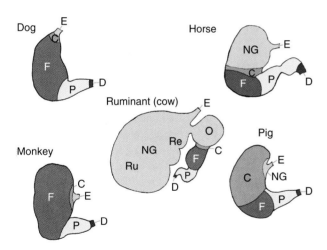

Figure 14-23. Diagram of the different mucosal regions among domestic species. *C,* Cardiac; *D,* duodenum; *E,* esophagus; *F,* fundic; *NG,* nonglandular; *O,* osmasum; *P,* pyloric; *Re,* reticulum; *Ru,* rumen.

branched but longer and straighter (Figure 14-25). The neck of each gland empties into a gastric pit. The cells of the neck portion are mucus secreting, as are the surface cells, and consequently are referred to as **mucous neck cells.** The surface cells including those lining the gastric pits are more columnar than the mucous neck cells (Figure 14-26). The surface cells

and mucous neck cells produce a protective layer of mucin that lines the internal surface of the stomach and may reduce autodigestive activities from injuring the gastric mucosa. Among the cells that continue from the gastric pits into the mucous neck cells are scattered stem cells **(regenerative cells)** that replace cells of the surface and proper gastric glands (see Figure 14-26). These cells contain fewer organelles than occur in the rest of epithelial cells in this region, and lack secretory vesicles. Gastric epithelial cells typically have a life span of 3 days after cell replication. One of the newly formed cells migrates either toward the surface or into the gastric gland to replace one of several cell types.

In addition to the mucous neck cells, the proper gastric glands are composed of three other cell types: parietal cells, chief cells, and enteroendocrine cells.

Parietal Cells

The parietal cell is the largest, somewhat pyramidally shaped, and located along the upper half of a gland (Figure 14-27; see also Figure 14-26). Parietal cells are larger than the other principal cell of the proper gastric gland, the chief cell, and produce hydrochloric acid and, except in cats and dogs, gastric intrinsic factor. The apical margin of this cell can be highly involuted, forming deep canaliculi that are lined by microvilli. The depth of these canaliculi can extend

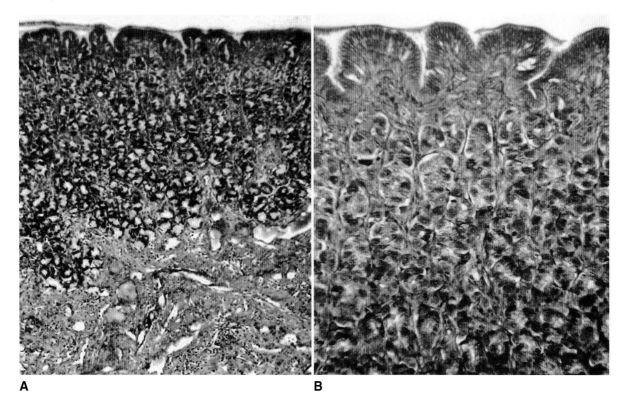

Figure 14-24. A, Light micrograph of the cardiac gastric gland region in a cat's stomach. (Hematoxylin and eosin [H&E] stain; ×15.) **B,** Apical portion of the cardiac region. (H&E stain; ×100.)

down to the level of the nucleus, which is round and centrally placed (Figure 14-28). Numerous eosinophilic vesicles, round and tubular, and mitochondria lie inside the apical cell membrane, giving the cell's cytoplasm a distinctly granulated appearance. The formation of the hydrochloric acid occurs actually outside the cell within the canaliculi. Carbonic acid is initially made by the enzyme, carbonic anhydrase, within the parietal cell. During this process hydrogen ions are actively transported by an H+, K+ ATPase pump out of the cell and into the intracellular canaliculi to combine with Cl⁻. In this manner, free hydrochloric acid is generated by the parietal cell and will move to the gastric lumen. The vesicles associated with these cells are believed to be involved in hydrochloric acid (HCl) production with regard to the generation of new microvilli with the active pump in place.

Chief Cells

Much of the rest of the gland is composed of **chief cells.** The chief cell is the most common cell type of proper gastric glands of domestic species, forming most of their lower halves. Their pyramidal/cuboidal shape is similar to that of the parietal cell, but smaller than

the latter. These cells contain numerous secretory granules that are positioned apically for their release and give this area of the cytoplasm a foamy appearance in traditional histological preparations (see Figures 14-26 and 14-27). The granules arise from an extensive rough endoplasmic reticulum and Golgi apparatus that surround the basally located round nucleus and cause this portion of the cytoplasm to react basophilically. When seen ultrastructurally, these secretory bodies can be easily distinguished from the rough endoplasmic reticulum and Golgi apparatus that give rise to them (Figure 14-29). The secretory granules contain the proenzyme **pepsinogen.** When the pepsinogen is exocytosed into the gland's lumen, it is converted into pepsin by HCl that has been also formed recently within the lumen. Pepsinogen release can be triggered by either neural stimulation via the vagus nerve or hormonally induced by the receptor binding of **secretin** at the base of the cell along the cell membrane. The secretory granules have been referred to previously as **zymogen granules,** and these cells have been called **zymogen cells.** If not preserved appropriately, the zymogen/secretory granules of the chief cells will appear vacuolar rather than granular, giving that part of the cell a foamy appearance.

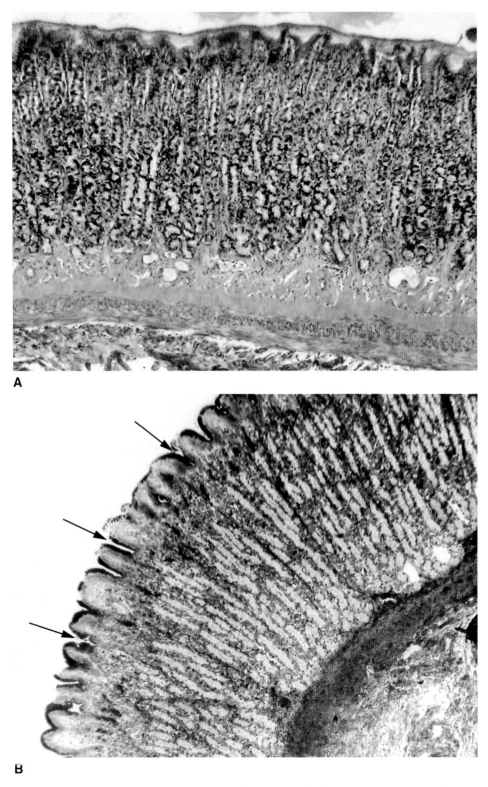

A

B

Figure 14-25. A, Light micrograph of the mucosa of the fundic gastric gland region in a cat's stomach. (Hematoxylin and eosin stain; ×15.) **B,** Light micrograph of the mucosa of the fundic region in a pig's stomach. Arrows point to gastric pits. (Plastic section, toluidine blue stain; ×20.)

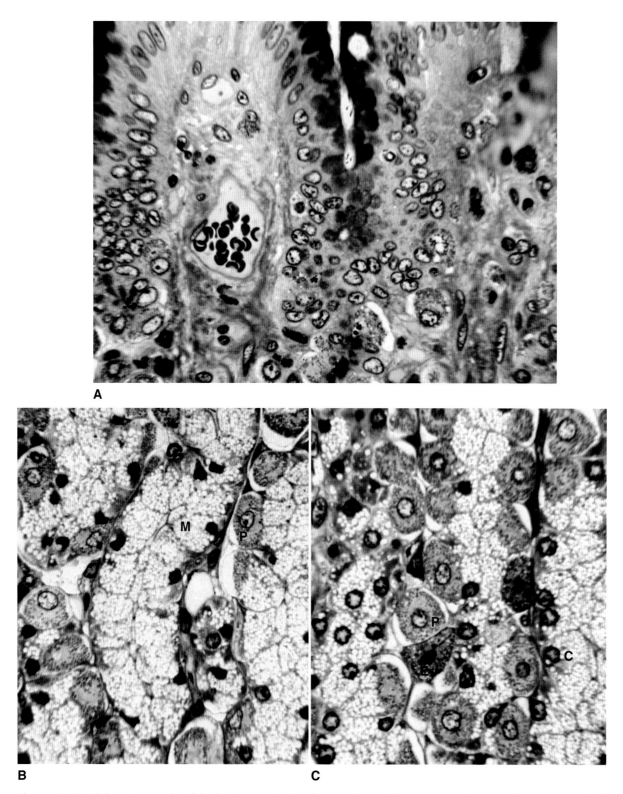

A

B

C

Figure 14-26. Light micrographs of the fundic gastric gland region in a pig's stomach. **A,** Portion of a gastric pit leading to the neck of the gastric gland. **B,** Apical portion of the gastric glands with numerous mucous *(M)* neck cells and parietal *(P)* cells. **C,** Basal portion of the gastric glands with chief *(C)* cells, parietal *(P)* cells, and occasional endocrine *(E)* cells. (Plastic section, toluidine blue stain; ×250.)

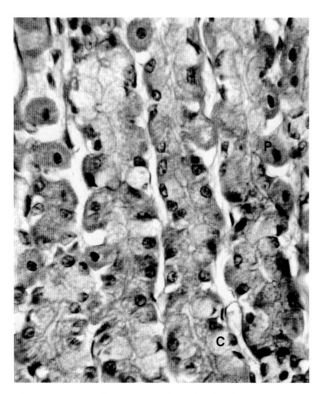

Figure 14-27. Light micrograph of the fundic gastric gland region in a cat's stomach with mostly chief *(C)* cells and parietal *(P)* cells. (Hematoxylin and eosin stain; ×250.)

Enteroendocrine Cell

The fourth and least common type of cell to compose the proper gastric glands is the **endocrine cell** or **enteroendocrine cell.** This cell type receives its name because it is housed in the alimentary or "enteric" canal and secretes hormones that enter adjoining blood and lymph vessels and can be spread systemically, an endocrine effect. These cells may also act upon other cells of the alimentary system because they are diffusely dispersed in a particular area—paracrine effect. The endocrine cell type actually consists of a group of small cells that are scattered throughout the epithelia of the gastric mucosae and are representatives of the **diffuse neuroendocrine system** (DNES). Some of these cells are involved in amine precursor uptake and decarboxylation and can be referred to as **amine precursor uptake and decarboxylation** (APUD) cells as well. The endocrine cells react with silver-bearing stains and for that reason are called **argentaffin** or **argyrophilic cells.** When trying to reveal their presence, the use of a silver treatment is preferred because these cells have a tendency to react inadequately to the traditional hematoxylin and eosin stain. The endocrine cells manufacture a variety of gastrointestinal hormones, which in the stomach include gastrin, glucagon (enteroglucagon), histamine, serotonin, and somatostatin. Most of the cells lie inside the basement membrane of the gland but do not reach its luminal surface. Some, however, do appear to have luminal contact and most likely respond directly to specific substances within the lumen. At least a dozen types of endocrine cells are known to exist, and for the most part, each has granules of a distinct size and is able to produce a single kind of hormone (Figure 14-30).

Pyloric Gland Region

Moving caudally from the cardiac gland region, ingested food materials within the stomach come into contact with the pyloric gland region, which can be considerable in area in the dog and cat or only a relatively small portion of the equine, porcine, and ruminant stomachs (see Figure 14-23). The pyloric glands are short, and more reminiscent of those seen in the cardiac gland region than the fundus gland region (Figure 14-31) of the stomach in domestic animals (Figure 14-32). The glands, which are simple, branched, coiled, and tubular, empty into the base of deep gastric pits. The cells of these glands are mucus secreting, filled with their stored, carbohydrate-rich product and causing the basally located nuclei to appear frequently more flattened than round.

Tunicae Submucosa and Muscularis Gastric Motility and Emptying of Contents

Although the mucosal portion of the stomach varies in the development of its glands, both with regard to form and location, the adjacent submucosa and muscularis tunics are less distinguishable when comparing one area of the stomach with another, being harmonious and confluent in their activities. The submucosa lies externally to the lamina muscularis mucosae of the stomach, which can be prominent, with smooth muscle cells organized into inner circular and outer longitudinal layers and occasionally a third, outermost longitudinal layer (see Figure 14-24). The submucosa consists of a dense, irregular connective tissue well infiltrated with blood and lymphatic vessels and nerves that serve the mucosa. Immediately outside the submucosa is a well-developed tunica muscularis, which can stay in motion even when emptied (see Figure 14-31). The tunica muscularis or **muscularis externa** has two or three layers of smooth muscle that embrace the submucosa and mucosa. The smooth muscle is oriented to form an inner longitudinal to helical layer, an outer or middle circular layer that can be more pronounced in the pyloric region where it

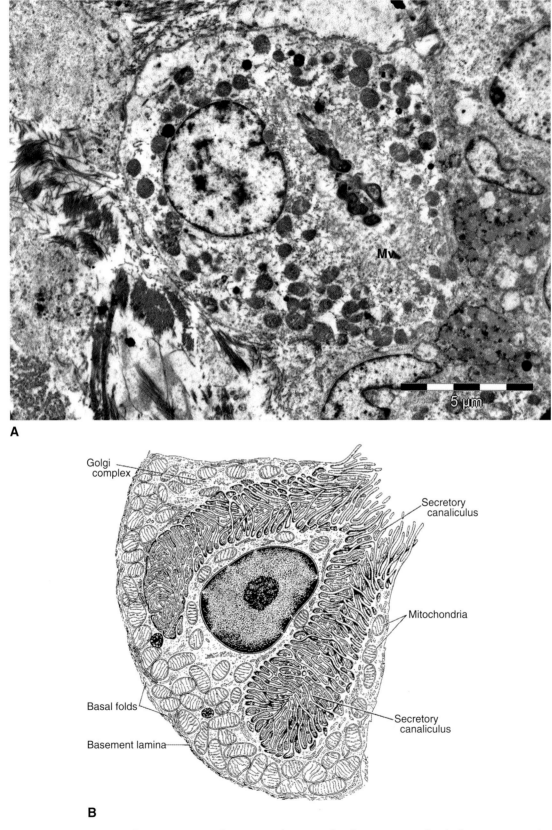

A

B

Figure 14-28. A, Transmission electron micrograph (×5000) of a parietal cell in a gastric gland of a pig's stomach. Microvilli *(Mv)* seen deep within the body of the cell represent extended intracellular canaliculi that are associated with the secretion of hydrochloric acid. **B,** Ultrastructurally based illustration of a parietal cell reveals depth of secretory canaliculi. *(From Fawcett DW:* Bloom and Fawcett: a textbook of histology, *ed 11, Philadelphia, 1986, Saunders.)*

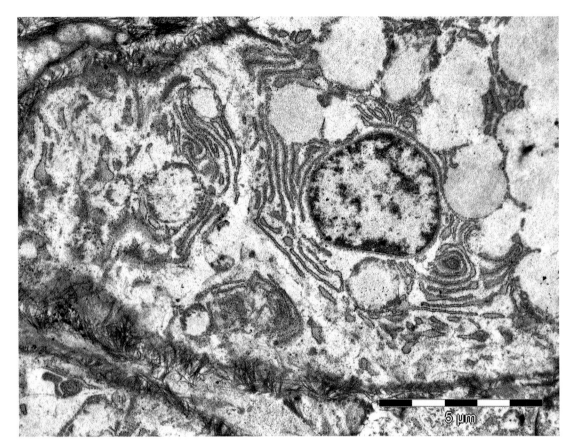

Figure 14-29. Transmission electron micrograph (×5000) of a chief cell in a gastric gland of a pig's stomach. Well-developed rough endoplasmic reticulum occupies much of the base of the cell; the apex is filled with secretory granules.

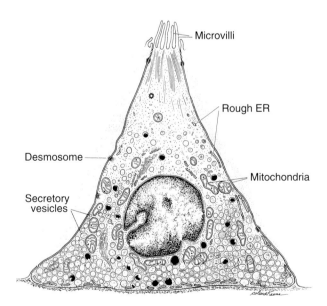

Figure 14-30. Diagram of an endocrine cell within the proper gastric glands of the stomach. *ER,* Endoplasmic reticulum. *(Modified from Fawcett DW:* Bloom and Fawcett: a textbook of histology, *ed 11, Philadelphia, 1986, Saunders.)*

thickens into the pyloric sphincter, and a variably developed outermost longitudinal layer. In addition a third layer may lie internal to the circular layer, arranged helically rather than longitudinally or circularly.

Whereas the musculature of the stomach remains active in its ability to contract, intensity of contraction can vary according to filling and emptying of this organ. In the dog when ingested materials enter the stomach, the musculature initially relaxes before gradual waves of peristaltic contraction occur, principally within the longitudinal layer of the fundic gland region, propelling food caudally. As the peristalsis continues, the most liquid portion of the ingesta is moved into the pyloric region and is propulsed or squirted into the anterior-most region of the small intestine, the duodenum. The circular layer of muscle within the externa muscularis of the pylorus broadens into the **pyloric sphincter muscle,** which causes the submucosa and mucosa to protrude into the lumen of the pylorus and assists in keeping the more solid food from entering the small intestine as long as possible, repulsing particles greater than 2 mm in diameter.

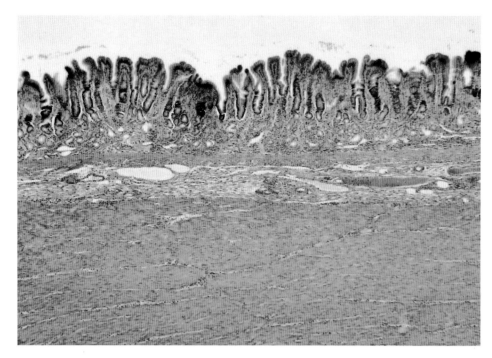

Figure 14-31. Light micrograph of the fundic gastric gland region in a dog's stomach. (Hematoxylin and eosin stain; ×15.)

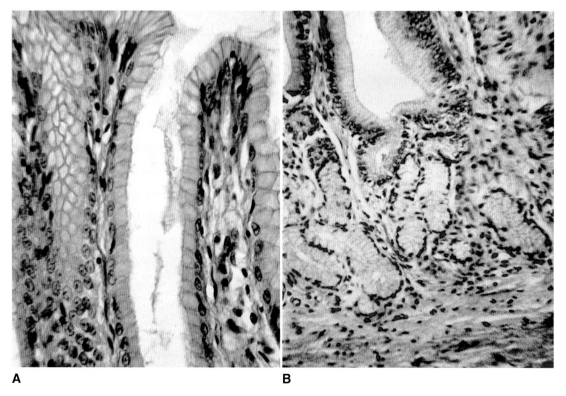

A   B

Figure 14-32. A, Light micrograph (×250) of the gastric pit within the pyloric gland region of the feline stomach. **B,** Light micrograph (×100) of the mucus-secreting pyloric glands in the canine stomach. (Hematoxylin and eosin stain.)

RUMINANT STOMACH (COMPOUND STOMACH)

The stomachs that are formed in ruminant species share some of the basic construction of other domestic animals, especially their posterior portions, which include cardiac, fundic and pyloric gland regions. However, these regions—collectively referred to as the **abomasum**—contribute only to a small portion of the ruminant stomach. The abomasum, which is the posterior-most portion of the ruminant stomach, is connected contiguously with three other chamber-like portions—**rumen, reticulum,** and **omasum**—that along with the abomasum form the compound stomach (see Figure 14-23).

The rumen, reticulum, and omasum originate from the esophageal region of the stomach and are referred to together as the **proventriculus** (forestomach). The proventriculus effectively facilitates the breakdown of the fibrous ingesta being ingested by this group of herbivores. It is essentially aglandular, consisting of tissues that allow ingesta to be further macerated by mechanical and chemical means.

Rumen

The proventriculus's largest chamber is the rumen, also known as the **paunch;** it is lined by keratinized stratified squamous epithelia that follow numerous mucosal papillae projecting into the lumen (Figure 14-33). The papillae can vary in size and shape, from tongue shaped to conical. In addition to lacking glands, the lamina propria is not subtended by a muscular layer, but instead blends with the submucosa, forming a lamina propria-submucosa, a partially condensed loose connective tissue that also lacks lymph nodules (Figure 14-34).

The cornified mucosal epithelium offers physical protection against potentially sharp fibers that an individual animal has consumed. Concomitantly, this epithelium facilitates volatile fatty acids to be metabolized and various metabolites (sodium and potassium ions, ammonia, etc.) to be absorbed. In effect, the mucosal epithelium provides the ideal lining to house a blend of suitable bacteria and protozoa that essentially ferment the ingested plant food. The fermentation process is responsible for the formation of the volatile fatty acids and other substances to be either metabolized or absorbed in the proventriculus. A byproduct of the anaerobic fermentation process is methane and carbon dioxide, which, as gases, have to be continuously expelled from the rumen by **eructation contractions.** These contractions allow the gases to move back through the esophagus into the lungs via the pharynx, where they are expelled during

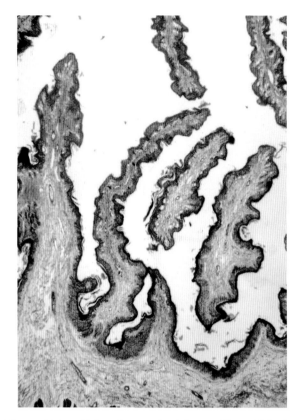

Figure 14-33. Light micrograph of the papillae within the bovine rumen. (Hematoxylin and eosin stain; ×15.)

normal expiration. The volatile fatty acids **(VFAs)** produced during fermentation include acetic, propionic, and butyric acids, consisting of approximately 60%, 25%, and 15%, respectively, of the VFAs absorbed by the proventriculus.

The tunica muscularis, which is composed of well-developed inner circular and outer longitudinal layers of smooth muscle, is responsible not only for the mechanical mixing of ingesta and the removal of gas through eructation contractions, but also regurgitation. After plant materials have been chewed, swallowed, and held in the proventriculus for a period of time, reverse peristalsis moves the partially digested food back to the oral cavity, where it can be masticated further and swallowed again.

Reticulum

The reticulum is a continuation of the rumen, similar both in structure and function. The principal morphological difference between the two portions of the proventriculus is the presence of mucosal primary folds, also referred to as **reticular crests** (Figure 14-35). As these crests project vertically into the lumen of the proventriculus, they fuse or anastomose with

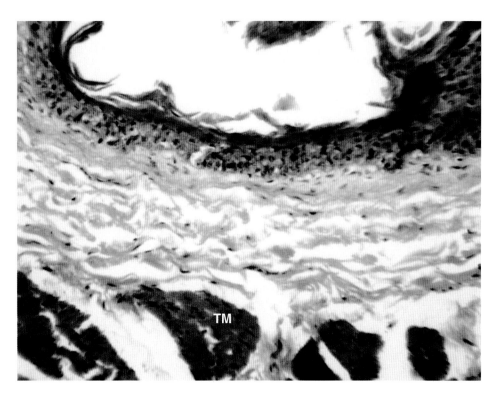

Figure 14-34. Light micrograph of the lamina propria-submucosa within the rumen portion of the bovine stomach. *TM,* tunica muscularis. (Hematoxylin and eosin stain; ×100.)

one another in a symmetrical manner, forming honeycomb-like ridges that give this portion a reticulate appearance. Apically within these primary crests or folds, is a lamina muscularis mucosae, which when contracted can reduce the heights of these crests (Figure 14-36). The smooth muscle within the primary crests remains essentially continuous throughout the reticulum and cranially is confluent with the lamina muscularis of the esophagus.

Secondary crests, which are shorter, can extend from the sides of the primary crests (see Figure 14-35). In addition, papillae, which can vary in size, can arise between the crests as well as extend from them. Except for the lamina muscularis within the primary crests, the lamina propria merges with the submucosa.

In addition to the reticular crests is the **reticular sulcus,** a groove that occurs ventrally along the medial wall of the reticulum. The groove is lined by broad extensions of the mucosa and submucosa that form folds or labia.

Omasum

Within this portion of the proventriculus, the internal surface has developed into numerous folds, or **laminae,** that are oriented along the longitudinal plane. The laminae, which can number up to roughly

100, project into the lumen mostly from the greater curvature of this portion of the proventriculus and consist of several orders. The first order is the largest and runs the greatest length within the omasum; the remaining orders (second, third, fourth, etc.) are respectively shorter and thinner (Figure 14-37). Along each lamina numerous papillae extend into the lumen, reducing the space for ingesta to fill.

As in the rumen and reticulum, the mucosal epithelium is cornified. However, the lamina propria mucosae is thinner and less developed than that of the rumen and reticulum; it is externally lined by a prominent lamina muscularis mucosae that extends into each omasal fold (Figure 14-38). This layer of smooth muscle is further bounded by internal extensions of the tunica muscularis, specifically extensions of its inner circular layer. The addition of the tunica muscularis within these folds occurs within the largest laminae (those of the first three orders). The submucosa that separates the lamina muscularis mucosae from the tunica muscularis is little developed.

As a result of the additional muscle, both from the mucosa and the tunica muscularis, the omasum is able to break down mechanically the fibrous diet very effectively. Collectively, the omasal laminae facilitate the fine maceration of the consumed plant materials. Concomitantly, the overall architecture of the omasal

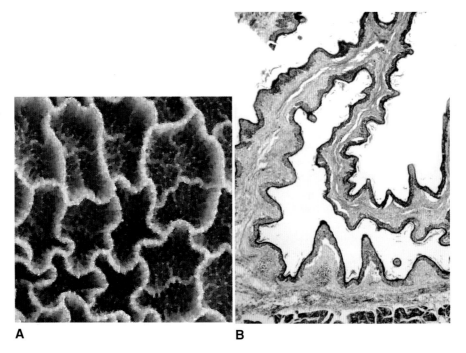

Figure 14-35. A, "Honeycombed" mucosal lining of the reticulum in the ruminant stomach. **B,** Light micrograph of the individual reticular crests in this portion of the bovine stomach, with numerous papillae. (Hematoxylin and eosin stain; ×15.)

A   B

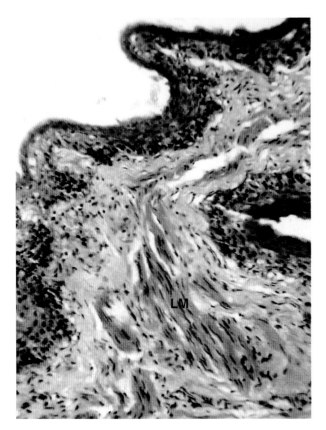

Figure 14-36. Light micrograph of a reticular crest with the presence of the lamina muscularis *(LM)* mucosae. (Hematoxylin and eosin stain; ×100.)

laminae and associated papillae direct the ground ingesta to abomasum through the interconnecting ostium.

Abomasum

The abomasum represents the glandular portion of the ruminant stomach, which is essentially identical to that previously described for the glandular portions of the stomachs of nonruminant domestic species.

SMALL INTESTINE

Throughout the digestive system, the ingesta has been mostly involved in the process of breaking down. Although this process continues in the small intestine, useful ingesta is absorbed here as well. To that end, the small intestine has features that enhance food digestion and absorption, such as its **extended length** and the presence of mucosal **plicae** and **villi.** All these modifications plus the development of **microvilli** along the apical surface of the luminal cells are designed to greatly expand the surface area for absorption (Figure 14-39).

Lengths of the small intestine vary according to the overall body size of the animal—in the dog roughly 3 to 3½ times longer than its body length and 5 times or greater in body length in the horse. The mucosal folds or plicae (also called the **plicae circulares**), are prominent semicircular extensions that

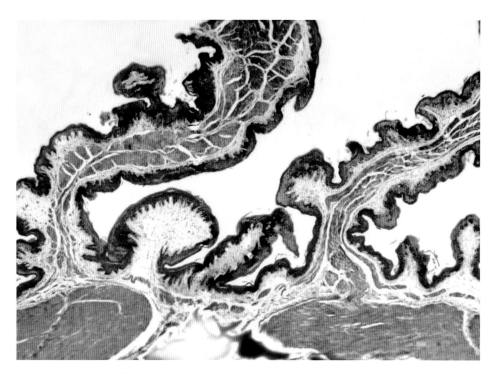

Figure 14-37. Light micrograph of different-sized laminae within the omasum of a cow. (Hematoxylin and eosin stain; ×20.)

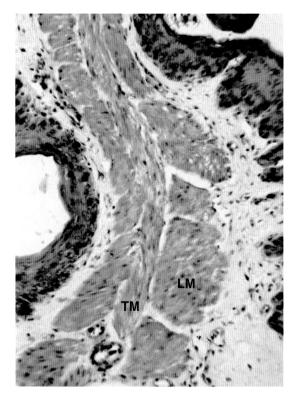

Figure 14-38. Light micrograph of the lamina muscularis *(LM)* mucosae and tunica muscularis *(TM)* within a large omasal fold of the bovine stomach. (Hematoxylin and eosin stain; ×100.)

project into the lumen and as a result more than double the surface area of the epithelial lining. In ruminant digestive systems, the plicae remain present, regardless of the amount of ingesta passing through, whereas in other domestic mammals they become stretched and difficult to observe in the presence of ingesta. Along the entire inner mucosa, extensions smaller than the plicae project into the lumen, forming the villi. The villi tend to be more developed within the proximal portion (the duodenum) than those located distally (the ileum) (Figure 14-40). Within a specific portion of the small intestine the shape of the villi among mammals can vary: short and conical in rodents, short and wide in ruminants, and long and fingerlike, anastomosing along their basal halves in primates and to a lesser extent in carnivores (Figure 14-41). Each villus has a core of lamina propria, consisting of capillary loops, lymphatic channels that end blindly, loose connective tissue with plasma cells and lymphocytes, corresponding extracellular matrix (ECM), and a line of smooth muscle fibers that extends its vertical length (Figure 14-42). The presence of villi easily increases the surface area by 10 times or more. In addition to the plicae and the villi, most of the cells that form the mucosal epithelium possess the peglike microvilli, cellular modifications that can increase further the surface area another 20 to 40 times or more (see Figure 14-39).

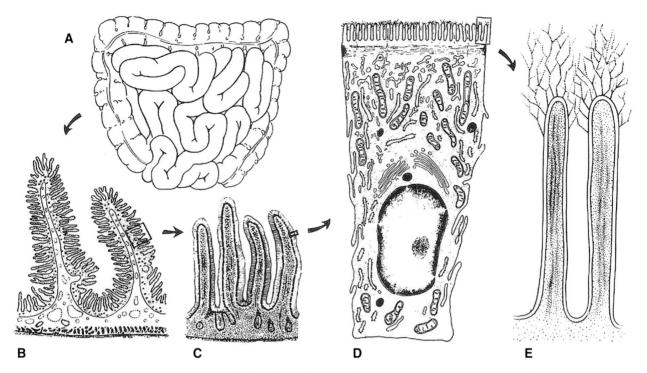

Figure 14-39. Diagram of the greatly amplified surface of the small intestinal mucosa beginning with the extended length of the small intestine *(A)* with regular large infoldings, plicae *(B)* lined by further variably shaped projections, and villi *(C)* that, in turn, are lined by microvilli along the epithelial surface *(D)*, which are coated with an extensive glycocalyx *(E)*. *(Modified from Fawcett DW:* Bloom and Fawcett: a textbook of histology, *ed 11, Philadelphia, 1986, Saunders.)*

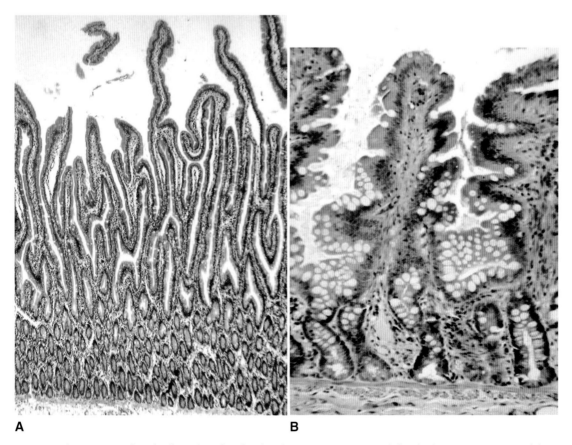

Figure 14-40. Light micrographs of villi within the duodenal portion (**A,** ×25) and the ileal portion (**B,** ×60) of the monkey small intestine. (Hematoxylin and eosin stain.)

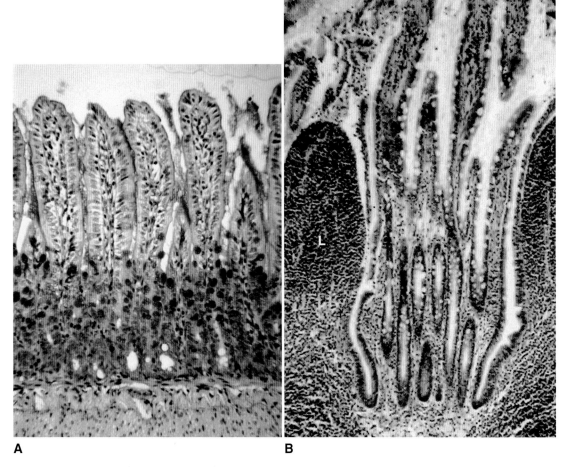

A   **B**

Figure 14-41. Light micrographs of the villi within the ileum of a rat intestine (**A,** periodic acid–Schiff [PAS] stain; ×100) and that of a cat along with raised lymph nodules *(L)* (**B,** hematoxylin and eosin stain; ×40). The PAS stain reveals the increased presence of goblet cells in this region.

Although the absorbing cells are able to provide some digestive materials (mostly enzymes) that enhance absorption, additional sources for enzymatic digestion occur along the small intestine. These consist of embedded, submucosal simple glands located efficiently between the plicae and villi, and the largest individual contributor for intestinal digestion, the pancreas, which is even more efficiently located, being entirely sequestered from the small intestine and connected only by a principal duct and an accessory duct.

The small intestine is divided into three regions: the **duodenum,** the **jejunum,** and the **ileum.** These regions share numerous common histological features throughout each of their four tunics. The anatomical differences that occur among the regions are discussed separately for each region.

Tunica Mucosa

The mucosal portion of the small intestine consists of the traditional three laminae: the epithelium, the lamina propria, and the lamina muscularis. The epithelium is simple columnar in type, lining villar and intervillar surfaces, with four cell types associated with it.

1. The primary cell is the **absorptive cell** or **enterocyte,** which in most species possesses the classic columnar shape (Figure 14-43). Absorptive cells easily form the largest cell population of the mucosal epithelium, each having an oval nucleus that is usually positioned basally within the cell and surrounded partially by mitochondria, free ribosomes, and rough endoplasmic reticulum (rER). Apically this cell forms numerous microvilli and a well-developed junctional complex, which together are associated with a highly developed cytoskeletal region known as the terminal web (see Figure 3-20). Light microscopically these modifications comprise the **striated border** (brush border) and the **terminal bar** (see Figure 14-43). The microvilli form an extensive glycocalyx, sometimes called the "fuzzy

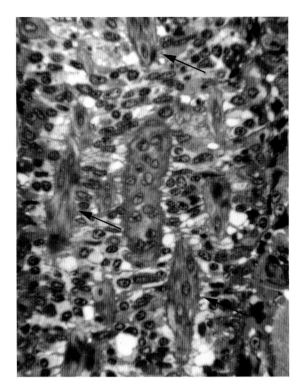

Figure 14-42. Light micrograph of the strands of smooth muscle *(arrows)* that compose the lamina muscularis mucosae within a villus of the small intestine of a pig. (Plastic section, toluidine blue stain; ×250.)

coat," which minimizes potential microbial invasion along this amplified surface of the cell, protects the expanded cell membrane from possible autodigestive injury, and offers a location for certain enzymatic elements and carrier proteins. Beneath the terminal web the absorptive cell possesses an extensive smooth endoplasmic reticulum (sER), which is involved in triglyceride synthesis and fat metabolism by reesterifying fatty acids into triglycerides and packaging emulsified fats into chylomicrons that then are released basally into the adjacent capillary bed.

2. The next most common cell of the epithelium that lines the small intestine is the **goblet cell.** Intermittently scattered between the absorptive cells, their density gradually increases toward the large intestine (see Figure 14-41). Although their heights exceeds their widths, these secretory cells become round as their cytoplasm becomes filled with **mucigen** (see Figure 4-2). When mucigen is released as mucin into the intestinal lumen, it becomes hydrated and better known as **mucus.** Mucus protects the mucosal epithelium as a whole and facilitates the movement of nonabsorbed ingesta and excrement toward the rectum and anus.

3. Another cell type that comprises the epithelium is the **enteroendocrine cell** (see Figure 14-30). Although not nearly as common as the absorptive and goblet cells, this cell is still nonetheless present, producing paracrine and endocrine hormones in a comparable manner as described previously for the proper gastric glands of the fundic gland region of the stomach.

4. The fourth cell type associated with the mucosal epithelium is called the **M cell (microfold cell),** with microfolds (microplicae) that project luminally from its apical surface (Figure 14-44). These cells, which are believed to be a part of the mononuclear phagocyte system, most likely are able to sample materials, including potential antigens, within the intestinal lumen and transport antigens directly to nearby lymphocytes. They can be flattened or squamous in appearance when apically lining lymph nodules that lie between villi.

The newest cells of the mucosal epithelium are formed at the base of the villi. Consequently, older cells are pushed to the tip of each villus where they are eventually shed by mechanical abrasion.

Between the base of adjacent villi the epithelium invaginates into the adjacent lamina propria, forming simple tubular glands, the **intestinal crypts** (crypts of Lieberkühn) (Figure 14-45). Like the epithelium, these glands are composed of a variety of cells. The upper half of each gland is lined by absorptive and goblet cells. The goblet cells in this portion are short lived, dying soon after releasing its contents. The absorptive cells continue to be pushed to the luminal surface and progress their way to the tips of the villi. The replenishment of the absorptive and goblet cells is provided by the continual proliferation of the **regenerative cells,** which are a part of the intestinal crypts as well, but lie more within the lower halves of the glands than in the upper halves. These cells represent the major stem cell for the intestinal mucosa and appear as narrow cells with oval, euchromatic nuclei. Toward the bottom of each crypt may be a fourth population of cells, the **acidophilic granule cells** (Paneth cells). They are not found in all mammals (absent in carnivores, for example), but are present in rodents, ruminants, equids, and primates (see Figures 14-40 and 14-45). These cells are typically pyramidal and have been shown to have antimicrobial capabilities (Figure 14-46). Much of the apical portion of their cytoplasm is filled with acidophilic granules that arise from a well-developed Golgi apparatus and rER.

The rest of the lamina propria of the intestinal mucosa is made up of well-vascularized loose connective tissue that forms the core of each villus and sur-

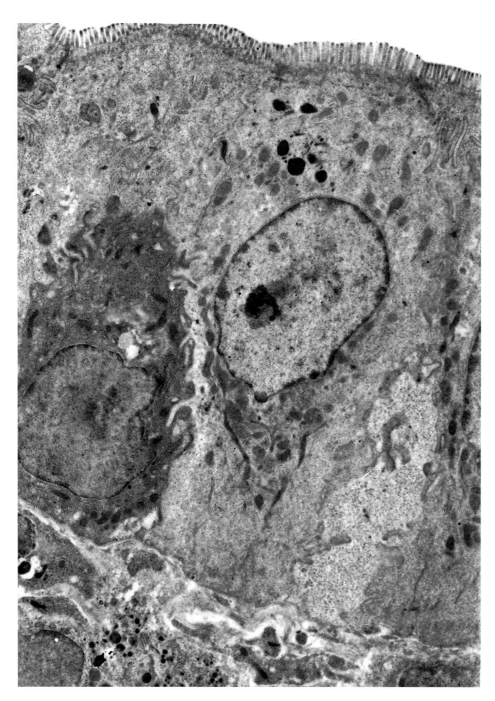

Figure 14-43. Transmission electron micrograph (×5000) of an absorptive cell in the small intestine of a mouse.

rounds each nearby crypt (see Figure 14-45). In addition to the extensive system of blood vessels, numerous cells of defense (plasma cells, lymphocytes, mast cells, and granulocytes) lie freely within the network of reticular fibers (see Figure 5-16). In addition to the blood vessels is also an extensive lymphatic system, consisting of lymph capillaries that empty into the **submucosal lymphatic plexus.** Those capillaries that end blindly near the tip of each villus are the **lacteals.** Eventually, the lymph is directed to the thoracic duct via a series of lymph nodules along the way.

The intestinal mucosa possesses a lamina muscularis that varies in amount regarding region and species. In those areas where it is well formed, the lamina muscularis can consist of two layers (inner circular and outer longitudinal). At the base of the villus, a small extension of the lamina muscularis branches vertically, running the full length of the villar core (see Figure 14-42). The contraction of this smooth muscle helps facilitate the movement of blood and lymph away from the villus after its vessels have become filled during digestion and absorption.

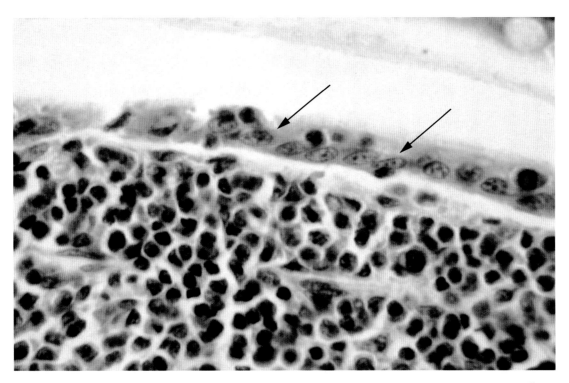

Figure 14-44. Light micrograph of the M cells *(arrows)* that line a lymph nodule within the small intestine of a cat. (Hematoxylin and eosin stain; ×400.)

Tunica Submucosa

This region of the small intestine houses the largest blood and lymph vessels that serve the mucosa. Dense irregular connective tissue is the major type present, and is best developed next to its inner and outer muscular perimeters, which comprise the lamina muscularis mucosae and tunica muscularis, respectively.

As in the mucosa, this region can also contain lymph nodules and glands. The lymph nodules can be few and isolated or clustered **(aggregated lymph nodules, Peyer's patch),** all part of the **gut-associated lymphatic tissue (GALT)** (see Figures 12-20 and 14-41). In response to the antigen-presenting cells, IgA is secreted from the plasma cells that differentiated from B lymphocytes, which had migrated from nearby mesenteric lumph nodes. The **submucosal glands** are branched tubuloalveolar and vary in their secretory content—serous in the porcine and equine intestinal tract, seromucous in the cat, and mucous in the dog and ruminant species (Figure 14-47). Although their amount varies among domestic animals, they tend to be most prominent within the proximal-most portion of the small intestine of smaller domestic species. However, in larger ruminants, pigs, and equids, these glands can exist throughout most of the length of the intestinal submucosa.

In addition to the blood and lymph vessels, lymph nodules, submucosal glands, and dense irregular connective tissue, are intrinsic parasympathetic nerve centers called the **submucosal plexi** that help direct submucosal activity, especially with regard to the glands.

Tunica Muscularis

As in many portions of the digestive system, the tunica muscularis is composed of two major layers of smooth muscle—the inner circular and the outer longitudinal (Figure 14-48). When contracting, this area of the small intestine is responsible for its peristaltic activity. Segmenting contractions of the inner circular muscle result in ringlike constrictions that aid in mixing the ingesta for further digestion and absorption. The actual propulsion of the ingesta farther down the intestinal tract is contributed by segmenting contractions of the outer longitudinal muscle. This contraction at a particular site is then followed by the inner circular layer. The peristaltic contractions move the luminal contents along in phase with slow waves. The slow-wave frequency is governed by the interstitial cells of Cajal, which are fibroblast-like cells located next to the cell bodies of the myenteric plexus and believed to form a gastroenteric pacemaker system. The **myenteric plexus** is located between the

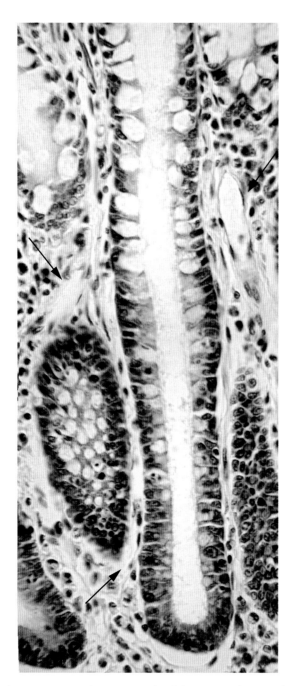

Figure 14-45. Light micrograph of the intestinal crypt of the cat. Arrows point to the network of blood vessels that surround each gland. (Hematoxylin and eosin stain; ×250.)

inner and outer layers of the tunica muscularis and functions to direct the outer longitudinal muscle (Figure 14-49).

Tunica Serosa

Except for areas where the small intestine connects directly with other organs by adventitial tissue, the tunica serosa is coated externally by a thin layer of connective tissue, which, in turn, is lined by a mesothelium (see Figures 3-3 and 14-48).

Duodenum

The initial portion of the small intestine is the duodenum, which of the three portions has generally the largest and most numerous villi. Concomitantly, its crypts are most numerous and best developed. Among domestic mammals, the submucosal glands also occur most frequently in this portion (see Figures 14-40 and 14-47).

Jejunum

The jejunum forms the middle portion of the small intestine, and although it is very similar histologically to the duodenum, it does have subtle differences. The villi are generally smaller and less dense in number when compared with those of the duodenum in the same animal. The submucosal glands are generally much less developed in the jejunum—absent in the dog, but present in the horse.

Ileum

The distal-most portion consists of the ileum, which shares the same basic histological construction as the jejunum, but generally is less developed with regard to the villi and glands and more developed with regard to lymph nodules, which can be larger and more aggregated than in the duodenum and jejunum (see Figures 14-40 and 14-41).

LARGE INTESTINE

The large intestine forms the caudal-most portion of the digestive tract, and beginning with its attachment to the small intestine by the ileocecal junction consists sequentially of the cecum, colon, rectum, and anus (or anal canal). For any particular animal, the microscopic anatomy of the cecum, colon, and rectum is quite similar from one to another. In fact, it is the appearance of the gross anatomy of the large intestine along with associated functional variations that are responsible for its subdivision into the four portions.

Cecum

The cecum forms the beginning of the large intestine and in nonruminant herbivorous mammals is the area within the alimentary canal responsible for the digestion and absorption of plant-rich ingesta. In horses,

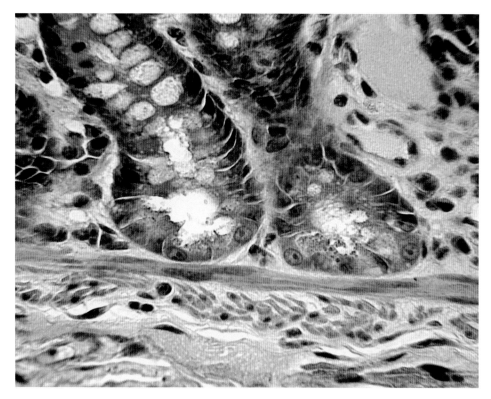

Figure 14-46. Light micrograph of acidophilic granule cells in intestinal crypts of the monkey. (Hematoxylin and eosin stain; ×400.)

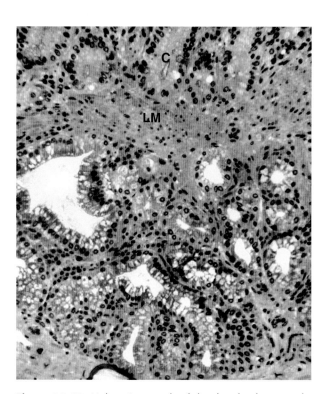

Figure 14-47. Light micrograph of duodenal submucosal glands. *C,* Crypts; *LM,* lamina muscularis mucosae. (Hematoxylin and eosin stain; ×100.)

rabbits, guinea pigs, and the like, the microfauna here as well as in the colon contribute to the fermentation and breakdown of cellulose in much the same way as in the forestomachs of ruminants. In fact, in these domestic animals the cecum is well developed. By comparison, it is less prominent in ruminants and comparatively small in carnivores.

The cecum, as in the entire large intestine, lacks the villar expansion of the mucosa seen previously in the small intestine. Much of the mucosa consists of long, simple unbranched tubular glands (Figure 14-50). Each gland is made up of goblet cells, lacking acidophilic granule cells altogether. The presence of lymphatic tissue is considerable here, with the mucosa and submucosa housing numerous lymph nodules, which tend to be variably concentrated according to the animal. In the dog, pig, and ruminant, the nodules are most conspicuous at the beginning of the cecum; they are more prevalent toward the end of the cecum in the cat and the horse.

Within the tunica muscularis of the horse and the pig, the outer longitudinal muscle forms flattened bundles or fascicles of smooth muscle and elastic fibers called **teniae ceci.** The outermost portion of the tunica muscularis is lined by the serosa, which is indistinguishable from the serosa of the small intestine.

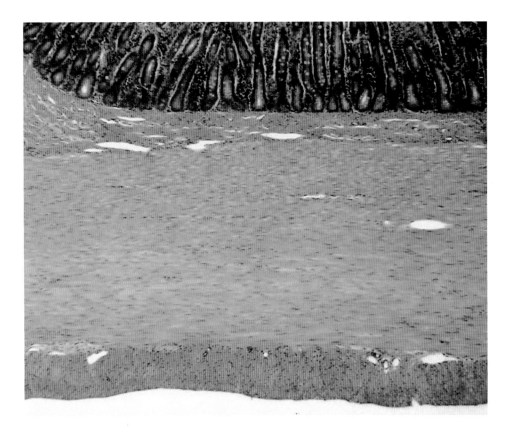

Figure 14-48. Light micrograph of the tunica muscularis of the canine duodenum oriented in cross section. (Hematoxylin and eosin stain; ×25.)

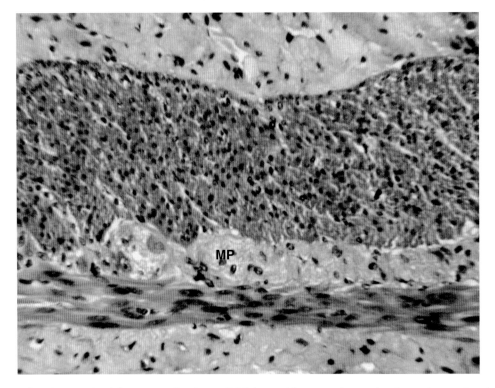

Figure 14-49. Light micrograph of the myenteric plexus *(MP)* located between inner circular and outer longitudinal layers of the tunica muscularis of the canine small intestine. (Hematoxylin and eosin stain; ×100.)

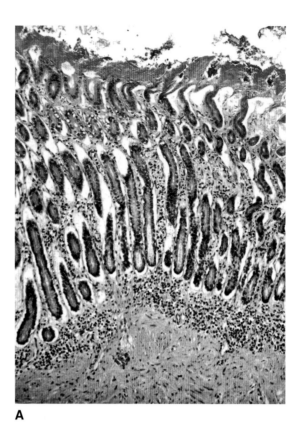

Figure 14-50. A, Light micrograph of the cecum of the manatee. Overall it is similar to those of domestic species but possesses a stratified squamous epithelium along the internal surface. (Hematoxylin and eosin [H&E] stain; ×100.) **B,** Light micrograph of the mucosal portion of the cecum in the pig viewed in cross section reveals the compact arrangement of the intestinal crypts. (H&E stain; ×100.)

A

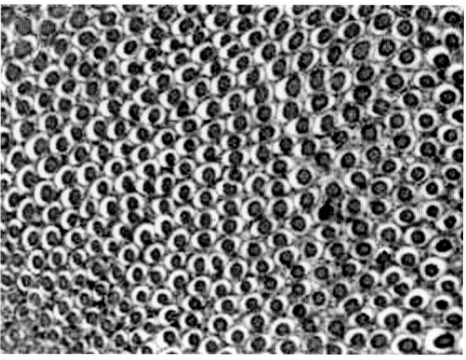

B

Colon

Histological differences between the colon and the cecum are few and subtle. The mucosal surface continues to be smooth, having numerous openings of the simple tubular glands that lie within its lamina propria (Figure 14-51). Within an individual, these glands are generally longer than those of the cecum, containing, as before, numerous mucus secreting cells and occasional enteroendocrine cells. The lamina propria and lamina muscularis of the mucosa and the submucosa are very similar to that of the cecum and that of the small intestine. However, the circular folds (plicae circulares) associated with the small intestine mucosae of different domestic animals do not occur in either the colon or the cecum. The ribbonlike fascicles of smooth muscle in the tunica muscularis of the cecum of the horse and the pig continue within the colon, forming the **teniae coli.**

Overall, the tunica muscularis provides motility for further mixing of the ingesta as well as the propulsion of nondigestible ingesta and excrement to the anus. The activity of the smooth muscle layers is in some ways like that seen in the small intestine, including peristaltic and antiperistaltic movements, but overall more complicated. These slow-wave contractions originate within the midportion of the colon and move cranially toward the cecum. By comparison, the removal of the waste or fecal materials begins cranially or distally, occurring as mass contractile movements that propel the luminal substances toward the anus.

Rectum

The tissue construction of this portion of the large intestine is again very similar to that of the cecum and colon, consisting of a smooth mucosa with numerous simple tubular mucus-secreting glands that possess even more goblet cells than the colon, and a similar tunica submucosa. The tunica muscularis of the rectum is generally more developed than that of the colon, and in the horse and the pig is made up of an intact outer longitudinal layer rather than bundles. As in the colon and the cecum before it, the tunica muscularis of the cranial rectum has a serosal lining. However caudally, the outermost part of the rectum is composed of adventitia.

Anal Canal

The anal canal forms the end of the large intestine as well as the end of the entire digestive tract. It fuses with the rectum, forming a mucocutaneous junction (the rectoanal junction) (Figure 14-52). At this junc-

tion the rectal glands become short and disappear, giving rise to a simple columnar epithelium. As this epithelium extends toward and merges with the epidermis of the surrounding cutaneous tissue, it becomes stratified squamous. The lamina muscularis mucosa disappears as well as the outer longitudinal layer of the tunica muscularis. The inner circular layer of the tunica muscularis, which has enlarged, forms the **inner anal sphincter muscle** and is surrounded by a fibroelastic coat, an extension of the outer longitudinal layer. The inner anal sphincter muscle and its fibroelastic coat are surrounded, in turn, by skeletal muscle, the **outer anal sphincter muscle,** that too is circularly oriented, arising from the pelvic floor.

In most large herbivorous domestic species, the anal canal is short in distance and free of glands. However, in dogs, cats, and pigs, the anal canal is more developed, having glands and associated specific zones. The zone closest to the rectum is the **columnar zone,** consisting of folds **(anal columns),** and intervening grooves that are oriented longitudinally. The columns and grooves end in the **intermediate zone,** which is shorter than the columnar zone. This zone and the columnar zone possess a nonkeratinized stratified squamous epithelium and modified sweat glands (the **anal glands**) that lie within the lamina subtending propria-submucosa. These glands are tubuloalveolar in form and vary in their product: mucus bearing in the pig and lipid rich in the dog and the cat. The intermediate zone fuses with the last portion of the anal canal—the **cutaneous zone**—which has a fully keratinized stratified squamous epithelium.

In the dog and the cat, paired invagination of the mucocutaneous lining between the intermediate and cutaneous zones results in diverticula known as **anal sacs.** Each sac has its own duct that empties its contents into the anal canal (Figure 14-53). Both the sac and the duct are lined by stratified squamous epithelia. In the dog these sacs temporarily hold the secretions of nearby apocrine sweat glands. The anal sacs of the cat store the secretions of apocrine sweat glands and sebaceous glands. In the dog the ducts of the anal sacs can be occluded, which may result in becoming infected if not expressed. The lack of sebum in these sacs in the dog may contribute to their occasional occlusion.

In the dog, within the propria-submucosa of the cutaneous zone are sebaceous-like glands not associated with hair—the **circumanal glands.** These glands, which also occur within the integument of the tail, loin, and prepuce, can be considerable in development. The superficial-most portion is sebaceous, whereas the deepest portion is more endocrine in appearance, consisting of secretory-like cells (a glandular parenchyma) that may have associated ducts,

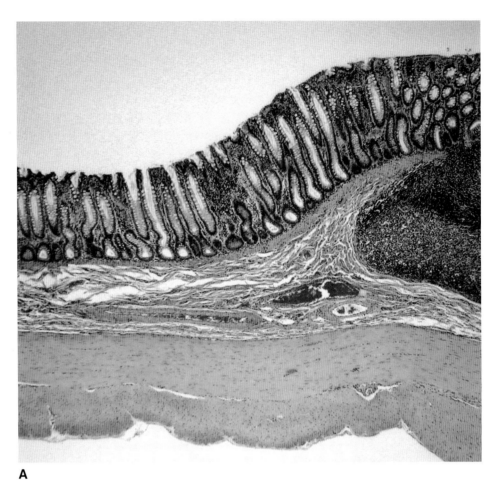

A

Figure 14-51. A, Light micrograph of the canine colon. (Hematoxylin and eosin [H&E] stain; ×15.) **B,** Light micrograph of the tunica mucosa consisting of simple tubular mucus-secreting glands. (H&E stain; ×100.)

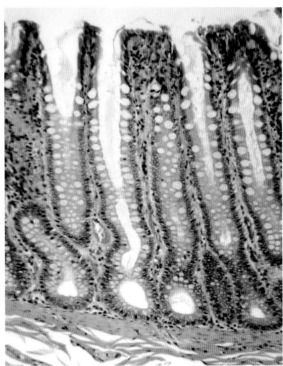

B

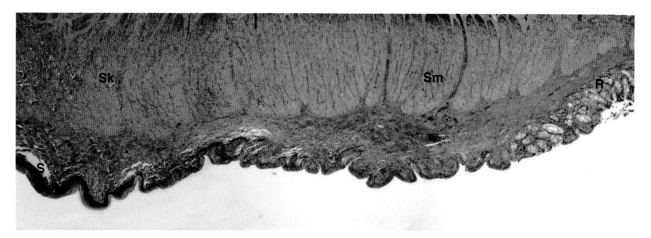

Figure 14-52. Light micrograph of the anal canal that extends from the gland-bearing rectum *(R)* to the stratified squamous epithelium of the skin *(S)*, composed internally of bundles of smooth muscle *(Sm)* that give way to skeletal *(Sk)* muscle. (Hematoxylin and eosin stain; ×10.)

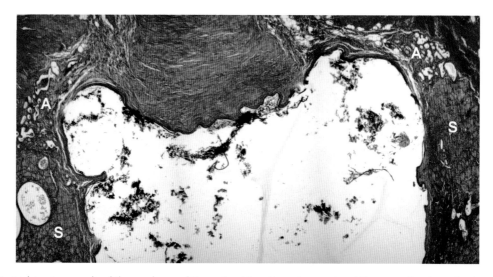

Figure 14-53. Light micrograph of the anal sac of the cat, with adjacent apocrine *(A)* sweat glands and sebaceous *(S)* glands. (Hematoxylin and eosin stain; ×10.)

which when present end blindly. The cells have a hepatocyte-like morphology and for that reason are sometimes referred to as **hepatoid.** Their function remains a mystery. Nevertheless, they have strong clinical significance in that these glands can become tumiferous.

AVIAN DIGESTIVE SYSTEM

The digestive tract of birds, including domestic fowl, is morphologically different from that of mammals in a number of ways. In place of lips and teeth, the entrance to the oral cavity is formed by a cornified beak attached to the upper and lower jaws. The oral cavity and the tongue are lined by kera-

tinized stratified squamous epithelia. Within the propria-submucosa of the oral cavity are numerous salivary-like glands that are not as developed as those in mammals, being simple branched tubular in their shape and mucous in their secretions. The avian tongue, which is narrow and tapered, has a core of skeletal muscle, mucus glands (lingual salivary glands), and bone, the **entoglossal bone,** which is positioned more caudally.

The epithelial lining of the esophagus continues to be keratinized stratified squamous. As in the oral cavity and the tongue, the propria-submucosa of the esophagus houses more simple branched mucus glands. The tubular secretory units of these glands in the upper portion of the avian digestive tract are arranged in a circular fashion, all emptying into a

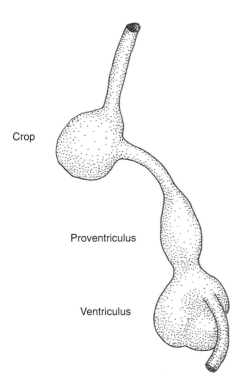

Crop

Proventriculus

Ventriculus

Figure 14-54. Diagram of the crop, proventriculus, and ventriculus of the chicken.

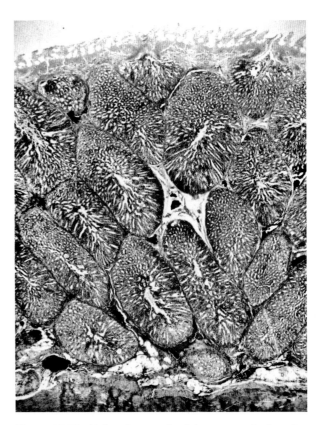

Figure 14-55. Light micrograph of the proventriculus of a chicken. (Hematoxylin and eosin stain; ×10.)

central lumen or duct that directs the secretions to this portion of the alimentary canal. Within the esophagus is a diverticulum (the **crop** or **ingluvies**), that temporarily stores ingesta so that it can be further moistened by its own glands (which vary in amount and shape according to the species, and even being absent in some, such as the turkey) as well as by the mucous secretions of the esophagus, tongue, and the oral cavity (Figure 14-54). Histologically, the crop is similar to the esophagus.

The esophagus directs the ingested food to the stomach, which in birds consists of two separate organs, the proventriculus and the ventriculus (see Figure 14-54). The esophagus is directly attached to the **proventriculus,** which is the glandular stomach within the avian digestive system. The mucosa is arranged in folds, or plicae, that lie on broad papillae, which can be seen grossly. The mucosal folds are lined by a simple columnar epithelium. Simple branched glands lie at the base of each mucosal fold. In addition to these glands is a large system of submucosal glands that empties at the tip of each papilla (Figures 14-55 and 14-56). The submucosal glands are much more elaborate in their development than those within the esophagus, crop, tongue, and oral cavity. These glands are considered to be compound, having a collection of numerous branching tubular adenomeres that empty into large central ducts, which

lead to a single duct opening at each papilla. The secretory cells of the submucosal glands are morphologically indistinguishable from one another and are believed to be composed of one type. This cell, which is low columnar in appearance but appears serrated due to the lack of any apical attachment along its lateral sides, has a round somewhat basally located nucleus within an acidophilic cytoplasm. It is believed to secrete enzymes and hydrochloric acid (HCl) similar to that formed by the glandular portion of the mammalian stomach. The thin tunica muscularis is made up of three layers of smooth muscle: inner and outer longitudinal layers sandwiching a middle circular layer. The outer longitudinal layer is then lined externally by a typical tunica serosa.

The proventriculus empties into the **ventriculus,** or **gizzard,** which is the muscular stomach. The obvious and distinguishing feature of the gizzard is the enormously developed tunica muscularis (Figure 14-57). This portion is composed of multiple bands of smooth muscle fibers that lie parallel to the lumen of the gizzard and is replaced by regular dense connective tissue along its lateral sides. Because birds lack the grinding capability that teeth, especially molars, offer, the muscle of the gizzard functions to mechanically break up ingesta before entering the small intestine.

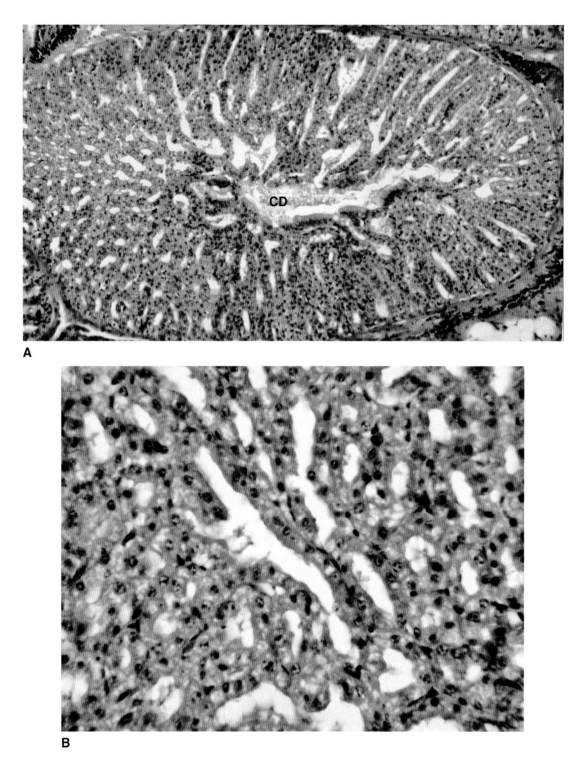

A

B

Figure 14-56. Light micrographs of the submucosal glands in the proventriculus of a chicken. **A,** Portion of an individual gland with a large central duct *(CD).* **B,** Close-up of the branching tubules that make up the submucosal gland. (Hematoxylin and eosin stain; **A,** ×50; **B,** ×250.)

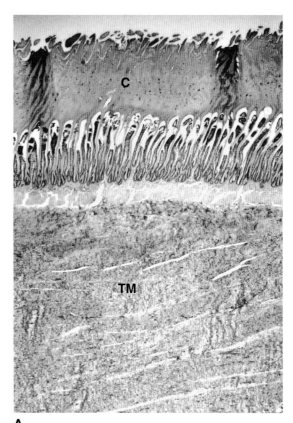

A

Figure 14-57. A, Light micrograph of the ventriculus of a chicken. *C,* cuticle; *TM,* tunica muscularis. (Hematoxylin and eosin [H&E] stain; ×10.) **B,** Light micrograph of the simple tubular gastric glands that branch basally. (H&E stain; ×100.)

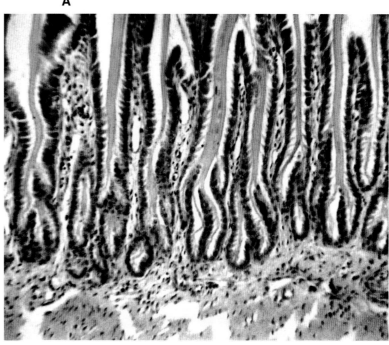

B

It is especially developed in herbivorous and granivorous (grain consuming) species, including the domestic chicken. Carnivorous and frugivorous (fruit consuming) species, such as carrion-consuming buzzards and fruit-eating tanagers, possess thin-walled gizzards. The mucosa of this organ has a simple columnar epithelium that is subtended by simple, straight tubular glands that produce a material called the **cuticle (keratinoid, koilen).** It is given this name due to its histological appearance and staining characteristics. This cornified-like secretion can occur in layers and react positively to stains that are used to reveal keratohyalin.

The small and large intestines of the avian digestive system are similar to those in mammals. However, the junction of the small and large intestines opens into two appended blind sacs: the **ceca.** Within each cecum, the villi shrink in size and disappear at the distal-most point. The lamina propria and submucosa are heavily infiltrated with both diffuse and nodular lymphatic tissues. The nodules are well established near the openings of the ceca and form the **cecal tonsils.**

Lymphatic tissue is generally present throughout the avian alimentary canal, consisting mostly of the diffuse form that is located within the propria-submucosa. However, nodular lymphatic tissue is also present in the small and large intestines and of course in the ceca.

The avian alimentary canal ends at the **cloaca.** The cloaca, a common orifice for the digestive, excretory, and reproductive tracts, is subdivided by transverse folds into three portions: the **coprodeum,** the **urodeum,** and the **proctodeum,** respectively. The mucosal lining of the cloaca is composed of a simple columnar epithelium.

SUGGESTED READINGS

Bergman RA, Afifi AK, Heidger PM Jr: *Histology,* Philadelphia, 1996, Saunders.

Boshell JL, Wilborn WH, Singh BB: Filiform papillae of the cat tongue, *Acta Anat* (Basel) 114:97, 1982.

Dougbag AS, Berg R: Morphological observations on the normal cardiac glands of the camel *(Camelus dromedarius), Anat Anz* 148:258, 1980.

Elias H: Comparison of the duodenal glands in domestic animals, *Am J Vet Res* 8:311, 1947.

Fawcett DW: *Bloom and Fawcett: a textbook of histology,* ed 11, Philadelphia, 1986, Saunders.

Flachsbarth MF, Schwarz R: The cytology of a highly specialized sebocyte, as demonstrated in the holocrine glands of anal sacs in the domestic cat, *Felis silvestris f catus, Zeit Saug Intern J Mam Biol* 57:144, 1992.

Gartner LP, Hiatt JL: *Color textbook of histology,* Philadelphia, 1997, Saunders.

Groenewald HB, Boot KK: A comparative thickness of the tunica muscularis in the forestomach and abomasum of grey, white and black Karakul lambs, *Onderstepoort J Vet Res* 59:225, 1992.

Hudson LC: Histochemical identification of the striated muscle of the canine esophagus, *Anat Histol Embryol* 22:101, 1993.

Junqueira LC, Carneiro J, Long JA: *Basic histology,* Los Altos, Calif, 1986, Lange.

Leeson CR, Leeson TS, Paparo AA: *Atlas of histology,* ed 2, Philadelphia, 1985, Saunders.

Merritt AM: Normal equine gastroduodenal secretion and motility, *Equine Vet J Suppl* 29:7, 1999.

Nishikawa S: Correlation of the arrangement pattern of enamel rods and secretory ameloblasts in pig and monkey teeth: a possible role of the terminal webs in ameloblast movement during secretion, *Anat Rec* 232:466, 1992.

Ojima K: Functional and angioarchitectural structure and classification of lingual papillae on the postero-dorsal surface of the beagle dog tongue, *Ann Anat* 183:19, 2001.

Ojima K, Takeda M, Matsumoto S, Nakanishi I: An investigation into the distributive pattern, classification and functional role of the conical papillae on the posterodorsal surface of the cat tongue using SEM, *Ann Anat* 179:505, 1997.

Pfeiffer CJ, Levin M, Lopes MA: Ultrastructure of the horse tongue: further observation on the lingual integumentary architecture, *Anat Histol Embryol* 29:37, 2000.

Prokopiw I, Hynna-Liepert TT, Dinda PK, et al: The microvascular anatomy on the canine stomach. A comparison of the body and the antrum, *Gastroenterology* 100:638, 1991.

Stevens CE, Hume ID: *Comparative physiology of the vertebrate digestive system,* ed 2, Cambridge, UK, 1995, Cambridge University Press.

Takayama I, Horiguchi K, Daigo Y, et al: The interstitial cells of Cajal and a gastroenteric pacemaker system, *Arch Histol Cytol* 65:1, 2002.

Titkemeyer CW, Calhoun ML: A comparative study of the structure of the small intestine of domestic animals, *Am J Vet Res* 16:152, 1955.

Warshawsky H: The teeth. In Weiss L, editor: *Histology: cell and tissue biology,* ed 5, New York, 1983, Elsevier Biomedical.

Digestive System II: Glands

KEY CHARACTERISTICS

- Mostly parenchymatous, secretory organs associated with the alimentary canal for the breakdown of ingesta and facilitation of nutrient metabolism, including salivary glands, pancreas, liver, and gallbladder

Along the connecting tubular organs that form the digestive system of domestic animals are a variety of associated parenchymatous structures that are mostly glandular in function, facilitating the breakdown and absorption of food.

SALIVARY GLANDS

The salivary glands consist of simple branched to compound tubuloalveolar glands that are housed within the propria-submucosa of the buccal cavity. These extensions of the mucosal epithelium vary considerably in development and can be separated into two groups: the **major salivary glands** and the **minor salivary glands.** The major salivary glands are the **mandibular, parotid, sublingual,** and **zygomatic glands,** and the minor glands are the **buccal, labial, lingual,** and **palatine glands.**

The major salivary glands contain lobules and lobes of numerous adenomeres and series of ducts that together are held, innervated, and nourished by the connective tissue stroma. Each adenomere or secretory portion is made up of a collection of mucus-secreting and/or serous cells (Figure 15-1; see also Figure 14-17). The distribution of the mucus and serous cells can vary considerably within each of these glands. Portions of lobules or even whole lobules can be exclusively serous. Mucous cell–bearing adenomeres, however, are rarely free of serous cells, having occasional crescent-shaped serous cells (demilunes) lying outside the mucous cells (see Figure 4-9). In some microlobules, the mixing of the two types of secretory cells can be nearly equal, with the serous cells, forming a continuous outer layer next to mucous cells, and resulting in bilayered adenomeres (see Figure 15-1).

In addition to the secretory cells, each adenomere is bounded by myoepithelial cells lying within its basal lamina. These cells are less distinctive than the demilunes, with small, flattened heterochromatic nuclei within similarly flattened cytoplasm (see Figure 15-1). Their cell processes occasionally branch, each partially enveloping a secretory end piece. Contraction of these cells facilitates the release and movement of the secretory product away from the adenomere.

Each adenomere empties into the **intercalated duct,** a small duct lined by a simple cuboidal epithelium (see Figure 15-1). At least several of the intercalated ducts come together to form a **striated duct** (Figure 15-2). Like the intercalated duct, the striated duct is lined by a single layer of epithelium that can be cuboidal to columnar. These cells possess marked basal infoldings of their cell membranes that extend apically toward the duct's lumen. With the presence of mitochondria within each infolding, the cells have a striated appearance. The infoldings are associated with Na^+, K^+ ATPase, which alters the ion concentrations within the secretory product by removing

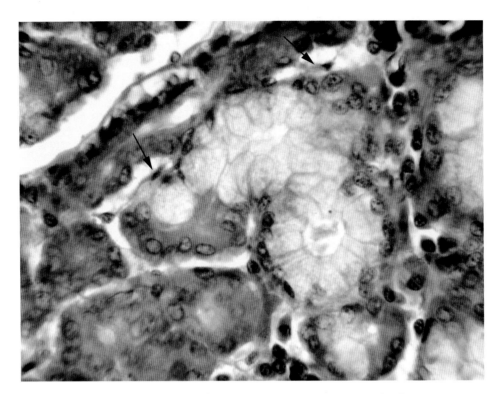

Figure 15-1. Light micrograph of seromucous adenomeres within the canine salivary gland. Arrows point to myoepithelial cells. (Hematoxylin and eosin stain; ×250.)

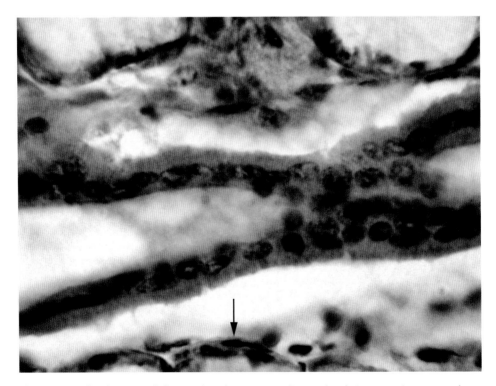

Figure 15-2. Light micrograph of a striated duct within the canine salivary gland. Arrow points to nearby myoepithelial cells associated with adjacent serous acini. (Hematoxylin and eosin stain; ×400.)

sodium and chlorine and replacing them with potassium and bicarbonate. Within lobules, striated ducts merge and form **intralobular ducts** that join with one another to form **interlobular ducts.** Intra- and interlobular ducts are bilayered with the intralobular ducts generally having stratified cuboidal epithelia and interlobular ducts having stratified columnar epithelia (see Figures 3-16 and 3-17). Interlobular ducts eventually empty saliva into **interlobar ducts,** which then empty the saliva into the terminal duct and then into the oral cavity.

The saliva that is delivered to the oral cavity contains enzymes, some of which enhance taste and begin the digestive process, such as salivary amylase and lipase. Another enzyme within saliva is lactoperoxidase, which acts as an antimicrobial agent. In fact, saliva contains a number of antimicrobial agents, including secretory immunoglobulin A (IgA), lysozyme, and lactoferrin. IgA is contributed by lymphocytes and plasma cells that have migrated into the stroma. Salivation is largely under the direction of the autonomic nervous system, being innervated parasympathetically by cranial nerves (CN) VII, IX and X and sympathetically. The senses of taste, smell, and sight as well as the process of mastication all can trigger salivation. Parasympathetic innervation leads largely to watery saliva, which is the release of saliva from serum-rich lobules, whereas sympathetic innervation directs mucus-rich lobules to release their mucin, resulting in a drier, more viscous saliva.

EXOCRINE PANCREAS

The second largest gland of the body is the pancreas, having both exocrine and endocrine components. The exocrine portion consists of an enormous number of oval to round adenomeres that form a compound tubuloacinar gland and secrete enzymes that like other glands of the digestive system facilitate the breakdown of ingesta. In addition to enzymes such as amylase and lipase, which are found also in saliva, others are contributed including carboxylases, collagenase, elastase, esterase, and trypsin. Because of their potentially disruptive actions, many of the enzymes are released in a proenzyme state, such as trypsinogen, which is transformed by enterokinase into its active form, trypsin; the enterokinase is provided by the intestinal mucosa. The secretory cells are reminiscent of the serous cells seen in the salivary glands; they are pyramidally shaped and have round nuclei surrounded by basophilic cytoplasm (Figure 15-3). Each cell has a well-developed Golgi apparatus that functions to package the enzymes and proenzymes into secretory

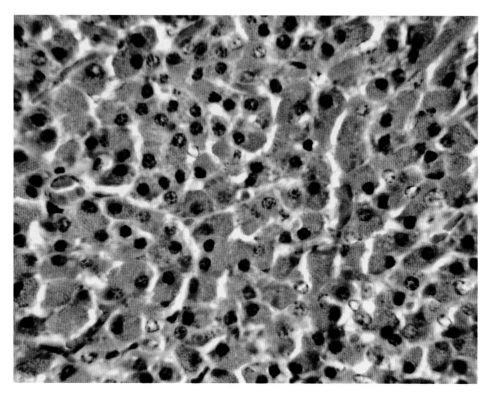

Figure 15-3. Light micrograph of the secretory cells of the equine exocrine pancreas. (Hematoxylin and eosin stain; ×250.)

Capillary   Acinar cells

Centroacinar
cells

Duct

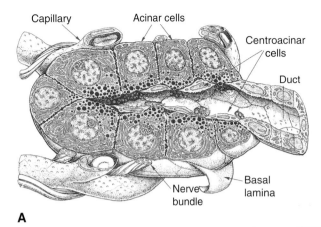

Basal
lamina

Nerve
bundle

A

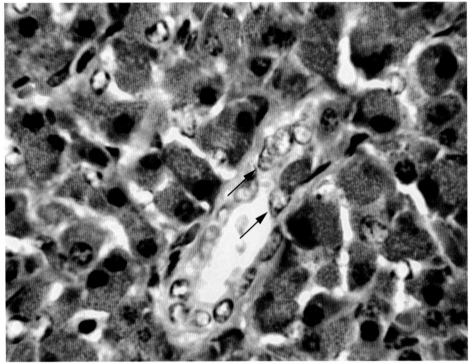

B

Figure 15-4. A, Illustration of an acinus within the exocrine pancreas. **B,** Light micrograph of the intercalated duct within the equine exocrine pancreas. Arrows point to centroacinar cells. (Hematoxylin and eosin stain; ×500.) *(A modified from Fawcett DW:* Bloom and Fawcett: a textbook of histology, *ed 11, Philadelphia, 1986, Saunders.)*

vesicles known as **zymogen granules.** The zymogen granules can be released individually or in small clusters that fuse with one another, emptying as a microcanal into the acinar lumen. As the secretions are emptied into the lumen of each acinus or tubuloacinus, they pass by flattened, porous cells that centrally line the secretory unit, the **centroacinar cells,** confluent extensions of the adjacent intercalated duct (Figure 15-4).

Although the centroacinar cells provide the initial conduit for the secretions, these cells along with those forming the intercalated ducts contribute bicarbonate and water to the secretions. By adding bicarbonate, the pH is elevated. In this way, the acidic chyme is neutralized and the secreted enzymes are allowed to

function more effectively. The secretory contributions of the centroacinar cells are controlled, in part, by the enteroendocrine cells of the small intestine. The enteroendocrine cells release **secretin,** a hormone that signals the centroacinus cells and cells of the intercalated ducts to secrete bicarbonate and water. This is usually done in response to increased acidity of the chyme.

The exocrine secretions of the pancreas—**pancreatic juice**—continue along the extensive system of ducts within and between the lobules of this gland. As the smaller ducts merge into larger ducts (e.g., intralobular ducts joining interlobular ducts) connective tissue elements that form the associated stroma increase concomitantly in size (Figure 15-5).

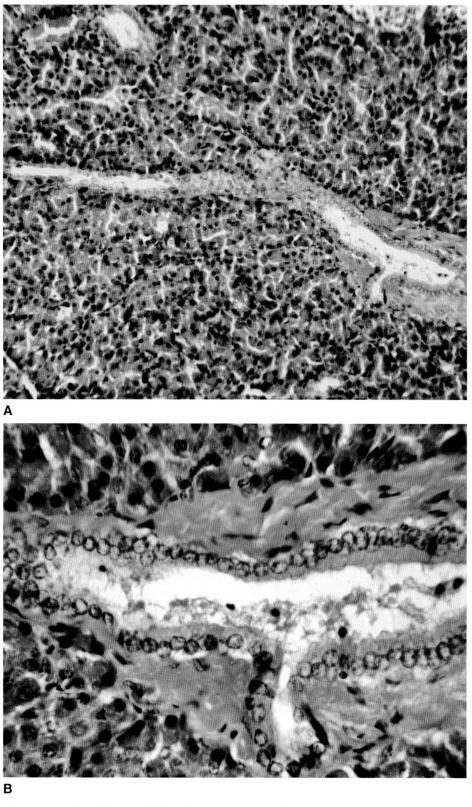

A

B

Figure 15-5. Light micrographs of the intralobular ducts (**A,** ×100) with increased thickened stroma (**B,** ×250) within the porcine pancreas.

The epithelial lining remains single layered but changes in shape, going from cuboidal to columnar. Eventually the secretions reach the largest ducts, the **main pancreatic duct** and the **accessory pancreatic duct,** which empty into the duodenum.

LIVER

The largest gland in the body of domestic species is the liver because it produces bile for the gastrointestinal tract. Although it has secretory capabilities, this organ also is able to excrete, provide storage, detoxify, metabolize, esterify, and phagocytize (Table 15-1). In short, it plays the role as the control center for the digestive system. The principal cell of the liver is the **hepatocyte,** which, as incredulous as it may sound, performs most of the activities listed in Table 15-1. The hepatocyte comprises the parenchyma of the liver and is organized by the stromal elements of the liver into structural units called **hepatic lobules** (Figure 15-6). The liver is encased by a serosal lining or peritoneum that contains a thin capsule of connective tissue that continues to subdivide the liver into lobes and to a lesser extent into lobules, providing physical support for the intrinsic lymph and blood vessels associated with hepatocytes.

HEPATIC LOBULE

Within the liver of domestic animals, the parenchyma is anatomically constructed into the hepatic lobule, also referred to as the **classic liver lobule** (see Figure 15-6). The stromal elements help clearly define this lobule in certain animals such as the pig. From a functional sense, blood flows from the periphery of each lobule toward its center where the **central vein** lies (Figure 15-7). Conversely, bile is secreted into canaliculi between hepatocytes, which then flows into **bile ducts** that lie at the periphery next to the **portal vein** and **hepatic artery.** The bile duct, portal vein, and hepatic artery collectively form the **portal triad** (Figure 15-8). To appreciate the hepatic lobule from its histological point of view, the liver parenchyma needs to be oriented in the appropriate plane so as to reveal the polygonal positioning of four to six sets of portal triads that surround the central vein.

TABLE 15-1	Key Morphological Characteristics of the Major Glands of the Gastrointestinal Tract of Domestic Species		
GLAND	**ARCHITECTURAL ORGANIZATION**	**CELLS (MORPHOLOGY AND ACTIVITY)**	**FUNCTION**
Salivary	Parenchyma arranged into compound tubuloalveolar adenomeres	Serous cells, including demilunes, secrete enzymes; mucous cells release water absorbing carbohydrate-laden secretion; mucous and serous cells except for demilunes (crescent shaped) are pyramidal to polyhedral shaped	Lubricates ingesta and begins digestive process with release of amylase and lipase and enhances taste; also contributes antimicrobial component
Exocrine pancreas	Parenchyma arranged into compound tubuloalveolar adenomeres	Serous cells secrete enzymes and are pyramidal to polyhedral shaped; centroacinus cells add bicarbonate and water at junction of intercalated duct; low cuboidal to flattened	Further facilitates digestive process by releasing numerous enzymes into the duodenum of the small intestine including trypsin, carboxylases, collagenases, elastase, and esterase
Liver	Parenchyma arranged into laminae associated with vasculature, which together form lobules	Hepatocytes are polyhedral shaped and receive, metabolize, and store materials absorbed from the small intestine and secrete bile; stellate macrophage defends against vascular-carried pathogens as well as removes debris and dying red blood cells; perisinusoidal cells are lipid-bearing stellate cells associated with retinol metabolism	Is the control center of the digestive system; involved in the metabolism, esterification, and storage of fats, proteins, and carbohydrates as well as secretion of bile for lipid absorption, and the detoxification of blood-borne toxins
Gallbladder	Tubular with simple columnar mucosa and minimal muscular development and scattered tubuloalveolar glands	Columnar-shaped light cells and occasional dark cells compose the mucosal epithelium; absorb water and salt of the bile; goblet cells also exist in cattle	Stores and concentrates bile before being released into the duodenum of the small intestine

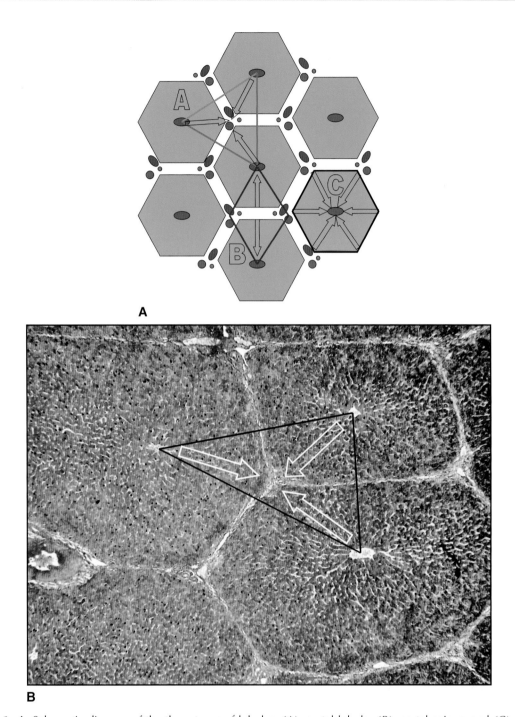

A

B

Figure 15-6. A, Schematic diagram of the three types of lobules: *(A)*, portal lobule; *(B)*, portal acinus; and *(C)*, classical lobule. Light micrographs of **B,** portal lobule, *Continued*

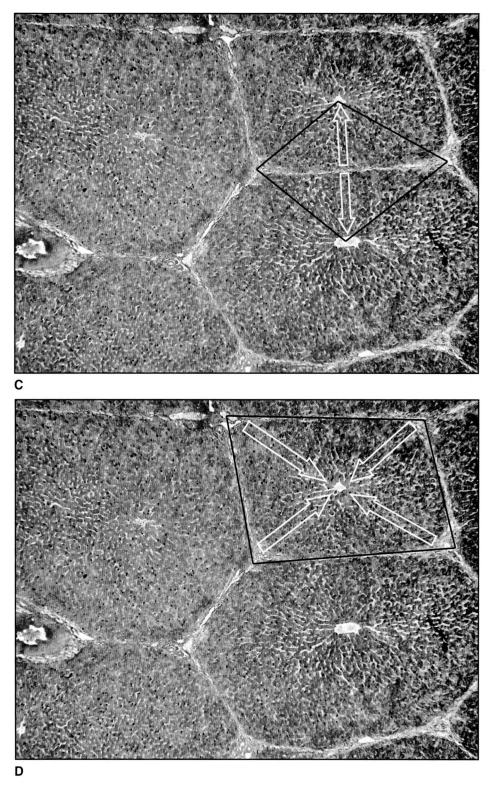

Figure 15-6, cont'd C, portal acinus, and **D,** classical lobule. (Hematoxylin and eosin stain; ×20.)

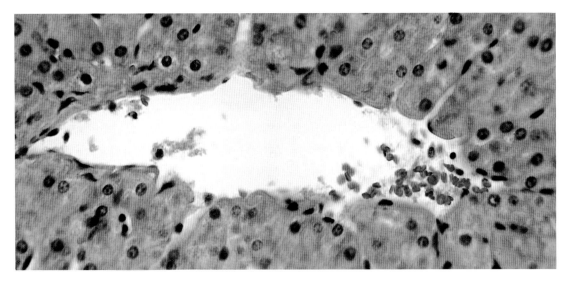

Figure 15-7. Light micrograph of the central vein within the lobule of porcine liver. (Hematoxylin and eosin stain; ×100.)

PORTAL LOBULE

As a secretory organ, the liver can be thought to have a different type of lobule, the **portal lobule.** In this instance, the focal point is directed to the primary lumen that the bile is deposited that being the bile duct. The bile duct then forms the central lumen of a secretory unit that consists of a triangular region with a central vein at each apex (see Figure 15-6). The portal lobule is an imagined entity that stresses the exocrine glandular function of the liver.

HEPATIC ACINUS

In addition to the use of stromal and glandular parameters, the parenchyma of the liver can be subdivided according to its angioarchitecture, resulting in the formation of the **hepatic acinus (portal acinus).** In this scheme of organization, the direction of blood flow is emphasized (see Figure 15-6). The focal points for the hepatic acinus are two adjacent central veins and nearby portal triads. Within the hepatic acinus three zones of vascular influence have been designated; zone one is the innermost area and is supplied by the greatest amount of oxygen, and zone three is the outermost area, with the least amount of oxygen. From a clinical perspective, the use of the hepatic acinus is warranted, especially with regard to liver damage that was the result of hypoxic or toxic insults.

HEPATOCYTE AND SINUSOID

The functional cell of the liver is the **hepatocyte.** Histologically, hepatocytes are similar among domestic species; they're polyhedral cells that possess one or two round nuclei. In uninucleated cells, the nucleus varies in size although many tend to be large and euchromatic, often possessing two or more nucleoli (Figure 15-9). Among the parenchyma, cells with smaller nuclei are diploid, whereas those with larger nuclei are polyploid.

Hepatocytes are metabolically active and possess an extensive body of mitochondria, ribosomes, rough endoplasmic reticulum, and Golgi apparatus (Figures 15-10 and 15-11). The Golgi apparatus is often located near the bile canaliculi. Peroxisomes are also frequently encountered in their cytoplasm, as well as variable amounts of smooth endoplasmic reticulum and lysosomes. The storage organelles, glycogen and lipid vacuoles, can be abundant, especially after feeding. When observing liver parenchyma of an individual, it is interesting to observe the variability in the amount of the different organelles that occurs between cells, particularly when comparing one hepatic lobule with another and one zone of an acinus lobule with another zone within the same lobule. This variability suggests that a heterogeneity of function is most likely occurring among the hepatocytes regardless of domestic species and that this possible heterogeneity may be directly influenced by vascular relationships.

Hepatocytes are linked in a way to form sheets or plates of cells; they are separated by **hepatic sinusoids** (see Figure 15-7). The hepatic sinusoids are capillaries that connect the interlobular vessels, the hepatic artery (arteriole), and the portal vein (venule) to the central vein (see Figures 15-5 and 15-6). All hepatocytes have one or more sides of their cells exposed to these sinusoids. The sinusoids are covered by a porous

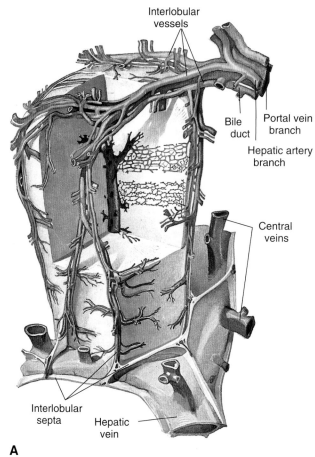

Interlobular
vessels

Bile
duct

Portal vein
branch

Hepatic artery
branch

Central
veins

Interlobular
septa

Hepatic
vein

A

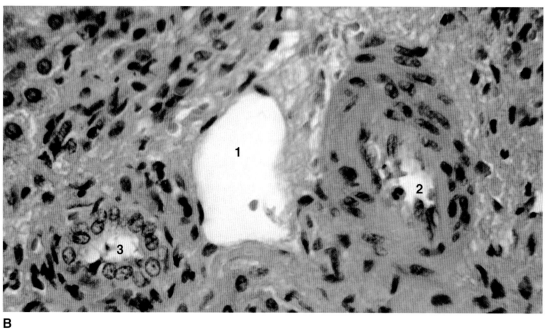

B

Figure 15-8. A, Illustration of the vascular components of the liver **B,** Light micrograph of the triad. *(1),* portal vein; *(2),* hepatic artery; *(3),* bile duct. (Hematoxylin and eosin stain; ×100.) *(**A** modified from Fawcett DW:* Bloom and Fawcett: a textbook of histology, *ed 11, Philadelphia, 1986, Saunders.)*

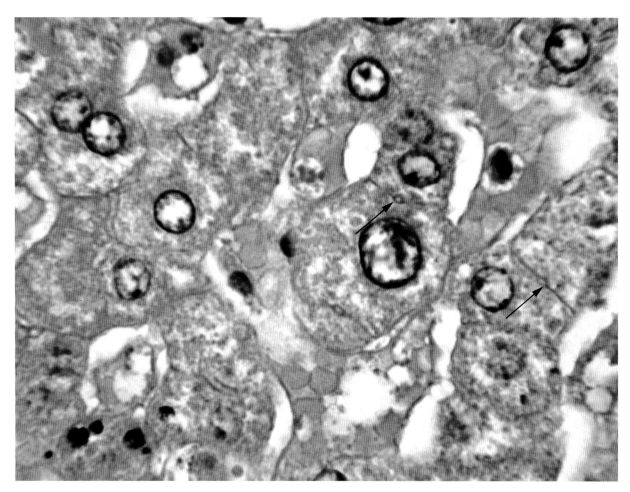

Figure 15-9. Light micrograph of hepatocytes with single large nuclei and multiple nucleoli and those with two small nuclei (binucleated) in the porcine liver. Arrows point to bile canaliculi. (Hematoxylin and eosin stain; ×15.)

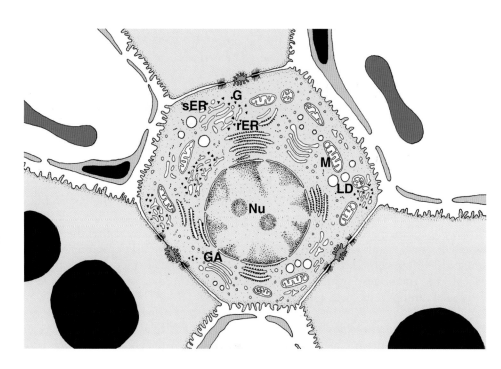

Figure 15-10. Illustration of the mammalian hepatocyte. *G,* Glycogen; *GA,* Golgi apparatus; *LD,* lipid droplets; *M,* mitochondrion; *Nu,* nucleus; *rER,* rough endoplasmic reticulum; *sER,* smooth endoplasmic reticulum.

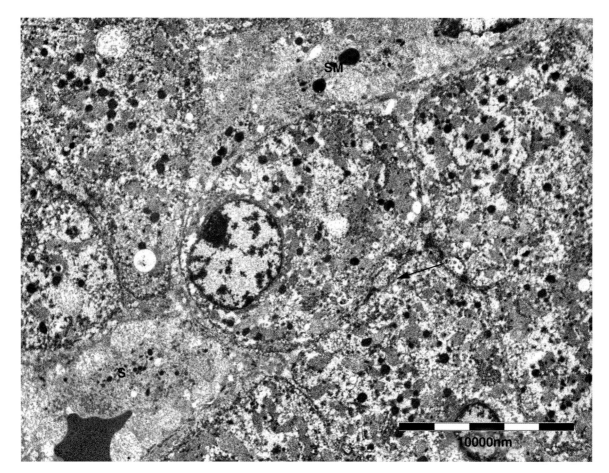

Figure 15-11. Transmission electron micrograph of a hepatocyte in the liver of a pig. *S,* Sinusoid; *SM,* stellate macrophage. Arrow points to bile canaliculus.

and fenestrated endothelium called the **sinusoidal lining cells (sinusoidal endothelial cells).** The sinusoidal lining cells are separated from the hepatocytes by a **perisinusoidal space (space of Disse).** The perisinusoidal space is usually occupied by numerous microvilli of adjacent hepatocytes (Figure 15-12). These microvilli can vary considerably in length, sometimes branch, and are flexous, lacking a core of actin seen in intestinal mucosa. Nevertheless, they amplify enormously the surface of the sides of the hepatocytes apposing the sinusoids. In this way, the exchange of materials to and from the hepatocyte is made without the influence of shearing forces associated with blood flow. Although there may be occasional collagen fibers (type III) within the perisinusoidal space, basal laminar development by the sinusoidal lining cells is minimal in most mammals except in ruminants, which possess nonporous sinusoidal lining cells that form continuous basal laminae.

In addition to the sinusoidal lining cells, sinusoids frequently contain a member of the monocyte-macrophage system, the **stellate macrophage (Kupffer cell)** (Figure 15-13). The stellate macrophage lies within the sinusoidal lumen and is flattened so as to reduce impedance to blood flow. In porous sinusoids, its cell processes (pseudopodia) often extend into the perisinusoidal space. Occasionally, they can lie entirely within the space. The stellate macrophage has complement and Fc receptors and is capable of removing foreign particulate matter as well as dying erythrocytes and cell debris. Because blood coming from the portal vein may contain microorganisms, especially bacteria, that have penetrated the mucosal lining of the gut and have entered the bloodstream, these cells provide an essential line of defense by phagocytizing the microorganisms that had been previously opsonized somewhere along the gastrointestinal tract. Besides the sinusoidal lining cells and the macrophages are **perisinusoidal cells,** also referred to as **Ito cells, lipocytes,** or **vitamin-rich cells** (Figure 15-14). These cells store the bulk of liver retinoids in lipid droplets and are very much involved in retinol dynamics within the body (see Figure 15-13).

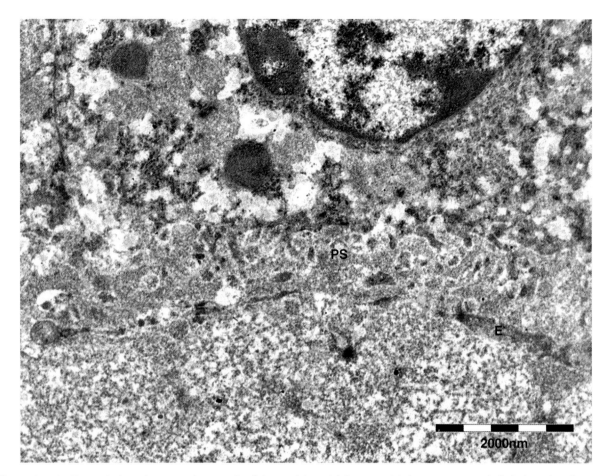

Figure 15-12. Transmission electron micrograph of the perisinusoidal space *(PS)* between an endothelial *(E)*-lined sinusoid and adjacent hepatocyte in the liver of a pig.

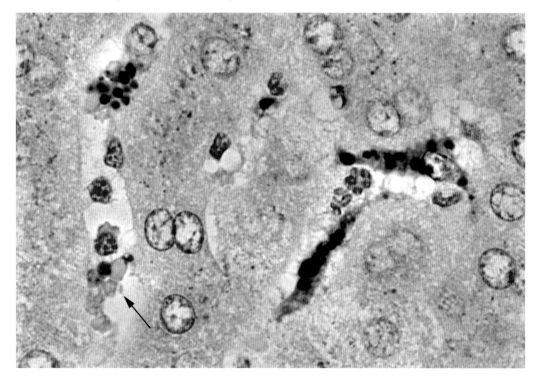

Figure 15-13. Light micrograph of active stellate macrophages and perisinusoidal cell *(arrow)* along the sinusoids of a porcine liver. (Iron stain; ×1000.)

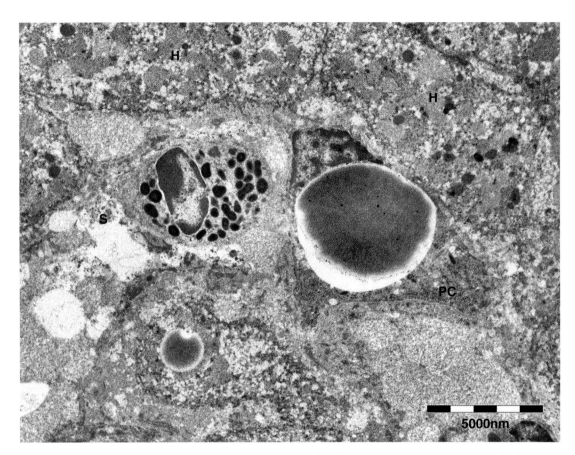

Figure 15-14. Transmission electron micrograph of a perisinusoidal cell *(PC)* next to a sinusoid *(S)* and adjacent hepatocytes *(H)* in the liver of a pig.

The lateral sides of the hepatocytes attach one cell to another, resulting in the plates that radiate from the central vein. Cell-to-cell attachment is facilitated by the cell junctions, gap junctions that are dispersed along the lateral cell membranes and provide communication between adjoining cells, and a fascia occludens that surrounds a discrete intercellular tunnel-like space called the **bile canaliculus** (Figure 15-15). The fascia occludens functions as a tight junction, keeping the secreted bile within the lumen of the bile canaliculus and preventing it from reaching the sinusoids and associated bloodstream. Each lateral side of the hepatocyte forms one of these microchannels that function to conduct bile from these cells to the periphery of the hepatic lobule. The apposing cell membranes that form the boundary of the bile canaliculus consist of irregular microvillus-like processes that serve to expand its surface area and enhance bile secretion.

Biliary System

One of the functions of the liver is to remove bilirubin from the blood (see Table 15-1). **Bilirubin** is a yellow-green pigment that is a byproduct of hemoglobin degradation. This water-insoluble toxic compound is bound to plasma albumin and circulates throughout the body's vasculature until it is eventually absorbed (endocytized) by hepatocytes. The bilirubin is conjugated with glucuronide within the smooth endoplasmic reticulum (sER) to form a water-soluble product **(bilirubin glucuronide)** that is released or excreted into the bile canaliculus. In addition to bilirubin glucuronide, bile salts, cholesterol, phospholipids, and plasma electrolytes are released into the canaliculi. The contents of the bile canaliculi flow to the portal triads, initially entering epithelial-lined (low simple cuboidal) **bile ductules** that then empty into the **interlobular biliary ducts** (see Figure 15-8). The interlobular biliary ducts, which are also lined by a single-layered epithelium (cuboidal to columnar), lead the bile to larger, merging **intrahepatic ducts** that further become consolidated into the **hepatic ducts,** which are lined by simple columnar epithelia. The hepatic ducts exit the liver from its lobes and in most domestic species is joined by the **cystic duct** that empties the gallbladder before entering the duodenum. In the horse, the hepatic ducts connect with the

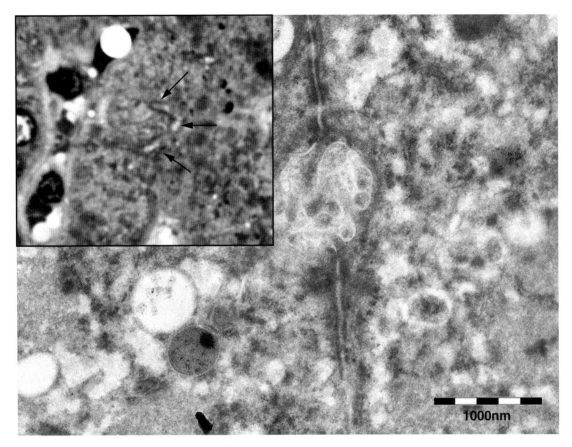

Figure 15-15. Transmission electron micrograph of the bile canaliculus between adjacent hepatocytes in the porcine liver. Light microscopy *(inset)* of the bile canaliculus *(arrows).* (Plastic section, toluidine blue stain; ×500.)

duodenum without any junction of a cystic duct because the gallbladder is absent in this animal.

Vascular Supply

It is important to understand the relationship of the vascular supply of the liver as it pertains to both the body and the digestive system (see Figure 15-8). The liver is provided with a dual blood supply; it is oxygenated by the **hepatic artery** and nourished nutrient-wise by the **portal vein.** The portal vein, which carries blood primarily from the intestines, and the hepatic artery enter the liver at a hilus, the **porta.** The portal vein accounts for nearly 80% of the blood flow to the liver, with the remainder arriving by the hepatic artery. Both the portal vein and the hepatic artery distribute their blood within the liver in a comparable manner. Each vessel branches and gives rise to tributaries—the inlet arterioles and venules that are the interlobular hepatic artery (or arteriole) and the interlobular portal vein (or venule)—that flow into the hepatic sinusoids (Figure 15-16). The sinusoids drain into the central vein, which, being perpendicular to the hepatic lobule,

empties into the **sublobular vein.** The sublobular veins then converge into the larger **hepatic veins,** which continue on to the vena cava.

GALLBLADDER

In most domestic species, after the bile leaves the liver it is first stored in the gallbladder before being delivered to the small intestine (Figure 15-17). While the bile is held in the gallbladder, it becomes further concentrated as water and salts are resorbed. It delivers bile to the small intestine as needed (after feeding), and is contained and restricted by a sphincter of smooth muscle that surrounds the common bile duct and closes it during fasting.

Histologically, the gallbladder consists of a mucosal epithelium; propria-submucosa, tunica muscularis, and serosa and adventitia (see Table 15-1). The mucosal epithelium is simple columnar, consisting of **clear or light cells** with less frequent **dark cells** (Figure 15-18). Apically, the cells possess microvilli and are

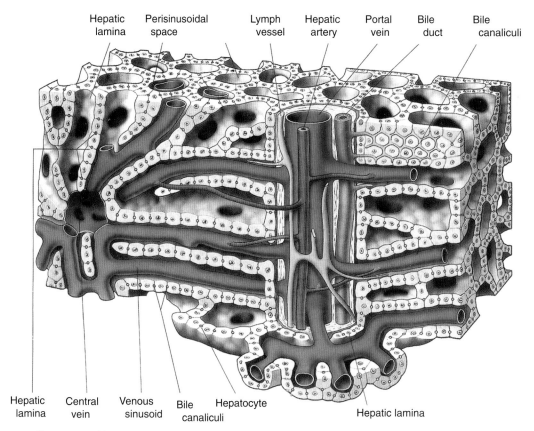

Hepatic lamina Perisinusoidal space Lymph vessel Hepatic artery Portal vein Bile duct Bile canaliculi

Hepatic lamina Central vein Venous sinusoid Bile canaliculi Hepatocyte Hepatic lamina

Figure 15-16. Illustration of hepatic sinusoids and their vascular components. *(Modified from Fawcett DW:* Bloom and Fawcett: a textbook of histology, *ed 11, Philadelphia, 1986, Saunders.)*

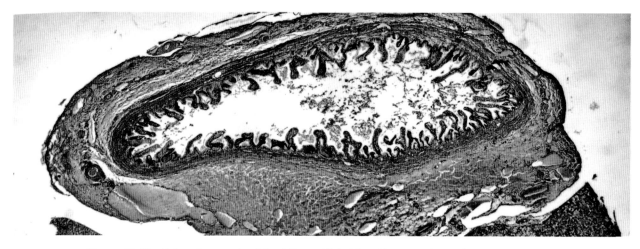

Figure 15-17. Light micrograph of the feline gallbladder. (Hematoxylin and eosin stain; ×10.)

laterally attached by tight junctions. In the bovine gallbladder, the mucosal lining also has goblet cells. The propria-submucosa is composed of loose connective tissue and scattered tubuloalveolar glands (Figure 15-19). Variations exist among domestic species with regard to the amount and location of the glands and their type of secretory material, being either mucous or serous. Nodular and/or diffuse lymphatic tissue also is present. After releasing the bile, the mucosa of the gallbladder can be greatly folded. When compared with other components of the digestive system, the tunica muscularis is weakly developed, consisting of muscle fibers that are directed in one plane of orientation (see Figure 15-17).

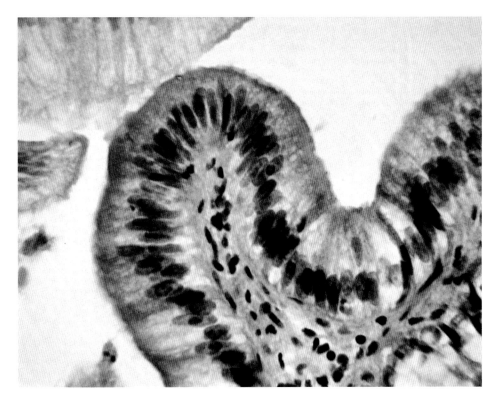

Figure 15-18. Light micrograph of the simple columnar epithelium that lines the gallbladder of a cat. (Hematoxylin and eosin stain; ×500.)

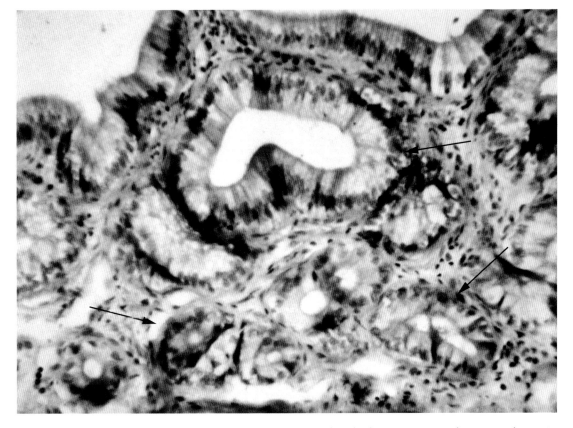

Figure 15-19. Light micrograph of tubuloalveolar glands *(arrows)* within the lamina propria-submucosa of a canine gallbladder. (Hematoxylin and eosin stain; ×250.)

SUGGESTED READINGS

Bartok I, Toth J, Remenar E, Viragh S: Ultrastructure of the hepatic perisinusoidal cells in man and other mammalian species, *Anat Rec* 194:571, 1979.

Bioulac-Sage P, Balabaud C: Proliferation and phenotypic expression of perisinusoidal cells, *J Hepatol* 15:284, 1992.

Fawcett DW: *Bloom and Fawcett: a textbook of histology,* ed 11, Philadelphia, 1986, Saunders.

Flaks B: Observations on the fine structure of the normal porcine liver, *J Anat* 108:563, 1971.

Forssmann A: The ultrastructure of the cell types in the endocrine pancreas of the horse, *Cell Tissue Res* 167:179, 1976.

Gartner LP, Hiatt JL: *Color textbook of histology,* Philadelphia, 1997, Saunders.

Kmiec Z: Cooperation of liver cells in health and disease, *Adv Anat Embryol Cell Biol* 161:III-XIII, 2001.

Kuijpers GA, Van Nooy IG, Vossen ME, et al: Tight junctional permeability of the resting and carbachol stimulated exocrine rabbit pancreas, *Histochemistry* 83:257, 1985.

Phillips CJ, Tandler B: Salivary glands, cellular evolution, and adaptive radiation in mammals, *Eur J Morphol* 34:155, 1996.

Pinzani M: Novel insights into the biology and physiology of the Ito cell, *Pharmacol Ther* 66:387, 1995.

Stevens CE, Hume ID: *Comparative physiology of the vertebrate digestive system,* ed 2, Cambridge, UK, Cambridge University Press, 1995.

Wahlin T, Bloom GD, Carlsoo B: Histochemical observations with the light and the electron microscope on the mucosubstances of the normal mouse gallbladder epithelial cells, *Histochemistry* 42:119, 1974.

Urinary System

KEY CHARACTERISTICS

- Continuous tract, originating as a pair of organs: the kidneys composed of a cortex and a medulla that can be unilobar or multilobar
- Enhanced luminal modifications for absorption and excretion include brush borders and basolateral infoldings
- Nephron is principal structural and functional unit, subdivided into renal corpuscle with glomerulus, proximal tubule, descending and ascending thin tubule of the loop of the nephron, and distal tubule
- Major cells: mesangial cells, podocytes, epithelial lining of the uriniferous tubule (simple squamous and cuboidal cells), interstitial cells, juxtaglomerular cells, principal and intercalated cells of the collecting ducts

Throughout the body, the cells and tissues of the organs and organ systems that they comprise are continually nourished by the absorbed nutrients that have entered the bloodstream. Concomitantly, waste materials are deposited back into the bloodstream by the same cells and tissues. The urinary system functions primarily to remove the metabolic wastes of the body in the form of **urine** and maintain a homeostasis of the essential ingredients that support the body by removing or conserving electrolytes, water, glucose, and proteins. The kidney is the major organ involved in these functions and is associated with other structures—the ureters, urinary bladder and the urethra—that facilitate the removal of urine by acting collectively to direct, store, and release urine to the outside of the body. In the process of filtering and removing materials from the bloodstream, the urinary system is involved in the body's acid-base balance, hemodynamics, and blood pressure regula-

tion, and can release substances in a hormonal manner that influence these and other activities within the body.

KIDNEY

Most of the activities of the urinary system are performed by the **kidneys,** which exist as a pair of organs regardless of species. Kidneys vary in size and shape according to the domestic animal. In carnivores and small ruminants, each kidney is smooth and bean shaped. Although smooth in the horse, the kidney is more heart shaped, and in large ruminants, it is oval and lobed or cobblestoned rather than smooth (Figure 16-1). Medially, each kidney indents, forming the **hilum,** an area where the ureter leaves the kidney and major blood and lymphatic vessels and nerves enter and exit. The kidney possesses a thin capsule of dense,

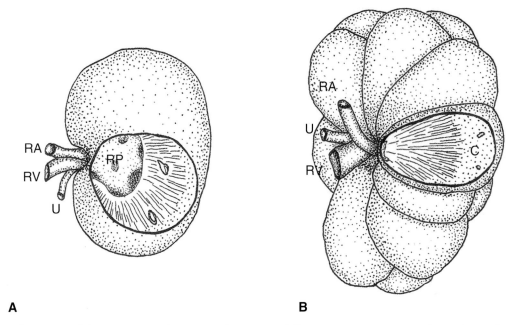

Figure 16-1. Illustration of the two principal patterns of corticomedullary organization among domestic species. **A,** Unilobar (dogs, cats). **B,** Multilobar (large ruminants). *C,* Cortex; *RA,* renal artery; *RP,* renal pelvis; *RV,* renal vein; *U,* ureter.

irregular connective tissue composed of collagen and elastic fibers along with occasional smooth muscle cells. Because the kidneys are retroperitoneally positioned along the posterior abdominal wall, they are lined in part by a smooth serosal mesothelium. The kidneys also are partially embraced by adipose tissue (perirenal fat) that covers their ventral borders and is present in the region of the hilum.

KIDNEY STRUCTURE

A partially dissected kidney reveals its general organization, which consists of a darker brown-red **cortex** and a lighter **medulla** (see Figure 16-1). In all domestic species, the cortex lies outside of the medulla. However, there is some variation in the development of both portions, which has resulted in the formation of unilobar kidneys with a unified cortex and medulla, as found in carnivores, horses, and small ruminants, and multilobar kidneys with either partially lobed or deeply lobed cortices and medullae, as seen in pigs and large ruminants, respectively. In the multilobar kidney, the medullary portion is always separated into pyramidally shaped lobes that point toward the hilum. The cortex also may be separated as in the ox and the cow or be fused into a single structure as in the pig.

URINIFEROUS TUBULE

The cortical and medullary components of the kidney are both made up of **uriniferous tubules (renal tubules)** that are the primary structure involved in performing the different functions of this organ and includes the drainage channels that empty into the renal pelvis. In the cortex these tubules originate and become oriented in a highly coiled, tortuous way. The portions that twist and wind are the **convoluted tubules** and compose the **cortical labyrinth** (Figure 16-2). At some point within the cortex, the tubules become straightened as they are directed both to and from the medulla. The clusters of straightened tubules form the **medullary rays,** referring to their imminent association with the medulla. In addition to the cortical labyrinth and medullary rays, the cortex contains numerous, small, dark red, spherical bodies called **renal corpuscles.** The proximal-most portion of the convoluted tubules originates from the renal corpuscle.

The medulla, likewise, consists of a portion of the same uriniferous tubules that extend to and from the medullary rays. Portions of these tubules can be further distinguished according to their location. The part that is closest to the cortex forms the **outer zone** and the part that approaches the ureter forms the

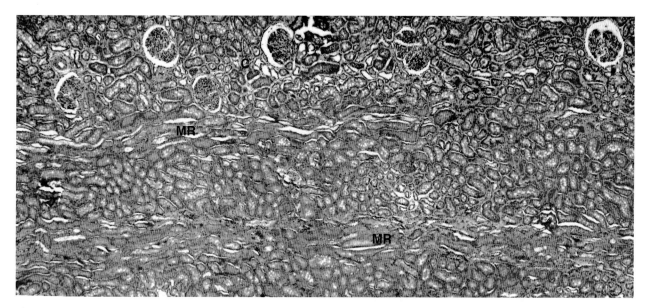

Figure 16-2. Light micrograph of the cortical labyrinth *(C)* and medullary rays *(MR)* within the porcine kidney. (Hematoxylin and eosin stain; ×10.)

inner zone. In multilobar kidneys, the tubules of the medulla of each lobe make up a **renal pyramid,** in which the base (outer zone) of the renal pyramid emanates from the adjoining cortex, and the tip (the **renal papilla**), of each renal pyramid lies next to the renal pelvis.

Nephron of the Uriniferous Tubule

Each renal corpuscle and its associated tubule comprises a **nephron,** the functional and structural unit of the kidney. At the beginning of a nephron, the renal corpuscle gives rise to the **proximal convoluted tubule** (Figure 16-3; see also Figure 16-2) that bends and twists before straightening into the **proximal straight tubule,** which is now a part of a medullary ray. The proximal straight tubule enters the medulla, and at a particular point within the medullary outer zone it narrows into the **thin tubule** that extends into the inner zone, then loops back to the outer zone, where it widens into the **distal straight tubule.** As the distal straight tubule enters the cortex, it returns to its renal corpuscle and from there once again twists and turns, becoming the **distal convoluted tubule.**

Collecting Duct System of the Uriniferous Tubule

The distal convoluted tubule of a nephron empties into a nearby **collecting duct** (collecting tubule) that is shared by other distal convoluted tubules of other

adjacent nephrons. The collecting duct lies within the same medullary ray that holds the proximal straight and distal straight tubular portions of the nephron. The collecting duct then empties into a **papillary duct,** which flows into the renal pelvis.

Nephron Type

Each kidney houses hundreds of thousands of nephrons that are, as one might imagine, more numerous in larger animals (and their larger kidneys). For example, 400,000 or more nephrons exist in the canine kidney, whereas nearly half of that many occur in the kidney of the domestic cat. Within the nephron population, different types have been classified according to either the location of the renal corpuscle within the cortex or the length of thin tubules as they loop within the inner medulla. Renal corpuscles distinguished by their location are **superficial, midcortical,** or **juxtamedullary** (deep cortical). Distinction based on thin tubular length divides nephrons into two types: **short looped** and **long looped** (see Figure 16-3). The short-looped nephron possesses a short thin tubule that loops or turns around within the outer zone of the medulla. In most domestic species the renal corpuscles that lie superficially or midcortically form the short-looped thin tubules. In contrast, the long-looped nephron possesses a long thin tubule that turns around in the inner zone of the medulla. In this instance, the renal corpuscle usually lies near the outer medulla, and thus this type generally fits the juxtamedullary type.

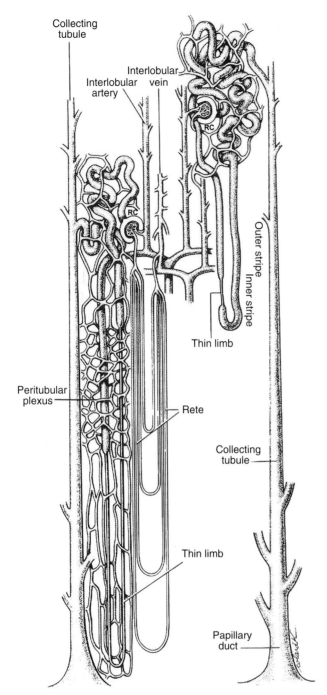

Collecting
tubule

Interlobular
vein

Interlobular
artery

RC

Outer stripe

Inner stripe

Thin limb

Peritubular
plexus

RC

Rete

Collecting
tubule

Thin limb

Papillary
duct

Figure 16-3. Drawing of the nephron and associated collecting ducts. *RC,* Renal corpuscle. *(Modified from Fawcett DW: Bloom and Fawcett: a textbook of histology, ed 11, Philadelphia, 1986, Saunders.)*

NEPHRON

RENAL CORPUSCLE

Each nephron begins with the **glomerulus,** a small, spherical plexus of capillaries and a surrounding cellular sheath and its remarkably thickened basement membrane, that together form the **glomerular capsule (Bowman's capsule)** (Figure 16-4). The glomerulus and its capsule then form the renal corpuscle. The point at which the capillary plexus or rete of the renal corpuscle is arterially supplied and drained is the **vascular pole.** Opposite to the vascular pole, the space between the capsule and the glomerulus is funneled into the attached proximal convoluted tubule and forms the **urinary pole** of the renal corpuscle (see Figure 16-3).

Glomerulus

At the vascular pole of the renal corpuscle is a cluster of anastomosing capillaries supplied by the **afferent glomerular arteriole** and drained by the **efferent glomerular arteriole** (Figure 16-5). The capillaries are lined by a simple squamous endothelium that is basically porous (large fenestrae, but without diaphragms) and designed to contain blood cells, platelets, and macromolecules. This tuft of capillaries (also called the **glomerular rete**) has a well-formed basement membrane within which is a body of pericyte-like cells, the **mesangial cells.** The mesangial cells (or collectively the **mesangium**) effectively replace connective tissue cells within the glomerular rete and occur for a short distance outside the glomerulus but within the vascular pole, referred to at this point as the **extraglomerular mesangium** (Figure 16-6; see also Figure 16-5). Mesangial cells can be phagocytic and may help maintain the basal lamina of the glomerulus, and may have vasoconstrictive properties and participate in the vasodynamics of the capillary blood flow.

The glomerular basement membrane consists of three layers, or laminae. Two of the layers are electron lucent, being those that lie immediately next to the endothelium and farthest away from it, and as a result are known as the **lamina rara interna** and **lamina rara externa,** respectively. These layers possess proteoglycans ladened with heparan sulfate and the usual basement membrane–associated glycoproteins, fibronectin and laminin (Figure 16-7). The middle layer is electron dense and thus called the **lamina densa.** The collagen type IV networks that partly compose the glomerular basement membrane normally undergoes a switch in alpha chains in the dog; if it fails to occur due to mutation or some other reason, it will result in an abnormal basement membrane and subsequently lead to renal failure.

Glomerular Capsule

Each glomerulus is surrounded by its own thickened periodic acid–Schiff (PAS)–positive capsule **(Bowman's**

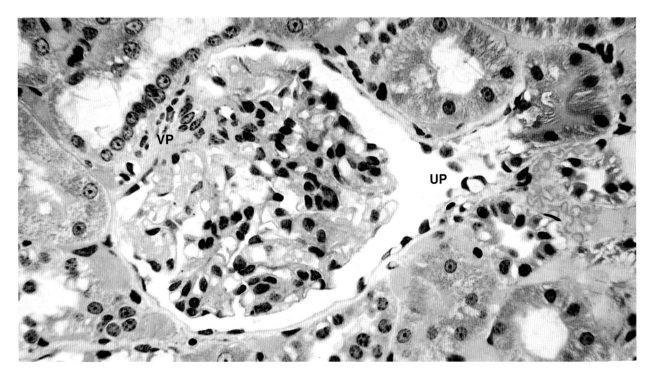

Figure 16-4. Light micrograph of the renal corpuscle of a monkey. *UP,* urinary pole; *VP,* vascular pole. (Plastic section, hematoxylin and eosin stain; ×100.)

capsule) (see Figure 16-7). The capsule is a dilated beginning of the proximal convoluted tubule and consists of a simple squamous epithelium (capsular epithelium). During the development of this cell-lined sphere, the forming glomerular rete pushes the distal end (at what will become the vascular pole) toward the tubule (what will become the urinary pole). In this way, a part of the capsule becomes tightly fitted over the glomerulus. This portion is the **visceral layer** of the glomerular capsule and is composed of a uniquely designed simple squamous epithelium (glomerular epithelium). Although the visceral layer of the glomerular capsule is tightly associated with the glomerular rete on one side, it is free of any contact on its other side, exposed to the **urinary space** that exists between the glomerular epithelium and the rest of the glomerular capsule. The outermost portion of the glomerular capsule, which remains free from any direct involvement with the glomerular rete, is the **parietal layer** (see Figures 16-4, 16-5, and 16-7). This layer consists of a single layer of squamous cells, which effectively holds the plasma filtrate formed by the glomerulus and guides the filtrate to the proximal tubule at the urinary pole. At the vascular pole the simple squamous epithelium becomes confluent with the glomerular epithelium.

GLOMERULAR EPITHELIUM

Cells of glomerular epithelium are **podocytes** (Figure 16-8; see also Figures 16-4 and 16-5). They are named after their principal morphological feature—the presence of numerous footlike or podial cellular processes. These processes extend from larger branches of their cell body and wrap their way around portions of individual capillaries (Figure 16-9). The small processes **(pedicels)** of one branch of the cell interdigitate with the small processes of another branch, leaving only thin spaces, **filtration slits,** between them. The filtration slits are 60 nm or less in width and covered by a thin (6 nm) electron-dense **filter diaphragm.** Cytologically the podocyte has the usual assortment of organelles that are scattered within the large processes or branches of the cell body and surround an oval to irregularly shaped nucleus. The pedicels generally lack organelles, having primarily cytoskeletal elements (filaments and microtubules).

Glomerular Filtration

As blood moves into the glomerular rete from the afferent glomerular arteriole, much of the plasma is able to pass through the capillary endothelium, its

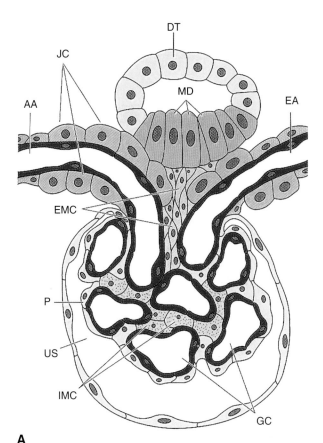

A

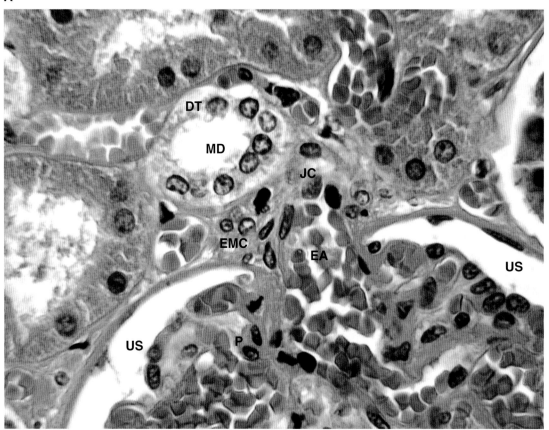

B

Figure 16-5. **A,** Schematic diagram of the vascular pole of the mammalian renal corpuscle. **B,** Light micrograph (×300) of the vascular pole within the porcine renal corpuscle. *AA,* Afferent arteriole; *DT,* distal tubule; *EA,* efferent arteriole; *EMC,* extraglomerular mesangial cells; *GC,* glomerular capillaries; *IMC,* intraglomerular mesangial cells; *JC,* juxtaglomerular cells; *MD,* macula densa; *P,* podocyte; *US,* urinary space.

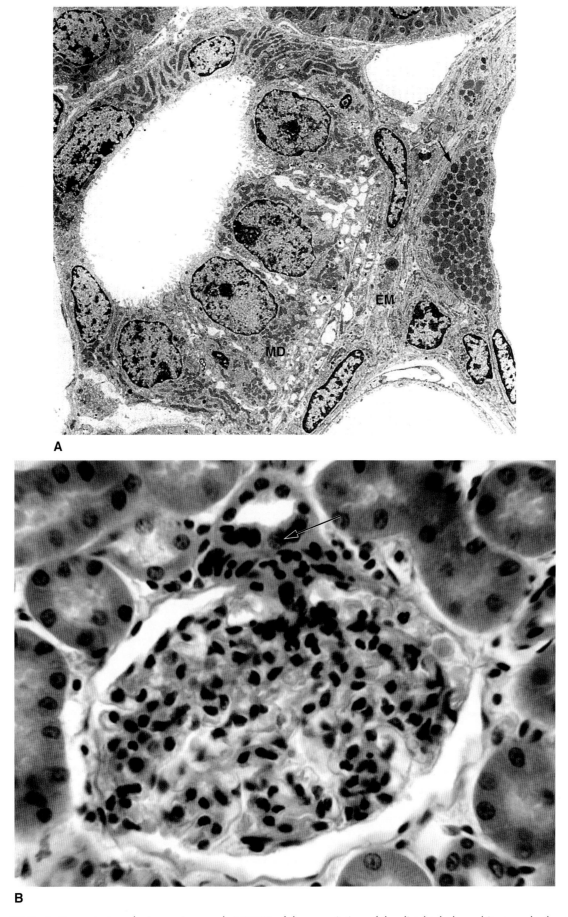

A

B

Figure 16-6. A, Transmission electron micrograph (×3500) of the association of the distal tubule and its macula densa *(MD)* with the extraglomerular mesangial cells *(EM)* along the renal corpuscle of a rat. Arrow points to a juxtaglomerular cell with renin-filled granules. **B,** Light micrograph of the canine renal corpuscle and associated distal tubule with macula densa *(arrow).* (Hematoxylin and eosin stain; ×100.) *(***A** *modified from Brenner BM, Rector FC Jr: The kidney, vol 1, ed 4, Philadelphia, 1991, Saunders.)*

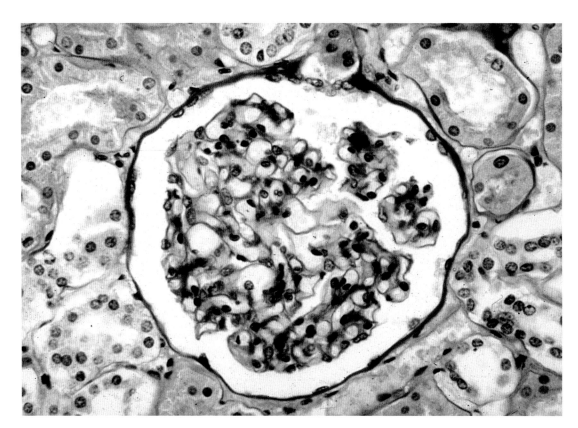

Figure 16-7. Light micrograph of a porcine renal corpuscle stained for carbohydrates to reveal the glomerular basement membrane including the glomerular capsule. (Periodic acid–Schiff stain; ×100.)

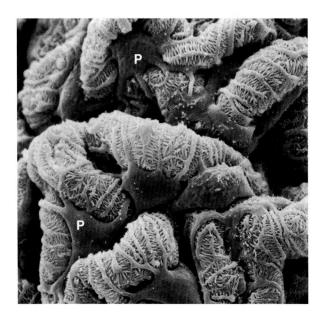

Figure 16-8. Scanning electron micrograph of the podocytes *(P)* that externally line the glomerular capillaries. *(From Brenner BM, Rector FC Jr: The kidney, vol 1, Philadelphia, 1976, Saunders.)*

basement membrane, and pass by the podocytes and their pedicels before entering the urinary space. Larger molecules, such as albumin, that weigh 70,000 daltons and greater have difficulty moving into the urinary space because they are trapped by the glomerular basement membrane. The filter slit and diaphragm of the podocytes, the glomerular basement membrane, and the pores of the capillary endothelium collectively filter blood plasma. The entire plasma supply of an individual is filtered daily in this manner approximately 100 times.

PROXIMAL TUBULE

The ultrafiltrate of plasma that entered the urinary space is immediately guided to the urinary pole and the proximal tubule (Figure 16-10; see also Figure 16-4). The tubules of the kidney, which begin with the proximal tubules, serve to collect, alter, and move the glomerular ultrafiltrate to a system of ducts for its eventual excretion. The first portion of the proximal tubule—the **proximal convoluted tubule**—bends and coils for a considerable distance within the cortex (see Figures 16-2 and 16-3). The proximal convoluted

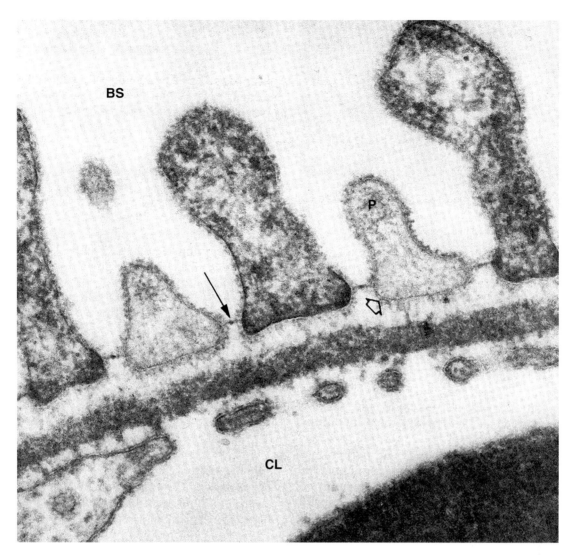

Figure 16-9. Transmission electron micrograph of the pedicels (P) that form filtration slits between them, each with filter diaphragm *(thin arrow)*. *BS,* Bowman's (urinary) space; *CL,* capillary lumen; *open arrow,* lamina rara externa. *(From Brenner BM, Rector FC Jr:* The kidney, *vol 1, Philadelphia, 1976, Saunders.)*

tubule is, in fact, the major component of the cortical labyrinth. When observed light microscopically, the proximal convoluted tubule is lined by a simple cuboidal epithelium (Figure 16-11; see also Figure 16-10). Each cell has a granular, eosinophilic cytoplasm and forms apically numerous long microvilli. Because this portion of the uriniferous tubule is highly tortuous, the characteristic morphology of its cuboidal cell is often difficult to appreciate. It is best to examine those parts of the proximal convoluted tubule that have been medially sectioned. With rapid fixation and proper tissue processing, the cells can be seen to have a brush luminal border. Inadequate preparation of this region of the kidney may cause the tubule to collapse and the lumen to disappear. The granular appearance of the cytoplasm seen histologically is largely due to

the presence of numerous mitochondria, many of which are elongated and oriented api-basally within the cell (Figure 16-12). Microbodies and lysosomes also are often encountered. At the base of most microvilli, caveoli are observed. The presence of the numerous microvilli and caveoli is an indication of the enormous transport activities that these cells perform. Adjacent cells are attached laterally by a well-developed system of interwoven processes. In addition, they are attached to one another by desmosomes, intermediate junctions, and tight junctions. The nucleus is round and positioned toward the base of the cell. The base of the cell forms many infoldings, which, in turn, are anchored to a basement membrane (see Figure 16-12). The infoldings, like the lateral processes, can be quite developed, extending nearly

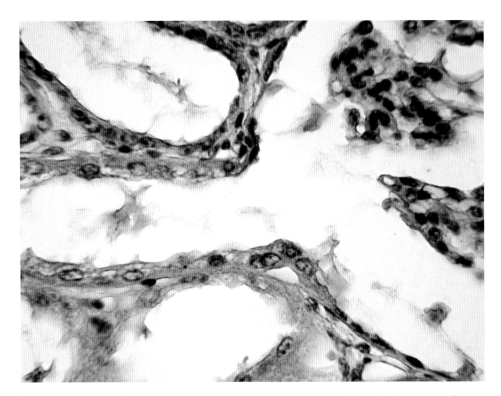

Figure 16-10. Light micrograph of the urinary pole and connecting proximal tubule of a bovine renal corpuscle. (Hematoxylin and eosin stain; ×250.)

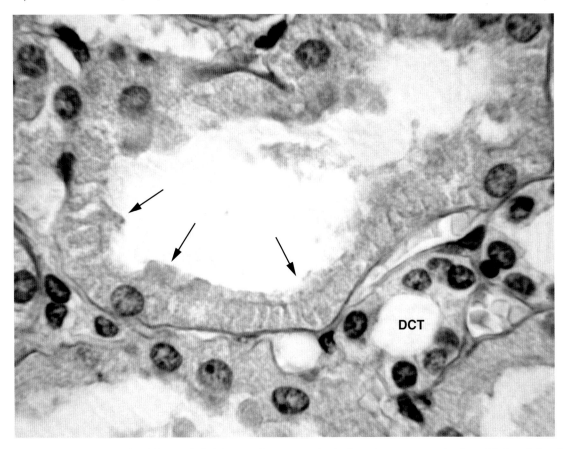

Figure 16-11. Light micrograph of the epithelial lining of a proximal tubule with pronounced microvilli (brush border, *arrows*) and basal infoldings. *DCT,* Distal convoluted tubule. (Periodic acid–Schiff stain; ×400.)

the length of the cell. As the glomerular ultrafiltrate passes through the lumen of the proximal tubule, most of its water and sodium chloride are resorbed and transported to the subjacent loose connective tissue that surrounds the different elements of the cortex and medulla.

When the proximal tubule enters a medullary ray it becomes straight and is referred to as the **proximal straight tubule** (see Figure 16-3). The proximal straight tubule forms the first part of the **loop of the nephron** (Henle's loop). The proximal straight tubule, also called the **descending thick limb** of the loop of the nephron, is composed of a simple cuboidal epithelium similar to that of the proximal convoluted tubule (see Figure 16-3). The cells, however, are not as developed cytoplasmically as those of the proximal convoluted tubule, with fewer organelles and less extensive apical canaliculi and caveoli, lateral intercellular processes, and basal processes. Overall, cells of the proximal straight tubule are shorter in height than those of the proximal convoluted tubule. In domestic carnivores, lipid droplets are variably associated with the cuboidal cells of the proximal tubule. In dogs, the droplets are formed primarily within the cells of the proximal straight tubule, whereas in cats, they occur within cells of the proximal convoluted tubule.

THIN LIMB OF THE LOOP OF THE NEPHRON

Within the medulla the proximal straight tubule narrows and becomes the **thin limb of the loop of the nephron** (Henle's loop), which at first continues toward the renal papilla as the **descending thin limb** and then turns back toward the cortex; it is now referred to as the **ascending thin limb** (Figure 16-13; see also Figure 16-3). At the point where the descending thick limb becomes the descending thin limb, the cuboidal cells are transformed into squamous cells. The lengths of the thin limbs vary; they are generally shorter in nephrons in which the renal corpuscles lie superficially within the cortex, which are the short-looped nephrons, and longer in nephrons in which the renal corpuscles lay juxtamedullarly, being the long-looped nephrons. In both instances, the descending thin limbs begin within the outer zone, resulting in

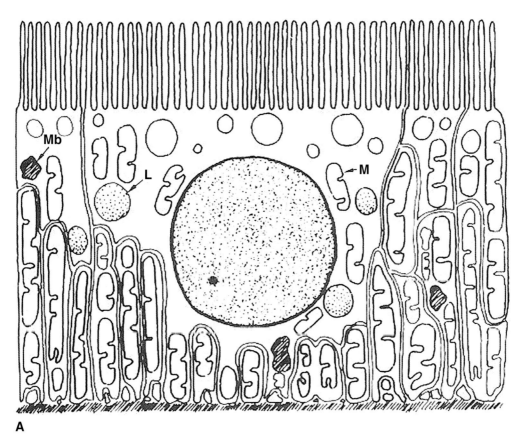

A

Figure 16-12. A, Diagram of the upper proximal tubule characterized in part by the presence of extensive basal infoldings filled with mitochondria *(M). L,* Lysosome; *Mb,* microbody. *Continued*

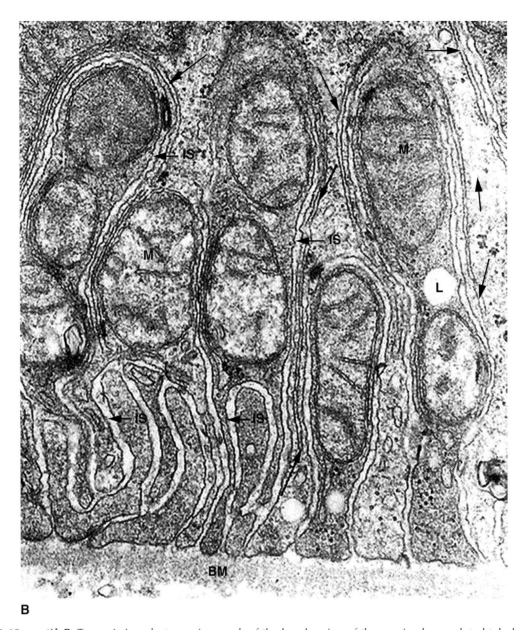

B

Figure 16-12, cont'd B, Transmission electron micrograph of the basal region of the proximal convoluted tubule with numerous mitochondria *(M)*. The arrows point to cell membrane infoldings. *BM,* Basement membrane; *IS,* intercellular space; *L,* lipid droplet. *(From Brenner BM, Rector FC Jr:* The kidney, *vol 1, Philadelphia, 1976, Saunders.)*

the formation of the **outer stripe,** which consists of proximal and distal straight tubules, and the **inner stripe,** consisting of the thin limbs and the remainder of the distal straight tubules (see Figure 16-3). The thin limbs of the short-looped nephrons stay within the inner stripe, the innermost portion of the outer zone of the medulla. The thin limbs of the long-looped nephrons move through the entire width of the outer zone and extend within most of the inner cortex of the medulla. When examined ultrastructurally, the squamous cells can be further distinguished and subdivided into different types on the combined basis of their location within the thin limb of the loop of nephron, their association with the type of nephron (short looped versus long looped), and their morphology, including cellular thickness, intercellular connections (number and extent of lateral interdigitating processes), and presence or absence of basal plasmalemma infoldings (Table 16-1, Figure 16-14). However, when seen histologically, the thin limbs look similar to one another, especially in cross section, where they may be mistaken for blood and lymph vessels that are frequent within this region of the kidney. The thin limbs, however, have thicker squa-

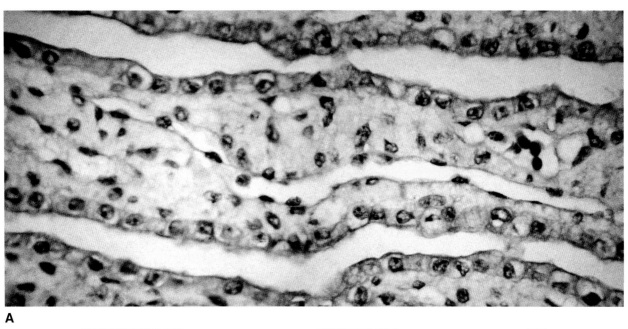

A

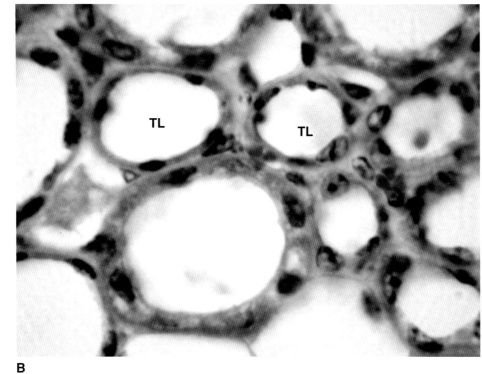

B

Figure 16-13. A, Light micrograph of a thin limb within the inner medulla of the canine kidney. (Hematoxylin and eosin [H&E] stain; ×200.) **B,** Light micrograph of thin limbs *(TL)* and collecting ducts within the medulla of the bovine kidney as seen in cross section. (H&E stain; ×250.)

mous cells and nuclei that protrude into the lumen more than those of vessels, and, of course, lack blood cells altogether (see Figure 16-14). Overall, the thin limbs are permeable to water, permeable within the descending thin limbs and becoming impermeable within the ascending limbs. The thin limbs closely

interact with adjacent interstitial vasculature and provide an osmolarity gradient that increases from the outermost portion of the outer zone of the medulla to the innermost portion of the inner zone. (Further details on the activities of this tissue are described later in this chapter.)

TABLE 16-1   Key Morphological and Functional Characteristics of the Nephron and Associated Collecting Duct System of Domestic Species

REGION	ARCHITECTURAL ORGANIZATION	CELLS (MORPHOLOGY AND ACTIVITY)	FUNCTION
Renal corpuscle: glomerulus	Capillary plexus fed by an afferent arteriole and emptied by an efferent arteriole at the vascular pole; the plexus is lined externally by modified squamous epithelial cells (podocytes)	Capillary endothelium is fenestrated; podocytes form pedicellate interdigitating processes with filtration slits that along with shared basal laminae of the podocytes and capillary endothelium form a filtration barrier; intermesangial cells: polyhedral clustered cells	Blood filtration
Renal corpuscle: glomerular capsule	Epithelium and its thickened basement membrane surround the glomerulus and are separated from it by urinary space	Simple squamous epithelium that reflexes at the vascular pole onto the capillary plexus as podocytes, and joins a cuboidal epithelium at the urinary pole, which drains the filtrate into the proximal tubule	Forms a physical outer shell to house the glomerular filtrate and lead it to the nephron tubule
Proximal convoluted tubule	Undulating thickened tubule that is the widest and longest component of the nephron, extending from the urinary pole to the proximal straight tubule	Simple cuboidal epithelium with long microvilli (brush border) and long basal infoldings with sodium pumps along the basolateral cell membrane; in cats epithelial cells contain lipid	Reabsorbs transcellularly and paracellularly most of the water, sodium and chloride, and all amino acids, glucose, and bicarbonate
Proximal straight tubule	Straightened thickened tubule that can extend within medullary rays either from the outer cortex or inner cortex to the outer medulla zone (outer stripe)	Simple cuboidal epithelium with long microvilli and basal infoldings though both less developed than those of the proximal convoluted tubule; in dogs epithelial cells contain lipid	Continued resorption that occurs in the proximal convoluted tubule
Descending thin tubule of the nephron loop	Narrowed straightened tubule extending from the proximal straight tubule to the inner zone of the medulla (inner stripe), where it continues toward the renal calyx before returning toward the cortex at the loop of the nephron	Simple squamous epithelium: type I within the cortical nephron lacks interdigitation or lateral processes between adjacent cells; type II within outer medullary zone possesses long interdigitating processes as well as basal infoldings; type III within inner medullary zone has less lateral interdigitation than type II	Permeable to water and to a lesser degree salts (sodium and chloride); the filtrate within the lumen becomes increasingly hyperosmotic as it continues to flow into an interstitial environment of high osmolality
Ascending thin tubule of the nephron loop	Narrowed straightened tubule extending from the loop of nephron to the distal straight tubule of the inner zone of the medulla (beginning of the inner stripe)	Simple squamous epithelium: type IV within inner medullary zone possesses long interdigitating processes between adjacent cells but lacks basal infoldings; active pumps occur basolaterally, directing salts to the interstitium	Impermeable to water but permeable to salts (sodium and chloride); the filtrate within the lumen becomes increasingly hypo-osmotic (hypotonic) as it returns to an interstitial environment of low osmolality
Distal straight tubule	Thickened straightened tubule that continues within medullary rays (inner stripe) at junction of inner and outer medullary zones	Simple cuboidal epithelium with shortened height and short apical processes, tight junction, and basal infoldings with numerous mitochondria; active pumps occur basolaterally directing salts to the interstitium	Impermeable to water but permeable to salts (sodium and chloride); the luminal filtrate continues to become increasingly hypotonic
Macula densa and associated region	Thickened tubule continues from the distal straight tubule after shortly entering the cortical labyrinth and contacts vascular pole of the renal corpuscle	Simple columnar epithelium with numerous microvilli, tight junction, and basally associated with the afferent artertiole, juxtaglomerular (JG) cells and extraglomerular mesangial cells; JG cells: modified smooth muscle of the arterial tunica media filled with renin-containing granules	Cells of the macula densa monitor volume and sodium content of luminal filtrate and initiate renin release by JG cells and subsequent formation of angiotensin II
Distal convoluted tubule	Undulating thickened tubule continues from the macula densa and joins the collecting duct directly when superficial or a connecting tubule when located midcortically or juxtamedullarily	Simple cuboidal epithelium with shortened height, apically positioned nuclei and short, few apical processes, tight junction, and long basal infoldings	Resorption of salts (sodium and chloride) when stimulated by aldosterone and resorption of water when exposed to antidiuretic hormone (ADH); maintains glomerular filtration rate when stimulated by prostaglandin
Collecting duct	Thickened straightened tubule with enlarged lumen that increases in width as it approaches the internal limit of the medulla, being joined cortically by distal convoluted tubules and connecting tubules	Simple cuboidal epithelium consisting of mostly principal cells, lightly stained cytoplasm and basally positioned nucleus, and scattered intercalated cells, more intensely stained cytoplasm with greater height and centrally placed nucleus	Resorption of water when exposed to ADH as well as changes in salt due to the increased osmotic pressure gradient within interstitium of the inner medulla

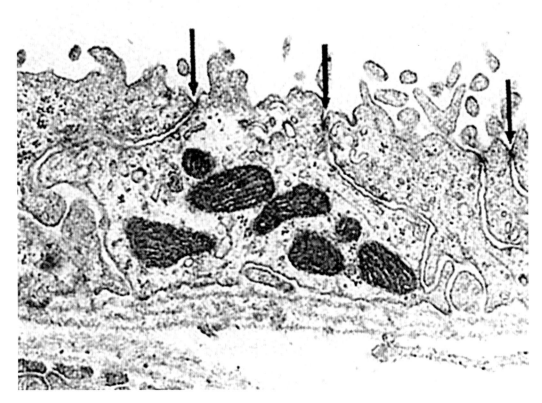

Figure 16-14. Transmission electron micrograph of one of the different epithelial types found along a descending limb of a long-looped nephron. Arrows point to the shallow tight junctions that apically seal the well-developed lateral interdigitations that occur between adjacent cells. *(From Brenner BM, Rector FC Jr: The kidney, vol 1, Philadelphia, 1976, Saunders.)*

DISTAL TUBULE

Regardless of the type of nephron, the ascending thin limb broadens into the **distal straight tubule** within the inner stripe, occurring at the junction of the inner and outer zones of the medulla (see Figure 16-3). As in the continuation of the proximal straight tubule into the descending thin limb, the transition from the ascending thin limb into the distal straight tubule can be gradual or abrupt (Figure 16-15). The distal straight tubule **(ascending thick limb)** consists of a cuboidal epithelium that is shorter than that of the proximal straight tubule. The cells of this epithelium possess numerous mitochondria and basal interdigitations and a well-developed tight junction with one another that enables this tissue to be impermeable to urea and water (see Figure 16-15). In short, this portion of the nephron is able to maintain the appropriate concentrations of water, urea, and salts within its lumen. The distal tubules return via the medullary rays to the renal corpuscles from which they had originated. When the distal straight tubules leave

the medullary rays and complete the loops of their respective nephrons, they enter the cortical labyrinth and become twisted and coiled, much like the proximal counterpart (Figure 16-16). At this point they are referred to as the **distal convoluted tubules.**

The distal convoluted tubule travels a short distance before coming into contact with its associated renal corpuscle near its vascular pole and then continues for a fairly short distance to contort its way to the collecting tubule, where its contents are emptied and the entire nephron has ended. The lengths of the distal convoluted tubules are considerably less than those of the proximal convoluted tubules. For that reason they occupy a much smaller portion of the cortical labyrinth than the proximal convoluted tubules. As in the distal straight tubules, the cuboidal cells of the distal convoluted tubules contain round apically located nuclei and a cytoplasm that contains numerous elongated and sometimes branching mitochondria that are often partitioned within long basal infoldings and scattered rough and smooth endoplasmic reticulum (see Figure 16-15). These cells also form relatively

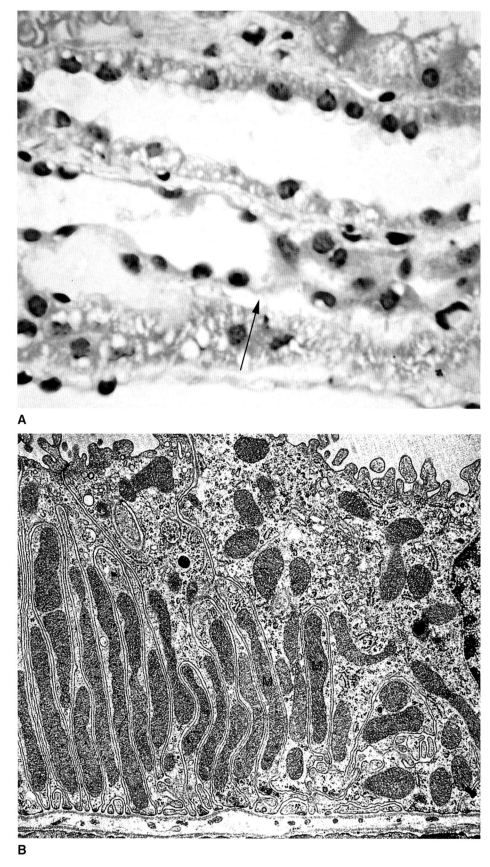

Figure 16-15. A, Light micrograph where a thin ascending limb becomes thickened *(arrow)* within the inner stripe of the pig. (Hematoxylin and eosin stain; ×250.) **B,** Transmission electron micrograph of the distal straight tubule from the kidney of a rat. Numerous elongated mitochondria *(M)* extend nearly the full height of the cell within basal infoldings. *(From Brenner BM, Rector FC Jr: The kidney, vol 1, Philadelphia, 1976, Saunders.)*

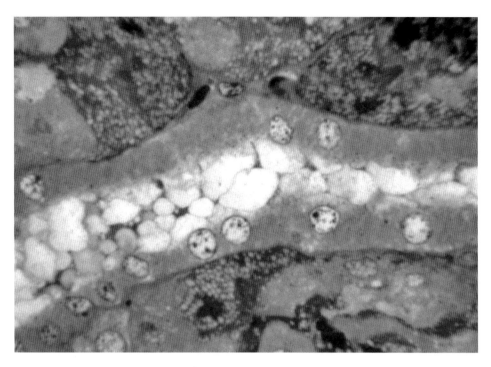

Figure 16-16. Light micrograph of the distal convoluted tubule surrounded by proximal tubules in the porcine kidney. (Toluidine blue stain; ×500.)

few, short apical processes, and, like the cells of the ascending thick limb (distal straight tubule), a junctional complex with a well-developed tight junction. When histologically distinguishing the distal convoluted tubules from the proximal convoluted tubules, the presence of the brush border in the cells of proximal convoluted tubules versus their absence in the cells of distal convoluted tubules is the most obvious feature to observe. In addition, the distal convoluted tubule cells are slightly smaller and stain more palely than their proximal convoluted tubule counterparts (see Figures 16-11 and 16-16).

JUXTAGLOMERULAR APPARATUS

Within a short distance after the distal straight tubule has left the medullary ray and has entered the cortical labyrinth, it comes into contact with vascular pole of its parent renal corpuscle and forms the **juxtaglomerular apparatus.** The portion of the distal tubule that is involved with juxtaglomerular apparatus is the **macula densa,** a cluster of cells that resides immediately adjacent to the vascular pole (see Figures 16-5 and 16-6). The cells of the macula densa tend to have a more crowded and taller appearance than the rest of the cuboidal cells of the tubule (Figure 16-17). As in columnar cells throughout the body, the cellular contents of these cells are arranged with greater

polarity than that of the rest of the distal straight tubule cells, having smooth and rough endoplasmic reticulum, a Golgi apparatus, and smaller and more dispersed mitochondria than that occurring in distal straight tubule cells (see Figure 16-6). Apically the cells have numerous microvilli and are laterally attached by tight junctions near the luminal surface. Basal to the tight junctions, considerable amounts of intercellular space can be encountered. The bases of the cells do not form the usual basal lamina/basement membrane found in most epithelia. Instead cells of the macula densa are intimately associated with the afferent arteriole and the extraglomerular mesangial cells of the renal corpuscle (see Figures 16-5, 16-6, and 16-17). Specifically, the cells of the macula densa lie directly against the outermost cells of the afferent arteriole, the outermost layer of the extraglomerular mesangium, and to a much lesser extent the outermost cells of the efferent arteriole. The arteriolar cells that the macula densa resides next to are modified smooth muscle fibers called **juxtaglomerular cells,** or simply **JG cells,** and comprise a part of the tunica media. The JG cells form variously sized granules that contain **renin,** a proteolytic enzyme (see Figure 16-6, A). These granules tend to be small and can be beyond the practical resolving range of the light microscope. Their abundance varies among species being sparsely populated in the dog. In addition to these cells, a fourth population, the **peripolar cells,** recently has

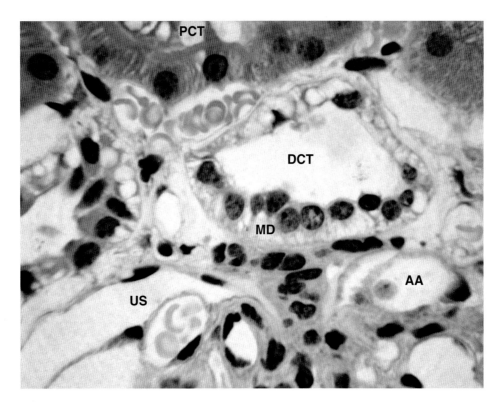

Figure 16-17. Light micrograph of the distal convoluted tubule *(DCT)* and its macula densa *(MD)*. *AA,* Afferent arteriole; *PCT,* proximal convoluted tubule; *US,* urinary space. (Hematoxylin and eosin stain; ×400.)

been determined to be associated with the juxtaglomerular apparatus. These cells are positioned at the point where the parietal and visceral layers of the glomerular capsule are joined. Though their function has yet to be determined, they are largest and most abundant in sheep and goats and least developed in dogs and cattle. The physiologic importance of the rest of the juxtaglomerular apparatus is described later.

COLLECTING DUCT SYSTEM

Each nephron empties its contents into the collecting duct system of the uriniferous tubule, consisting of connecting tubules, collecting ducts, and papillary ducts (see Figure 16-3). The distal convoluted tubules of nephrons with superficially located renal corpuscles become joined as **connecting tubules** that empty directly into the **collecting ducts** (straight collecting tubules). By comparison, one or more distal convoluted tubules of nephrons with midcortical and juxtamedullary located renal corpuscles join **arched connecting tubules** (arched collecting ducts) before their contents are directed into the collecting ducts. In the cortex the collecting ducts are housed within the medullary rays and run along the same axes of the

coexisting descending and ascending limbs of the nephrons (Figure 16-18; see also Figure 16-2). As the collecting ducts continue into the medulla, they fuse and become larger in diameter. The epithelia lining the tubules and ducts are simple cuboidal among domestic species. Two types of cells compose this epithelium: **principal cells** (light cells), with scattered, small mitochondria, and rough and smooth endoplasmic reticula that lie mostly above basally placed round nuclei; and **intercalated cells** (dark cells), which as the name implies are intercalated between the principal cells, being taller, more intensely stained, and generally less numerous than the adjacent principal cells (Figure 16-19). The intercalated cells contain many vesicles and mitochondria and round, centrally placed nuclei. The vesicles lie apically near the luminal surface and are involved in the release of hydrogen ions. These cells are important in maintaining the body's acid-base balance. Outside of guiding the glomerular ultrafiltrate toward the excretory passages, the function of the principal cells is unknown. The principal cell and the intercalated cells together form a well-developed tight junction near the luminal border. Thus, as in the distal tubule, the collecting ducts are impermeable to water. The lateral borders of the principal and

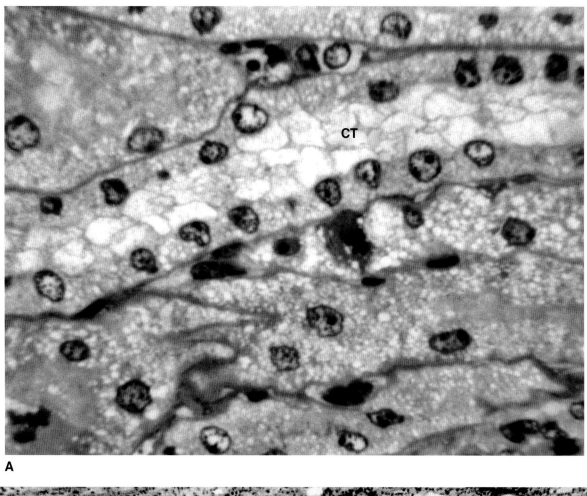

A

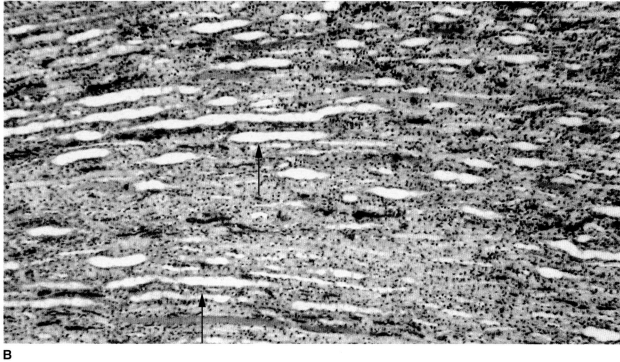

B

Figure 16-18. A, Light micrograph of a collecting tubule *(CT)* within the outer cortex of a pig. (Plastic section, toluidine blue stain; ×400.) **B,** Light micrograph of the numerous collecting ducts *(arrows)* within the medulla of the bovine kidney. (Hematoxylin and eosin stain; ×35.)

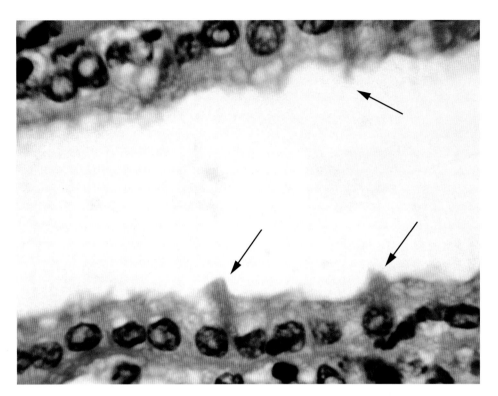

Figure 16-19. Light micrograph of a collecting duct from a bovine kidney. Arrows point to intercalated cells. (Hematoxylin and eosin stain; ×400.)

intercalated cells are well defined and not plicated nearly as much as that occurring within the tubule of the nephron. Neither cell type possesses many microvilli, having instead microplicae.

As the collecting ducts move within the inner zone of the medulla toward the renal crest, they join to form the **papillary ducts** (see Figure 16-3). The papillary ducts are lined by a simple columnar epithelium that consists of tall principal cells. These ducts travel a short distance before opening into the **area cribrosa** at the renal crest or the tips of the pyramids. This is the point where the papillary ducts connect with the renal pelvis or minor calyces, and the simple layered epithelium of the papillary ducts becomes transformed into a transitional epithelium (Figure 16-20).

STROMAL COMPONENTS

RENAL INTERSTITIUM

The uriniferous tubules are supported by a loose connective tissue that is very sparsely developed in the cortex and moderately developed in the medulla. The cortical labyrinth contains only a fine shell of connective tissue elements (fibrocytes and collagen

fibers) that are involved with the basement membranes of the different components of the nephron and its associated vascular bed. In the medulla is a fair amount of connective tissue elements between the limbs of the loops of nephrons, the nearby vessels, and the collecting ducts (see Figure 16-18). In addition to fibrocytes, two other cell types are encountered: macrophages and interstitials cells. **Interstitial cells** are fibroblast-like in appearance, with small branched processes that attach one cell to another and contain lipid droplets. These cells can be found between collecting ducts, loops of the nephrons, and nearby vessels (Figure 16-21).

RENAL CIRCULATION

Both kidneys of the body receive their arterial supply from the abdominal aorta. The renal artery enters the hilum of each kidney and in that vicinity branches into **lobar arteries** and then into **interlobar arteries.** The interlobar arteries move radially along the longitudinal axis of each pyramid until they reach the corticomedullary junction. At that point, they split into **arcuate arteries** that bend or arch their way along the inner margin of the cortex (Figure 16-22). Tributaries of the arcuate arteries, called the **interlobular arteries,** extend outwardly toward the superficial

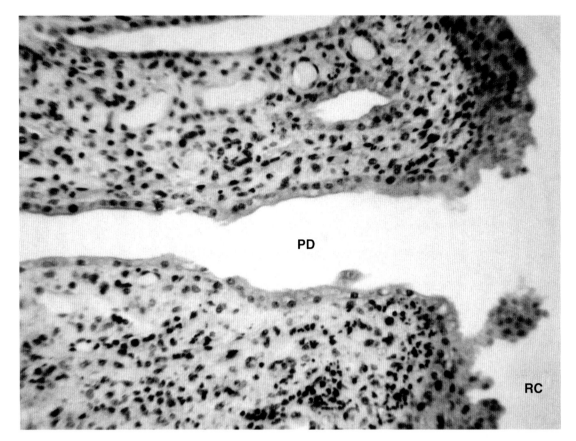

Figure 16-20. Light micrograph of a papillary duct *(PD)* in a bovine kidney. *RC,* Renal calyx. (Hematoxylin and eosin stain; ×100.)

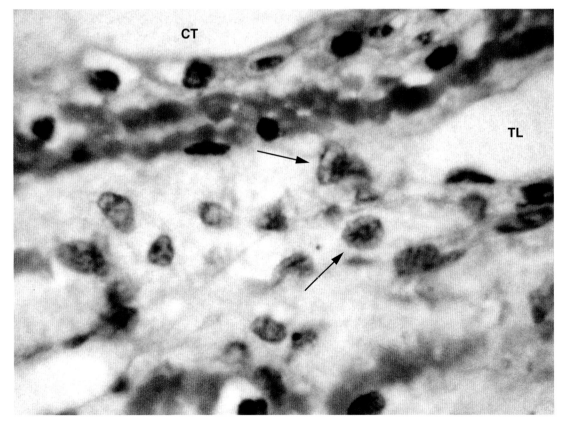

Figure 16-21. Light micrograph of interstitial cells *(arrows)* within the bovine medulla. *CT,* Collecting tubule: *TL,* thin limb. (Hematoxylin and eosin stain; ×400.)

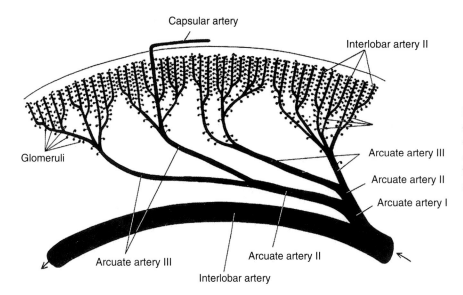

Capsular artery

Interlobar artery II

Glomeruli

Arcuate artery III

Arcuate artery II

Arcuate artery I

Arcuate artery III

Arcuate artery II

Interlobar artery

Figure 16-22. Schematic diagram of the arterial branching in the canine kidney. *(From Fawcett DW:* Bloom and Fawcett: a textbook of histology, *ed 11, Philadelphia, 1986, Saunders.)*

cortex. As each interlobular artery moves toward the kidney surface, smaller branches extend from it, forming the **afferent arterioles** that course their way to the renal corpuscles (see Figure 16-3). At the vascular pole of each renal corpuscle, an afferent arteriole extends inside the capsule of the corpuscle, divides into a small capillary cluster, and becomes the vascular bed of the glomerulus (see Figure 16-5). The capillaries reunite to form the **efferent arteriole** at the base of the vascular pole. From that point, the fate of the efferent arterioles differs according to their location within the cortex. Efferent arterioles of the superficial and midcortical renal corpuscles continue to form the **peritubular plexus** of fenestrated capillaries that surround the uriniferous tubules of the cortex. By comparison, efferent arterioles arising from the juxtamedullary corpuscles move or descend into the adjacent outer zone of the medulla (see Figure 16-3). These arterioles **(descending vasa recta)** become straight and branch within the outer stripe, each following the course of the loop of nephron. Branches of the descending vasa recta form a peritubular plexus or network around the uriniferous tubules of the medulla and empty into venules that return or ascend to the cortex called the **ascending vasa recta.** The distribution of the capillaries between the descending vasa recta and the ascending vasa recta is fairly even along the length of both limbs of the loop of nephron, playing an integral role in the physiology of urine formation. The capillaries of the peritubular plexus of the medulla as well as the venules are fenestrated.

The ascending vasa recta empties into the **arcuate veins** that basically follow the same path as the arcuate arteries. The arcuate veins also collect blood from the **stellate veins** of the cortex. The stellate

veins receive their blood from the peritubular plexus within the cortex. These veins lie superficially beneath the capsule of the kidney and appear star shaped when viewed tangentially. In most domestic species, the stellate veins empty into interlobular veins, which drain into the arcuate veins. The arcuate veins, in turn, flow into the **interlobar veins,** which essentially parallel the interlobar arteries (see Figure 16-22). The interlobar veins join one another before emptying into the **renal vein,** which then leaves the kidney at the hilum to connect to the caudal vena cava. In the cat, the stellate veins, which are more capsular than subcapsular in location, come together at the hilum and drain into the renal vein in a direct manner rather than pass through the interlobular, arcuate, and interlobar veins.

RENAL NERVES AND LYMPHATICS

Each kidney is innervated both afferently and efferently. The nerve fibers, which are mostly sympathetic and unmyelinated, enter the region of the hilum, following a similar course as that of the renal artery. It is generally believed that the smooth muscle component of the arteries and arterioles within the cortex and the medulla is innervated. Other portions of the kidney that are innervated include the juxtaglomerular cells at the vascular pole of the renal corpuscle and the interstitial cells along the loop of nephron.

Like the nervous tissue and the vasculature, the largest lymph vessels lie in the region of the hilum, where they exit the kidney. Smaller lymph vessels exist superficially within the cortex as well as deep within the medulla. Lymph that leaves the kidneys is generally received by lymph nodes near the abdominal aorta and the vena cava.

KIDNEY FUNCTION

The kidney functions to control the body fluid in terms of both its amount and content. Specifically, water, major ions—including hydrogen, sodium, potassium, chloride, and bicarbonate, and various solutes such as sugars and amino acids—can be retained or removed. The conservation of essential metabolites and the removal of metabolic wastes are the two principal activities that the kidneys perform for the body and its fluid. The direct result of these activities is the formation of urine. Besides body fluid conservation and waste removal, the kidneys regulate blood pressure and calcium transport, and can act as organs of secretion, releasing renin, prostaglandins, erythropoietin, and other substances into the bloodstream.

URINE FORMATION

Approximately one fifth of the blood that leaves the heart to enter the general circulation is received by the kidneys. Of that nearly one fifth becomes the glomerular filtrate as the blood passes through the vascular poles of the renal corpuscles. During a 24-hour period, the entire blood supply circulates through the kidneys several hundred times. As one can imagine, an enormous amount of glomerular filtrate is generated daily. However, of that amount only 1% is actually removed or excreted. The following section and Table 16-1 briefly describe the process of urine formation along the uriniferous tubule.

Glomerular Filtration

When blood flows from the afferent arteriole into the tuft of glomerular capillaries, its intracapillary pressure is greater than that of the surrounding environment, being the opposing hydrostatic pressure within the urinary space of the glomerular capsule, as well as the colloid osmotic pressure of the plasma proteins. Because of the combined presence of the basal lamina, the pores of the endothelium, and the slits of the podocytes (all creating the **filtration barrier**) (see Figure 16-9), the blood that normally enters the urinary space of the glomerular capsule is free of cells and restricts molecules according to size, shape, and charge. As a result, molecules that are generally large (macromolecules) and negatively charged (because of the repelling force of the anionic basal lamina and glycocalyx of the endothelial cells and podocytes) are

prevented from passing through the filtration barrier. That portion of the blood that has passed into the urinary space of the glomerular capsule is the **glomerular filtrate,** or the **ultrafiltrate.** Materials continually caught in the filtration barrier are believed to be removed by both podocytes and nearby mesangial cells.

Proximal Tubule

As ultrafiltrate leaves the urinary space of the glomerular capsule and enters the proximal portion of the renal tubule (the proximal tubule) at the urinary pole of the renal corpuscle, it immediately becomes modified. The cuboidal cells lining the proximal tubule resorb much of the ultrafiltrate that flows distally within the tubular lumina. All of the protein and glucose, nearly all of the bicarbonate, and approximately three quarters of the water and the sodium and chloride ions are resorbed along the proximal tubule and subsequently enter the adjacent interstitium (Figure 16-23). Much of the materials resorbed do so by paracellular routes rather than across the cell membranes of the tubular epithelium. This is due to the absence of a well-formed tight junction complex among this epithelium. Movement by the sodium and chloride ions as well as by water is facilitated by Na^+, K^+ ATPase pumps located within their basolateral cell membranes. Similar pumps occur within the apical cell membrane of the tubular epithelium and facilitate the movement of sodium and cotransport amino acids and glucose into these cells. While resorption is occurring, these cells concomitantly release hydrogen (offsetting the bicarbonate resorption), ammonia, and various organic ions into the lumen. As a result, the ultrafiltrate, even though it is continually altered, progresses iso-osmotically to the thin tubule of the loop of the nephron.

Thin Tubule of the Nephron

While the ultrafiltrate travels through the remainder of the loop of the nephron, a differential in the osmotic pressure occurs. From the junction of the cortex and the medulla to the deep inner zone of the medulla is an increasing osmolarity gradient (hypertonicity) maintained by the surrounding interstitium (see Figure 16-23). As the thin limb descends, its simple squamous epithelium remains highly permeable to water and less permeable to sodium, causing water to leave the tubular lumen but making the solute that is still within progressively more concentrated (see Table 16-1). In effect, the intraluminal contents have come into balance with the osmotic gradient of the adjacent interstitium. However, as the

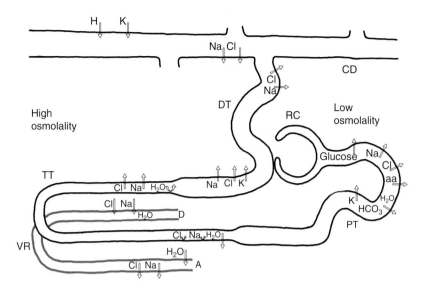

Figure 16-23. Diagram of the histophysiological activity of the nephron within the mammalian kidney. Within the body of the kidney, the medulla is kept at high osmolality by the vasculature, specifically the vasa recta *(VR)*, which establishes an osmotic gradient within the medullary and cortical interstitium. *A,* Ascending; *aa,* amino acids; *CD,* collecting duct; *D,* descending; *DT,* distal tubule; *PT,* proximal tubule; *RC,* renal corpuscle; *TT,* thin tubule.

luminal fluid of what now has high osmolarity moves into the ascending portion of the loop of the nephron, the simple squamous and simple cuboidal epithelia that line both of the thin and thick limbs, respectively, are impermeable to water. Nevertheless, they still remain permeable to salts. This is in part due to the presence of active pumps, such as that for chloride, that direct salts from the lumen to the interstitium. In this way, the level of osmolarity of the fluid within the ascending limbs remains comparable with the neighboring interstitial gradient, while a constant volume is kept within this part of the loop of the nephron. Because the flows of the ascending and descending portions of the loop have essentially countered one another, the mechanism at work here is known as the **countercurrent multiplier system.** The actual driving force behind this system is the occurrence of the increasing osmolarity gradient within the interstitium. To achieve this, a second countercurrent system is established as well, but in this instance involving the vasculature. The vasa recta is important in establishing the osmotic gradient of the interstitium. In this system, the endothelial lining of the descending (arteriola) vasa recta and the ascending (venula) recta are permeable to water and salts (see Figure 16-23). Because the lumen of the arterial component is considerably smaller than that of the venous component, water leaves the descending vasa recta and concomitantly receives salts, while in an opposite manner water enters the ascending vasa recta and concomitantly loses salts. One should keep in mind that the vascular countercurrent system is passive, relying on the forces of osmosis, whereas the countercurrent system of the loop of the nephron is passive and active.

Distal Tubule and Collecting Duct

As the ultrafiltrate reaches the cortex and then enters the cortical labyrinth, it has progressively become hypotonic. The level of osmolarity, however, can vary considerably from one time to another. When the ultrafiltrate reaches the juxtaglomerular apparatus, the cells of the macula densa are believed to monitor the volume of the ultrafiltrate and its sodium content. If critical levels are exceeded, neighboring JG cells are directed to release renin in the vasculature. Renin is an enzyme that converts blood-borne angiotensinogen into angiotensin I, a vasoconstrictor. Angiotensin I, however, is able to be converted into angiotensin II, a hormone that can produce a variety of responses, including potent vasoconstriction, stimulation of the production and release of aldosterone, antidiuretic hormone (ADH, or vasopressin), and prostaglandins, as well as inhibit renin release and increase thirst. Each of these responses affects renal activity. Aldosterone release stimulates the resorption of salts (sodium and chloride) from the lumina of distal convoluted tubules. The release of ADH increases water resorption from the lumina of distal convoluted tubules and collecting ducts. And prostaglandin release maintains the glomerular filtration rate by causing the afferent glomerular arteriole to become vasodilated. Although the conversion of angiotensin I into angiotensin II (by the converting enzyme) can occur in the kidneys, it can occur in other parts of the body, especially the lungs and the lungs' vascular bed.

When the ultrafiltrate or urine reaches the collecting duct, it can become hypotonic (low osmolality). The urine will stay hypotonic unless the collecting duct (and the distal convoluted tubule) is

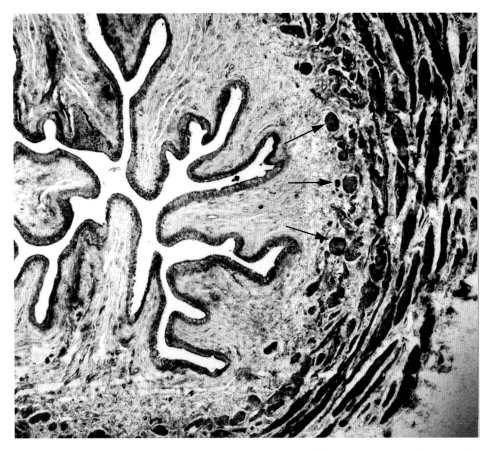

Figure 16-24. Light micrograph of the bovine ureter viewed cross sectionally. Arrows point to the inner layer of the longitudinally oriented smooth muscle within the tunica muscularis. (Hematoxylin and eosin stain; ×15.)

stimulated by ADH to resorb water. Specifically, as the ultrafiltrate moves within the collecting duct toward the inner medulla, it is influenced by the increasing osmotic pressure gradient that has been established by the countercurrent systems of the loop of the nephron and the vasa recta. As a result, water once more leaves the lumen of the uriniferous tubule, entering the hypertonic interstitium. If ADH is absent, water permeability of the collecting duct is lost and the urine remains diluted. In addition, differences that occur in medullary organization among domestic species affect the ability to concentrate urine.

EXCRETORY PASSAGES

Urine that leaves the papillary ducts and in effect has left the uriniferous tubule, enters the excretory passages of the urinary system. The excretory passages consist of the calyces, the pelvis, the ureter, the urinary bladder, and the urethra. The general organization of each structure is consistent with that of tubular organs and the tunica mucosa, propria-

submucosa, muscularis and adventitia and serosa are formed.

When the urine leaves the duct system of each renal papilla, it first enters a funnel-like receptacle, the **calyx,** which then merges and expands into a larger receptacle, the **pelvis.** The mucosal lining of the calyces and the pelvis as well as the rest of the excretory passages consists of a transitional epithelium (see Figure 16-20). In the horse, mucus secreting glands (simple and branched tubuloalveolar) are housed in the propria-submucosa of the pelvis.

Extending from the kidney, the **ureter** guides the urine to the urinary bladder through a lumen lined by a plicated or folded mucosa that continues to be lined by a transitional epithelium and subjacent loose connective tissue, comprising the lamina propria-submucosa (Figure 16-24). This tissue is surrounded by a two- or sometimes three-layered tunica muscularis. Unlike organization of the gastrointestinal tract, the outer layer is oriented in a circular manner, and the inner layer is oriented longitudinally. As the ureter approaches the urinary bladder, an additional layer of muscle, which is also longitudinally oriented, externally covers the circular layer. Peristalsis of these layers results in moving the urine to the urinary bladder. The tunica muscularis is then lined either by an adventitia or a thin tunica serosa.

Urine that drains into the **urinary bladder** is stored there until the internal pressure within the bladder reaches a point that initiates the need for micturition. Histologically, the urinary bladder differs to some extent from that of the ureter. Although it has an internal lining consisting of a transitional epithelium, only the cat possesses a propria-submucosa. Among the rest of the domestic species, the submucosa is distinguished from the mucosa by the mucosa's lamina muscularis. The smooth muscle comprising the tunica muscularis (the detrusor muscle) is more oblique and interwoven and lacks specific circular layers. The transitional epithelium of the urinary bladder is able to undergo a considerable transformation in shape (see Figures 3-18 and 3-19). When the urinary bladder has been emptied, the epithelium thickens and the mucosa becomes folded. Emptying or voiding of the bladder is referred to as **micturition** and is the result of voluntary caudal brainstem activity, which in turn is under cerebellar and cortical control. In order for the urinary bladder to fill, parasympathetic innervation of the detrusor muscle has to be inhibited while the sympathetic innervation of the detrusor is stimulated, inhibiting contraction, along with stimulation of the pudendal nerve, which closes the urethral sphincter. Histological description of the urethra is presented in the male reproductive system (see Chapter 18).

SUGGESTED READINGS

Bankir L, De Rouffignac C: Urinary concentrating ability: insights from comparative anatomy, *Am J Physiol* 249:R643, 1985.

Brenner BM: *The kidney,* Philadelphia, 1996, Saunders.

Brenner BM, Rector FC Jr: *The kidney,* vol 1, Philadelphia, 1976, Saunders.

Brenner BM, Rector FC Jr: *The kidney,* vol 1, ed 4, Philadelphia, 1991, Saunders.

Eisenbrandt DL, Phemister RD: Postnatal development of the canine kidney: quantitative and qualitative morphology, *Am J Anat* 154:179, 1979.

Fawcett DW: *Bloom and Fawcett: a textbook of histology,* ed 11, Philadelphia, 1986, Saunders.

Gartner LP, Hiatt JL: *Color textbook of histology,* Philadelphia, 1997, Saunders.

Gibson IW, Gardiner DS, Downie I, et al: A comparative study of the glomerular peripolar cell and the renin-secreting cell in twelve mammalian species, *Cell Tissue Res* 277:385, 1994.

Harvey SJ, Zheng K, Sado Y, et al: Role of distinct type IV collagen networks in glomerular development and function, *Kidney Int* 54:1857, 1998.

Spangler WL: Ultrastructure of the juxtaglomerular apparatus in the dog in a sodium-balanced state, *Am J Vet Res* 40:802, 1979.

Yadava RP, Calhoun ML: Comparative histology of the kidney of domestic animals, *Am J Vet Res* 73:958, 1958.

Endocrine System

KEY CHARACTERISTICS

- Glandular system with close vascular association
- Secretes chemicals called *hormones* into adjacent bloodstream, targeted for various organs throughout the body

The **endocrine system** regulates the metabolism of many organs and their tissues throughout the body, and in doing so provides corporal homeostasis in tandem with the central nervous system (CNS). Whereas the CNS governs the activities of different components of the body rapidly through the transmission of electrical signals, the endocrine system directs activities in a slower and more sustained way by releasing secretions known as **hormones** that are guided by the vascular system to their destinations— **target organs.** We will see that even though the endocrine system and the CNS operate in different ways they are intertwined and interdependent.

The endocrine system consists of a collection of glands that are dispersed throughout the thorax and the head and range from collections or nests of cells within organs to individual organ entities. Those that comprise organs include the **pituitary** (hypophysis), **pineal, thyroid, parathyroid,** and **adrenal glands.** Portions of the endocrine system that exist as collections of cells within other glands include the **pancreatic islets** (islets of Langerhans), **neurosecretory neurons of the hypothalamus,** and endocrine cells associated with the male and female reproductive systems, known as **interstitial cells of the testes,** and **endocrine-secreting cells of the interna theca, granulosa, and corpus luteum,** respectively.

HORMONES

The singular common feature that places each component of the collection of glands within the endocrine system is their ability to synthesize a compound that is released into an adjacent vascular bed and is subsequently targeted for specific receptor(s). The receptor can be either on or within specific cells. If on a targeted cell, the receptor is associated directly with the cell membrane. If the receptor is within the cell's cytoplasm, the hormone should be able to diffuse through the cell membrane.

Hormones can be separated initially based on whether they are water soluble or insoluble. Those that are **water insoluble** are lipid soluble and composed of steroid and fatty acid derivatives. Water-insoluble hormones are able to diffuse through the cell membrane and connect with cytoplasmic-borne receptors. Hormones of this type include testosterone, estradiol and progesterone. Upon binding with the respective receptor, the hormone-receptor complex moves into the nucleus and binds to a portion of a strand of deoxyribonucleic acid (DNA) near a promoter site for gene transcription.

By comparison, **water-soluble hormones** can bind to receptors at the level of the cell membrane. Hormones of this type consist of polypeptides and proteins, such as insulin and follicle-stimulating hormone. The binding of the hormone to the cell-surface receptor can result in the phosphorylation of specific regulatory proteins (such as cyclic adenosine monophosphate [AMP] and cyclic guanosine monophosphate [GMP]) by a protein kinase. The regulatory proteins then act as second messengers that initiate a signal transduction. In addition to polypeptides and proteins, water-soluble hormones can include amino acid derivatives such as epinephrine. As epinephrine binds to its receptor, it also associates with guanosine triphosphate–binding proteins (G proteins) needed for the appropriate hormone-induced signal induction.

After successful activation of a target cell, an inhibitory signal is usually formed. This signal is responsible for providing a feedback mechanism that directly or indirectly stops the production and secretion of the hormone.

PITUITARY (HYPOPHYSIS CEREBRI)

The **pituitary (hypophysis)** lies in a fossa within a recess, the sella turcica, of the sphenoid bone. In a number of ways this structure can be considered the single-most important gland of the endocrine system, providing hormones for the control of growth, metabolism, and reproduction. Embryologically derived from the oral ectoderm and neuroectoderm, the pituitary consists of two portions, the **adenohypophysis** and the **neurohypophysis.** The adenohypophysis originates from an epithelial evagination (Rathke's pouch) of the cranial portion (the developing pharynx) of the developing digestive tract that moves dorsally toward the cranium. Concomitantly, the developing diencephalon protrudes or evaginates in a similar manner, moving ventrally toward Rathke's pouch. This extension of the CNS forms the embryonic neurohypophysis. As the two extensions meet and join one another, the epithelial evagination (the developing adenohypophysis) loses its connection altogether from the pharynx. The rates of develop-

ment of the two portions of the pituitary during embryonic growth vary among domestic species. As a result, the shape and amount of tissue for each portion differ considerably (Figure 17-1).

Because of their different embryonic origins, the two portions of the pituitary contrast sharply in both their histological construction and physiological activities. The adenohypophysis, which is epithelial in appearance and glandular in function, is composed of three parts: the pars distalis, the pars intermedia, and the pars tuberalis. The **pars distalis (pars anterior)** in most instances makes up the largest portion of the adenohypophysis, being positioned anterior and ventral within the pituitary. In the horse and the dog, the pars distalis can encircle much of the neurohypophysis as well as another portion of the adenohypophysis, the pars intermedia (Figure 17-2; see also Figure 17-1). The **pars intermedia** is the part of the adenohypophysis that with regard to its location is most intimately associated with the neurohypophysis, being immediately apposed to it. The third part of the adenohy-

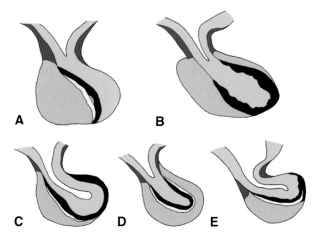

Figure 17-1. Schematic diagram of the pituitary glands (hypophyses) of domestic species along their midline. *(A)*, large ruminants; *(B)*, horse; *(C)*, pig; *(D)*, dog; *(E)*, cat; light blue, pars distalis; dark blue, pars tuberalis; black, pars intermedia; green, neurohypophysis with infundibular recess; beige, hypophyseal cleft.

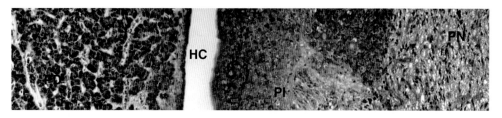

Figure 17-2. Light micrograph of a narrow portion of the canine pituitary gland, extending externally from the pars distalis (PD) to its internal-most region, the pars nervosa (PN) with the pars intermedia (PI) and hypophyseal cleft (HC) in between. (Hematoxylin and eosin stain; ×100.)

pophysis, the **pars tuberalis,** lines the base of the neurohypophysis as the latter extends away from the brain (see Figure 17-1).

The neurohypophysis can be separated into three parts: the median eminence, the infundibulum, and the pars nervosa, each a continued extension of the other (Figure 17-3; see also Figure 17-1). The three confluent parts have morphologic features not dissimilar to those found within the CNS in that they consist of nerve fibers and glia. Likewise, each part is externally lined by the same protective capsule of dense connective tissue. The **median eminence** is the proximal-most portion, extending from the hypothalamus and lying next to the third ventricle. The median eminence leads into the next part of the neurohypophysis, the infundibulum. The **infundibulum** forms the middle portion of the neurohypophysis, extending from the median eminence to the pars nervosa. The **pars nervosa (lobus nervosus)** is the distal-most portion of the neurohypophysis that may end in a lobelike body.

VASCULATURE

The pituitary, like all endocrine glands, possesses a well-developed vascular bed. Although the vascular tree that supplies the blood vessels of the pituitary varies among domestic species, the trees within the pituitary form the same basic pattern. The hypophyseal arteries supply vascular beds for both the adenohypophysis and neurohypophysis (see Figure 17-3). Its superior or rostral-most portion gives rise to an extensive primary capillary bed within the median eminence and supplies the infundibulum and adjacent pars tuberalis. The capillaries of the median eminence coalesce and drain into the pars distalis via a portal system of veins that branch and form a secondary capillary bed throughout the pars distalis (see Figure 17-3). The vessels descending from the primary capillary bed to form the secondary one comprise the **hypophyseal portal system.** It is through the hypophyseal portal system that the neurohypophysis and associated neurons of the hypothalamus are able to direct the

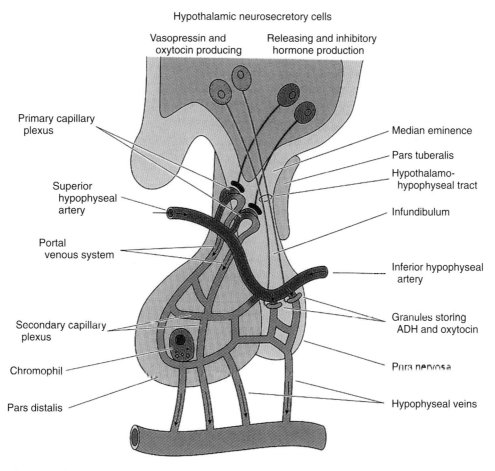

Figure 17-3. Schematic diagram of the vasculature associated with the mammalian pituitary gland. *ADH,* Antidiuretic hormone.

adenohypophysis, especially the pars distalis, and its secretory activities.

The hypophyseal arteries also provide a vascular bed for the pars nervosa of the neurohypophysis. Specifically, the inferior hypophyseal arteries and collateral vessels originating from the hypophyseal portal system contribute to the formation of this bed, which serves to receive neurosecretory granules released by the axonal terminations or endings of the neurons of the hypothalamus (see Figure 17-3).

ADENOHYPOPHYSIS

Pars Distalis

The **pars distalis** is composed of secretory cells arranged in cords and clusters separated by sinusoids that form the secondary capillary bed previously described. Traditionally, the secretory cells of this portion of the pituitary have been characterized and distinguished by classic histochemical means into chromophobic and chromophilic categories. Chromophobic cells, as the name implies, have little reaction with traditional stains and dyes. Chromophilic cells have been separated further on the affinities that the granules have for acidic or basic stains or dyes into two subgroups or populations: **acidophils** and **basophils.**

More recently, the cells have been characterized by immunohistochemical methods, revealing subpopulations involved in the production of specific hormones (Table 17-1). As a result, the cells of the pars distalis are presently described by both histochemical and immunohistochemical means.

Acidophils. These cells of the pars distalis possess granules that react positively when stained with an acidic stain such as eosin (Figures 17-4 and 17-5). These small, rounded cells form the most numerous population of secretory cells within the pars distalis. Immunolabeling methods have further characterized and subdivided acidophils into two subtypes: somatotropes and lactotropes.

Somatotropes store evenly sized granules 300 to 400 nm in diameter formed and interspersed by extensive rough endoplasmic reticulum and a moderately developed Golgi apparatus. These cells produce the **growth hormone (GH),** also called **somatotropin** or **somatotropic hormone (STH)** that induces cell division and enlargement, hyperplasia and hypertrophy to occur among somatic cells. The effects of GH are usually facilitated by additional proteins **(somatomedins)** that are released elsewhere, such as the liver and kidney, and can have a profound influence on specific tissue development of long bones, for example. The secretion of GH is governed by its own

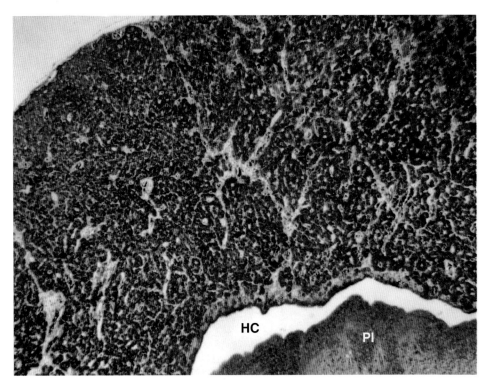

Figure 17-4. Light micrograph of the pars distalis in the dog. *HC,* Hypophyseal cleft; *PI,* pars intermedia. (Hematoxylin and eosin stain; ×20.)

TABLE 17-1 Key Morphological and Functional Characteristics of the Glands of the Endocrine System among Domestic Species

GLAND	ARCHITECTURAL ORGANIZATION	CELL MORPHOLOGY	FUNCTIONAL CORRELATION (AND SPECIES VARIATIONS)
Pituitary: adenohypophysis	Pars distalis: parenchymal cords with reticular fibers and sinusoidal capillaries	Secretory cells are generally polyhedral, usually with granules and divided histochemically into types: **acidophils**—granules positively react with acidic stains, consisting of somatotropes with 300- to 400-nm granules of STH (GH) and lactotropes with 600-nm granules of prolactin; **basophils**—granules react with positive stains, consisting of corticotropes with 200- to 400-nm granules of ACTH and β-LPH, thyrotropes with 150-nm granules or less of TSH, and gonadotropes with 200-nm granules or more of FSH or LH; **chromophobes**—granular to agranular weakly staining cells without known function(s)	STH increases metabolic rates of most cells and stimulates somatomedin release for cartilage and long bone development; prolactin promotes mammary gland development during pregnancy and milk production after parturition; ACTH stimulates corticosteroid production; TSH stimulates thyroglobulin production; FSH stimulates secondary ovarian growth and estrogen production
	Pars intermedia: parenchymal cords, clusters and small follicles and sinusoidal capillaries	Secretory cells are generally polyhedral and basophilic (basophils) with a subpopulation of melanotropes with granules of MSH	Well developed in the horse and pig; least developed in ruminants; MSH stimulates melanin synthesis
	Pars tuberalis: parenchymal clusters and small follicles	Cells with mildly basophilic granules, may or may not be secretory; occasionally basophils of the pars distalis may occur	
Pituitary: neurohypophysis	Hypothalamohypophyseal tract: axons from supraoptic and paraventricular nuclei of the hypothalamus	Axons remain unmyelinated extending from the two nuclei toward the pars nervosa containing small granules filled with either ADH (from the supraoptic nerve) or oxytocin (from the paraventricular nerve) within infundibular stalk	ADH conserves body water through renal resorption, and can contract arterial smooth muscle (raising blood pressure); oxytocin causes uterine smooth muscle contraction during conception and parturition, and assists in milk let-down by stimulating myoepithelial cell contraction within mammary glands
	Pars nervosa: axonal endings surrounded by a fenestrated capillary bed	Axons dilate at their endings next to the blood vessels; pituicytes with astrocyte-like processes support axons and their endings	
Pineal	Parenchymal cords, clusters and small follicles and sinusoidal capillaries	Secretory cells (pinealocytes) contain vesicles of melatonin and serotonin; are somewhat stellate with prominent round nuclei within their cell bodies with scattered radiating processes contacting nearby pinealocytes or blood vessels; support cells consist mostly of astrocytic glia; calcium-ladened concretions (corpora arenacea) develop with age extracellularly	Melatonin is released at night and serotonin during the day and together facilitate the body's biological clock and circadian rhythms
Thyroid	Small to large follicles, each lined by a capillary bed	Follicular cells form a simple cuboidal epithelium with short, variably numbered microvilli, centrobasally placed round nuclei, and surrounded by acidophilic cytoplasm with well-developed Golgi apparatus and involved in T_4 and T_3 production; additional parenchymal cell is the parafollicular cell, being round to polyhedral, lying singly or in clusters with large round nucleus surrounded by pale cytoplasm containing calcitonin-filled granules	T_4 and T_3 increase metabolism and rate of growth, stimulate carbohydrate and fat metabolism, decrease cholesterol and triglycerides and increase fatty acids, increase heart rate and respiration, decrease body weight; calcitonin suppresses bone resorption and lowers plasma calcium level

Continued

TABLE 17-1 Key Morphological and Functional Characteristics of the Glands of the Endocrine System among Domestic Species—cont'd

GLAND	ARCHITECTURAL ORGANIZATION	CELL MORPHOLOGY	FUNCTIONAL CORRELATION (AND SPECIES VARIATIONS)
Parathyroid	Parenchymal cords and clusters intertwined closely with capillaries	Major type of secretory cell, the principal cell (chief cell), can possess lightly eosinophilic cytoplasm with presence of lipids, glycogen, and lipofuscin (inactive state) or darkly stained cytoplasm filled with parathyroid hormone–bearing secretory granules (active state)	Parathyroid hormone increases calcium level in body fluids; light and dark principal cells are randomly configured in most domestic species, but separated in small ruminants with the active (dark) cells located centrally
		An additional secretory cell in some species, the oxyphil cell is twice the size or greater than the principal cell with an eosinophilic cytoplasm with few granules and occurs singly or in small clusters	The function of the oxyphil cell is unknown; found in large ruminants and horses (and humans)
Adrenal	Outer cortex: parenchyma forms irregular clusters or glomeruli (zona glomerulosa) or arcades (zona arcuata)	Secretory cells are usually rounded to polyhedral in zona glomerulosa and columnar in zona arcuata, mildly acidophilic with smooth ER, mitochondria, some lipid droplets, and few to no granules, and secrete mineralocorticoids (aldosterone)	Mineralocorticoids stimulate the excretion of K$^+$ and the resorption of Na$^+$ within the renal distal tubules and in doing so, regulate balance of electrolytes and body fluid volume
	Middle cortex: parenchyma forms radially oriented cords or fascicles (zona fasciculata)	Secretory cells are cuboidal to polyhedral, mildly acidophilic with smooth ER, mitochondria, many lipid droplets, and secrete glucocorticoids (cortisol and cortisone)	Glucocorticoids help regulate carbohydrate, protein and fat metabolism, provide anti-inflammatory activity, reduce capillary permeability, and suppress immune response
	Inner cortex: parenchyma forms reticulated cords (zona reticularis)	Secretory cells are cuboidal to polyhedral, acidophilic with smooth ER, mitochondria, lipid droplets (though fewer than those seen in the zona fasciculata), and lipofuscin, and secrete androgens (dehydroepiandrosterone) as well as glucocorticoids	In addition to the glucocorticoid functions, the androgens can provide weak male-related characteristics and may be metabolized to other sex hormones
	Medulla: irregular parenchymal cords and clusters intermingled with sinusoidal capillaries	Secretory cells are large, polyhedral or columnar, with chromaffin-positive granules containing catecholamines (epinephrine and norepinephrine), numerous mitochondria and well-developed Golgi apparatus; in domestic herbivores larger, often columnar cells containing epinephrine form an outer region, whereas smaller, polyhedral cells containing norepinephrine form an inner region	Epinephrine generates "fight or flight" in response to sudden fear or stress by a variety of effects including the increase in heart rate and cardiac output, release of glucose from liver and skeletal muscle, and vascular shunting and blood flow augmentation to organs; norepinephrine constricts blood vessels and elevates blood pressure
Pancreatic islets	Irregular parenchymal clusters intermingled with sinusoidal capillaries	Secretory cells are generally polyhedral, usually with granules and divided histochemically into four types: A (α) cells have numerous Gomori aldehyde fuchsin red-positive granules containing glucagon; B (β) cells have numerous Gomori aldehyde fuchsin purple-positive granules containing insulin; C cells have few or no granules and may represent developing A, B, or D cells; D (δ) cells are generally smaller and have a heterogeneous population of granules containing somatostatin	Glucagon increases blood sugar levels; insulin decreases blood sugar levels; somatostatin inhibits the release of hormones by A and B cells within the islets, and reduces smooth muscle contractility within the alimentary canal and gallbladder; A cells are positioned along islet periphery in cattle, centrally in the horse

ACTH, Adrenocorticotropic hormone; *ADH,* antidiuretic hormone; *β-LPH,* lipotropic hormone; *ER,* endoplasmic reticulum; *FSH,* follicle-stimulating hormone; *GH,* growth hormone; *LH,* luteinizing hormone; *MSH,* melanocyte-stimulating hormone; *STH,* somatotropic hormone; *TSH,* thyroid-stimulating hormone.

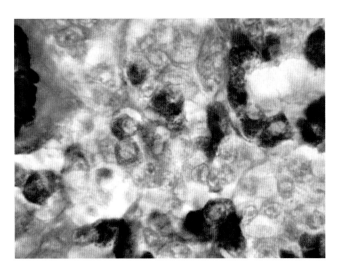

Figure 17-5. Light micrograph of distinctly stained acidophils within the pars distalis of the horse. (Mallory stain; ×400.)

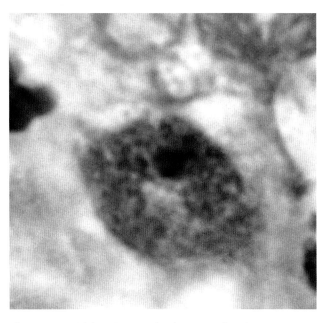

Figure 17-6. Light micrograph of an occasional lactotrope within the pars distalis of a mare. (Mallory stain; ×1000.)

releasing and inhibiting factors, somatotropin-releasing hormone and somatostatin, respectively.

Lactotropes form and store larger—600 nm or more in diameter—granules than those of somatotropes. The large granules, in fact, consist of smaller granules that have fused together. The granules hold the hormone **prolactin,** which during pregnancy promotes the development of the mammary glands and after pregnancy promotes lactation. As one might surmise, these cells are most developed in females, especially those that are pregnant or recently were pregnant. Among the females of domestic species, such as mares, lactotropes (Figure 7-6) and somatotropes are comparable in number. However, in males, lactotropes are fewer and more isolated than somatotropes and are seen singly rather than in clusters.

Basophils. Basophils are much more sparsely populated within the pars distalis than acidophils (Figure 17-7). However, these cells are generally larger than acidophils. As in acidophils, the cytoplasm of this population of cells contains granules, but in this instance react basophilically with stains such as hematoxylin (see Figure 17-7). They also can react positively with periodic acid–Schiff (PAS) reagent because of the strong carbohydrate component of the glycoproteins stored within these granules. With the assistance of immunohistochemistry, three subtypes have been identified: corticotropes, thyrotropes, and gonadotropes.

Corticotropes are widely scattered throughout the pars distalis and possess small to moderately sized granules, 200 to 400 nm in diameter, that contain the hormones **adrenocorticotropic hormone (ACTH)** and

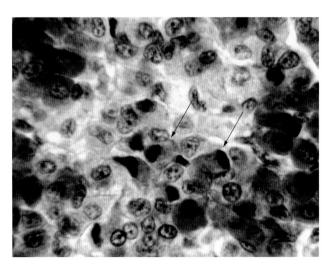

Figure 17-7. Light micrograph of scattered basophils *(arrows)* within the pars distalis of a rat. (Mallory stain; ×400.)

beta-lipotropic hormone (β-LPH). ACTH activates the release cells' secretory products within the adrenal cortex, specifically cortisol and corticosterone. The release of ACTH into the bloodstream by the corticotropes is, in turn, stimulated by the corticotropin-releasing hormone (CRH). Depending on the species, the shape of corticotropes can vary from round to oval or even stellate.

Thyrotropes by comparison are concentrated within the midventral portion of the pars distalis. These cells, which lie within parenchymatous cords, form small granules (150 nm in diameter or less) that hold **thyroid-stimulating hormone (TSH),** also called **thyrotropin,** which is responsible for thyroid hormone production. Although the production of TSH is stimulated by **thyrotropin-releasing hormone (TRH),** it is inhibited by the negative feedback of the thyroid hormones, **triiodothyronine (T_3)** and **thyroxin (T_4).**

Gonadotropes, which make up the last subtype of basophil, are indistinctive round cells dispersed within the pars distalis. These cells possess an extensive rough endoplasmic reticulum and associated Golgi apparatus, which produce small granules approximately 200 nm or greater in diameter. Each granule stores either **follicle-stimulating hormone (FSH)** or **luteinizing hormone (LH)** and can be stimulated to be released by the **gonadotropin-releasing hormone (GnRH).** In the female, FSH stimulates the growth of secondary follicles within the ovary, and estrogen secretion. In the male, it stimulates sustentacular cells (Sertoli cells) to form androgen-binding protein. LH assists FSH in ovarian development, causing the follicle to attain its full size and help promote ovulation, corpus luteal development, and secretion of progesterone as well as estrogen. In the horse it recently has been found that gonadotropes consist of several subpopulations of cells that are able to produce and release either FSH or LH or both at a specific time.

Chromophobes. In addition to acidophils and basophils is another population of parenchymatous cells within the pars distalis. This population has little to no affinity for most stains and dyes that are used to histochemically reveal and characterize cells of the body, and as a result has been referred to as **chromophobes** (see Figures 17-4 through 17-7). Some of the chromophobes can be found to stain weakly. These cells, which are small and possess some granules, may represent chromophils that either have lost or secreted most of their granules or are newly forming chromophils that have recently arisen from stem cells. Some chromophobes lack granules altogether. Whereas some of these cells are likely to be stem cells, some of the cells line follicles (i.e., follicular cells) and appear to be secretory. However, functional activities of these cells have remained a mystery. Some of the agranular, nonstaining chromophobes have a stellate shape. These cells are widely dispersed throughout the pars distalis and are in contact with one another by the formation of gap junctions along their interconnecting long processes. It is unknown whether these cells provide physiological and/or physical support for secretory cells of the pars distalis.

Pars Intermedia

The **pars intermedia** lies between the pars distalis and the pars nervosa (see Figures 17-1 and 17-2). In keeping with its origin from the evaginating oral ectoderm, the pars intermedia comes into immediate contact with the pars nervosa and is separated from the pars nervosa by a tenuously thin sheath of connective tissue. In fact, it is not unusual to have some of the cells of the pars intermedia migrate into the pars nervosa (Figure 17-8). This portion of the adenohypophysis is well developed among domestic mammalian species, enveloping the neural lobe of the neurohypophysis in many instances, including carnivores, the pig, and the horse (see Figure 17-1). In contrast with its direct connection with the neural lobe, the pars intermedia of most mammals is separated from the pars distalis by a remnant space, the **hypophyseal cleft** (Rathke's cleft), that resulted from the early embryological development of this organ.

The parenchyma of the pars intermedia is arranged in clusters, cords, and small follicles or cysts that store colloidal material. Basophils comprise the major cell type of this portion of the adenohypophysis (Figure 17-9). Immunohistochemical testing has revealed many of these cells to be **melanotropes**—cells that form granules containing the **melanocyte-stimulating hormone (MSH)** that stimulates melanin synthesis. Other types of parenchymatous cells vary from species to species and can include those types usually found in the pars distalis.

Pars Tuberalis

The **pars tuberalis** is the thinnest portion of the adenohypophysis that extends from the pars distalis and wraps around the infundibular stalk (see Figure 17-1). The parenchymatous cells form clusters and small follicles. Although they can possess granules that are mildly basophilic, their function as secretory cells has not been revealed (Figure 17-10). On occasion, some of the basophils of the pars distalis—thyrotropes and gonadotropes—have been identified in this area.

NEUROHYPOPHYSIS

As described, the neurohypophysis consists of the median eminence, the infundibulum, and the pars nervosa. During the early development of the pituitary, the neurohypophysis originated as a part of the central nervous system, evaginating ventrally from the hypothalamus. As adenohypophyseal components come into contact with the forming neurohypophysis and the two become intimately linked by their

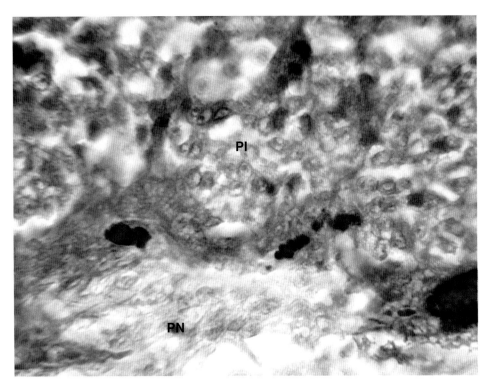

Figure 17-8. Light micrograph of the thin layer of connective tissue that separates the pars intermedia (PI) from the pars nervosa (PN) in the equine pituitary gland. (Mallory stain; ×250.)

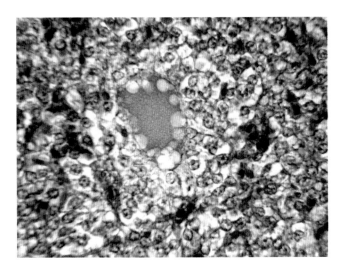

Figure 17-9. Light micrograph of the equine pars intermedia with a small follicle. (Mallory stain; ×250.)

intertwining vasculature as previously described (see Figure 17-3), the neurohypophysis retains its original ties with the hypothalamus. As a result when referring to the pituitary, the neurohypophysis and the hypothalamus can be described as one entity: the **hypothalamohypophyseal tract.**

Hypothalamohypophyseal Tract

The hypothalamohypophyseal tract consists of axons derived from neurons and their cell bodies, which are housed in the **supraoptic** and **paraventricular nuclei** of the hypothalamus (see Figure 17-3). These neurons are actually neurosecretory cells that produce the hormones **oxytocin** and **antidiuretic hormone (ADH),** also known as **vasopressin.** Oxytocin stimulates contractions of smooth muscle within the myometrium of the uterus during conceptus and in pregnant individuals causes contractions of the uterus at parturition. After birth it is secreted upon response to suckling and facilitates myoepithelial cell contraction within the mammary gland and subsequent release of milk (milk let-down). ADH increases resorption of water by the kidneys and as a result conserves body water and causes smooth muscle contraction in arteries. Neurosecretory cells of supraoptic nuclei synthesize ADH, whereas those of paraventricular nuclei make oxytocin.

In addition to the two hormones, **neurophysin** (a carrier protein) is made by each neurosecretory cell. Specific neurophysin binds to each hormone as the hormones are transported within each axon to the neural lobe of the pituitary. The axons, which remain unmyelinated, initially enter the posterior

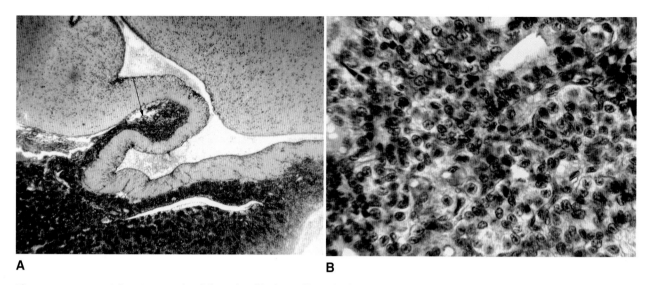

A   **B**

Figure 17-10. A, Light micrograph of the infundibular stalk and adjacent pars tuberalis *(arrows)* of a rat. (Hematoxylin and eosin [H&E] stain; ×20.) **B,** Light micrograph of the pars tuberalis of a rat. (H&E stain; ×250.)

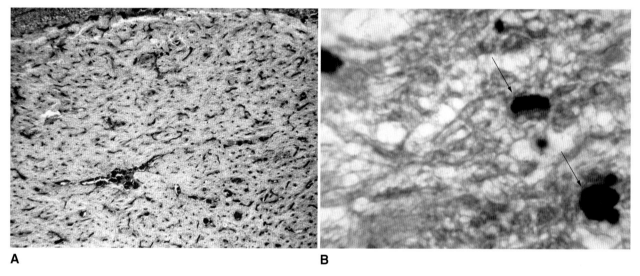

A   **B**

Figure 17-11. Light micrographs of the pars nervosa within the pituitary gland of the horse. Within the distal portion of the equine pars nervosa, blood vessels *(arrows)* are surrounded by axonal endings and pituicytes. (Mallory stain; **A,** ×20; **B,** ×400.)

neurohypophysis at the median eminence and continue on to form the body of the infundibular stalk before ending anteriorly in the pars nervosa (neural lobe). The hormones are contained within secretory vesicles, also known as *secretory granules*, and may be seen to accumulate within the axons along the hypothalamohypophyseal tract.

Pars Nervosa

The axons terminate in the distal or anterior portion of the neurohypophysis known as the **pars nervosa.**

The ends of the axons dilate as they come into proximity with the bed of fenestrated blood vessels that course through the pars nervosa (Figure 17-11). Accumulations of secretory granules occur similarly here as that seen more proximally within the hypothalamohypophyseal tract. When the neurosecretory cells are signaled to secrete their hormones, the secretory granules are exocytosed into a perivascular space that lies between the axonal ending and the adjacent blood vessel. In addition to the blood vessels and the axons and their endings, is a fairly extensive population of neuroglia referred to as **pituicytes.** These cells, which can also be found along the rest of the hypothalamo-hypophyseal tract, ensheathe each axon and most likely provide both physical and physiological support.

PINEAL GLAND (EPIPHYSIS CEREBRI)

Another component of the endocrine system that has close affiliation with the CNS is the pineal gland. In mammalian species, the pineal gland originates from the roof of the diencephalon before projecting dorsally from its midline during development. In non-mammalian species, the pineal gland does not form a stalk, but instead retains its ventral position close to the surface of the brain and possibly receptive to light that can pass diffusely through a thin skull. In lower vertebrate animals, this structure is able to function as a true photoreceptor structure, forming a third eye called the **pineal eye.** As one can surmise, the relationship between the pineal gland and light has weakened during the evolutionary progression of vertebrates, but nevertheless still exists in mammals. Instead of being directly influenced by light, the pineal gland receives light-generated information from the eyes that passes through the midbrain to the cervical spinal cord and cranial cervical ganglion, where sympathetic nerves terminate within the pineal gland.

The principal secretory cell is the **pinealocyte,** which can be organized into cords and follicles (Figure 17-12). Pinealocytes possess round nuclei with prominent nucleoli, smooth endoplasmic reticulum (sER),

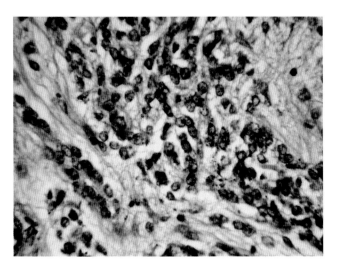

Figure 17-12. Light micrograph of the canine pineal gland with pinealocytes arranged in irregular cords separated by astrocytes. (Hematoxylin and eosin stain; ×250.)

rough endoplasmic reticulum (rER), and associated Golgi apparatus and secretory vesicles. These cells are involved primarily in the synthesis of **melatonin.** The formation and release of this hormone is believed to be responsible for the circadian rhythm among animals, especially as it pertains to sexual activity and seasonal breeding. Longer photoperiods result in a lowered production of melatonin, whereas shorter photoperiods (longer nights) cause melatonin production to rise. Additional parenchyma consists of the glial cells, **astrocytes (interstitial cells),** not unlike the astrocytes found within the CNS. These cells have long, cytoskeletal-rich processes that envelope and support the pinealocytes. Although scattered throughout the gland, they are the predominant parenchyma within the stalk that attaches the gland to the diencephalon. The gland is partially lobulated by meningeal septae that invaginate from a pia mater lining that forms a thin capsule. The septae form conduits for the sinusoidal network that collects and sends the pinealocyte secretions throughout the rest of the body.

Among the parenchyma are concentric deposits of calcium phosphates and carbonates within an organic matrix, which together constitute **corpora arenacea,** or **brain sand.** Both the origin and function for the existence of these concretions have remained a mystery. Also present are pineal pigment granules, which are histochemically identified as melanin granules in the cat, and in the horse can be influenced seasonally with regard to their development.

THYROID GLAND

In mature domestic mammals the thyroid gland is located dorsolaterally next to the trachea near (inferior to) the level of the larynx. During embryogenesis it originates as an evagination or outpocketing of the oral cavity, which eventually becomes united with the fifth pharyngeal pouch. The parenchyma of the thyroid is encased externally by a capsule of dense irregular connective tissue that internally branches into very narrow septae (Figure 17-13). The septae, which consist of a capillary network surrounded by sparsely populated fibrocytes and their thinly developed extracellular matrix (ECM), separate most of the parenchyma into **thyroid follicles** (Figure 17-14). Among domestic species and mammals overall, follicular size increases generally with increasing body size, with a corresponding decrease in parenchyma percentage. The thyroid parenchyma is composed of two cell types: the follicular cell, which lines each follicle, and the parafollicular cell, which exists between adjacent follicles.

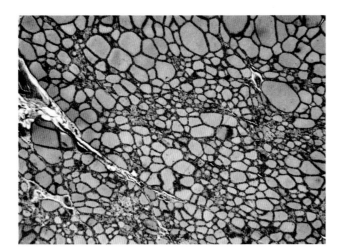

Figure 17-13. Light micrograph of a canine thyroid. (Hematoxylin and eosin stain; ×20.)

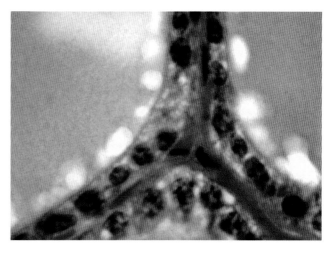

Figure 17-15. Light micrograph of follicular cells in the horse. (Hematoxylin and eosin stain; ×600.)

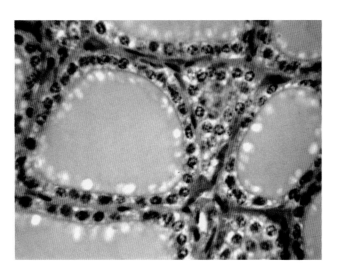

Figure 17-14. Light micrograph of follicles lined by follicular cells and separated by a thin vascular network. (Hematoxylin and eosin stain; ×250.)

FOLLICULAR CELL

The **follicular cell (thyrocyte)** is cuboidal, with a basally positioned round nucleus that is surrounded by acidophilic cytoplasm (Figure 17-15). The cytoplasm contains fairly extensive rough endoplasmic reticulum, Golgi apparatus, and lysosomal systems that collectively work to produce the hormones **thyroxine (T$_4$)** and **triiodothyronine (T$_3$)** (Figure 17-16). The principal functions of these hormones include raising cellular metabolic activities and growth rates, increasing endocrine gland activity, stimulating carbohydrate and fat metabolism, decreasing body weight, and increasing heart rate, respiration and muscle action. The production and release of T$_4$ and T$_3$ are not

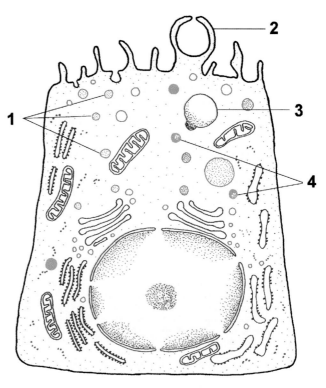

Figure 17-16. Illustration of the follicular cell and its organelles associated with thyroxin production. The left side of the cell is involved in the process of synthesis and iodination of thyroglobulin, whereas the right side is involved in its reabsorption and digestion and subsequent release of T$_3$ and T$_4$. *(1)*, Secretory vesicles; *(2)*, endocytotic uptake of colloid; *(3)*, coalescence of colloid droplet with lysosome; *(4)*, lysosomes.

immediate events, but instead require their storage within **thyroglobulin,** the large glycoproteinaceous molecule. Thyroglobulin is complexed with iodine along the apical surface of these cells, which possess numerous microvilli. As the thyroglobulin is being iodinated, it is exocytosed into a follicular chamber. The resulting storage material within the follicle is called **colloid.** The size of the thyroid follicle, which depends directly on the amount of colloid that is held at a particular time, can vary greatly, but generally ranges from 50 to 200 μm in diameter (see Figures 17-13 and 17-14). When the secretion of T_4 and T_3 is called upon, the follicular cell ingests the colloid by phagocytosis (see Figure 17-16). Lysosomes will fuse with the phagosomes basally within the cell and the secondary lysosomes will hydrolyze the thyroglobulin into T_4 and T_3, which will then be actively secreted into the adjacent capillary bed at the base of the cell.

Stimulation of T_4 and T_3 production and their release is provided by TSH, which, as described, is formed by basophil cells of the adenohypophysis. The TSH binds to specific receptors along the basal portion of the cell membrane of the follicular cell and subsequently causes the follicular cell to ingest the colloidally stored thyroglobulin. As the T_4 and T_3 are being enzymatically liberated from the thyroglobulin, an excess or residual amount of iodine is left behind within the cytosol. This iodine, which is initially bound to tyrosine (monoiodotyrosine and diiodotyrosine), is recycled eventually for future iodination of freshly stored colloidal thyroglobulin. Cells that are active in colloid production or the release of T_4 and T_3 have greater height than those that remain metabolically inactive.

Because the lysosomal system within the follicular cell is critically involved in hormone synthesis, lipofuscin accumulation during age progression may signify decreased thyroid function, which generally accompanies advancing age. However, this correlation may not occur consistently among domestic species because lipofuscin buildup in the horse varies greatly with regard to age.

PARAFOLLICULAR CELL

A second glandular cell of the thyroid is the **parafollicular cell** that, as its name implies, lies around or nearby thyroid follicles (Figure 17-17). Parafollicular cells can exist individually or in small clusters within the basal lamina of follicular cells, being most common where three or more adjacent follicles abut one another. These cells are also referred to as **C cells** or **clear cells** because of their pale staining cytoplasm, which surrounds a comparably large, round nucleus. Whereas the cells often measure twice the diameter of that of follicular cells, they represent only a small fraction of the total parenchyma of the thyroid. The cytoplasm of the parafollicular cells contain numerous small granules filled with the hormone **calcitonin,** a peptide that inhibits osteoclastic absorption of bone and as a result lowers blood calcium level. The granules are formed by a well-developed Golgi apparatus and rER. The granules are released when calcium levels within the blood are high.

PARATHRYOID GLANDS

In most domestic species, the parathyroid glands consist of two pairs of endocrine glands—the external and internal parathyroids—each pair derived from the third and fourth pharyngeal pouches, respectively. In pigs and domestic fowl (and birds in general) only the external pair are formed. In animals with internal parathyroids, these glands are either immersed within the thyroid or lie next to it. Like the thyroid, the parathyroid glands are encased by a thin capsule of dense irregular connective tissue, which, in the instance of internal parathyroids, can blend with the stroma of the thyroid (Figure 17-18). Two cell types are associated with the parenchyma of the parathyroid glands: the principal cell and the oxyphil cell.

PRINCIPAL CELL

The major cell type and in many animals the only cell type is the **principal cell,** also known as the **chief cell.** The principal cells are arranged in cords or clusters, separated and supported by thin stromal septae. These septae include the necessary vascular bed, lymphatic channels and nerve fibers that serve these glands. Normally, the majority of the principal cells are observed in a quiet or inactive state of physiological activity. These cells can be referred to as **light cells** because of their mildly eosinophilic cytoplasm, and with stored lipid, glycogen, and even lipofuscin they are usually larger than their active counterpart, the **dark cells** (Figure 17-19). Dark cells represent physiologically active cells, having cytoplasm filled with secretory granules and the organelles that make them. Cytoplasmically, these cells are polar having some rER basally with the Golgi apparatus and secretory granules apically located. As a result of this polar arrangement, the secretory granules are exocytosed along the apicolateral domain into the extracellular space. The principal cells produce **parathyroid hormone (PTH),** which functions to raise the calcium level in body fluids and along with calcitonin regulates calcium metabolism within the body. The rise in calcium is normally the result of a combination of increased calcium absorption at the intestinal level, release of bone calcium through osteoclastic activation and subsequent bone resorption, and renal calcium retention.

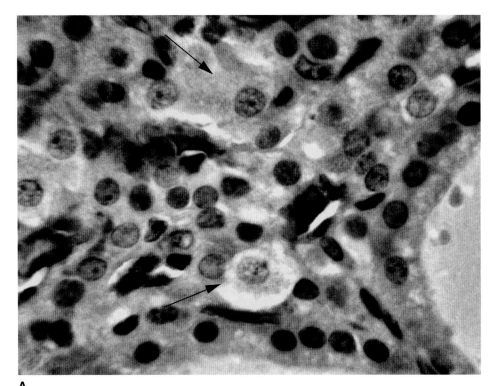

A

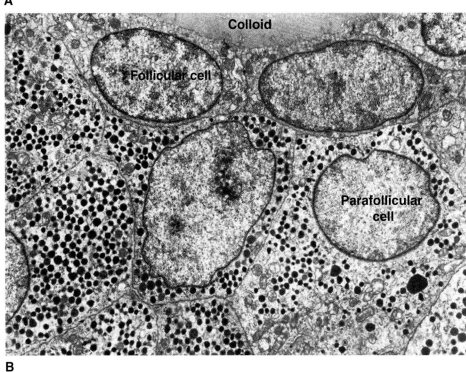

B

Figure 17-17. A, Light micrograph (×400) of the parafollicular cell *(arrows)* within the equine thyroid. Hematoxylin and eosin stain. **B,** Transmission electron micrograph of parafollicular and follicular cells in the thyroid of a cat. *(From Fawcett DW:* Bloom and Fawcett: a textbook of histology, *ed 11, Philadelphia, 1986, Saunders.)*

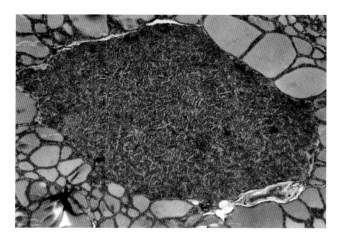

Figure 17-18. Light micrograph of a parathyroid gland located within the thyroid of a dog. (Hematoxylin and eosin stain; ×20.)

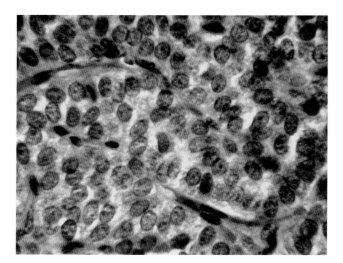

Figure 17-19. Light micrograph of the canine parathyroid with its clusters of principal cells. (Hematoxylin and eosin stain; ×400.)

OXYPHIL CELL

In some species, such as the ox and other large ruminants as well as the horse, there is a second secretory cell type, the **oxyphil cell.** This cell can be considerably larger in diameter than the principal cell (25-30 µm vs. 5-10 µm for principal cells) and has a mildly eosinophilic, granular cytoplasm that contains numerous mitochondria and glycogen and only a few granules. The oxyphil cell can occur singly or in small clusters, and collectively form only a small portion of the entire parenchyma of the parathyroids. The function of this cell type has yet to be revealed. It may represent a different physiological state of the principal cell because there can be an additional presence of "intermediate" or "transitional" cells that share histological similarities of both oxyphil and principal cells.

ADRENAL (SUPRARENAL) GLANDS

In the thoracic cavity are a pair of endocrine glands (the **adrenal glands**) positioned cranially to the kidneys near or at their anterior poles. These glands are derived from two germ layers resulting in a cortex of mesodermal origin that surrounds a medulla of ectodermal neural crest origin. The cortex is covered by a capsule of dense irregular connective tissue that is well penetrated by an extensive arterial supply, forming a highly developed subcapsular system of blood vessels for an organized arrangement of parenchyma. Arteries providing for the adrenal glands originate from three sources: the inferior phrenic arteries, which give rise to the **superior suprarenal arteries;** the aorta, which gives rise to the **middle suprarenal arteries;** and the renal arteries, which give rise to the **inferior suprarenal arteries.** The subcapsular system of blood vessels branches internally and becomes a sinusoidal network that is directed centripedally toward the medulla, emptying into medullary veins (Figure 17-20).

ADRENAL CORTEX

The adrenal cortex forms the bulk of the adrenal gland and possesses a level of parenchymatous architecture that is unmatched in organization among the other endocrine glands. In domestic mammals, the cortex can be subdivided into at least three regions or zones. Avian adrenal glands, however, lack the ordered arrangement of the parenchyma found in mammalian cortices. In fact, the adrenal glands of domestic fowls and birds, in general, do not possess parenchyma that is separated into cortical and medullary regions.

In ruminants (and primates), the outermost portion is referred to as the **zona glomerulosa.** The parenchyma in these animals is arranged in cords and clusters (Figure 17-21; see also Figure 17-20). In most other domestic species including dogs, cats, horses, and pigs, the parenchyma forms arcades just beneath the capsule (Figure 17-22). Consequently, in those animals this portion of the cortex is referred to as the **zona arcuata.** In horses, the secretory cells of the zona arcuata are distinctly columnar, whereas in most other domestic animals they can be rounded to polyhedral to low columnar. Light microscopically, the cytoplasm within this parenchyma is most often mildly eosinophilic with only a suggestion of vacuoles and vesicles. Ultrastructural observations have reported

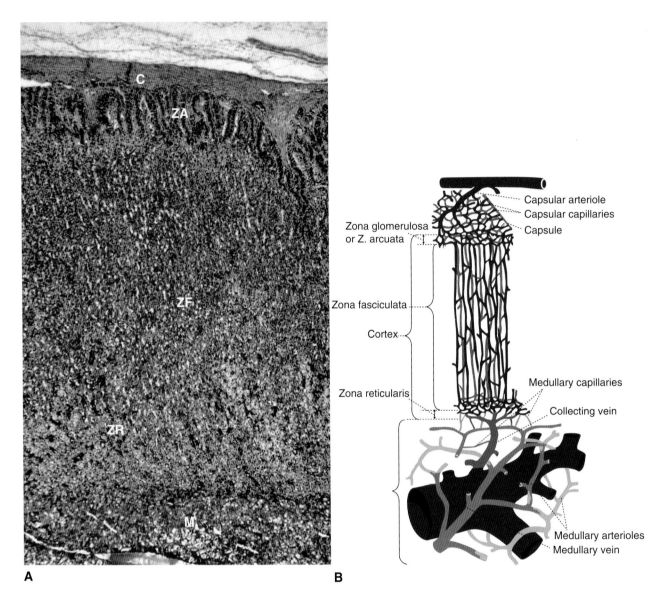

Figure 17-20. A, Light micrograph of the canine adrenal gland. *C,* capsule; *M,* medulla; *ZA,* zona arcuata; *ZF,* zona fasciculata; *ZR,* zona reticularis. (Hematoxylin and eosin stain; ×15.) **B,** Diagram of the vascular network within the mammalian adrenal gland. *(Modified from Fawcett DW:* Bloom and Fawcett: a textbook of histology, *ed 11, Philadelphia, 1986, Saunders.)*

the usual presence of mitochondria and sER, but with less rER and only few lipid droplets. Granules also have been found in ruminants, but their number is comparatively few and their function unknown. The endocrine cells of the zona glomerulosa/arcuata secrete **mineralocorticoids,** including **aldosterone,** a hormone that influences the activities of the renal tubules and maintains the necessary balance of electrolytes within the body fluids.

In most domestic species, the parenchyma of the zona glomerulosa and zona arcuata end internally, joining a short region of undifferentiated cells, the **zona intermedia.** From the outermost zones, the parenchyma becomes radially aligned, forming single layers of cords or fascicles that are separated by sinusoidal capillaries, which also are directed toward the medulla (Figure 17-23). This next portion of the cortex is aptly named the **zona fasciculata.** The secretory cells of the zona fasciculata have a foamy appearance as a result of the presence of numerous lipid droplets, and because of that morphological trait are called **spongiocytes.** Interspersed between the many lipid droplets is a well-developed network of sER and rounded mitochondria. The endocrine cells of the

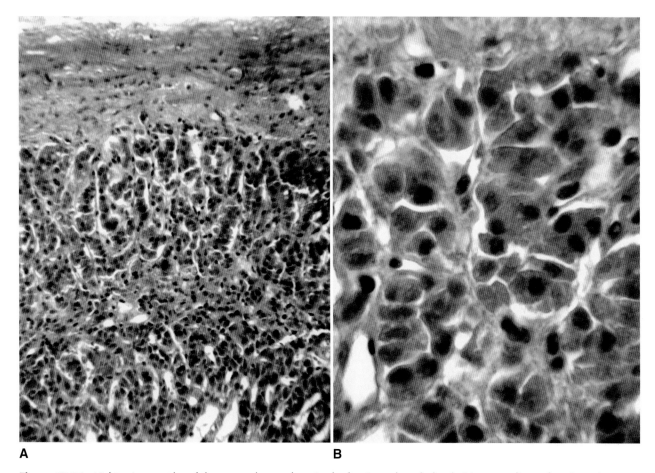

A   **B**

Figure 17-21. Light micrographs of the zona glomerulosa in the bovine adrenal gland. (Hematoxylin and eosin stain; **A,** ×100; **B,** ×400.)

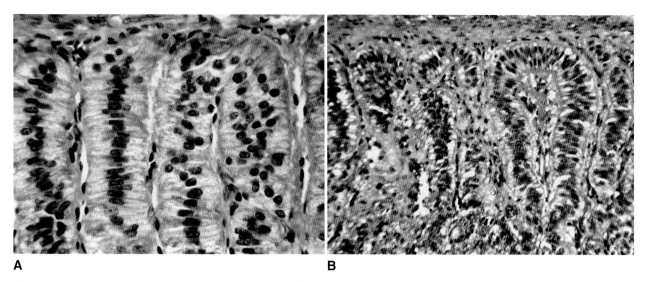

A   **B**

Figure 17-22. Light micrographs of the zona arcuata in the dog and the horse. (Hematoxylin and eosin stain; **A,** ×250; **B,** ×100.)

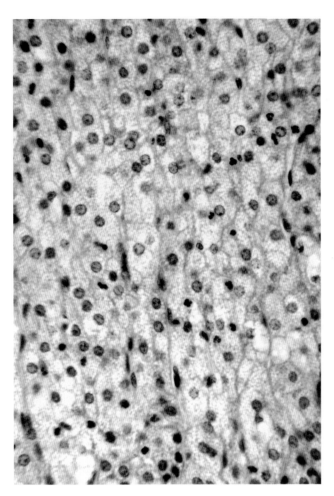

Figure 17-23. Light micrograph of the zona fasciculata in the dog. (Hematoxylin and eosin stain; ×250.)

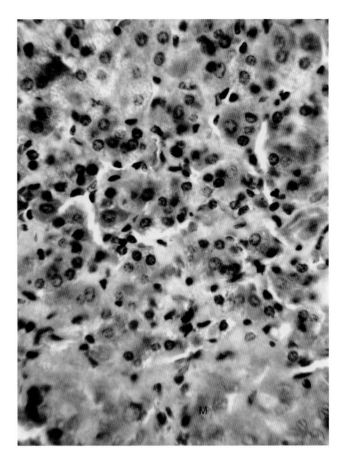

Figure 17-24. Light micrograph of the zona reticularis in the dog. *M,* medulla. (Hematoxylin and eosin stain; ×250.)

zona fasciculata are involved in the production of hormones known as **glucocorticoids,** which include **cortisol** and **corticosterone.** Glucocorticoids help direct the metabolism of carbohydrate, protein, and fat. They are able also to reduce inflammatory response by lowering the number of circulating cells of defense, especially eosinophils and lymphocytes.

The cells of the zona fasciculata end internally next to the innermost zone of the cortex, the **zona reticularis.** As the name implies, the parenchyma of the zona reticularis appears to anastomose and form reticulated chains of cells (Figure 17-24). For the most part, these cells stain more acidophilically than spongiocytes of the zona fasciculata, having fewer lipid droplets (some have lipofuscin). Occasionally, cells with pyknotic nuclei are encountered in this portion of the cortex. Like the zona fasciculata, the zona reticularis produces glucocorticoids, but considerably fewer. With the presence of the senescent and degenerating cells, the zona reticularis may represent the

oldest portion of the cortex, at least regarding cells involved in glucocorticoid synthesis.

ADRENAL MEDULLA

In domestic mammals, the center of the adrenal gland consists of the **adrenal medulla.** Whereas the adrenal cortex is characterized by an organized arrangement of its parenchyma, the adrenal medulla features a disorganized parenchyma that is composed of two types of secretory cells: the chromaffin cell and the sympathetic ganglion cell, both of ectodermal neural crest origin.

The epithelioid **chromaffin cell,** which is the principal endocrine cell of the medulla, forms small clusters and chains surrounded by sinusoidal vessels (Figure 17-25). These polyhedral cells contain sER and rER and well-developed Golgi apparatus that lie next to the nuclei and are involved in the production of small granules. When exposed to chromic acid, the granules turn brown, forming a chromaffin reaction, which historically led to the name of these cells. The granules can hold the catecholamine

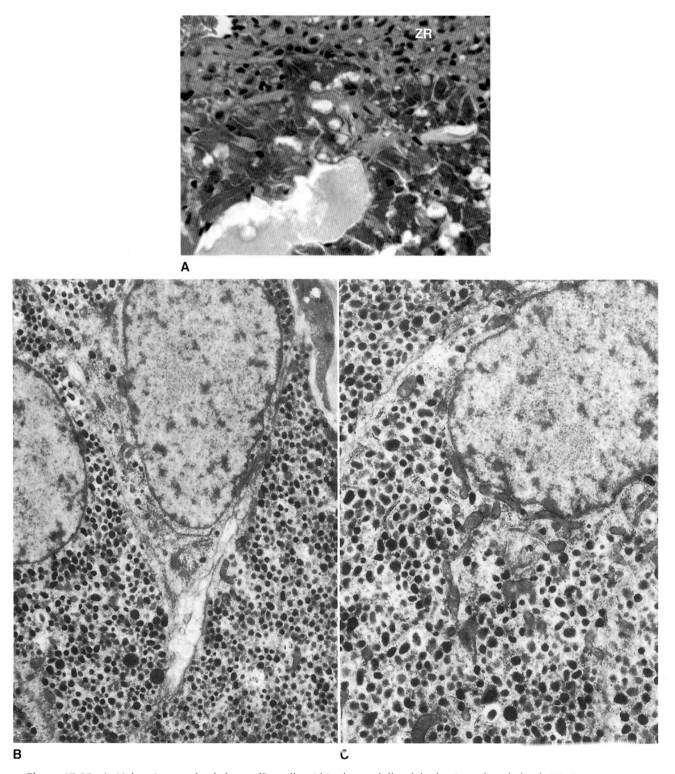

Figure 17-25. **A,** Light micrograph of chromaffin cells within the medulla of the bovine adrenal gland. *ZR,* Zona reticularis. (Chromaffin stain; ×250.) **B** and **C,** Transmission electron micrographs of catecholamine-bearing cells in the medulla of a cat. *(From Fawcett DW:* Bloom and Fawcett: a textbook of histology, *ed 11, Philadelphia, 1986, Saunders.)*

neurotransmitters—epinephrine and norepinephrine. However, an individual chromaffin cell will produce only one of these substances, and for that reason the chromaffin cell can be divided into two types: epinephrine secreting and norepinephrine secreting. Although most cells secrete epinephrine, the two types are generally randomly distributed throughout the medulla. Among the herbivorous domestic species, such as ruminants, horses, and pigs, the chromaffin cells are largest along the outer portion of the medulla and smallest within its inner portion. In the horse, the cells within the outer portion are also somewhat columnar. The two types of chromaffin cells represent modified sympathetic neurons that are stimulated by preganglion sympathetic splanchnic nerves during circumstances that lead to anxiety and as a result prepare the body for "fight or flight." When the chromaffin cells are called upon, the release of their granules increases the movement of blood throughout the organs of the body and elevates the level of blood glucose, which together makes an individual more alert and ready for physical activity than previously (see Table 17-1).

PANCREATIC ISLETS (ISLETS OF LANGERHANS)

Within the pancreas—the largest exocrine gland of the body—is the smallest endocrine gland, consisting of clusters of cells known as the **pancreatic islets** or the **islets of Langerhans.** The pancreatic islets originate from the same endoderm that gives rise to the rest of the exocrine pancreas (see Figure 4-1). The size and arrangement of cells within each islet are not as random as once supposed and are now understood to vary according to location within the pancreas, species, and age.

Histologically, the cells within each islet appear pale in contrast with the surrounding highly stained serous secreting cells, being arranged in irregular disseminating clusters intertwined with a network of blood vessels (Figure 17-26). In most domestic animals, the clusters consist of four cell types based on a combination of morphological and histochemical features, being: A (α), B (β), C, and D (δ).

A, or **alpha (α) cells,** form the second-most numerous type of endocrine cell within the islet. These cells are involved in **glucagon** production, which counteracts insulin by increasing glucose release from the liver and is released when blood glucose levels are low. They possess secretory granules that do not dissolve in alcohol, allowing them to be recognized as red cells by the Masson trichrome stain or Gomori aldehyde

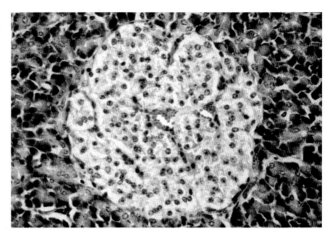

Figure 17-26. Light micrograph (×250) of a pancreatic islet in the dog.

fuchsin reaction. In cattle, A cells are positioned mostly along the periphery of the pancreatic islet, whereas in the horse they comprise the central region.

B, or **beta (β), cells** comprise the largest population of secretory cells within the pancreatic islets. These cells form and release granules filled with **insulin.** The granules can be very distinctive among domestic species, especially in the dog and cat, which possess granules that contain dense crystals. Except for the horse, crystalloid structures can be found in other animals as well. When secreted, insulin lowers blood glucose levels primarily through the cellular uptake of glucose, especially by skeletal muscle fibers and adipose tissue, and inhibiting the liver release of glucose. Deficiency in insulin production leads to sustained hyperglycemia and glycosuria and result in **diabetes mellitus,** a life-threatening disorder of carbohydrate metabolism. Other subcellullar features are nearly identical to those of A cells. The nuclei of B cells are often slightly smaller than those of A cells.

C cells form a relatively small portion of the total population of cells within the pancreatic islet. They either have few granules or lack them altogether and are most likely young developing cells that will eventually mature into one of the other secretory cells within the islet. Their occurrence was only determined by transmission electron microscopy.

D, or **delta (δ), cells** form another small population of cells within the pancreatic islet. These cells possess granules more heterogeneous in size and density than those occurring in A and B cells. The granules contain the hormone **somatostatin,** which is able to inhibit the release of glucagon and insulin by A and B cells, respectively. Somatostatin also lowers gastric motility within the digestive tract.

SUGGESTED READINGS

Booth KK, Goshal NG: Angioarchitecture of the canine thyroid gland, *Anat Anz* 145:32, 1979.

Calvo JL, Boya J, Garcia-Maurino JE, Rancano D: Presence of melanin in the cat pineal gland, *Acta Anat* 145:73, 1992.

Cozzi B: Cell types in the pineal gland of the horse: an ultrastructural and immunocytochemical study, *Anat Rec* 216:165, 1986.

Dalefield RR, Palmer DN, Jolly RD: Lipofuscin and abnormalities in colloid in the equine thyroid gland in relation to age, *J Comp Pathol* 111:389, 1994.

Fawcett DW: *Bloom and Fawcett: a textbook of histology,* ed 11, Philadelphia, 1986, Saunders.

Furuoka H, Ito H, Hamada M, et al: Immunocytochemical component of endocrine cells in pancreatic islets of horses, *Nippon Juigaku Zasshi* 51:35, 1989.

Gartner LP, Hiatt JL: *Color textbook of histology,* Philadelphia, 1997, Saunders.

Gelberg H, Cockerel, GL Minor RR: A light and electron microscopic study of a normal adrenal medulla and a pheochromocytoma from a horse, *Vet Pathol* 16:395, 1979.

Gensure RC, Gardella TJ, Juppner H: Parathyroid hormone and parathyroid-related peptide, and their receptors, *Biochem Biophys Res Commun* 328:666, 2005.

Grandi D: The pineal body of the mink and the horse with special reference to the reproductive cycle. An ultrastructural and immunocytochemical study, *Ital J Anat Embryol* 100(suppl 1):231, 1995.

Ives PJ, Haensly WE, Maxwell PA, McArthur NH: A histochemical and ultrastructural study of lipofuscin accumulation in thyroid follicular cells of aging domestic cats, *Mech Ageing Dev* 4:399, 1975.

Okada H, Capen CC, Rosol TJ: Immunohistochemical demonstration of parathyroid hormone-related protein in thyroid gland of sheep, *Vet Pathol* 32:315, 1995.

Rahmanian MS, Thompson DL, Melrose PA: Immunocytochemical localization of prolactin and growth hormone in the equine pituitary, *J Anim Sci* 75:3010, 1997.

Rahmanian MS, Thompson DL, Melrose PA: Immunocytochemical localization of luteinizing hormone and follicle-stimulating hormone in the equine pituitary, *J Anim Sci* 76:839, 1998.

Saadeh FA, Babikian LG: A comparative histologic study of thyroid follicular size and epithelium percentage in certain animals, *Anat Anz* 143:96, 1978.

Tan JH, Nanbo Y, Oikawa M, et al: Immunocytochemical differences in adenohypophyseal cells among Mongolian pony mares, stallions and geldings, *Am J Vet Res* 59:262, 1998.

Wieczorek G, Pospischil A, Perentes AG: A comparative immunohistochemical study of pancreatic islets in laboratory animals (rats, dogs, minipigs and nonhuman primates), *Exp Toxicol Pathol* 50:151, 1998.

Wild P, Setoguti T: Mammalian parathyroids: morphological and functional implications, *Microsc Res Tech* 32:120, 1995.

Male Reproductive System

KEY CHARACTERISTICS

- System designed for the production, sustenance, and transport of spermatozoa; consisting of a tubular tract with accessory glands, and emptying (connecting) into the distal portion (urethra) of the urinary system.

Among domestic animals, the male reproductive system is composed of the **testes** and their investments: **genital ducts, accessory glands,** and **penis.** These structures function collectively to produce and transport spermatozoa to the female reproductive tract and ultimately fertilize ova. In addition, the penis forms the external-most portion of the male urinary tract and serves as the last conduit for the excretion of urine.

TESTES

The male of each domestic mammal possesses a pair of testes that lie in a pouch of skin known as the **scrotum.** As the testes develop they evaginate from the abdominal cavity along its posterior wall, and in doing so, descend into the scrotum. During this process, a part of the peritoneum is brought along with the anterolateral portion of each testis, resulting in the formation of the **tunica vaginalis.** The tunica vaginalis attaches the testes to the scrotum but concomitantly separates them with a thin serous cavity, allowing mobility of the testes within the confines of the scrotum.

Each testis is covered by a capsule of dense irregular connective tissue called the **tunica albuginea,** which has its own serosal lining (Figures 18-1 and 18-2). The tunica albuginea houses a vascular bed that feeds and drains the testis. This bed or layer can be deep in some animals, including boars and stallions, and sometimes is referred to separately as the **tunica vasculosa.** Septae of the tunica albuginea (the **septula testis**) project inwardly and divide the testis into lobules, the **lobula testis.** The septula testis converges posteriorly in equine, feline, and rodent species and centrally in canine, porcine, and ruminant species to form the **mediastinum testis.** The mediastinum testis, which is actually a thickened portion of the tunica albuginea, contains the rete testis as well as larger lymphatic and vascular vessels.

The lobules of the testis vary in number according to species. Each lobule holds the parenchyma, which consists of one to four looping **seminiferous tubules.** Seminiferous tubules are the site of spermatozoa production (spermatogenesis). The ends of each tubule are connected to short, straight ducts called the **tubule recti** that guide the developing spermatozoa to the rete testis. The **rete testis** is a labyrinth of anastomosing channels that collects spermatozoa from all of the seminiferous tubules and their respective tubule recti. This rete, in turn, empties by way of short ducts (the **ductuli efferentes**) into a highly convoluted collecting channel, the **ductus epididymidis.** Together, the ductuli efferentes and the ductus epididymidis

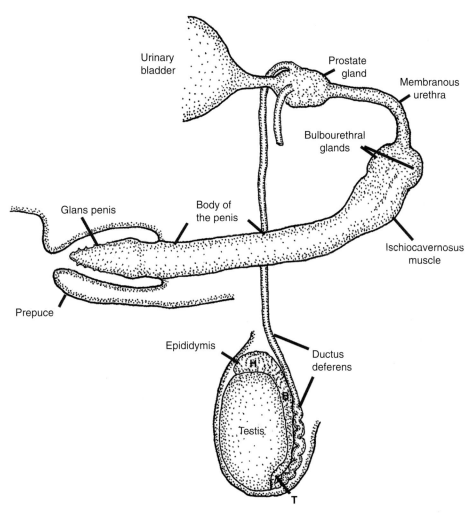

Figure 18-1. Schematic diagram of the male reproductive tract of the cat. In noncarnivorous domestic species, the ductus deferens leads first to a vesicular gland, which lies immediately before the prostate gland. *H,* Head; *B,* body; *T,* tail of the epididymis.

constitute the **epididymis,** which stores spermatozoa while they fully mature (see Figure 18-1).

SEMINIFEROUS TUBULES

The seminiferous tubules can be likened to a highly coiled tubular gland that is holocrine in secretion (see Figure 18-2). Each tubule is lined by the **seminiferous epithelium,** a germinal stratified epithelium that is the site of spermatogenesis. This epithelium forms a basal lamina that is attached to a thin wall of connective tissue, the lamina propria, consisting of collagen (types I and IV), fibrocytes, and occasional blood vessels and nerve fibers (Figure 18-3). In many species, including the bull, cat, dog, rabbit, and stallion, the cells within this connective tissue are myofibroblastic. The myofibroblasts lie next to the germinal epithelium, whereas the fibrocytes lie more

peripherally. During contraction, the lumen of the seminiferous tubule narrows, moving the spermatozoa into the adjacent system of ducts for their eventual maturation and subsequent release.

As animals such as stallions age, atrophy of seminiferous tubules occurs. Concomitantly, the lamina propria thickens, with an increase in collagen type IV and elastic fibers, resulting in interstitial fibrosis.

Sustentacular Cell

The seminiferous epithelium is composed of two cell types: the sustentacular cell and the spermatogenic cell. The **sustentacular cell (Sertoli cell)** is a support cell that extends from the basal lamina to the tubular lumen and, as a group, occupies much of the volume of the seminiferous epithelium (Figure 18-4). The lateral sides of adjacent sustentacular cells form

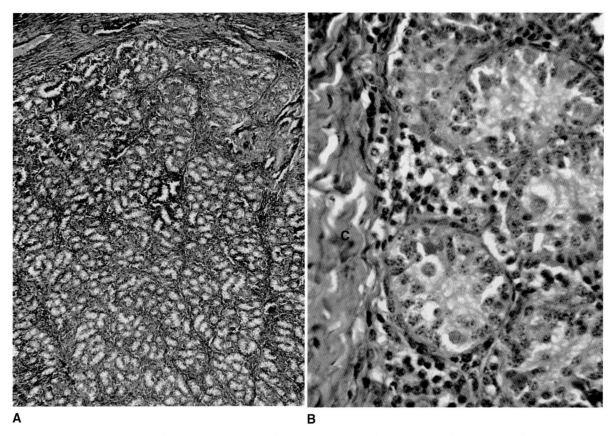

A   **B**

Figure 18-2. Light micrograph of the seminiferous tubules in an immature boar. *C*, Capsule. (Hematoxylin and eosin stain; **A,** ×20; **B,** ×100.)

numerous infoldings as well as tight junctions (zonulae occludentes) and consequently are difficult to see without the assistance of special stains or transmission electron microscopy. Because of the presence of the tight junctions, the contents of the blood vessels beneath the basal lamina of the seminiferous epithelium cannot freely mix or communicate with contents of the lumen of the seminiferous tubule without passing through the sustentacular cells. As a result, a **blood-testis barrier** is formed by these cells.

The nucleus of the sustentacular cell is oval, but can be variably indented, and located toward the basal lamina. The cytoplasm is filled with polysomes (free ribosomes), smooth endoplasmic reticulum, some rough endoplasmic reticulum, associated Golgi apparatus and vesicles, many of which are endolysosomal in origin, mitochondria, and a well-developed cytoskeleton, consisting of microtubules, actin, and the intermediate filament, vimentin. The relative amounts of these organelles vary according to ongoing spermatogenic activities.

The relationship of the lateral sides of adjacent sustentacular cells is tightly linked to the development and activity of the spermatogenic cell (see Figure 18-4). To begin with, the establishment of the blood-testis barrier is needed to protect the spermatogenic process from being attacked by the immune system. The first production of spermatozoa occurs well after the development of the immune system and would result in an immunological response if not for the presence of the blood-testis barrier. As germ cells develop, the lateral sides of the sustentacular cells offer an excellent location for both physical and physiological support. Moreover, as the spermatogenic cells proceed in their development, portions of their cytoplasm are extruded and removed. These pieces of cell debris are readily phagocytized and recycled by the neighboring sustentacular cells. Eventually, adjacent sustentacular cells release the developing male gametes into the lumen of the seminiferous tubule, a process referred to as **spermiation.**

In addition to these roles, the sustentacular cells are able to control the influence of the hormones, testosterone and follicle-stimulating hormone (FSH), and by doing so, help synchronize spermatogenic activities. These cells also synthesize and secrete their own substances, including androgen-binding protein, transferrin, and inhibin. **Androgen-binding protein** acts

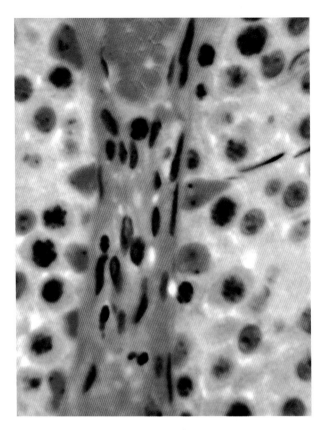

Figure 18-3. Light micrograph of the connective tissue surrounding seminiferous tubules in the equine testis. (Hematoxylin and eosin stain; ×250.)

to increase testosterone concentration within the seminiferous tubules by binding to testosterone and in this way preventing testosterone from leaving this area. **Transferrin,** or **testicular transferrin,** is an apoprotein that binds iron, which is carried in the plasma, and transports the metal to the developing gamete. **Inhibin** is a hormone that is released luminally by the sustentacular cells to be absorbed by the epithelium of the efferent ductules and contiguous epididymis so that it can enter the bloodstream and subsequently inhibit the secretion of FSH by the pituitary. In addition to these secretions, sustentacular cells produce the **antiparamesonephric hormone (antimüllerian hormone)** during the early (embryonic to prepubertal) development of the male. This hormone functions to suppress the development of the female reproductive system and as a result secure the "maleness" of the individual until the arrival of sexual maturity. During this period of early development, the sustentacular cells remain in a germinative and relatively undifferentiated state.

During the aging of stallions, sustentacular cells decline substantially in number even though testicu-

lar development continues in animals as old as 12 to 13 years. During this period of development the sustentacular cells are able to accommodate increased numbers of germ cells despite their dwindling population.

Spermatogenic Cell

In terms of both purpose and number, the chief cell of the seminiferous epithelium is the spermatogenic cell. The spermatogenic cell that gives rise to the rest of this cell population is the **spermatogonium** (Figure 18-5). Spermatogonia lie next to the basal lamina of the seminiferous epithelium between adjacent sustentacular cells. The blood-testis barrier lies adluminally to these cells, as zonulae occludentes are formed above their apical boundary (see Figure 18-4). The presence of these tight junctions distinguishes and divides the cytoplasm of the sustentacular cell into two regions: the **basal compartment,** which lies beneath the tight junction and is reduced in height, and the **adluminal (apical) compartment,** which extends to the lumen of the seminiferous tubule and is involved with the different stages of spermatogenic cell development.

The spermatogonium is a small cell with a diploid oval nucleus and at puberty can be influenced by testosterone, causing it to enter a cycle of cell division. Not all spermatogonia enter this cycle. There are those that remain quiet or resting and do not divide often, having heterochromatic nuclei and relatively little cytoplasm, and are referred to as **reserve cells,** also known as **dark type A spermatogonia** (see Figure 18-4). Those that have entered the cycle consist of two types: **light type A spermatogonia** and **type B spermatogonia.** Light type A cells are similar morphologically to the dark type A except for the presence of pale or euchromatic nuclei. Type B cells are similar to the light type A cells, but have round instead of oval nuclei (see Figure 18-5). Type A spermatogonia are induced by testosterone to divide mitotically again and again, resulting not only in the production of more pale type A cells, but also type B cells. Type B cells are influenced to divide as well, but result in the formation of spermatocytes (Figure 18-6). With the cell division of each spermatogonium, whether it be light type A or type B, the resultant cells remain connected by intercellular bridges. Because of these connections, the different generations of spermatogonia and spermatocytes effectively constitute a syncytium.

SPERMATOCYTE MEIOSIS

Cells derived from type B spermatogonia move from the basal compartment to the adluminal com-

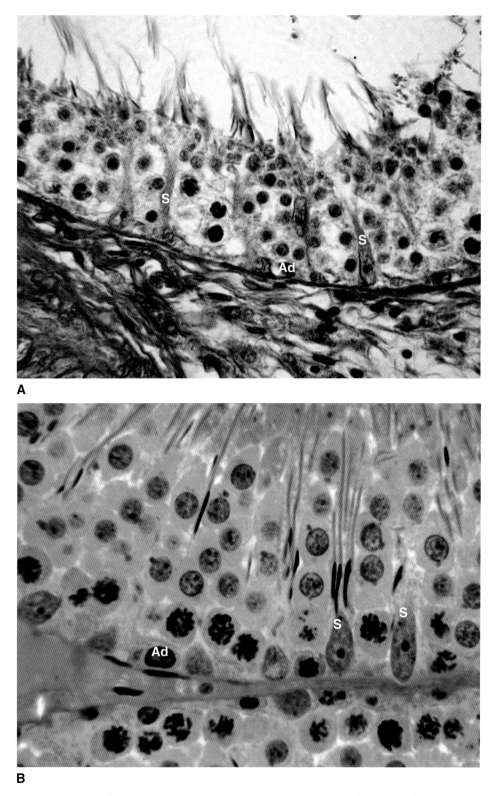

A

B

Figure 18-4. Light micrographs of a portion of the **A,** equine and **B,** murine seminiferous tubules revealing sustentacular cells *(S)* between the numerous developing spermatocytes. *Ad,* Dark type A spermatogonium. (Hematoxylin and eosin stain; **A,** ×250; **B,** ×300.)

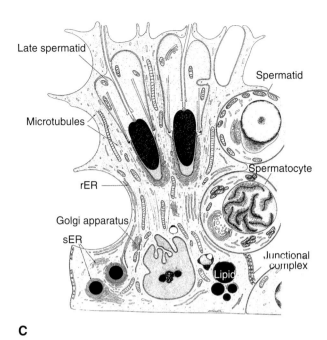

Late spermatid

Microtubules

rER

Golgi apparatus

sER

Spermatid

Spermatocyte

Junctional complex

Lipid

C

Figure 18-4, cont'd C, Schematic diagram of the sustentacular cell. *rER,* Rough endoplasmic reticulum; *sER,* smooth endoplasmic reticulum. *(Modified from Fawcett DW: Bloom and Fawcett: a textbook of histology, ed 11, Philadelphia, 1986, Saunders.)*

partment. These cells are **primary spermatocytes,** and as they pass into the adluminal compartment, they form tight junctions (zonulae occludentes) with the sustentacular cells. The tight junctions produced here help establish the blood-testis barrier. The primary spermatocytes become the largest cells of the spermatogenic population (Figure 18-7; see also Figure 18-6). Their nuclei are notable for both their size and appearance, being big and vesicular due to the presence of condensed chromosomes. Soon after the primary spermatocyte has moved into the adluminal compartment, the diploid nucleus increases its deoxyribonucleic acid (DNA) content to 4N. Subsequent to further cell division, which occurs twice (both involving meiosis rather than mitosis), the primary spermatocytes remain primary spermatocytes for an extended period (16 days in the bull). The extended length of time is due to the prolonged prophase **(prophase I)** of the first meiotic division (first maturation division), which includes four stages: leptotene, zygotene, pachytene, and diakinesis.

Leptotene, the first stage of prophase I, is recognized by the initial condensation of the chromosomes, which become threadlike in appearance. During **zygotene** the chromosomal homologs are now seen as pairs (four chromatids). As prophase continues into

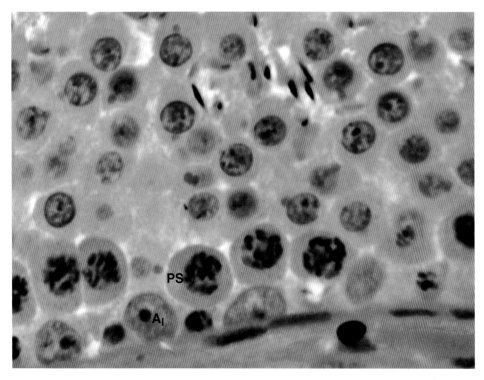

Figure 18-5. Light micrograph of a portion of the seminiferous tubule of a rat with light type A spermatogonium (A$_l$) and primary spermatocytes (PS). (Hematoxylin and eosin stain; ×300.)

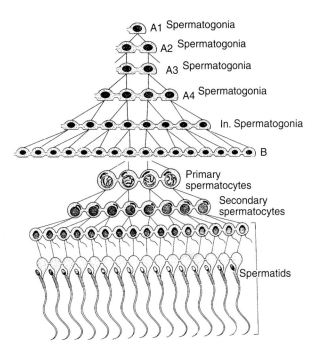

A1 Spermatogonia

A2 Spermatogonia

A3 Spermatogonia

A4 Spermatogonia

In. Spermatogonia

B

Primary spermatocytes

Secondary spermatocytes

Spermatids

Figure 18-6. Schematic diagram of spermatogenesis demonstrates the clonal nature of each male germ cell and the resulting intercellular bridges that create a syncytium during the development of the spermatocytes and subsequent spermatids. Most of the mass proliferation of these cells occurs during the mitotic divisions of the spermatogonia, which include the A₁-A₄ generations of the pale spermatogonia, subsequent intermediate (In.) spermatogonia, and B spermatogonia. The primary spermatocytes are the largest of the reproductive cells, having recently formed 4N content of DNA that becomes meiotically divided to 2N when secondary spermatocytes are subsequently formed. *(Modified from Fawcett DW: Bloom and Fawcett: a textbook of histology, ed 11, Philadelphia, 1986, Saunders.)*

the **pachytene** stage, the chromosomal pairs condense further into shortened and thickened tetrads. At this point prophase enters **diakinesis** and segments of the homologs are exchanged or crossed over, resulting in genetic recombination. As a result of the crossing over, each gamete receives a different, unique blend of genomic material. The surrounding nuclear envelope has now disintegrated. With the end of prophase the first meiosis enters **metaphase I** and the paired homologs move to the equatorial plate. During **anaphase I** the chromosomes migrate to each pole and enter **telophase I,** with the cell dividing into two but incompletely forming the same type of cytoplasmic bridge that occurred during previously mitotic divisions.

The newly formed cells are **secondary spermatocytes,** and each cell now has one-half of the number of chromosomes that the primary spermatocyte possesses, but each chromosome consists of two chromatids or dyads. These cells are small when compared with the primary spermatocytes and spend only a short time within the seminiferous epithelium, and for that reason are not usually encountered when examining the testis histologically. Within a short time the secondary spermatocytes enter the second meiotic division (second maturation division), which includes a relatively brief prophase II, followed by metaphase II, anaphase II, and telophase II. The subsequent cells formed from this division are **spermatids,** each containing a haploid complement of DNA. As before, the spermatids remain attached to one another by cytoplasmic bridges.

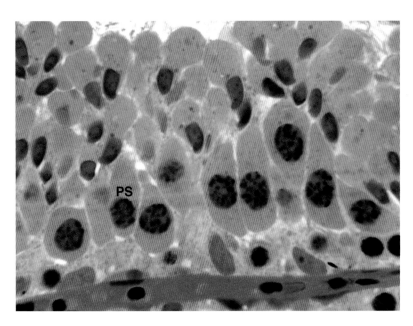

PS

Figure 18-7. Light micrograph of a portion of the seminiferous tubule of a rat with primary spermatocytes *(PS)* in the pachytene phase. (Hematoxylin and eosin stain; ×300.)

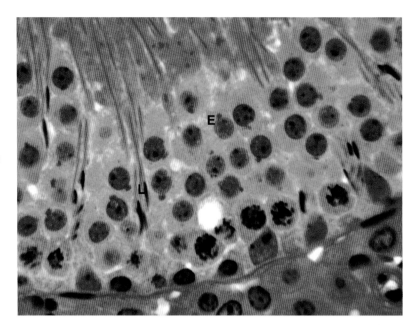

Figure 18-8. Light micrograph of the seminiferous tubule of a rat with early- *(E)* and late- *(L)* forming spermatids. (Hematoxylin and eosin stain; ×300.)

SPERMIOGENESIS

At the end of the second division, the newly formed spermatids undergo a remarkable transformation known as **spermiogenesis.** These cells are now located near the lumen of the seminiferous tubule. Initially, the young spermatid possesses a small haploid nucleus that is placed centrally within the cytoplasm (Figure 18-8; see also Figure 18-4, B). Although small in amount, this cytoplasm is filled with mitochondria, rough endoplasmic reticulum, and associated Golgi apparatus. From this point, the spermatid metamorphoses into a spermatozoon by going through a four-phase process that includes the Golgi phase, the cap phase, the acrosomal phase, and the maturation phase (Figure 18-9).

During the first phase, the **Golgi phase,** small vesicles, referred to as **preacrosomal granules,** are produced by the Golgi apparatus. The granules, which contain hydrolytic enzymes, fuse with one another to form the **acrosomal granule** contained within a single vesicle. That vesicle fuses with the nuclear envelope at the portion that will become the anterior pole of the mature spermatozoon nucleus. With the development of the acrosomal vesicle and its granule, the pair of centrioles that lie within the cytocentrum are repositioned toward the posterior pole of the nucleus. One of the centrioles, the distal centriole, forms the base of a developing axoneme that, in turn, forms the core of a developing flagellum.

The next phase, the **cap phase,** involves further development of the acrosomal vesicle, which contin-ues to form a cap, the **acrosome,** over the anterior portion of the still rounded nucleus (Figure 18-10; see also Figure 18-9).

During the acrosomal phase, the spermatid elongates along its anteroposterior axis. The chromatin within the nucleus begins to become tightly condensed and the nucleus begins to lengthen and become narrow (Figure 18-11). The histones usually associated with the DNA are replaced by protamines (basic proteins) that allow the nuclear material to be condensed even further. The acrosome covers the anterior half of the nucleus, forming the **head cap** (see Figure 18-9). The cytoplasm in front of the anterior pole of the nucleus has migrated posteriorly toward the flagellum. A cylindrical sheath of microtubules appears near the nucleus, just caudal to the head cap. This sheath, which is called the **manchette,** facilitates the elongation of the spermatid at this point. Eventually, the microtubules disassemble and are replaced by a short ring of electron-dense material called the **annulus** that lies next the cell membrane and caudal to the proximal centriole that acts as the principal basal body for the flagellar axoneme. Mitochondria are then moved next to the annulus, lying anterior to it. As mitochondria become repositioned around the axoneme of the flagellum, the annulus is moved posteriorly, delineating the flagellum into the mitochondrial portion known as the **middle piece** and the rest of the flagellum, consisting of the **principal piece** and the **end piece.** As the flagellum continues to develop, nine columns of **dense fibers** line the axoneme externally. Within the principal piece of the flagellum, the

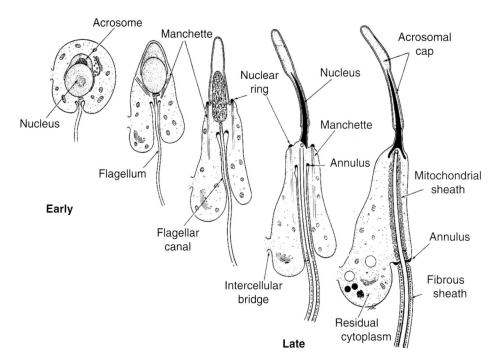

Figure 18-9. Schematic diagram of spermatid differentiation before spermiation, illustrating early stages, involving initial development of the acrosome and manchette, and late stages, including formation of the mitochondrial and fibrous sheaths. *(Modified from Fawcett DW:* Bloom and Fawcett: a textbook of histology, *ed 11, Philadelphia, 1986, Saunders.)*

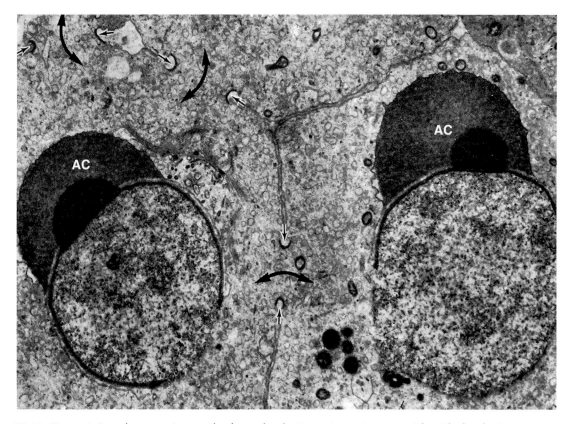

Figure 18-10. Transmission electron micrograph of two developing guinea pig spermatids with developing acrosomes *(AC)*. Curved arrows indicate intercellular bridges between the same generation of cells. Small arrows point to expansions of the cell membrane at the broad cellular connections. *(Modified from Fawcett DW:* Bloom and Fawcett: a textbook of histology, *ed 11, Philadelphia, 1986, Saunders.)*

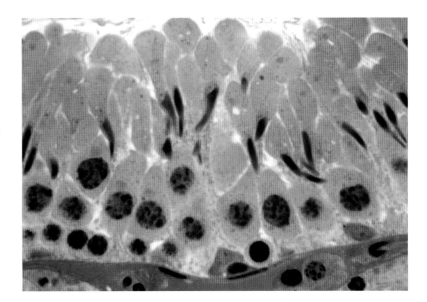

Figure 18-11. Light micrograph (×300) of spermiogenesis within the murine seminiferous tubule of the acrosomal phase with manchette.

axonemal core and outer dense fibers are surrounded by an additional ribbing of fibers. This fibrous ribbing consists of dense, ringlike structures that begin distal to the annulus and forms the **fibrous sheath.** The cell has become rotated so that the tail or flagellum extends into the lumen of the seminiferous tubule (see Figure 18-9).

With the **maturation phase** spermiogenesis is complete. During this phase, the spermatid continues to be further elongated and streamlined. Within the middle piece, the mitochondria are fully assembled in a helical manner, forming a mitochondrial sheath and distally encircling the base of the flagellum and its axoneme to the point at which the annulus meets the remainder of the flagellum (see Figures 18-8 and 18-9). Separation between adjacent spermatids occurs in this phase, resulting in the termination of the syncytium that occurs throughout much of the seminiferous epithelium. Concomitantly, a portion of the spermatid cytoplasm, that has been distally displaced along the flagellum and becomes the **residual body,** is removed and digested by the neighboring sustentacular cells. With the separation of the spermatids from one another and the phagocytosis of the excess cytoplasm, the reproductive cells become disengaged from the sustentacular cells and enter the lumen of the seminiferous tubule, a process referred to as **spermiation.** These cells have become spermatozoa.

SPERMATOZOON STRUCTURE

Newly formed spermatozoa are incapable of movement and lie motionless within the male reproductive tract. They will remain motionless and unable to fertilize oocytes until they have entered the female reproductive tract and become capacitated. Each spermatozoon consists of a head and a tail, which together make this cell long, ranging from 60 to 70 μm among domestic species (Figure 18-12).

Head

Because the head houses the nucleus, the size and shape of the deeply heterochromatic nucleus primarily influences the size and shape of the head for any particular species. In all instances the anterior portion of the nucleus, including its pole, is covered by the acrosomal cap. The cap contains enzymes needed to penetrate the oocyte's zona pellucida.

Tail

Posteriorly, the cap ends and the nucleus lies next to the **neck,** a short narrowed portion of the spermatozoon that joins the head to the tail. The pair of centrioles is located here. One of the centrioles forms the base of the axoneme and becomes the origin of the nine electron-dense fibers that run longitudinally along the axis the tail (see Figure 18-12).

Extending from the neck, the **middle piece** contains the proximal portion of the axoneme, the adjacent dense fibers, and an external layer of mitochondria that are oriented in a helical manner around the dense fibers. The caudal base of the middle piece narrows in its diameter as the mitochondria cease to wrap around the dense fibers and subjacent axoneme.

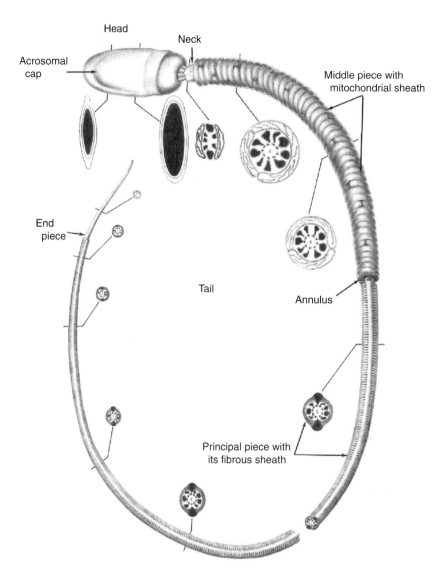

Figure 18-12. Illustration of the mature mammalian spermatozoon. *(Modified from Fawcett DW:* Bloom and Fawcett: a textbook of histology, *ed 11, Philadelphia, 1986, Saunders.)*

Instead an **annulus** is formed in their place, consisting of a short dense ring that is attached to the cell membrane (see Figure 18-12).

The **principal piece** begins at the end of the annulus and continues caudally as the longest portion of the tail. As in the middle piece, the flagellar axoneme is lined externally by the dense fibers that vary in size and are, in turn, surrounded by the **fibrous sheath** (see Figure 8-12). In this portion of the tail, the dense fibers that flank the axoneme are reduced to seven, as two of the original nine fibers terminate in the annulus of the middle piece. Throughout the length of the principal piece, its diameter gradually tapers before joining the last portion of the tail, the end piece. The tapering of the principal piece is due to the gradual reduction in size of the dense fibers and

associated fibrous sheath until they finally disappear altogether.

The **end piece** constitutes the final portion of the tail, consisting of only the microtubular axoneme of the flagella surrounded by the cell membrane.

SPERMATOGENIC CYCLE

During the continuous events of one spermatogenic cycle that ultimately result in the production of newly formed spermatozoa, several or more stages of spermatogonial development will be encountered among the seminiferous tubules as well as within an individual seminiferous tubule. Altogether, the specific number of stages that transpire during a single spermatogenic cycle vary from one species to another

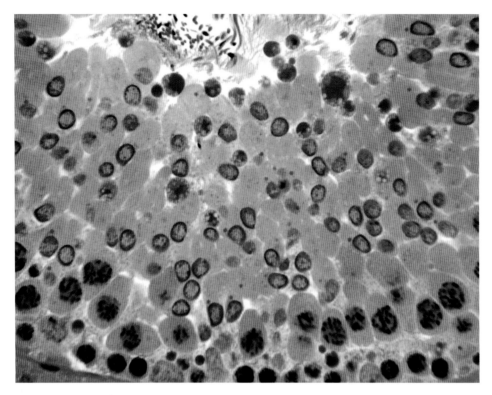

Figure 18-13. Light micrograph of an early stage of spermatogenesis in the seminiferous tubule of a rat. (Hematoxylin and eosin stain; ×250.)

(8 in the boar vs. 14 in the rat for example) and not unexpectedly, the duration of spermatogenic cycles among mammals varies as well (8.6 days in the boar vs. 12.9 in the rat). At early stages during the beginning of the cycle, round early spermatids line the lumen, followed externally by two layers of primary spermatocytes and a layer of spermatogonia (Figure 18-13). In progressive stages, the spermatids and their nuclei become elongated, and the primary spermatocyte layers or generations progress to old pachytene and young leptotene stages of meiosis (see Figure 18-7). As the spermatids continue to elongate, they appear burrowed well within the sustentacular cells. The primary spermatocytes have progressed to diplotene and zygotene stages. In the next stages, the more mature generation of primary spermatocytes has become transformed into a new generation of round early spermatids. The older, elongated spermatids have become distinctly clustered within the apical portion of the sustentacular cells (Figure 18-14). In the later stages, the clustered elongated spermatids continue to mature and move toward the seminiferous lumen (see Figure 18-8). More spermatogonia (types A and B) have formed in the outermost layers. The last stages include the spermiation stage, in which the initial generation of spermatids has ended the maturation process. After separating from their resid-

ual bodies, the newly formed spermatozoa enter the lumen, unattached to the seminiferous epithelium (see Figure 18-13).

The different stages occur in succession along the seminiferous tubule, forming a spermatogenic wave. However, segments of spermatogenic waves can also occur; for example, the first four stages may be found repeatedly along a portion of the seminiferous tubule. Variations in the amount of complete spermatogenic waves and their segmented forms are likely to be species specific. Among different species are those that can produce spermatozoa throughout the year and those that are seasonal breeders, spermiating at certain times or seasons of the year. In the latter instance, during the nonbreeding season the seminiferous epithelium is poorly developed, having few spermatogonia.

INTERSTITIAL CELL

Within the lamina propria surrounding the seminiferous tubules are clusters of endocrine cells, the **interstitial cells (cells of Leydig),** that form the hormone, **testosterone.** Although varying to some extent in size among domestic species, these cells are polyhedral and uninucleated, possessing cytoplasm filled with smooth endoplasmic reticulum and interspersed mitochondria (Figure 18-15). The interstitial

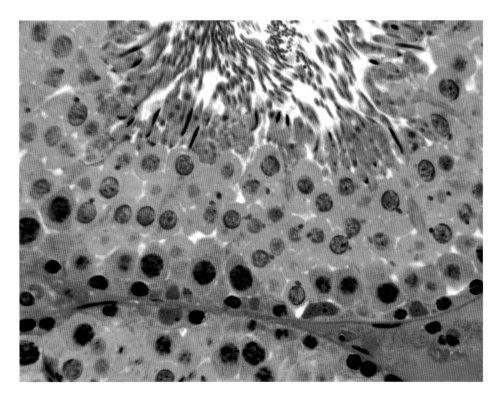

Figure 18-14. Light micrograph of a later stage of spermatogenesis in the seminiferous tubule of a rat. (Hematoxylin and eosin stain; ×250.)

cells can be especially well developed in the stallion and the boar, occupying considerable portions of the interstitial tissue that lie between adjacent tubules.

GENITAL DUCTS

The seminiferous tubules empty into a system of ducts that exist within the testes, the intratesticular ducts, and outside the testes, the extratesticular ducts. The intratesticular ducts consist of the tubuli recti and the rete testis, and the extratesticular ducts consist of the ductuli efferentes, the ductus epididymis, and the ductus deferens.

INTRATESTICULAR DUCTS

Tubuli Recti

The **tubuli recti** receive the spermatozoa formed by the seminiferous tubules. These tubules vary in length and although generally straight can be tortuous as they progress distally toward the rete testis. As the terminal segments of the seminiferous tubules join the tubuli recti, they narrow in diameter and are lined by sustentacular cells that become replaced distally by a simple squamous to cuboidal epithelium (Figure 18-

16). While the tubuli recti progress toward the rete testis, the epithelial lining may become more columnar in shape. The cells of the epithelium, which are apically modified with microvilli and occasional cilia, can house many lymphocytes and macrophages.

Rete Testis

The tubuli recti empty into the **rete testis,** which as a labyrinth-like network of anastomosing channels functions to receive via the tubuli recti the inactive spermatozoa produced by the numerous seminiferous tubules (Figure 18-17). Concomitantly, this portion of the intratesticular ducts creates the testicular fluid for the temporarily held spermatozoa. The rete testis continues to be lined by the same type of epithelium found within the distal portions of the tubuli recti with similar apical modifications. The network of channels is surrounded and held together by a substantial amount of dense connection tissue, which contains scattered myofibroblasts that lie beneath the epithelium.

EXTRATESTICULAR DUCTS

The first two types of the extratesticular ducts, the ductuli efferentes and the ductus epididymis, form the

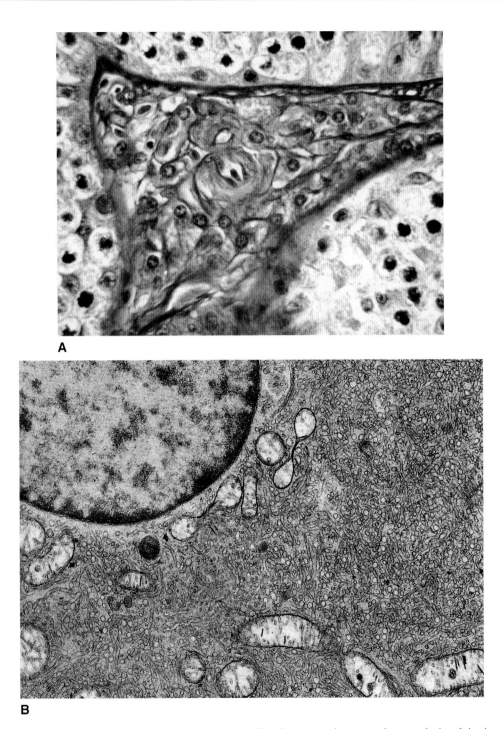

Figure 18-15. A, Light micrograph (×300) of the interstitial cells adjacent to the seminiferous tubule of the horse. **B,** Transmission electron micrograph of an interstitial cell within the testis of an opossum. *(Gartner LP, Hiatt JL: Color textbook of histology, Philadelphia, 1997, Saunders.)*

accessory structure known as the **epididymis.** The epididymis stores the spermatozoa, which continue to remain inactive within the male reproduction tract, and provides its own substance, replacing the testicular fluid formed by the rete testis.

Ductuli Efferentes

From the rete testis, 8 to 20 or so short tubules, known collectively as the **ductuli efferentes,** lead the spermatozoa to the ductus epididymis. These tubules or

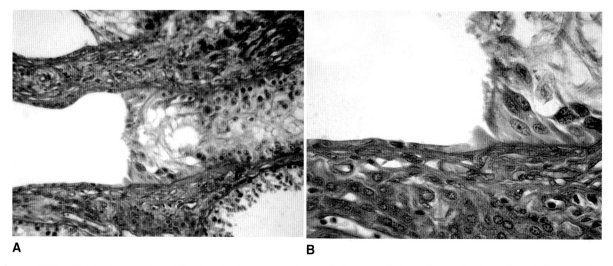

Figure 18-16. Light micrographs of the terminal segment of a seminiferous tubule as it empties into the tubuli recti of a horse. (Hematoxylin and eosin stain; **A,** ×100; **B,** ×300.)

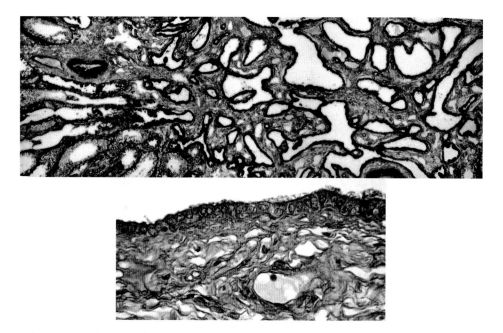

Figure 18-17. Light micrograph (×15) of the equine testis rete. Each channel is lined by low columnar ciliated epithelium (inset, ×250). (Hematoxylin and eosin stain.)

ductules are lined once again by a simple epithelium, simple cuboidal to low columnar, that is either ciliated or nonciliated. Those that are nonciliated are usually equipped apically with microvilli. Typically, those that are ciliated and those that are nonciliated are clustered from one another, resulting in alternating ciliated and nonciliated regions within the ductules. The nonciliated portions are most likely involved in the absorp-

tion of the testicular fluid, whereas the ciliated portions facilitate the movement of the spermatozoa toward the ductus epididymis. The underlying connective tissue is composed of collagen and elastic fibers and intermittent layers of contractile cells (myofibroblasts) that encircle each ductule and are innervated sympathetically and parasympathetically by nonmyelinated fibers in the cat.

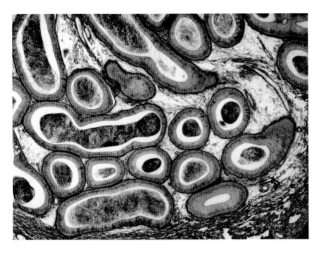

Figure 18-18. Light micrograph of the body region of an equine epididymis. (Hematoxylin and eosin stain; ×20.)

Ductus Epididymis

The **ductus epididymis** consists of a long, highly convoluted tubule that, for reference purposes, is subdivided into three portions: the head, body, and tail (see Figure 18-1). The length of the entire duct varies greatly among domestic species and can reach up to 70 meters in the stallion. The **head** (caput) is the portion that receives the contents contained within the ductuli efferentes. This portion, which immediately becomes highly coiled, and the **body** (corpus) possess a simple epithelium of considerable height, having at least two cell types: the tall columnar **principal cell** and the short polygonal **basal cell** (Figure 18-18; see also Figure 3-13). The principal cells of this pseudostratified columnar epithelium form the long, often branched microvilli, also known as **stereocilia** (see Figure 3-23). Much of their cytoplasm is filled with rough endoplasmic reticulum, that is located more basally, and Golgi apparatus and smooth endoplasmic reticulum, that are positioned apically. At the base of the stereocilia, pinocytotic and coated vesicles can be frequently observed. The principal cells function both to absorb and secrete. The secretions include enzymes, such as phosphatases and glycosidases, and the glycoprotein, **glycerophosphocholine,** which serves to keep spermatozoa from fertilizing secondary oocytes by inhibiting their capacitation (an event discussed in Chapter 19). The basal cells, which are comparatively few in number, contain sparse amount of organelles within a small cytoplasm and are believed to be stem cells for the principal cell population. In addition to these cell types, other cell types may be encountered in different species, including apical cells and clear cells. Lymphocytes and macrophages assist in removing cytoplasmic remnants that were not entirely removed by the sustentacular cells. It is within the head and the body of the ductus epididymis that the spermatozoa complete their maturation, including loss of the residual cytoplasmic droplets and initiation of flagellar motility. These final stages of sperm differentiation are likely the result of sequential interactions with epididymal fluid as the spermatozoa are moved through the head, body, and tail of this structure. With the coordinated activities of absorption and secretion, the spermatozoa mature as they become concentrated, protected, and stored.

The epithelial basement membrane of the ductus epididymis is attached to a thin layer of connective tissue, which, in turn, is encircled by a thin layer of smooth muscle (Figure 18-19). Contraction of the smooth muscle assists in moving the maturing spermatozoa to the caudal portion of the ductus epididymis. This portion—referred to as the **tail** (cauda) of the ductus epididymis—stores the mature spermatozoa for extended periods if necessary. The height of the principal cells within the pseudostratified epithelium becomes reduced as the tail moves toward the ductus deferens. The surrounding smooth muscle thickens.

Changes in normal hormone exposure of estrogens and quite possibly progestins and androgens during prepubertal development of dogs can result in alterations of both the epithelium and surrounding peritubular tissue that could alter the functional capability of the epididymis. As animals become aged, epithelial hyperplasia of the epididymis appears to be a normal feature.

Ductus Deferens

The ductus epididymis ends, emptying into the **ductus deferens** (vas deferens). At this junction, the coiled tail abruptly straightens, indicating the beginning of the ductus deferens (see Figure 18-1). The epithelial lining continues to be pseudostratified columnar with short stereociliated principal cells. Like the ductus epididymis, the base of the epithelium is attached to a thin layer of a well-vascularized loose connective tissue. This tissue is encircled by a very well-developed layer of smooth muscle that is additionally lined by another, external layer of smooth muscle oriented along the longitudinal axis of the ductus deferens; together they comprise a well-developed tunica muscularis (Figure 18-20). In large herbivorous species, the tunica muscularis of the ductus deferens includes obliquely positioned smooth muscle that intermingles with the circular and longitudinal layers. Externally, a usual serosal lining completes the construction of this part of the extratesticular duct system. Toward the end

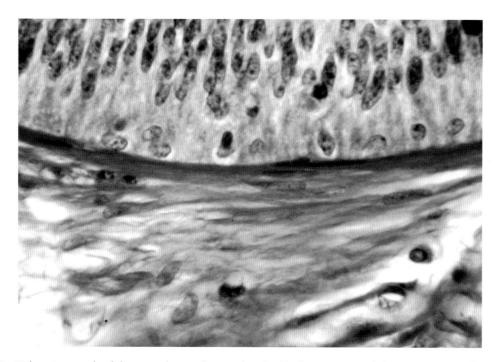

Figure 18-19. Light micrograph of the smooth muscle associated with the equine epididymis. (Hematoxylin and eosin stain; ×400.)

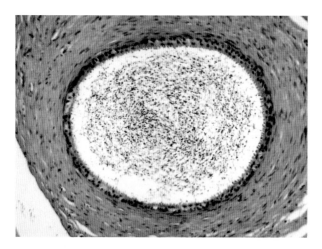

Figure 18-20. Light micrograph of the ductus deferens of the cat. (Hematoxylin and eosin stain; ×15.)

of the ductus deferens, the first accessory gland of the male reproductive tract is formed, consisting of simple branched tubuloalveolar mucus glands that lie within the propria-submucosa. In some domestic animals, such as the dog, ram, bull and stallion, this portion is extensive and forms an ampulla. The cat and the boar lack ampullae, but still possess this accessory gland.

The termination of the ductus deferens varies from species to species. In the bull, ram, and stallion, the ductus deferens joins the excretory duct of the vesicular gland to become an ejaculatory duct that empties into the urethra. In the boar, the ductus deferens does not join the excretory duct of the vesicular gland because each duct empties into the urethra separately. In the dog and cat, the ductus deferens leads directly to the urethra as well, but for a different reason than that of boars. Male carnivores do not form vesicular glands.

ACCESSORY GLANDS

In addition to the glands of the ductus deferens, spermatozoa are bathed in secretions that form the seminal plasma of the ejaculate or semen. In most domestic animals, the seminal plasma is made by the **accessory glands,** which include the ductus deferens, the vesicular gland, the prostate, and the bulbo-urethral gland (Table 18-1). Only carnivores lack the vesicular gland, and the dog lacks the bulbo-urethral gland as well. The seminal plasma is both mucous and serous in composition and functions to nourish and provide the necessary energy source for spermatozoa motility, lubricate the urethra, and create a volume of ejaculate that helps move the spermatozoa from the male into the female as a bolus and plug the vagina.

TABLE 18-1 Key Morphological Characteristics of the Glands Associated with the Male Reproductive Tract of Domestic Species

GLAND	ARCHITECTURAL ORGANIZATION	CELLS (MORPHOLOGY AND ACTIVITY)	FUNCTION AND SPECIES VARIATIONS
Terminal portion of the ductus deferens	Well-developed muscular tunic, especially in the boar, bull, and stallion; thins distally; simple, branched tubuloalveolar glands within lamina propria submucosa form ampullae in the dog, ruminant, and stallion	Secretory cells are columnar to cuboidal with basally located oval to round nuclei; release serous secretion; presence of scattered basal cells	Function is unknown; secretory cells can be glycogen-ladened in ruminants, and in the bull contain lipid droplets that can fuse into one, including basal cells
Vesicular	Muscular tunic can consist of inner circular and outer longitudinal, which may or may not be intertwined; compound tubuloalveolar or tubular glands within well-vascularized lamina propria submucosa that can develop into stromal partitions for lobe and lobule formation; secretory ducts empty centrally	Secretory cells are columnar to high columnar shaped, interspersed with occasional basal cells that can possess single lipid droplets; secretions released have high concentrations of sugars (fructose); secretory ducts consist of simple columnar to simple cuboidal	Provide energy source for spermatozoa; this gland is absent in carnivores; glands form vesicular outpocketings in the horse with ducts of stratified columnar epithelium; in the bull, stromal septae separating lobules contain smooth muscle
Prostate	Stromal capsule with considerable amount of smooth muscle that continues into stromal septae; glandular parenchyma consists of compound tubuloalveolar glands that comprise two portions: the body (external portion) and the disseminate (internal) portion; ducts can be widely sacculated, allowing considerable storage of secretory material	Secretory cells as well as duct cells are cuboidal to low columnar shaped; occasional basal cells occur; secretion is serous to seromucoid	Secretions increase motility of spermatozoa and facilitate vaginal plug formation; in the bull secretion contains citrate and fructose; bilaterally lobed in the dog encircling proximal pelvic urethra, whereas in the cat the lobes lie laterally and dorsally along the urethra; the body is less developed in ruminants (nonexistent in rams)
Bulbourethral	Stromal capsule with fibroelastic tissue and some smooth muscle as well as skeletal muscle (from the bulbocavernous and urethral muscles); glandular parenchyma consists of compound tubuloalveolar (ruminants and stallion) or tubular (boar and cat) glands	Secretory cells are high columnar shaped; occasional basal cells occur; secretion is mostly mucus; duct system is present, beginning with simple cuboidal to columnar epithelia that line small ducts and empty into pseudostratified columnar epithelial-lined larger ducts that flow into one or more principal bulbourethral duct(s)	Clears penile urethra of urine and assists lubrication of vagina as a preejaculatory fluid; in the cat, it has glycogen, which may provide energy source for spermatozoa; absent in the dog, but well developed in the boar

The accessory glands are largely targets of androgens, which can control activities of epithelial tissue as well as direct the development and regression of stromal cells, including smooth muscle elements.

VESICULAR GLAND

Anatomically, boars form a pair of vesicular glands, whereas carnivores lack this gland. In most domestic animals, the **vesicular gland** (seminal vesicles) consists of a lobulated compound gland that has a central duct surrounded radially by branching tubular to tubuloalveolar adenomeres (Figure 18-21). In the stallion, glandular epithelium lines a collection of vesicle-like outpocketings. The duct system is lined by a simple cuboidal epithelium that in the stallion, for example, can be stratified columnar. However, the glandular epithelium is pseudostratified columnar with round, short basal cells scattered between the columnar cells. The basal cells can contain single prominent lipid droplets that are rich in cholesterol and triglycerides and occupy most of the cytoplasm. Smaller lipid droplets occur within the cytoplasm of the columnar cells that also store extensive amounts glycogen, often near their apices. As the principal secretory cell, the columnar cells secrete large amounts of fructose that

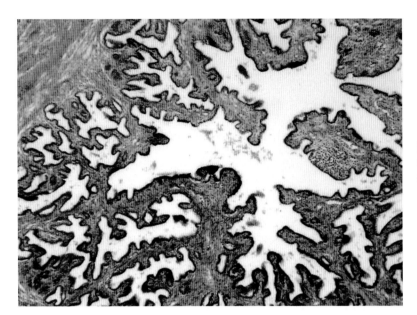

Figure 18-21. Light micrograph of the equine vesicular gland. (Hematoxylin and eosin stain; ×30.)

provides energy for the spermatozoa and makes this portion of the ejaculate viscous. The glandular epithelium also may be able to release lipochrome pigment into its secretion, giving it a pale yellow appearance. The propria-submucosa is made of well-vascularized loose connective tissue that becomes dense where the stroma separates the secretory portions into lobules and lobes. The tunica muscularis can vary in amount and orientation—either interwoven or layered circularly and longitudinally.

PROSTATE GLAND

The next accessory gland, the **prostate,** surrounds the pelvic urethra in two parts: an outer, compact **body (corpus prostatae)** that completely or partially covers an inner **disseminate part (disseminata prostatae).** The body of the prostate is externally lined by a capsule of dense irregular connective tissue that becomes continuous with the rest of the stroma, being primarily the propria-submucosa. Much of the glandular parenchyma of the prostate is located within the body, consisting of multiple compound tubuloalveolar secretory segments that individually wind through the propria-submucosa and its disseminate part and empty by their secretions directly into the urethra. The disseminate part is much like the body, but only less so, having fewer tubuloalveolar segments (Figure 18-22). The glandular epithelium as well as the ducts can range from cuboidal to columnar in shape. The secretory material is generally serous among domestic animals, but can have mucous adenomeres, such as that in the bull, which forms seromucoid secretions (see Table 18-1).

The body and disseminate part of the prostate are often variably developed among the males of different domestic species. In ruminants, the body is less pronounced than that of other domestic animals. In the bull, the glandular tissue exists intermittently among the bundles of smooth muscle within the tunica muscularis, whereas in the ram it is essentially nonexistent. By comparison, the disseminate part is considerably more developed in these males. Only the ventral portion of the propria-submucosa in the ram is void of any secretory segments.

The glandular parenchyma of the stallion is arranged in nearly an opposite manner of that in ruminants and is formed solely in the outer portion rather than internally. Here the gland is bilobed, with right and left portions interconnected dorsally by an isthmus.

The carnivorous prostate is well developed, and like the horse is best formed within the body or corpus prostatae, consisting of two lobes. However, both the cat and the dog possess the disseminate part, which is lobular and scattered.

BULBOURETHRAL GLAND

As the urethra progresses into the copulatory organ, the penis, another accessory gland usually exists, that being the **bulbourethral gland,** which consists of a paired structure that lies dorsolaterally to the pelvic urethra. The secretory units are arranged as either compound tubuloalveoli (in the stallion and ruminants) or compound tubuli (in the cat and the boar), being absent in the dog. The secretory epithelia are generally simple columnar and produce a

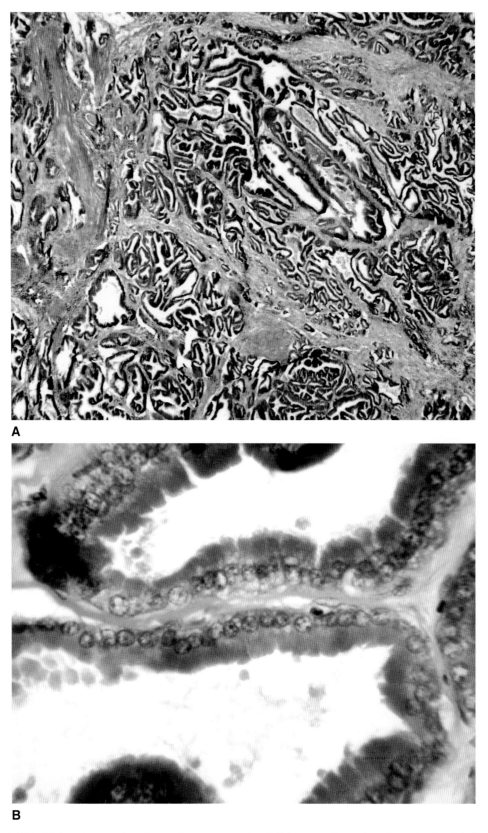

A

B

Figure 18-22. Light micrographs of a canine prostate gland. (Hematoxylin and eosin stain; **A,** ×20; **B,** ×250.)

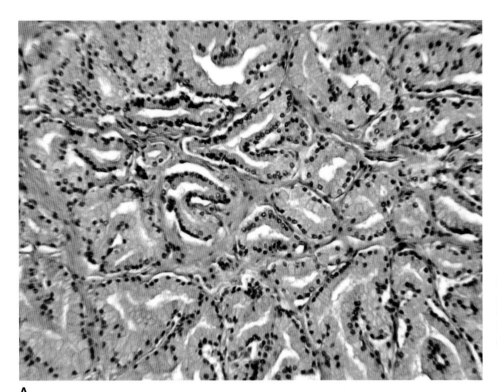

A

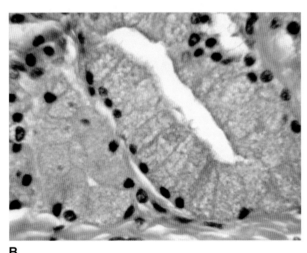

B

Figure 18-23. Light micrographs of a feline bulbourethral gland. (Hematoxylin and eosin stain; **A,** ×100; **B,** ×400.)

mucus-rich product in most species, but can contain serous material in ruminants as well (Figure 18-23). For the most part, the secretion of the bulbourethral gland, which is released before ejaculation, serves initially to clear the urethra of urine and subsequently aid in lubricating the vagina.

The adenomeres empty into a duct system, which initially consists of simple cuboidal or simple columnar epithelia (lining the collecting ducts). As these ducts join one another, the epithelial lining becomes pseudostratified columnar, eventually emptying into a single large duct that is lined by a transitional epithelium before connecting with the urethra.

The bulbourethral gland is externally covered by a capsule of fibroelastic connective tissue with smooth and skeletal muscle cells, the latter originating from adjacent bulbocavernous and urethral muscles. From the capsule, septae of thin dense to loose connective tissue support segments of the gland as they lie within the propria-submucosa. Smooth and skeletal muscle cells can be included within the septae.

URETHRA

As a part of the excretory duct system of the urinary tract, the **urethra** connects the urinary bladder

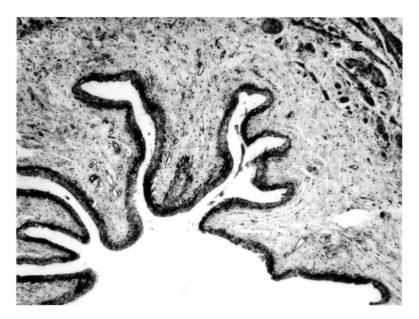

Figure 18-24. Light micrograph of a bovine pelvic urethra lined by transitional epithelium. *E,* Erectile tissue. (Hematoxylin and eosin stain; ×30.)

to the body surface, ending at the prepuce in most species or glans penis in the dog and the stallion, where it forms the external urethral opening. The entire urethra can be divided into several regions, beginning with the prostatic region, which extends from the urinary bladder to the **colliculus seminalis,** an area that becomes slightly enlarged and has openings of ducts from the ductus deferens, the prostate, and the vesicular gland. Folds lined by transitional epithelium, including the dorsomedial urethral crest, extend along the longitudinal axis of the urethra, projecting into its lumen. The propria-submucosa contains **erectile tissue,** consisting of endothelial-lined sinus-like caverns that can be engorged with blood. The tunica muscularis is composed of skeletal muscle, intermingling initially with smooth muscle in the region of the urinary bladder.

From the prostatic region, the urethra continues toward the base of the penis, forming the membranous (pelvic) urethra (Figure 18-24; see also Figure 18-4). The membranous urethra is lined by a transitional epithelium. The dorsomedial urethral crest seen within the prostatic region ceases to exist in the membranous region. The propria-submucosa contains loose connective tissue housing smooth muscle, many simple glands (mostly tubular and mucus secreting), and erectile tissue.

As the urethra enters the bulb of the penis, the membranous portion ends and the spongiose portion begins. The epithelial lining continues to be predominantly transitional with areas or patches of simple columnar, stratified columnar, and stratified cuboidal epithelia. At or near the urethral opening, the epithelium becomes stratified squamous. In the propria-submucosa, the erectile tissue is more pronounced, having larger vascular caverns than those encountered in the prostatic and membranous portions. This portion of the erectile tissue is the **corpus spongiosum.**

PENIS

The penis of domestic species functions as a shared outlet for the excretion of urine and the deposition of spermatozoa into the respective female reproductive tract. Consequently this structure can be considered a portion of both the urinary and reproductive systems in males. Although shared by both systems, the penis is designed for the copulatory ejaculation of semen and spermatozoa. For that reason, much of the penis consists of erectile tissues required for copulation. This structure then is composed of the paired corpora cavernosa penis, the corpus spongiosum penis, and the glans penis.

The **corpora cavernosa penis,** which makes up much of the body of the penis, consists of two dorsal columns of erectile tissue that are lined by a dense connective tissue, the tunica albuginea. The tunica albuginea may become discontinuous and allow the vascular cavernous spaces to join one another or, in the dog and stallion, form a connective tissue septum. The erectile tissue consists primarily of vascularized connective tissue that can be ladened with elastic fibers and/or smooth muscle (Figure 18-25). The vasculature is composed of sinuses that become engorged during erection, especially within a vascular-type penis, in cats, dogs, and horses.

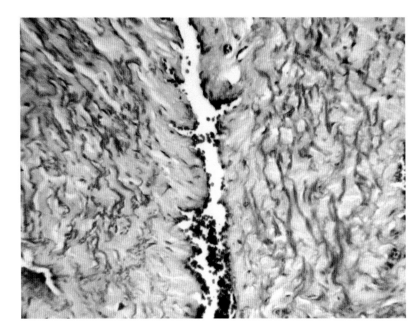

Figure 18-25. Light micrograph of the erectile tissue within the canine penis. (Hematoxylin and eosin stain; ×100.)

In pigs and ruminants, the penis enlarges to some extent with vascular engorgement. However, in these animals the tunica albuginea is well developed, consisting of dense connective tissue and forming a fibrous-type penis.

Distally the body becomes the glans, which is externally lined by a reflection of the integument, the prepuce, and ends as a slitlike aperture for the urethra. The **glans,** which is best developed in the dog and the stallion, contains a variety of tissues, depending on the species. In carnivores, the glans consists of erectile tissue, bone, **os penis,** and fibrocartilage (Figure 18-26), whereas in the bull it consists of dense connective tissue with an erectile venous plexus that surrounds the urethra, as well as forms much of the tunica albuginea.

The **prepuce** is an external layer of integument that is confluent with abdominal skin with associated hair and glands, and continues at the preputial opening to reflect or invaginate inwardly (see Figure 18-1). The internal layer may contain fine hairs and their sebaceous glands and sweat glands for some distance before reflecting onto the penile surface.

MECHANISM OF ERECTION

In the vascular-type penis, erection is the result of engorgement of the blood vessels within the erectile tissues. During stimulation, blood flow increases through the helicine arteries, which, in turn, causes the vessels within the cavernous tissues to fill. As the cavernous tissue surrounding the urethra (the corpus spongiosum) becomes engorged, this region will also

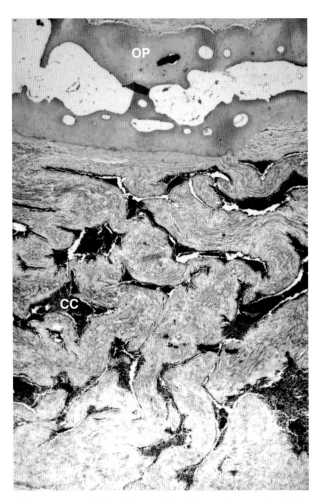

Figure 18-26. Light micrograph of the canine penis. *CC,* Corpus cavernosum; *OP,* os penis. (Hematoxylin and eosin stain; ×10.)

increase in size but without occluding the urethra and inhibiting ejaculation. In the fibrous-type penis, with the filling of the spaces within the erectile tissue, the length of the penis increases as it extends from the prepuce.

With the contraction of the smooth muscle of the helicine arteries as well as smooth muscle within the erectile tissues and tunica albuginea, the usual flaccid tone of the penis occurs. This process, which is known as *detumescence*, results in the marked reduction of blood flow into the cavernous tissues of the penis and a return to its normal circulation. In the boar, bull, and ram, a retractor penis muscle facilitates the retraction of the penis into the prepuce.

SUGGESTED READINGS

Arighi M, Singh A, Horney FD: Histology of the normal and retained equine testis, *Acta Anat* 129:127, 1987.

Christl HW: The lamina propria of vertebrate seminiferous tubules: a comparative light and electron microscopic investigation, *Andrologica* 22:85, 1990.

Connell CJ, Donjacour A: A morphological study of the epididymides of control and estradiol-treated prepubertal dogs, *Biol Reprod* 33:951, 1985.

Dacheux JL, Castella S, Gatti JL, Dacheux F: Epididymal cell secretory activities and the role of proteins in boar sperm maturation, *Theriogenology* 63:319, 2005.

Fawcett DW: *Bloom and Fawcett: a textbook of histology,* ed 11, Philadelphia, 1986, Saunders.

Fukuda T, Kikuchi M, Kurotaki T, et al: Age-related changes in the testes of horses, *Equine Vet J* 33:20, 2001.

Gartner LP, Hiatt JL: *Color textbook of histology,* Philadelphia, 1997, Saunders.

Hess RA: Spermatogenesis overview. In Knobil E, Neill JD, editors: *Encyclopedia of reproduction,* vol 4, San Diego, 1999, Academic Press.

James RW, Heywood R: Age-related variations in the testes and prostate of beagle dogs, *Toxicology* 12:273, 1979.

Jones JS, Berndston WE: A quantitative study of Sertoli cell and germ cell populations as related to sexual development and aging in the stallion, *Biol Reprod* 35:138, 1986.

Niu YJ, Ma TX, Zhang J, et al: Androgen and prostatic stroma, *Asian J Androl* 5:19, 2003.

Tsukise A, Yamada K: Histochemistry of cycloconjugates in the secretory epithelium of the goat bulbourethral gland, *Acta Anat* 129:344, 1987.

Wrobel KH, Gurtler A: Morphology and innervation pattern of the feline urogenital junction, *Anat Histol Embryol* 33:317, 2004.

Female Reproductive System

KEY CHARACTERISTICS

- Designed for the production, sustenance, and transport of ova and its subsequent fertilization and development
- Has endocrine components and fully interacts with the endocrine system
- Consists of a tubular tract (uterine tube, uterus, and vagina) with accessory glands, and connects with the caudal portion (urethra) of the urinary system
- In mammals, a portion of the system is involved in zygote implantation and subsequent placentation; in nonmammals the comparable portion is involved in eggshell formation

Among domestic animals, the female reproductive system forms a tract that is composed internally of **ovaries, uterine tubes, uterus, cervix,** and **vagina,** and externally of the **vulva** (Figure 19-1). Collectively, these components receive the male gametes and spermatozoa and facilitate their transportation as well as produce and transport the female gametes (ova) for fertilization. After fertilization the conceptus of mammals continues to develop within the tract until birth. In concert with birth and development of an organism, the **mammary gland** is included within the female reproductive system.

OVARY

Among domestic species, the ovary is oval to round and can vary in appearance and size according to different points along the cyclic production of ova, otherwise known as the reproductive cycle. As in the testes of the male reproductive system, ovaries are paired and involved in endocrine activities concomitant with ova production. Each ovary can be refer-

enced by cranial and caudal poles as well as its dorsal and ventral surfaces and medial and lateral borders.

In the adult female, the surface of an ovary is lined by a simple low cuboidal to squamous serosal epithelium. This epithelium is subtended by a layer of little vascularized, dense irregular connective tissue that forms the **tunica albuginea,** the capsule of the ovary. In most species the tunica albuginea covers the **cortex,** the first of two zones that comprise the body of the ovary in most species. The second zone is the **medulla,** which lies centrally within the ovary, surrounded by the cortex (Figure 19-2). In the horse, the cortex lies centrally, surrounded by the medulla.

CORTEX

The cortex contains a somewhat loosely arranged framework of connective tissue that forms the stroma and surrounds follicles of various stages of development. Cells within the stroma include clusters of fibroblasts, also known as **stromal cells,** that can vary in their morphology (often having an epithelioid appearance), and consist of interstitial gland cells and thecal cells associated with follicular development.

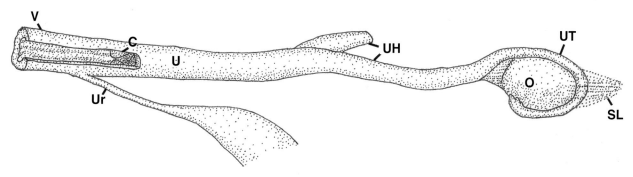

Figure 19-1. Schematic diagram of the female reproductive tract of the cat. *C,* Cervix; *O,* ovary; *SL,* suspensory ligament; *U,* uterus; *UH,* uterine horn; *UT,* uterine tube; *Ur,* urethra; *V,* vagina.

The interstitial gland cells are endocrine and can form cords in bitches, queens, and rodents.

Most of the cortex consists of follicles, which are ova-bearing structures that originate during fetal development with the production of the female gametes. The first formed follicles, the **primordial follicles,** consist of a **primary oocyte** and surrounding **follicular cells,** which at this time is a simple squamous epithelium with its own basal lamina (Figure 19-3). Having originated from oogonia, the primary oocyte has begun the first meiotic division and progressed through the leptotene, zygotene, pachytene, and diplotene stages of prophase. Completion of prophase will not occur until ovulation, which can take place many years later. Hundreds of thousands to millions of primary oocytes are initially formed in the fetus and held within primordial follicles located within the outer periphery of the cortex next to the tunica albuginea. Many of these degenerate fetally and continue to degenerate thereafter throughout the lifetime of the individual. Ultimately, only hundreds of primordial follicles will advance to ovulation during the normal course of an animal's life span. The remainder are stopped at various stages of development and subsequently break down in a process known as **follicular atresia.**

Ovarian Follicles

Follicles within the cortex of each ovary consist of a primary oocyte and surrounding supportive cells, the follicular cells, which in turn become surrounded by specialized stromal cells. Each follicle has the potential to undergo a progressive series of changes that result in four specific stages of development, comprising the formation of primordial follicles, primary follicles, secondary follicles and tertiary follicles.

Primordial Follicles. The first follicle formed is the **primordial follicle,** the most numerous fetally or soon postnatally as in canine species. Initially oogonia

develop from internal epithelial cell masses. Among the cell masses, clusters of cells separate from one another. Within each cluster a central cell differentiates into an oogonium, which subsequently enters the prophase of the first meiosis while concomitantly becoming larger—it thus becomes the primary oocyte. Morphologically, the primary oocyte possesses a large, round euchromatic nucleus, $10\,\mu m$ or greater in diameter with a distinct single nucleus (Figure 19-4; see also Figure 19-3). The cytoplasm is composed mostly of mitochondria, rough endoplasmic reticulum (rER), Golgi apparatus, and small vesicles that are most likely derived from the Golgi apparatus. The primary oocyte is entirely encased by a single layer of follicular cells that are flattened or squamous at this time. Laterally, adjacent follicular cells are attached to each other by desmosomal junctions, and basally these cells form a basal lamina. In large herbivores, primordial follicles tend to be evenly distributed throughout the outer cortex. By comparison, in carnivores these follicles are more clustered.

Primary Follicles. On reaching sexual maturity, from resting primordial follicles individual follicles will continue to develop into **primary follicles,** also referred to as being **preantral** and **unilaminar** (Figure 19-5). The primary oocyte grows larger, resulting in multiple Golgi complexes, extensive rER and polysomes, and further proliferation of mitochondria, all dispersing fairly evenly throughout the cytoplasm or ooplasm of the oocyte. Vesicles, which remain usually small, and multivesicular bodies build up as well. During this stage of development, the oocyte will increase its size by two or more times. Concomitantly, the adjacent follicular cells become distinctly cuboidal to low columnar and still comprise a single surrounding layer.

Secondary Follicles. The primary oocyte continues to enlarge appreciably in the same manner described for the primary follicles (Figure 19-6). The encircling follicular cells divide and give rise to a stratified

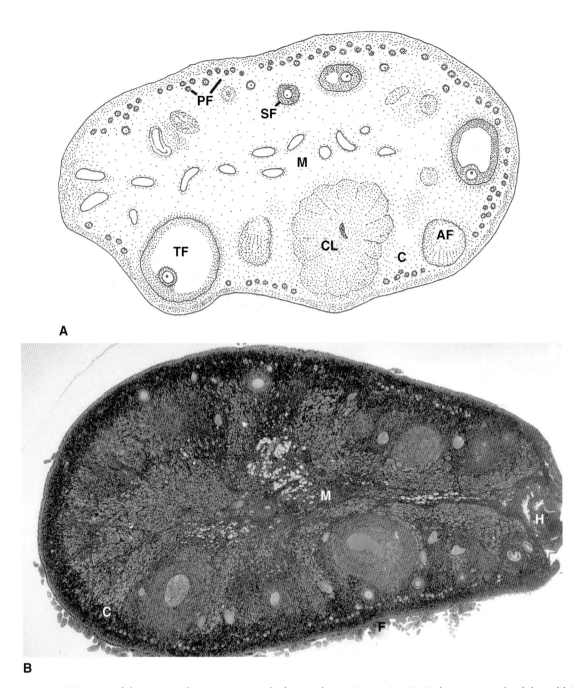

A

B

Figure 19-2. A, Diagram of the mammalian ovary typical of most domestic species. **B,** Light micrograph of the rabbit ovary. (Hematoxylin and eosin stain; ×6.) *AF,* Atretic follicle; *C,* cortex; *CL,* corpus luteum; *F,* fimbriae of the infundibulum; *H,* hilus; *M,* medulla; *PF,* primordial follicle; *SF,* secondary follicle; *TF,* tertiary follicle.

epithelial lining. As a result, a secondary follicle becomes formed, which can still be referred to as pre-antral, but is now **multilaminar** due to the multiple layers of follicular cells. The follicular cells are known at this stage of development as **granulosa cells.** Basally, the granulosa cells remain attached to the adjacent stroma by a thickened basal lamina, **membrana limitans externa.** Apically, the granulosa cells become separated from the oocyte by a space called

the **zona pellucida** (see Figure 9-6). The zona pellucida consists of an amorphous material produced by the secretions of the primary oocyte. Along the cell membrane of the oocyte, vesicles release a variety of glycoproteins, which result in the formation of this highly refractile layer. However, the zona pellucida does not form a true barrier as numerous microvilli-like processes extend from the oocyte and attach to filopodial extensions of the internal-most granulosa

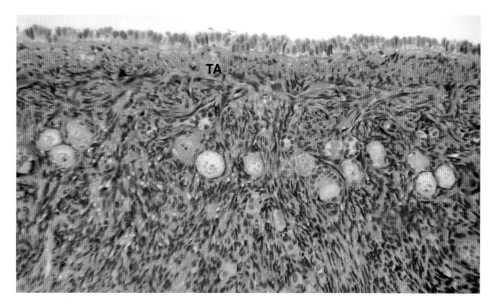

Figure 19-3. Light micrograph of the outer cortex in the rabbit ovary. *TA,* Tunica albuginea. (Plastic section, hematoxylin and eosin stain; ×100.)

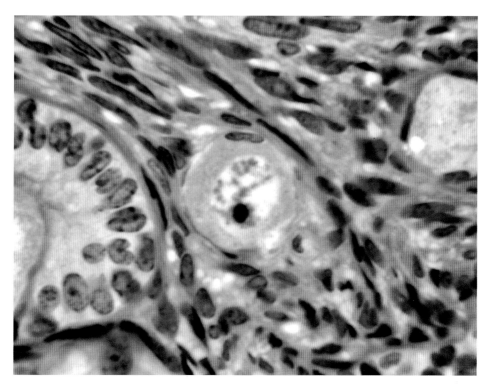

Figure 19-4. Light micrograph of a primordial follicle within the outer cortex. (Plastic section, hematoxylin and eosin stain; ×400.)

cells. The two sets of adjacent processes are further connected by gap junctions, thus allowing direct communication between the oocyte and the granulosa cells.

During the development of the secondary follicle, surrounding stromal cells become organized. These cells continue to divide and become concentrically oriented around the follicle with concomitant developed vascularity.

Tertiary Follicles. As granulosa cells continue to proliferate and a large spherical follicle takes shape, the **tertiary follicle** is formed (Figure 19-7). Spaces

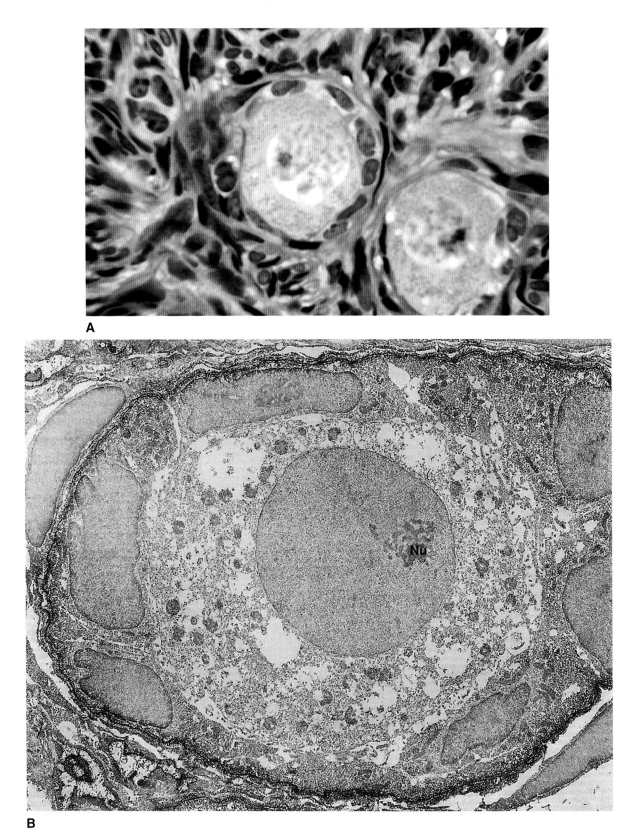

Figure 19-5. A, Light micrograph of a primary follicle in the rabbit ovary. (Plastic section, hematoxylin and eosin stain; ×400.) **B,** Transmission electron micrograph of a primary follicle in a rat ovary. (×7000.) *Nu,* Nucleolus of the primary oocyte. *(Modified from Gartner LP, Hiatt JL:* Color textbook of histology, *Philadelphia, 1997, Saunders.)*

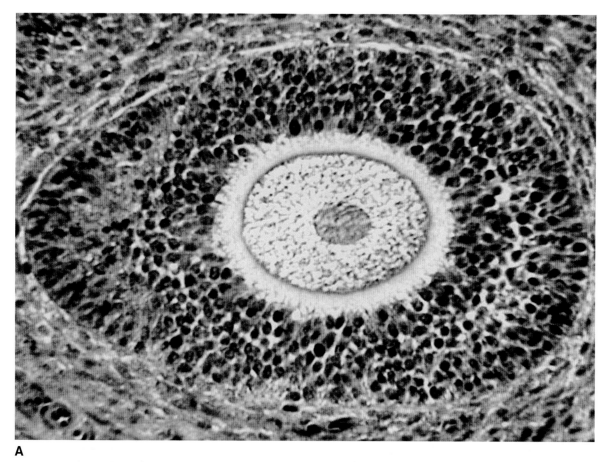

A

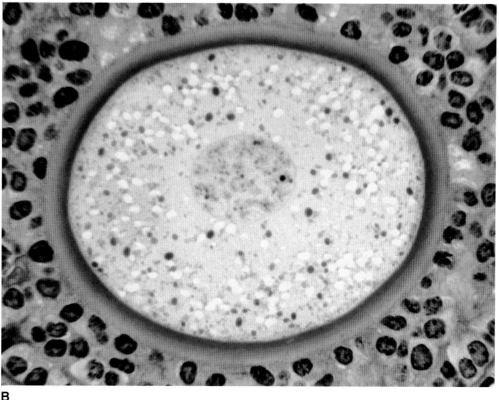

B

Figure 19-6. A, Light micrograph of a secondary follicle with the zona pellucida surrounding the primary oocyte in the canine ovary. (Hematoxylin and eosin [H&E] stain; ×100.) **B,** Light micrograph of the zona pellucida within a late secondary follicle in the rabbit ovary. (Plastic section, H&E stain; ×250.)

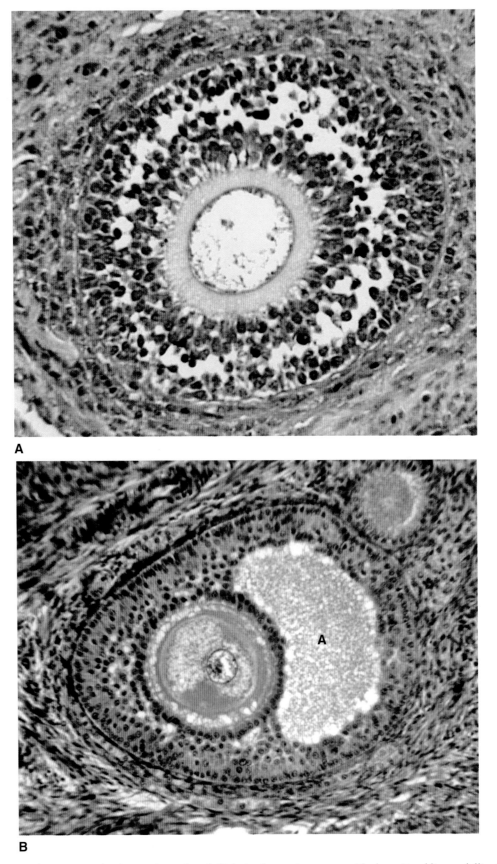

A

B

Figure 19-7. A, Light micrograph of an early tertiary follicle in the canine ovary with deposits of liquor folliculi between granulosa cells. (Hematoxylin and eosin [H&E] stain; ×100.) **B,** Light micrograph of a tertiary follicle with a developing antrum *(A)* in the feline ovary. (H&E stain; ×100.)

between granulosa cells arise, forming the **liquor folliculi,** a fluid of plasma origin in part, consisting of glycosaminoglycans and steroid-associated protein. The spaces, which become clefts, soon fuse into a single large cavity, the **antrum.** With the occurrence of this structure, the tertiary follicle is sometimes referred to as the **antral follicle.** With the development of the antrum, the primary oocyte is displaced off to one side. The surrounding layers of granulosa cells become the **cumulus oophorus.** The granulosa cells immediately adjacent to the oocyte increase in their height and become radially oriented around the oocyte, resulting in the formation of the **corona radiata** (Figure 19-8). These cells have a direct role in supporting the primary oocyte. During the course of the development of the tertiary follicle, most of the growth involves the antrum because the size of the oocyte does not progress much beyond 300 μm in diameter, being smaller than that in most species. Granulosa cells can occasionally be associated with round periodic acid–Schiff (PAS)–positive bodies (Call-Exner bodies) that contribute to the liquor folliculi (Table 19-1). Eventually the tertiary follicles increase to prominent sizes that can reach at ovulation 2 cm or greater in the cow and mare; in most domestic species they range between 6 and 11 mm, with the queen possessing the smallest at 3 to 4 mm. As the follicle reaches maturation, the cumulus oophorus with its primary oocyte and associated corona radiata breaks from the rest of the granulosa cells and moves freely within the antrum.

Within the surrounding stroma, the thecal cells further develop into two portions: an inner well-vascularized layer, the **theca interna,** and an outer fibrous connective tissue, the **theca externa** (Figure 19-9). The cells of the theca interna become less spindly than those of the theca externa during the development of the tertiary follicle. As the follicle matures, these cells, which form reticular fibers early in their development, become epithelioid as they build up metabolic machinery typically found in steroid-producing cells. Ultrastructurally, their cytoplasm is filled with smooth endoplasmic reticulum, mitochondria with tubular cristae, small lipid droplets, and a well-formed Golgi apparatus, with only a scattering of rER. These cells become responsible for the production of the precursor of estrogens—the female sex hormones. Cells of the theca externa remain fibroblastic and form a thin rim of loose connective tissue around the theca interna, housing the larger vessels that give rise to the capillary bed, which feeds the theca interna.

Once the tertiary follicle has completed its development, it has become a **mature follicle,** ready to rupture and release the oocyte, a process called **ovulation.** In most domestic species as ovulation

approaches, the primary oocyte is able to complete the first meiotic division. At this time two daughter cells are formed, each containing a complement of chromosomes, originating from both parents. One of the daughter cells becomes the **secondary oocyte,** and the other becomes the **polar body,** sharing little of the cytoplasm after cytokinesis and is subsequently given off (Figure 19-10). The secondary oocyte immediately undergoes the **second meiotic division** to be arrested once more, but in this instance in the metaphase stage. In canine and equine species, completion of the first meiotic division does not occur until shortly after ovulation.

Ovulation. As the tertiary follicle fully matures (except for the bitch and the mare in which the primary oocyte becomes the secondary oocyte), the mature follicle presses against the tunica albuginea of the ovary. As this process occurs, the compressed region loses vasculature, thins, and becomes transparent. This compressed region is called the **stigma** and will soon become the site of ovulation. The connective tissue of the stigma as well as the wall of the mature follicle at the site of the stigma break down. At this point, an opening is formed between the antrum of the mature follicle and the tissue within the abdominal cavity that lines the ovary.

A principal factor responsible for the series of events that have been just described is the change in the levels of the endocrine secretion known as **luteinizing hormone (LH)** (see Table 19-1). The surge of LH causes the primary oocyte to complete the first meiotic division and the secondary oocyte to enter the second meiotic division. With the rise of LH, histamine is elevated as well, causing blood vessels within the theca to dilate and the stroma of the maturing follicle to become edematous. A concomitant release of prostaglandins results in elevated **matrix metalloproteinase (MMP)** activities, which include collagenases and other enzymes involved in **extracellular matrix (ECM)** degradation and remodeling of the ovarian connective tissue. Specifically, the prostaglandins stimulate the follicular cells to secrete selected MMPs, principally, collagenases that contribute greatly to the breakdown of the follicular wall at the stigma and a concomitant inflammatory response as leukocytes penetrate this region. The combination of these activities results in the effective removal of both the follicular wall and the tunica albuginea, causing the oocyte with its corona radiata and other cells of the cumulus oophorus along with follicular fluid to be released from the ovary into the peritoneal cavity. At this point, the oocyte enters into the **fimbriated infundibulum** of the uterine tube. If the oocyte does not flow into the uterine tube, but remains at the ovary and becomes fertilized there, an

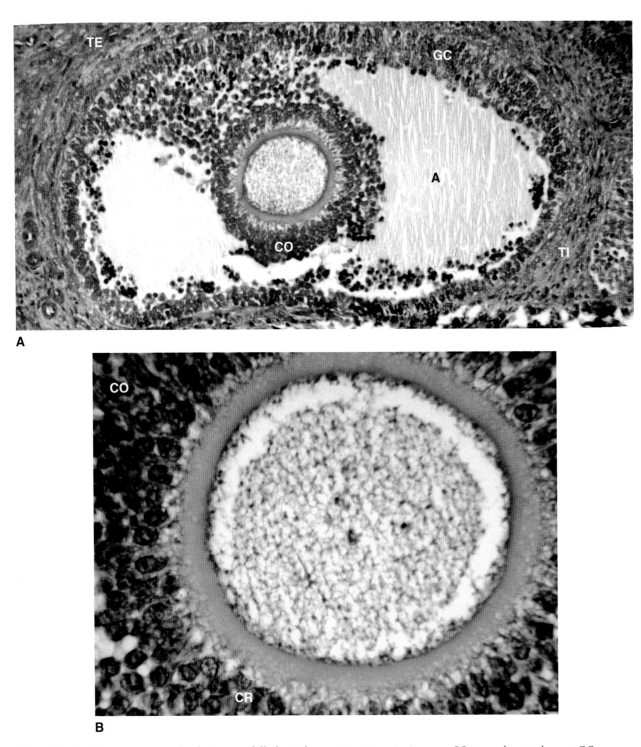

Figure 19-8. A, Light micrograph of a tertiary follicle in the canine ovary. *A,* Antrum; *CO,* cumulus oophorus; *GC,* granulosa cells; *TE,* theca externa; *TI,* theca interna. (Hematoxylin and eosin (H&E) stain; ×50.) **B,** Light micrograph of the cumulus oophorus *(CO)* and corona radiata *(CR)* surrounding the primary oocyte. (H&E stain; ×250.)

ectopic pregnancy will ensue, an event that fortunately is quite rare. Once the oocyte has entered the uterine tube, it has less than 24 hours to be fertilized. If the oocyte is not fertilized within that time, it will degenerate and be phagocytosed.

The amount of stromal remodeling that occurs for ovulation varies to some extent among domestic species, being most extensive in the mare. In this animal, the cortex is located centrally and for that reason the developing follicle has to travel a

TABLE 19-1 Morphological Events and Associated Glandular Activity of the Follicular Development in Domestic Mammalian Ovaries

FOLLICLE	MORPHOLOGY	GLANDULAR ACTIVITY	SPECIES VARIATIONS
Primordial	Large, round primary oocyte with distinct nucleus and surrounded by single layer of flattened follicular cells	None	Clustered in carnivores within outer cortex; evenly distributed within outer cortex in ungulates
Primary (preantral, unilaminar)	Primary oocyte enlarges by two or more times; surrounding layer of follicular cells becomes cuboidal to low columnar	Plasma (pituitary released) follicle-stimulating hormone (FSH) begins to rise	Rise in plasma FSH in does, ewes, and mares results in synchronous follicular wave development that can result up to four waves per cycle, the last two being ovulatory
Secondary (preantral, multilaminar)	Primary oocyte continues to enlarge and forms zona pellucida; surrounding follicular cells multiply and become multilayered granulosa cells; stroma cells increase in number and start to become organized	Raised FSH	
Tertiary (antral, multilaminar)	Granulosa cells continue to divide and surround primary oocyte forming cumulus oophorus and corona radiata as well as form antrum filled with liquor folliculi; stroma forms vascularized theca interna and fibrous theca externa	FSH declines; estrogens rise coming from granulosa cells and interstitial gland	Granulosa cells can contain Call-Exner bodies in the cow and ewe
Mature (late tertiary) and ovulation	Follicle and oocyte have reached full size; the follicle presses against tunica albuginea, which becomes avascular stigma; cumulus oophorus floats freely within antrum; stigma and follicular wall at stigma degenerate, resulting in follicular rupture	Estrogen level is sufficient to shut off FSH; surge in plasma (pituitary released) luteinizing hormone (LH) results in prostaglandin release and collagenase activity	First meiotic division is completed, forming secondary oocyte in all but bitch and mare, which occurs after ovulation
Corpus luteum (luteinization)	Ruptured follicle collapses, folds, and temporarily hemorrhages; granulosa cells become large luteal cells, and internal thecal cells become small luteal cells	Progesterone level rises due to luteal cell activity; during late estrous cycle progesterone level lowers	Presence of the yellow pigment lutein within luteal cells in most domestic species but absent in the ewe and sow
Corpus albicans	In the absence of fertilization, the luteal cells degenerate and are replaced by connective tissue	With continued lowering of progesterone is a gradual rise of FSH	

considerable distance before ovulation can take place

Corpus Luteum. On release of the oocyte and associated cells and fluid, the mature ruptured follicle collapses into a folded state. Vasculature of the adjacent theca has ruptured during ovulation as well and has resulted in the formation of a blood clot within much of the remaining antrum, forming the **corpus hemorrhagicum,** which is especially developed in large

domestic herbivores. Eventually the clot is removed and the vasculature along with connective tissue elements extends from the theca interna into the granulosa cells. The connective tissue elements consist mostly of small reticular fibers. The granulosa cells expand in size and number as they become transformed into lutein cells, specifically the **granulosa lutein cells,** also referred to as **large luteal cells** (Figure 19-11). At this same time, the adjacent cells

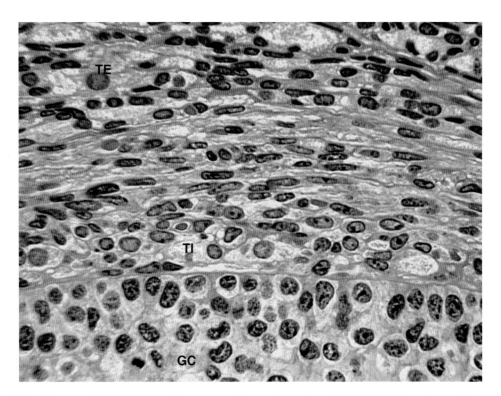

Figure 19-9. Light micrograph of the surrounding stroma of a canine tertiary follicle. *GC,* Granulosa cells; *TE,* theca externa; *TI,* theca interna. (Hematoxylin and eosin stain; ×250.)

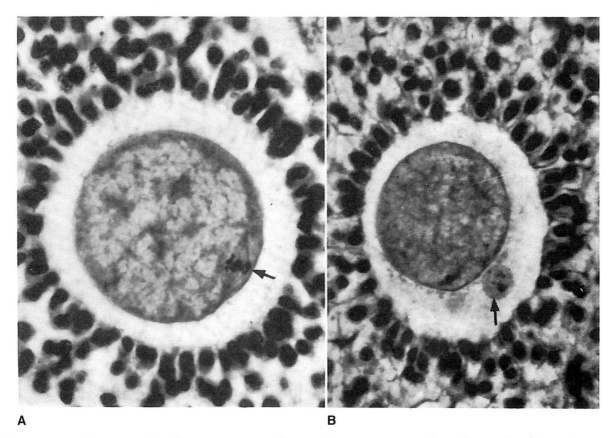

A   **B**

Figure 19-10. Light micrographs of rat ova: **A,** near ovulation with arrow pointing to first polar spindle, and **B,** after ovulation, but before fertilization with first polar body *(arrow)* lying within perivitelline space. *(Modified from Fawcett DW: Bloom and Fawcett: a textbook of histology, ed 11, Philadelphia, 1986, Saunders.)*

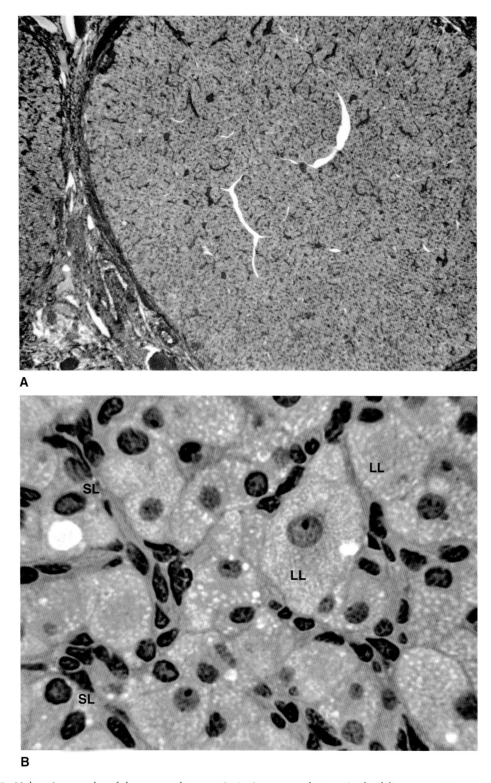

Figure 19-11. Light micrographs of the corpus luteum. **A,** Active corpus luteum in the feline ovary. (Hematoxylin and eosin [H&E] stain; ×20.) **B,** Rabbit corpus luteal tissue with many large luteal cells *(LL)* and scattered small luteal cells *(SL)*. (H&E; ×400.)

Continued

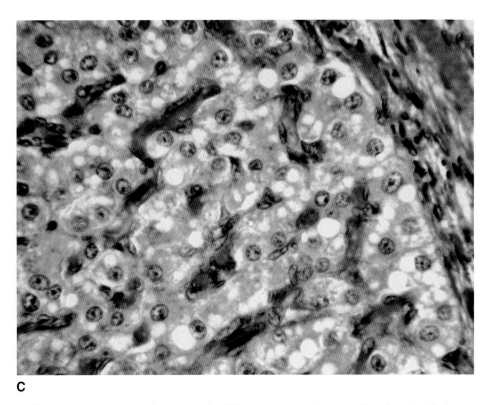

C

Figure 19-11, cont'd C, Regressing corpus luteum in the feline ovary. (H&E; ×250.) Most luteal cells have a preponderance of single large lipid bodies.

of the theca interna similarly divide and are converted into luteal cells, the **theca lutein cells,** which are also referred to as **small luteal cells** because they failed to increase in size comparable to those originating from the granulosa population.

The process of transforming both populations of cells into lutein cells is called **luteinization.** In bitches and queens as well as cows and mares, the yellow pigment lutein accumulates within the lutein cells. However, in ewes and sows this pigment is absent. The basal lamina that previously separated the granulosa cells from the theca cells has depolymerized during luteinization. As the granulosa cells become large luteal cells, they form abundant organelles to form steroids. Their cytoplasm, which histologically appears pale, is filled with smooth endoplasmic reticulum (sER), Golgi complexes, mitochondria, and some rER and lipid bodies. The large luteal cells become involved primarily in the production of **progesterone** and are able to convert androgens made by the small luteal cells into estrogens. As cells of the theca interna become small luteal cells, the same organelles that occur in the large luteal cells are formed in these cells, but are not nearly as abundant in their amount with the exception of the lipid bodies, which are numerous in these cells. The small luteal

cells produce progesterone and androgens and some estrogens. On the whole, the large luteal cells comprise the major portion of the corpus luteum.

During the formation of the corpus luteum from the corpus hemorrhagicum, the level of the LH remains high (see Table 19-1). As the luteal cells of the corpus luteum produce progesterone and estrogens, these hormones are able to inhibit the secretion of LH and FSH.

Corpus Albicans. If the secondary oocyte is not fertilized, the corpus luteum gradually degenerates, becoming the **regressive corpus luteum.** The regression is seen morphologically during late diestrus, as lutein pigment condenses among the luteal cells (see Figure 19-11). This regression begins approximately 2 weeks after ovulation in cows and sows. Connective tissue elements of the corpus luteum further develop and the corpus luteum becomes transformed into the **corpus albicans.** The luteal cells break down as they undergo autolysis and their remains are removed by macrophages. As remnants of a previous ovulatory event, the corpus albicans persists within the ovary as scar tissue for some time. With age, the presence of these scars become more abundant.

Atretic Follicles. As primordial follicles progress through different stages of development, most never

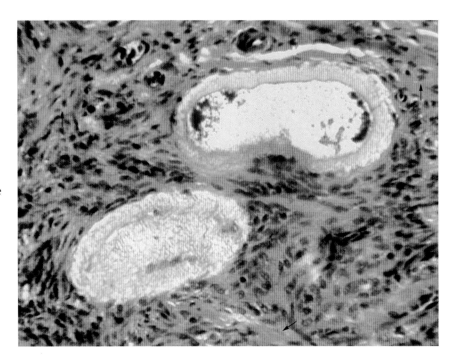

Figure 19-12. Light micrograph of two atretic follicles in the canine ovary. Arrows point to connective tissue scar of a corpus albicans–like region. (Hematoxylin and eosin stain; ×100.)

reach maturity, having degenerated at some point along the way (Figure 19-12). Before ovulation multiple follicles have become tertiary. However, as soon as one has matured and ruptured, the rest of the maturing follicles begin the process of degeneration or **atresia.** Morphological signs of atresia include nuclear pyknosis and chromatolysis of the granulosa cells of the follicular wall, whereas the cells of the theca layer fibrose. The intervening basal lamina thickens, folds, and hyalinizes, forming an undulating **glassy membrane** (Figure 19-13). The resulting **atretic follicles** become subsequently resorbed by macrophages in much the same manner that occurs to the corpus luteum as it becomes the corpus albicans. Cells of the theca interna may atrophy or enlarge and luteinize in a manner comparable with that seen in the corpus luteum. In those instances, the hypertrophied cells form cords around the regressing central portion of the atretic follicle.

In the bovine ovary, atresia of primary and secondary follicles occurs differently from that of tertiary follicles in that the oocyte is first to degenerate, whereas during atresia of the tertiary follicles, the oocyte degenerates after the regression of the follicular cells.

In atretic follicles of carnivores and rodents, epithelioid steroid-producing cells originate principally from the theca interna cells of tertiary follicles and from hypertrophied granulosa cells of primary and secondary follicles. Collectively, these cells comprise the **interstitial endocrine cells** or **interstitial gland** of their ovaries and generally are little seen in the adult ovaries of other domestic species.

Medulla

Except in the horse, the region known as the **medulla** is located centrally within the ovary (see Figure 19-2). It consists primarily of large blood vessels, nerve fibers, and lymph vessels surrounded by loose connective tissue that contains ample amounts of elastic and reticular fibers. The nerve fibers are mostly unmyelinated and vasomotor in function, though some have sensory capability. The medullary vasculature gives rise to the necessary capillary supply for follicular and subsequent corpus luteal development and regression. At the hilus of the ovary, the medulla becomes confluent with the mesovarium (Figure 19-14; see also Figure 19-2.) The **mesovarium** is a foldlike extension of the peritoneum that attaches and suspends each ovary within the pelvic region of the abdominal cavity and provides the site where vessels and nerve enter the ovary (see Figure 19-1).

Within the medulla, tubular cords or channels of epithelial cells form the **rete ovarii,** a homolog to the rete testis. These anastomosing tubules may be closed or, in the instance of ruminant species, open directly into the infundibulum of the uterine tube near its attachment to the ovary. Although the function of these cells remains speculative, they may contribute to the formation of granulosa cells of developing follicles as well as play a role in governing meiosis within the maturing oocyte. While associated with the medulla, the rete ovarii is most often found within the hilus of the ovary. It also can be found within the mesovarium.

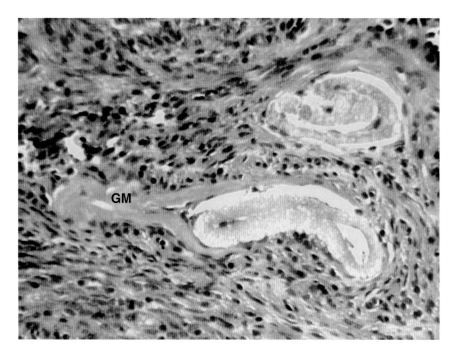

Figure 19-13. Light micrograph of follicular atresia with glassy membrane *(GM)* in the bitch. (Hematoxylin and eosin stain; ×100.)

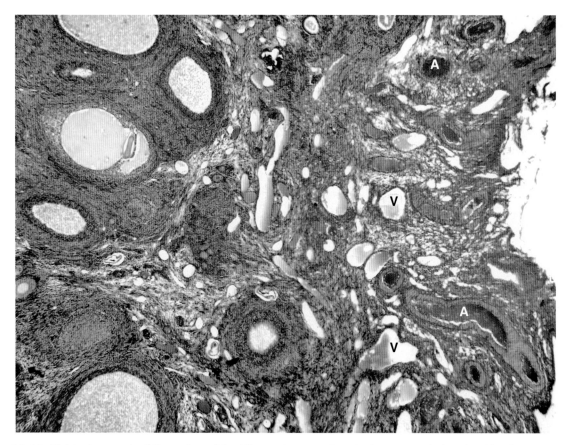

Figure 19-14. Light micrograph of the region of the hilus and mesovarium in the queen. *A,* Arteries; *V,* veins. (Hematoxylin and eosin stain; ×15.)

UTERINE TUBE

From each ovary, the ruptured oocyte flows into a **uterine tube** or **oviduct,** which consists of an open-ended undulating tubular structure that directs the female gamete toward the uterus while permitting the opposite flow of spermatozoa for successful fertilization (see Figure 19-1). The uterine tube is composed of three regions: infundibulum, ampulla, and isthmus.

The **infundibulum** is a funnel-like portion of the uterine tube that lies closest to the ovary. Its proximal-most or cranial portion forms a radiating fringe of projections called the **fimbriae** that lie next to the ovary and function to enhance the capture of the oocyte after leaving the ovary (see Figure 19-2). At the base or distal end of the infundibulum, the fimbriae coalesce into a single tubular structure before joining the ampulla. The **ampulla** forms the thin-walled portion of the uterine tube that contains numerous mucosal-submucosal folds and is the region where fertilization most likely occurs. The ampulla leads to the **isthmus,** which has a thicker muscular wall than that of the ampulla and fewer and less branched mucosal-submucosal folds than those of the ampulla.

Histologically, uterine tubes of many species are internally lined by a simple columnar epithelium. In the cow and the sow, the internal lining consists of pseudostratified columnar epithelia. Typically, the height of the epithelial cells shorten as the uterine tubes progress toward the uterus. Whether simple columnar or pseudostratified columnar, these epithelial cells can possess kinocilia and microvilli or just microvilli (Figure 19-15). **Ciliated cells** are especially prevalent within the infundibulum, where they facilitate the movement of ova into the uterine tubes. This movement is likewise contributed by the well-ciliated cranial portion of the ampulla. The cilia of the epithelia that line the uterine tube beat in unison not unlike that seen in respiratory epithelia, causing each ovum to be propelled to the uterus. Smooth muscle within the wall of the uterine tube also plays a role in moving ova to the uterus. In fact during ovulation, as smooth muscle contracts within the infundibulum, which at that time possess engorged veins that as a result become distended, the fimbriae are able to extend onto the ovary and help collect the soon-to-be-released oocyte.

In addition to ciliated columnar cells, nonciliated columnar cells exist within the epithelial lining (Figure 19-16; see also Figure 19-15). Although having some microvilli, these cells are believed to be secretory and provide nutritional support for the gametes moving through this portion of the reproductive tract. These secretions help the maturation

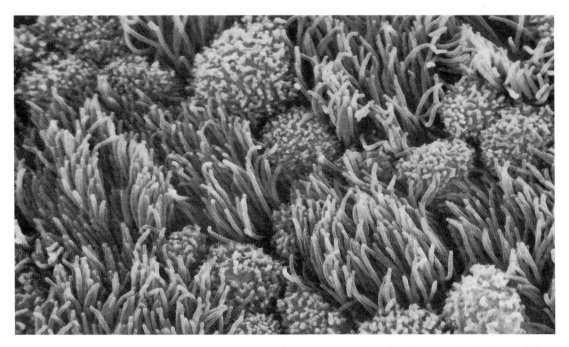

Figure 19-15. Scanning electron micrograph of the internal lining of the epithelial cells lining the fimbriae of the infundibular portion of the rabbit uterine tube and possessing either cilia or microvilli. *(From Fawcett DW: Bloom and Fawcett: a textbook of histology, ed 11, Philadelphia, 1986, Saunders.)*

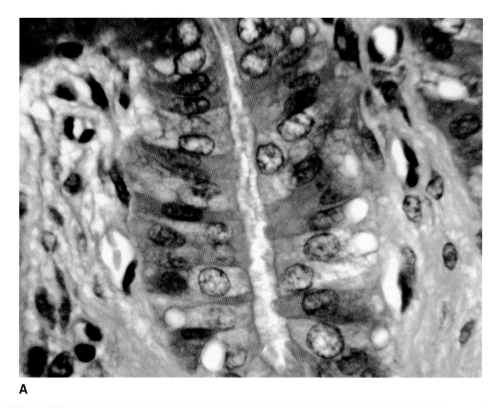

A

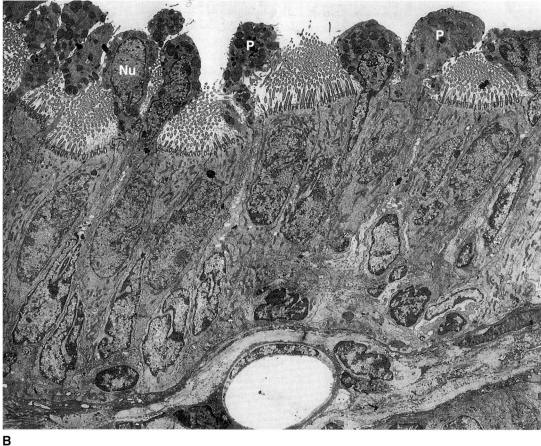

B

Figure 19-16. A, Light micrograph of the mucosal epithelium along the ampulla of uterine tube of the bitch. (Hematoxylin and eosin stain; ×100.) **B,** Transmission electron micrograph terminal segment of the mucosal epithelium along the uterine tube of the ewe. Peg *(P)* cells protrude between the ciliated columnar cells, sometimes bearing nuclei *(Nu)*. (×4000.) *(Modified from Gartner LP, Hiatt JL: Color textbook of histology, Philadelphia, 1997, Saunders.)*

process of spermatozoa known as **capacitation.** In this process, spermatozoa fully mature and only then are able to fertilize ova. As oocytes are released during ovulation, the nonciliated columnar cells become metabolically more active and typically increase in their height, being sometimes referred to as **peg cells.**

The epithelium is surrounded externally by a propria-submucosa, not possessing a lamina muscularis. The propria-submucosa consists mostly of loose connective tissue that is best developed within the folds of the ampulla and to a lesser extent those of the isthmus. In addition to primary folds, secondary and tertiary folds also are formed within the ampulla (Figure 9-17). Except for the epithelium, no glandular tissue occurs within this area of the uterine tube. The loose connective tissue is composed primarily of small collagen and elastic fibers that are interspersed with fibrocytes, occasional lymphoid cells, and less frequent mast cells.

The propria-submucosa is, in turn, surrounded by smooth muscle of the tunica muscularis. The tunica muscularis consists of two layers of smooth muscle: an inner circular, which can also be spiral, and outer longitudinal. Overall, the two layers are least developed within the infundibulum and ampulla with the inner circular layer more pronounced than the outer longitudinal layer and able to form radial bands that project into the propria-submucosa. Within the isthmus, the tunica muscularis increases in size while approaching the uterus. The tunica muscularis of each uterine tube is externally lined by a tunica serosa that is made of loose connective tissue and a simple squamous epithelium. The connective tissue of the tunica serosa houses the immigrating and emigrating vasculature and autonomic innervation that serve the uterine tube.

UTERUS

The paired uterine tubes direct the fertilized ovum or **conceptus** to the **uterus,** which is the site of implantation and subsequent fetal development. The uterus is composed of three regions: a pair of **horns (uterine horns)** in most domestic species or **fundus** in the single-tubed uterus of primates **(uterus simplex)** that guides the conceptus to the principal structure or **body** of the uterus (also known as the **corpus**), which is the site of implantation and, in turn, leads to the neck region, called the **cervix.** In all species the uterus becomes the portion of the female reproductive tract involved in embryonic and fetal development, but it is also the site for semen deposition in the mare (in the corpus) and the sow (in the cervix).

UTERINE HORNS AND BODY

The uterine wall of the body and uterine horns is composed of the **endometrium,** the **myometrium,** and the **perimetrium.**

Endometrium

The endometrium forms a tunica mucosa–submucosa that surrounds the luminal cavity and internally contains a simple columnar epithelium in canine, feline, and equine species along with areas of pseudostratified columnar epithelia in porcine and ruminant species. Small patches or isolated areas of simple cuboidal epithelia also can exist. The height of the epithelia and degree of cytoplasmic development among the epithelial cells will vary cyclically according to the stage of estrus.

The epithelium is subtended by a propria-submucosa that houses numerous glands surrounded by variably developed vasculature and connective tissue elements (Figure 19-18). The portion of the propria-submucosa next to the epithelium along with the epithelium make up the region known as the **functionalis** or **functional zone.** The propria-submucosa in this zone is composed of reticular fibers, numerous cells, and many helically **coiled arteries** that come from the **arcuate arteries** positioned within a vascular stratum within the myometrium. These coiled arteries form an extensive capillary bed that supplies the glands. The cells within the connective tissue of the functional zone consist of fibrocytes that can be stellate (mesenchymal-like), leukocytes, macrophages, and mast cells. Beneath (external to) the functional zone of the propria-submucosa is a thin region called the **basalis** or **basal zone,** which consists of a loose connective tissue that is less cellular than that of the functional zone and **straight arteries** that also are derived from the arcuate arteries. The straight arteries are considerably shorter than the coiled arteries of the functional zone.

Extending from the epithelium into the propria-submucosa and even into the myometrium are the uterine glands, which consist of simple or branched tubular glands that are generally coiled. The amount of the coiling seen in these glands is directly associated with the secretion of progesterone within the estrous cycle, being most pronounced during the later phases of the estrous cycle, late metestrus, and diestrus and during pregnancy (Figure 19-19). Phases of the estrous cycle and morphological changes that occur within the uterus are covered later in this chapter.

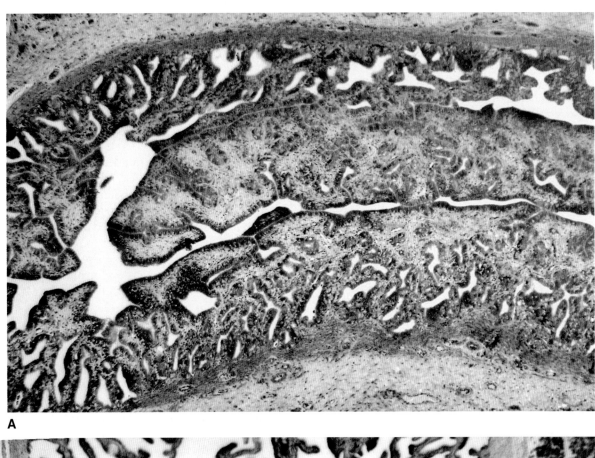

A

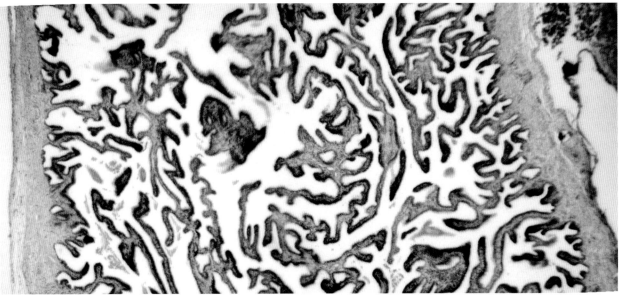

B

Figure 19-17. A, Light micrograph of the ampulla of the bitch. (Hematoxylin and eosin [H&E] stain; ×15). **B,** Light micrograph of the ampulla of the sow. (H&E stain; ×10.)

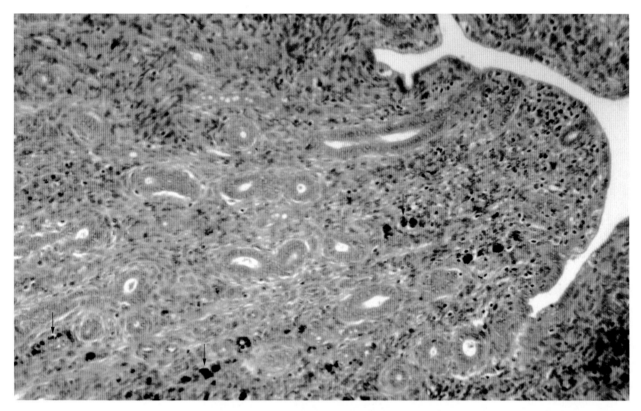

Figure 19-18. Light micrograph of the functional zone of the canine endometrium during late diestrus. Arrows point to coiled arteries. (Hematoxylin and eosin stain; ×50.)

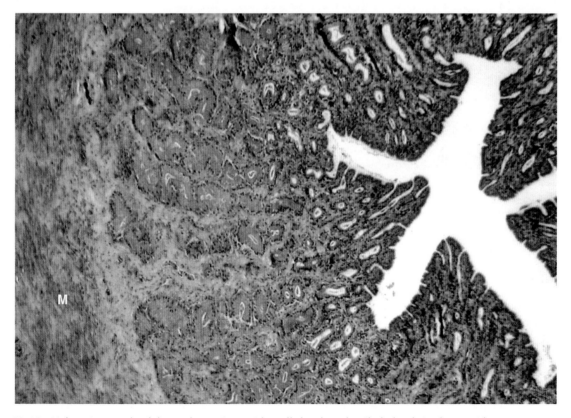

Figure 19-19. Light micrograph of the endometrium with well-developed coiled glands in the gravid queen. *M,* myometrium. (Hematoxylin and eosin stain; ×15.)

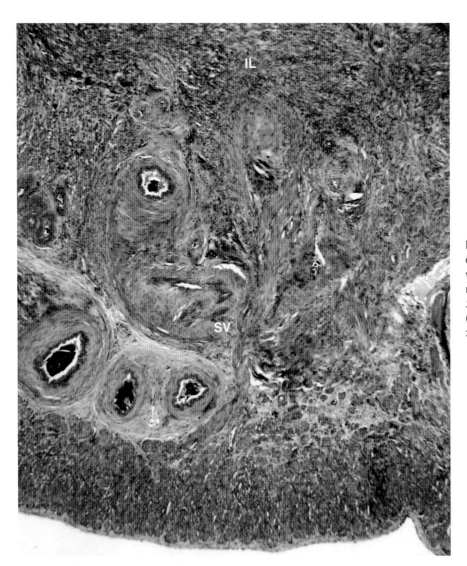

Figure 19-20. Light micrograph of the smooth muscle associated with the myometrium of the nongravid bitch. *IL,* Inner layer; *SV,* stratum vasculare. (Hematoxylin and eosin stain; ×20.)

Within the uterine horns of ruminants are regions of the propria-submucosa called **caruncles.** Caruncles can appear as rounded (cow) or cup-shaped folds (ewe) that lack any tubular glands but are well vascularized. These structures form the eventual sites of the maternal placenta, where the maternal tissues contact the extraembryonic membranes.

Myometrium

The myometrium comprises the tunica muscularis of the uterine horns and body. Most of it is composed of a thick inner layer of smooth muscle, which is externally covered by a comparatively thin outer layer of smooth muscle. The inner layer is oriented in a circular direction and can contain the basal portions of the endometrial glands. Deep within this layer, as it blends with the outer layer, the muscle fibers intermesh with a vascular layer, sometimes referred to as

the **stratum vasculare** or **vascular stratum** of the myometrium (Figure 19-20). This stratum gives rise to the arcuate arteries, which in turn give rise to the coiled and straight arteries of the endometrium, and houses large veins and lymph vessels as well. The outer layer of smooth muscle runs longitudinally with the axis of the uterus and along its inner margin blends with bundles of smooth muscle fibers of the inner layer. In both layers the smooth muscle cells are arranged in bundles that are attached to one another by thin sheaths of connective tissue that consist of fibrocytes, including those that are mesenchymal-like, histiocytes, mast cells and collagen and elastic fibers.

During pregnancy, the myometrium undergoes pronounced development (see Figure 19-19). The smooth muscle cells hypertrophy up to 10 times their nongravid length. This increase is due to the raised levels of estrogen (Table 19-2). The absence of estrogen leads to their atrophy. In addition to smooth

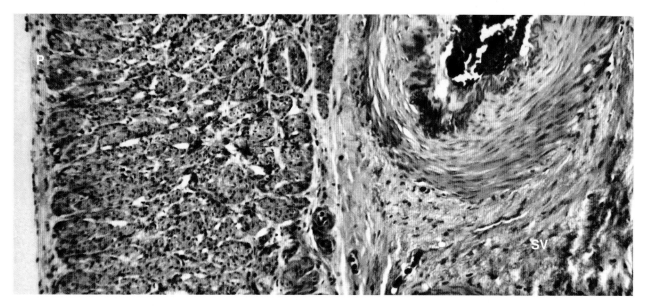

Figure 19-21. Light micrograph of the perimetrium *(P)* in the bitch. *SV,* Stratum vasculare. (Hematoxylin and eosin stain; ×100.)

TABLE 19-2 Morphological Events and Associated Glandular Activity of the Mammalian Uterus during the Estrous Cycle		
STAGE OF ESTROUS CYCLE	UTERINE MORPHOLOGY	GLANDULAR ACTIVITY/SPECIES VARIATIONS
Proestrus	Within the endometrium, the mucosal epithelium hypertrophies with neutrophil infiltration; propria-submucosa increases vascularization and congestion as well as edema	Glands remain straight with some lengthening
Estrus	Mucosal epithelium continues to thicken with mononuclear leukocyte infiltration; propria-submucosa reaches maximal vascularization, congestion, and hemorrhage as well as edema	Glands continue to elongate in the cow; heightened edema with maximal mast cell presence; microscopic hemorrhaging, metrorrhagia, just before ovulation
Metestrus	Blood vessels become less congested and edema lessens appreciably	Glandular growth progresses to point of coiling
Diestrus	Continued less vascular congestion and connective tissue edema	Glandular development reaches peak with branching and further coiling; in the absence of fertilization, glands gradually involute
Anestrus	Both mucosal epithelium and propria-submucosa are appreciably thin; epithelium becomes simple cuboidal	Glandular regression results in scattered simple tubular and sometimes branched adenomeres

muscle hypertrophy, new smooth muscle cells are formed. As the result of the increased size and number of smooth muscle cells of the myometrium, the uterus increases its mass many times during pregnancy.

Perimetrium

The perimetrium forms the tunica serosa for most of the uterine horns and the body of the uterus. It is composed mostly of loose connective tissue lined exter-

nally by a simple squamous epithelium. Small blood and lymph vessels and nerve fibers occur in this layer as well (Figure 19-21). In the gravid animal, smooth muscle occupies most of this layer.

CERVIX

The uterus ends caudally in the structure known as the cervix or neck region, which extends or protrudes into the vagina (see Figure 19-1). During pregnancy this portion of the uterus becomes valve-like and seals the uterus from the vagina. It generally lacks glands within the propria-submucosa, but can possess a mucus-producing epithelium that is especially laden with goblet cells and other mucus-producing cells within ruminant species. In the gravid animal, the mucigenous cells form a seal or plug that separates the lumen of the uterus from that of the vagina, protecting the developing fetus from harmful agents.

The propria-submucosa, consisting of dense irregular connective tissue, forms major folds with extending secondary and even tertiary folds, each lined by simple columnar epithelia. The propria-submucosa is externally embraced by a well-developed tunica muscularis that is a continuation of the myometrium of the uterine body, having an inner circular layer and an outer longitudinal layer of smooth muscle. Among the layers are well-developed elastic fibers that along with the muscularis help return this portion of the uterus to its normal shape after parturition. The tunica muscularis is surrounded by the tunica serosa, which consists of loose connective tissue.

VAGINA

The **vagina** is a muscular tube that connects the uterus to the vestibule and receives the male copulatory organ for the eventual fertilization of the ova within the uterine tubes. For the most part, the internal epithelial lining of the mucosa consists of a nonkeratinized stratified squamous epithelium. In most species the mucosa and submucosa form low folds or ridges that lie along the longitudinal axis of this structure (Figure 19-22). Mucous secretions found here arise originally from the cervix and increase in amount during estrus concomitant with the increased thickness of the epithelium (see Table 19-3 on p. 468). In the cow, mucus can be formed by clusters of goblet cells within the cranial portion of the vaginal mucosa.

The propria-submucosa is composed of loose or dense irregular connective tissue that lacks glands but contains scattered lymphoid tissue in the form of nodules. Externally surrounding the propria-submucosa, the tunica muscularis is composed of at least two layers of smooth muscle: the inner circular layer, which is made up of bundles held together by connective tissue; and the outer longitudinal layer, which is comparatively thinner than the thickness of the inner circular layer. In the bitch and sow is a thin inner longitudinal third layer.

Except cranially, most of the tunica muscularis is externally encased by adventitia of loose connective tissue that houses the larger vascular elements and nerve that serve the vagina. Cranially, the muscularis is enveloped by a tunica serosa that may have a thin longitudinal layer of smooth muscle, the **muscularis serosae.**

VULVA

The caudal-most and external ending of the female reproductive tract is referred to as the **vulva,** which is composed of the labia, vestibule, and clitoris. The **labia** consists of folds of skin that possess the basic components of the integument including hair and associated sebaceous and apocrine glands as well as loose to dense connective tissue with an extensive elastic fiber network.

The **vestibule** is the area that forms the cleft or space associated with the orifices of the vagina and urethra. The construction of the vestibule is comparable with that of the caudal vagina except it has more-developed lymphatic and vascular tissues. Blood vessels in this region are numerous, forming venous plexuses and cavernous erectile tissue, which during estrus becomes congested. The vestibule is externally lined by a nonkeratinized stratified squamous epithelium. In feline and ruminant species, the epithelium is lubricated by mucus-secreting compound tubuloacinar glands known as the **major vestibular glands** and are homologous to the bulbourethral glands of males. These glands are located well within the propria-submucosa; stratified squamous epithelia line their large ducts. During coitus they lubricate both the vestibule and the caudal portion of the vagina. In addition to the major vestibular glands are the mucus-secreting **minor vestibular glands.** These glands occur ubiquitously among domestic species and consist of simple branched tubular adenomeres that lie more superficially within the propria-submucosa than the major glands.

The last component of the vulva and a part of the vestibule is the **clitoris,** homolog of the male penis, that has a paired body, glans, and preputial covering. The body of the clitoris consists of dense connective tissue that surrounds the **corpus cavernosum clitoridis,** which is a paired erectile cavernous tissue, smooth muscle, adipose and lymphoid tissue. In the bitch and the mare, the cavernous tissue extends into the **glans clitoridis.** Only in the mare does this tissue become erectile. In other species this area can be well vascularized but lacks the cavernous tissue. Externally, the clitoris is lined by the **preputial covering,** a

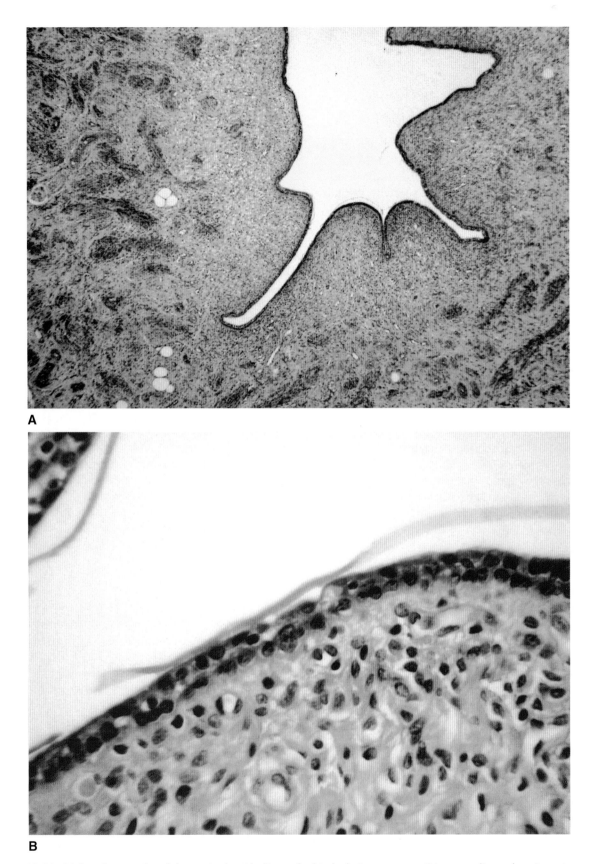

A

B

Figure 19-22. Light micrographs of the vaginal epithelium of a bitch during anestrus. (Hematoxylin and eosin stain; **A,** ×20; **B,** ×250.)

nonkeratinized stratified squamous epithelium that possesses numerous sensory nerve endings.

ENDOCRINE ASSOCIATIONS AND CYCLICAL CHANGES

The ovary operates under the guidance of endocrine physiology. The hormones involved in this operation are produced by the ovary, although other organs of the endocrine system, especially the pituitary, influence ovarian activity. It is through the combination of ovarian hormones and those of the hypothalamus and adenohypophysis within the pituitary that the female reproductive tract, and to some degree the entire body, undergoes periodical changes that result in the estrous cycle.

The estrous cycle consists of five stages: proestrus, estrus, metestrus, diestrus, and anestrus.

Proestrus is the portion of the cycle involved in both the development of follicles and uterine lining. During proestrus, progesterone decreases, allowing some follicles to progress rapidly toward maturation as follicle-stimulating hormone (FSH) is released. A concomitant regrowth of the endometrium follows the previous cycle. Before the next stage (estrus), FSH declines while estrogens rise, reaching their peak at estrus.

Estrus is the stage when the follicle fully matures and ruptures in most domestic species as the result of a sharp rise in luteinizing hormone (LH) release. The peaked levels of estrogen at the beginning of this stage steadily decline. This stage is also referred to as the period of **heat,** when the female is receptive to the male.

Metestrus is the period when the corpus luteum develops and results in the beginning of progesterone secretion as estrogens continue to lower.

Diestrus is the last active stage of the estrous cycle involving the continued development of the corpus luteum and progesterone release. Endometrial glands reach the height of their activity during this period, which becomes prolonged with ova fertilization and subsequent pregnancy. Toward the end of diestrus, involution of the corpus luteum and endometrium occurs.

Anestrus follows diestrus; in this stage fertilization does not occur and the female reproductive tract becomes sedentary.

When examining the histology of the estrous cycle among domestic species, it is important to understand the variety of events involved with the tissues and hormones that occur during oocyte development, ovulation, and fertilization. These events include follicle development, corpus luteum development, ovum fertilization, uterine changes, and vaginal changes (see Tables 19-1 through 19-3).

FOLLICLE DEVELOPMENT

The development of follicles, from primary through tertiary stages, is governed by the **gonadotropins,** hormones that are secreted by the pituitary's adenohypophysis. The influence of these gonadotropins is especially pronounced during late secondary and early tertiary follicular development during proestrus. At these stages of development, the granulosa cells of the follicles and the thecal cells of the surrounding stroma form hormone receptors. Specifically, the granulosa cells form **FSH receptors,** and the thecal cells form **LH receptors**. As these follicles continue to develop, the granulosa cells form LH receptors as well. During tertiary follicular development, LH is now able to stimulate thecal cells (theca interna) to produce and release the androgens, testosterone, and androstenedione, as well as some estradiol. Concomitantly, the granulosa cells have been stimulated by FSH to have their aromatase system upregulated so that as the androgens are formed and secreted by the nearby thecal cells, these steroidal compounds are taken in by the granulosa cells and converted to estrogens, estradiol-17 and estrone. These estrogens are then released as follicular fluid into the antrum.

As follicles mature and approach ovulation during estrus, a surge of LH stimulates the granulosa cells to trigger the events that result in ovulation. Specifically, in most species the primary oocyte is induced to complete its first meiosis.

CORPUS LUTEUM DEVELOPMENT

Upon rupture of the mature follicle, LH-sensitive follicular cells develop into luteal cells that comprise the corpus luteum and become involved in progesterone secretion. As metestrus progresses, the newly converted cells of the granulosa and internal theca produce and release progesterone, which continues throughout most of diestrus. As the end of diestrus approaches, the corpus luteum regresses. The luteal cells, once filled with small, even-sized lipid bodies, begin to accumulate greater amounts of lipid, consisting primarily of large, unevenly sized cholesterol bodies (see Figure 19-11). The regression of the corpus luteum is facilitated by the release of a luteolytic factor by the uterus in some domestic herbivores, including cows, ewes, and sows.

With successful fertilization and pregnancy, the corpus luteum remains active during gestation. However, eventually the placenta becomes the principal source of progesterone production during pregnancy.

FERTILIZATION AND IMPLANTATION

Upon rupture of the mature follicle, the secondary oocyte and adjacent follicular cells move into the infundibulum and then to the ampulla by the combined assistance of rhythmic beating of the mucosal cilia and contraction of the muscularis of these portions of the uterine tube. If the female reproductive tract has received spermatozoa, the sperm cells propel themselves en masse into the uterine lumen, moving into the isthmus of each uterine tube to meet the migrating secondary oocyte at some point within the ampulla. The secondary oocyte still is enveloped by the zona pellucida and surrounding granulosa cells that form the corona radiata. As spermatozoa burrow among these cells and reach the zona pellucida, one will successfully cause an **acrosome reaction,** whereby receptor protein at the acrosome of the sperm connects with a complementary glycoprotein of the oocyte within the zona pellucida, which in turn causes the fusion of the cell membranes of both gametes to occur. The sperm nucleus then enters the oocyte's cytoplasm and soon afterward meiosis of the secondary oocyte is completed, resulting in two uneven-sized cells with their own haploid nuclei: the large **ovum** and the small **second polar body** (see Figure 19-10). The sperm nucleus remains with the ovum and fuses with the nucleus of the ovum to form a **zygote** with a now diploid nucleus.

As in the case of the secondary oocyte, the zygote continues to move caudally toward the uterus. By the time it reaches the uterus, the zygote has undergone numerous divisions, having first become a solid sphere of cells (the **morula**) and then a hollow ball of cells, the **blastocyst,** which consists of **trophoblasts** and a few cells held inside called **embryoblasts.** It is at this point in development that no further movement along the female reproductive tract is required and the blastocyst becomes anchored along the uterine's endometrium. The trophoblasts trigger a series of reactions that result in **implantation.** Initially, the stellate stromal cells of the endometrium can become transformed in the bitch and queen into **decidual cells** that most likely serve to nourish the developing embryo. The trophoblasts continue to divide and form the fetal portion of the placenta and the amniotic sac.

UTERINE CHANGES

The hormone-based changes associated with the ovary during the estrous cycle have a dramatic effect on the function and structure of the uterus, especially its endometrium. If fertilization and implantation should occur, then the influence of hormones on the uterus is largely produced by the placenta. The changes and duration of changes that occur within the estrous cycle vary among domestic species. Moreover, the frequency of the estrous cycle varies. In domestic carnivores (bitches and queens), the anestrus period is usually quite extended and results annually in one to two estrous cycles during the normal adult reproductively active years. In these animals, particularly the bitch, the cycling activity is referred to as **monestrous,** indicating the long periods between functionally active cycles. In other domestic animals, there can occur either continuous estrous cycling with no inactive periods, as in bovine and porcine species, or seasonal estrous cycling, as in equine and ovine species, which collectively are referred to as **polyestrous.** In polyestrous animals, the degenerative and regenerative morphological changes that take place during the estrous cycle are not as remarkable as those in monestrous animals.

During proestrus, the endometrium regenerates much that had regressed during late diestrus (see Table 19-2). The epithelial lining and associated tubular glands enlarge but remain relatively straight. The adjacent propria-submucosa or functional zone becomes more vascularized and congested. The release of blood outside of the blood vessels **(hemorrhaging)** into the extracellular matrix (ECM) of the functional zone may occur to some extent at this time.

During estrus, the epithelial portion continues to grow and become more active in its mucus secretion. Vascular congestion, edema, and hemorrhage within the connective tissue reach a peak level.

During metestrus, the edema within the functional zone along with the vascular congestion and hemorrhage all lessen. The hyperplasia associated with the epithelium continues with coiling and branching of the tubular glands.

During diestrus the glandular hyperplasia reaches it maximal state. The tubular glands become highly coiled and branched. If fertilization has occurred, this level of activity will continue, otherwise the well-developed glandular and vascular tissues will degenerate and involute along with the concomitant degeneration of the corpus luteum (and loss of progesterone). The amount of involution and associated loss of vasculature are more exaggerated in monestrous animals than polyestrous animals.

VAGINAL CHANGES

In domestic animals vaginal changes occur during the estrous cycle, especially with regard to the vaginal

TABLE 19-3 Morphological Changes of the Vaginal Epithelium of the Bitch During the Estrous Cycle

STAGE OF ESTROUS CYCLE	HISTOLOGICAL MORPHOLOGY	SMEAR PREPARATION
Proestrus	Mucosal epithelium increases thickness and becomes cornified stratified squamous epithelium with a thin keratinized layer that continues to develop	Mostly large cornified epithelial cells with straight borders and with and without pyknotic nuclei; presence of occasional neutrophils that disappear by the middle of proestrus, and erythrocytes
Estrus	Mucosal stratified squamous epithelium contains numerous layers; many become keratinized	Many large cornified epithelial cells with pyknotic nuclei; during late estrus pyknotic nuclei disappear and erythrocytes lessen in number with an increase in cellular debris and bacteria
Metestrus and diestrus	Mucosal stratified squamous epithelium decreases the number of layers substantially; the outer layers do not become cornified	Decrease in the large nonnucleated cornified epithelial cells with gradual increase of nucleated noncornified epithelial cells; neutrophils become numerous, especially during diestrus; by late diestrus neutrophils become few; cellular debris and erythrocytes disappear
Anestrus	Mucosal epithelium remains appreciably thin with two to four layers of stratified cuboidal cells	Mostly small noncornified epithelial cells with rounded borders interspersed with a few neutrophils and lymphocytes

epithelia. These changes can be used both to ascertain the health of the uterus and vagina and determine the present stage of the estrous cycle, which can be very helpful for breeding purposes. In bitches and queens an effective method to monitor the progression of the cycle through cytological changes of the epithelial cells is to use vaginal smears (Table 19-3). In general, the epithelium thickens substantially during proestrus due to the influence of rising levels of estrogens. In the bitch the outermost cells become cornified and appear on smears as well as erythrocytes derived from the uterus. During estrus, cornification has reached its peak and keratinized cells are most frequently observed at this stage, whereas the erythrocytes lessen in number (Figure 19-23). During metestrus and diestrus less keratinization is seen and outer epithelial cells become smaller and more rounded than in the earlier stages. Neutrophils appear during metestrus and along with erythrocytes slowly disappear during diestrus. By anestrus, the highly stratified squamous epithelium that occurred during estrus has now become reduced to a stratified squamous to cuboidal epithelium consisting only of three or four layers of cells.

In the cow, comparable changes occur to the vaginal epithelium. However, as the epithelium thickens during the time of high estrogen secretion, the superficial cells do not become fully keratinized. The rate of development also varies according to location so that during early estrus, the cranial portion of the vaginal epithelium becomes its thickest, whereas by comparison, the caudal portion achieves its maximal thickness after estrus.

PLACENTATION

Following fertilization, the zygote becomes implanted, as previously discussed, at some point along the inner uterine wall. As the embryo develops at this location, a series of events occurs that culminates in the formation of the placenta. Between the second and third week after fertilization in most domestic species except for the mare, which is several weeks later, the gradual attachment of the embryo to the endometrium begins. With the progression of implantation, the integration of fetal and maternal tissues continues so as to provide the necessary mechanism for the dynamics of respiration, nutrition, and waste removal. In addition, as the placenta forms, it develops endocrine activity and is involved in the production of progesterone and relaxin.

During trophoblast expansion, the inner proliferating embryonic cells or embryoblasts become a lengthened mass and form the three basic germ layers, beginning initially with the **ectoderm,** which is directed toward the uterus, and the **endoderm,** which faces the center, followed by the intervening **mesoderm.** As the embryo is developed by these layers, the ectoderm continues on to compose the

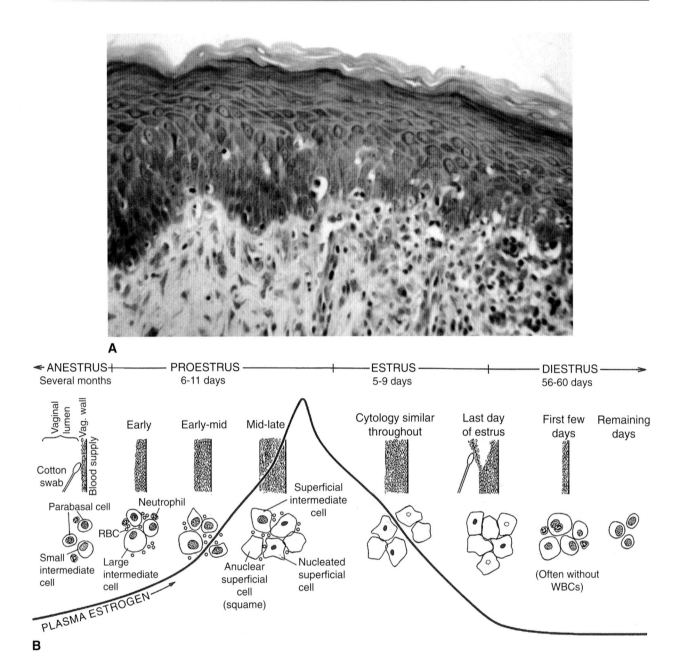

Figure 19-23. A, Light micrograph of the vaginal epithelium of a bitch during estrus. (Hematoxylin and eosin stain; ×125.) **B,** Illustration of vaginal changes including epithelial thickness and cytology and estrogen levels during the canine estrous cycle. *(From Feldman EC, Nelson RW: Canine and feline endocrinology and reproduction, ed 3, St. Louis, 2004, Saunders).*

amnion, a vascular free, translucent, single-layered epithelium with its own external, fibrous membrane that together surround the embryo (Figure 19-24). Meanwhile, the endoderm extends beyond the embryo to form its own cavity, the **yolk sac,** which is directly connected to the region that will become the midgut of the fetus, and the **allantois,** which similarly is an extension or diverticulum of the hindgut. The mesoderm also continues to proliferate beyond the embryo and a portion, the **somatic mesoderm,** grows along the inner cavity of the shell of trophoblasts to become the **chorion.** Another portion, the **splanchnic mesoderm,** grows along the yolk sac and allantois. Blood vessels arise first in the extraembryonic splanchnic mesoderm of the yolk sac, followed by that of the allantois. The chorion only becomes later vascularized when the allantoic mesoderm fuses with the chorionic mesoderm. At the point where the extraem-

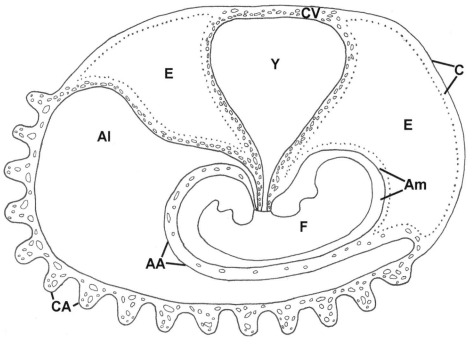

A

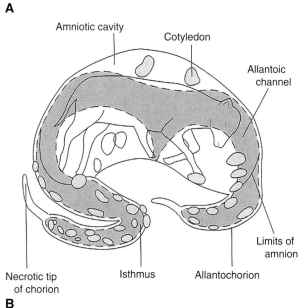

B

Figure 19-24. A, Diagram of the fetal membranes associated with placentation in domestic species. *Al,* Allantois cavity and endoderm with vascular mesoderm; *Am,* amnion; *AA,* allantoamnion; *C,* chorion; *CA,* chorioallantoic placenta; *CV,* choriovitelline placenta; *E,* exocoelom; *F,* fetus; *Y,* yolk sac. **B,** Diagram of a bovine conceptus during early pregnancy showing the arrangement of the fetal membranes including the cotyledons where the chorionic tissue interacts with the uterine caruncles. *(**A,** Redrawn from Dellmann HD, Carithers JR:* Cytology and microscopic anatomy, *Philadelphia, 1996, Williams & Wilkins;* **B,** *from Noakes DE:* Development of the conceptus. *In Noakes DE, Parkinson TJ, England GC, editors:* Arthur's veterinary reproduction and obstetrics, *London, 2001, Saunders.)*

bryonic membranes extend from the embryo, the mesoderm condenses and forms the body stalk that eventually is transformed into the **umbilical cord** with further development of the vasculature.

Placentation varies a great deal with regard to fetal-maternal circulation, fetal membrane development and organization, and the overall construction of the placenta, and for these reasons is classified in a number of ways. Types of classification include general and specific organization of chorionic structures; fetal extraembryonic membrane construction; and circula-

tion at the maternal and fetal interface and differences in tissues involved (Table 19-4).

CHORIONIC ORGANIZATION

The principal function of the chorion is to provide an effective interface between fetal and maternal tissues for necessary gaseous and nutrient-waste exchange. Being an avascular tissue, it derives vasculature from the fetus in part from the extraembryonic mesoderm associated with the allantois or the yolk

TABLE 19-4 Classifications of Placentation among Domestic Species

TYPE	PLACENTAL SHAPE	CHORIONIC SHAPE	CIRCULATION	CIRCULATORY PATTERN	DEGREE OF IMPLANTATION
Sow	Diffuse	Plicate (folded)	Epitheliochorial	Crosscurrent	Nondeciduate
Mare	Diffuse	Villous	Epitheliochorial	Countercurrent	Nondeciduate
Carnivores	Zonary	Lamellar	Endotheliochorial	Crosscurrent	Deciduate
Ruminants	Cotyledonary	Villous	Epitheliochorial	Crosscurrent	Nondeciduate
Others	Discoidal in primates and lab rodents	Trabecular (form of villous) in primates, labyrinthine in lab rodents and lagomorphs	Hemochorial in lab rodents, lagomorphs, and primates	Countercurrent in lab rodents and lagomorphs, multivillous (combination of concurrent and crosscurrent) in primates	Deciduate in primates

sac, forming either a chorioallantoic or choriovitelline placenta, respectively.

Chorioallantoic Placenta

Domestic species and most mammals in general possess chorioallantoic placentae in which the fetal placenta is supplied by blood vessels associated with the allantois. This developing diverticulum of the hindgut, which varies in size and is substantial in large animal herbivores, possesses well-formed vasculature. When joined with the chorion, a very efficient exchange structure between the mother and the fetus, the chorioallantoic placenta, is formed. Further classification and description of placentae are based on this form of placentation.

Choriovitelline Placenta

Before the allantois takes shape, the yolk sac is formed, which like the allantois has its own developing vasculature. The fusion of the vasculature of the yolk sac with the chorion forms the **choriovitelline placenta** (see Figure 19-24). Among most mammals, early placentation uses the vasculature associated with the yolk sac as it fuses with the chorion. However in most of these instances, this union is relatively short lived because the yolk sac is quite transient and involutes. The placentation in these animals becomes dependent on the chorioallantoic relationship. There are species, principally rodents and lagomorphs, with yolk sacs that remain during gestation. In these animals the yolk sac becomes inverted (i.e., the **inverted yolk sac placenta**), and the breakdown of the

adjacent chorion and outer wall of the yolk sac allows direct exposure of the endoderm to uterine tissue, including its glands. In this latter instance, the choriovitelline placenta is not vascularized.

PLACENTAL SHAPE

Among chorioallantoic placentae, the next way to distinguish and appreciate anatomical differences is to compare placental morphology based primarily on the location of maternal-fetal interaction along the chorionic sac. Among domestic species, these interactions usually involve highly vascularized chorionic villi or folds that form from the extraembryonic membrane and extend into the endometrium.

In the sow and the mare, the interaction occurs essentially over the entire sac without discrete areas and for that reason is called the **diffuse placenta.**

In ruminants, the maternal-fetal interaction is restricted to the caruncles, the nonglandular areas along the endometrium that vary in number, size, and shape according to the species. The chorionic tissue that interacts with the caruncles forms vascular tufts called **cotyledons;** the placentae are referred to as **cotyledonary** (see Figure 19-24). The cotyledons and caruncles together form **placentomes.** Between the placentomes, the chorion lacks vascular projections and is referred to as being smooth.

In the bitch and queen, the maternal-fetal interaction occurs as an equatorial belt around the chorionic sac. The beltlike structure creates an interactive zone, and consequently these placentae are known as being **zonary.** As between the placentomes in cotyledonary placentae, the chorion outside the interactive zone is smooth.

And in lagomorphs, rodents, and primates, the maternal-fetal interaction occurs in one or two round areas. Because of their disk shape, these placentae are referred to as **discoid.**

CHORIONIC SHAPE

In addition to differences in placental shape are morphological variations in the way the maternal and fetal tissues interact. The simplest form is the **folded placenta,** which occurs in the sow and consists of macroscopic folds, called **primary folds** or **plicae,** of the endometrium (Figure 19-25). As the chorion covers these folds during gestation, smaller, secondary folds (rugae) develop at the chorionic-uterine interface. These secondary folds cause considerable expansion of the surface area at the sites of maternal-fetal interaction. In carnivores the secondary folds can be well developed, slender, and elaborate, forming **lamellae** that result in the **lamellar placenta** (Figure 19-26).

In ruminants, fetal tissues form arborescent chorionic villi with extensive vascular beds that specifically are associated with the caruncles and can be referred to as **villous placentae** (Figure 19-27). The mare and humans also possess villous placentae.

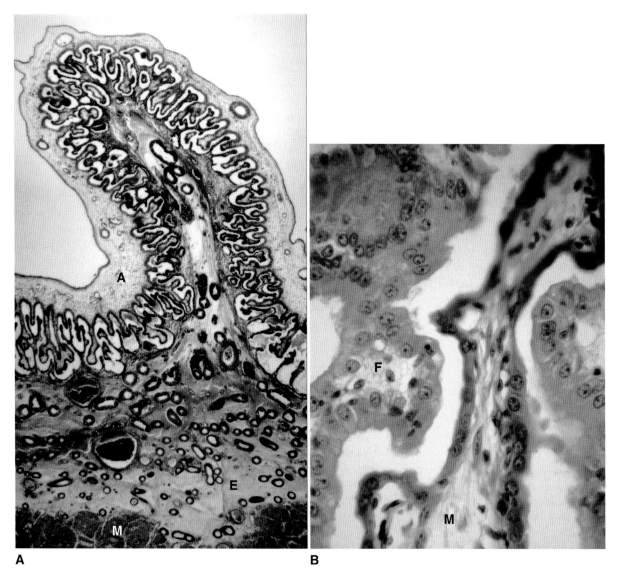

A   **B**

Figure 19-25. A, Light micrograph of primary folds that make up the folded placenta of the sow. *A,* Allantochorion; *E,* endometrium; *M,* myometrium. (Hematoxylin and eosin [H&E] stain; ×15.) **B,** Light micrograph of secondary folds or rugae that constitute the epitheliochorial placenta of the pregnant sow. *F,* Fetal; *M,* maternal. (H&E stain; ×250.)

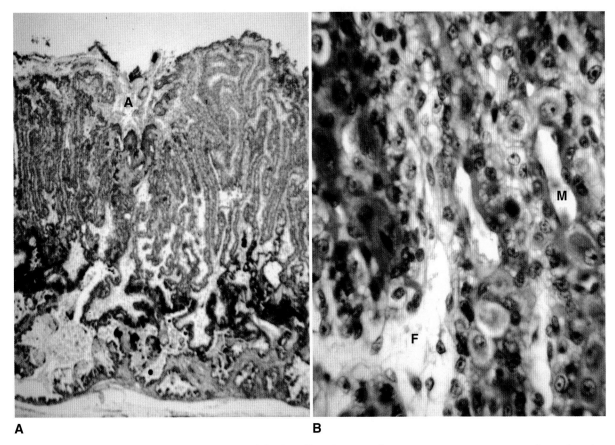

Figure 19-26. A, Light micrographs of a portion of the lamellar placenta of a pregnant queen. (Hematoxylin and eosin [H&E] stain; ×10.) **B,** Decidual cells stand out among the layers or lamellae that hold the maternal *(M)* and fetal *(F)* blood vessels. *A,* Allantochorion. (H&E stain; ×250.)

CIRCULATION

The tissues involved at the level of the chorion between the mother and the fetus for physiological exchange vary considerably in terms of invasiveness and result in further subdividing and classifying mammalian placentation. In the horse, ruminants, and pig, the trophoblast becomes implanted within the uterine tissues with little to no destruction of maternal tissues. This type of placenta is called **epitheliochorial** (see Figure 19-25, *B*). Fetal and maternal capillaries are separated by the endothelia of both capillaries as well as the chorionic epithelium and the uterine epithelium (Figure 19-28, *A*). Within the ruminant allantochorion, large, binucleated trophoblasts, known as **giant cells,** form and can move into the endometrial epithelium and fuse with the cells of the endometrial epithelium (Figure 19-28, *B*).

Another type, the **endotheliochorial placenta,** involves the loss of uterine epithelial tissue so that the trophoblast is now exposed directly to maternal capillaries. Trophoblasts frequently fuse to form multi-nucleated syncytiotrophoblasts. This type occurs in dogs and cats and other carnivores, as well as rodents, insectivores, and bats (see Figure 19-28, *C*).

The last type, the **hemochorial placenta,** involves the complete breakdown of maternal tissue layers so that the trophoblast is directly exposed to maternal blood without endothelial interference. There may be up to three layers of trophoblasts in this type, with one of the layers forming a syncytium where trophoblasts unite into a single entity, syncytic trophoblast or syncytiotrophoblast (see Figure 19-28, *D*). Hemochorial placentae occur in rodents, lagomorphs, and primates.

Deciduate

As the blastocyst has come to rest and become implanted, trophoblasts penetrate the endometrium at the site of implantation to varying degrees among hemochorial placentae and infiltrate the decidual cell population, while proliferating circumferentially. Some of the trophoblasts advance into the maternal vascular walls, continuing within these spaces into the

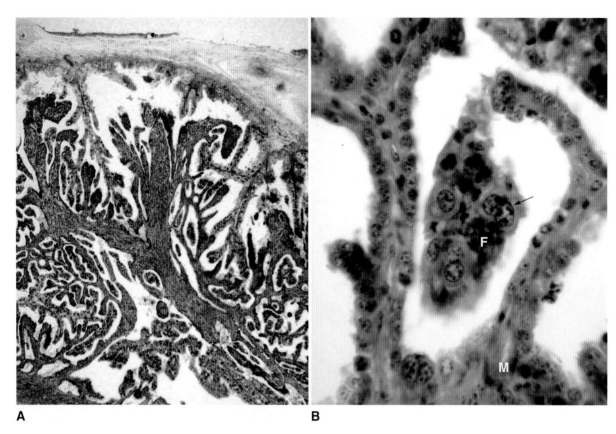

A   **B**

Figure 19-27. A, Light micrograph of a portion of the villous placenta of the pregnant cow. (Hematoxylin and eosin [H&E] stain; ×20.) **B,** Close-up of **A,** showing maternal *(M)* and fetal *(F)* components, separated by an artifactual space. Arrow points to binucleated trophoblast. (H&E stain; ×250.)

myometrium. The structure of these vessels can become remarkably altered as smooth muscle elements are destroyed and replaced by fibrin deposits, making these vessels more rigid. The degree of penetration by the trophoblasts varies among placental mammals. These placentae are referred to as being **deciduate** because both the fetal and the decidual portions are shed after parturition.

Nondeciduate

Placentae with less invasive trophoblastic activity, as seen in those species in which the uterine tissues remain intact such as cows, does, ewes, and mares, can be referred to as **nondeciduate.** In these instances, there is little loss of uterine tissue after parturition.

CIRCULATORY PATTERNS

In addition to the number of tissue layers present and the depth that fetal capillaries invaginate into the chorionic epithelium, the nutrient and gaseous exchange along the interhemal barrier is influenced by blood flow within adjacent maternal and fetal vascular networks. The rate of diffusion within the chorion depends in part on the size and number of vessels within a specific area as well as the direction of blood flow, which include concurrent flow, countercurrent flow, and crosscurrent flow. In concurrent flow, both maternal and fetal blood flow occurs in the same direction, is the least efficient, and does not exist in any species by itself. Countercurrent flow involves maternal and fetal blood flow occurring in opposite directions and is considered to be the most efficient because it allows arteriovenous equilibration in horses and rabbits. Crosscurrent involves a combination of both concurrent and countercurrent flow and occurs in ruminants.

MAMMARY GLAND

When active, the **mammary gland** is a large compound tubuloalveolar gland that functions to secrete milk, which is composed of a mixture of appropriate nutrients needed to sustain and protect the newborn. These nutrients include lactose, lipids, proteins, min-

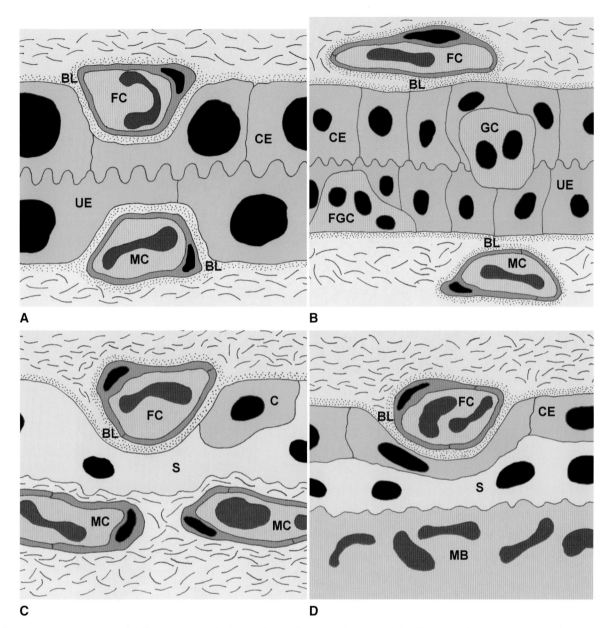

Figure 19-28. Diagram of different types of placental circulation and maternal-fetal barriers that occur among domestic species. **A,** Epitheliochorial—sow, mare. **B,** Synepitheliochorial—ruminants. **C,** Endotheliochorial—bitch, queen. **D,** Hemochorial (hemodichorial)—rabbit. *BL,* Basal lamina; *C,* cytotrophoblast; *CE,* chorionic epithelium; *FC,* fetal capillary; *FGC,* fused giant cell; *GC,* giant cell (binucleated trophoblast); *MB,* maternal blood; *MC,* maternal capillary; *S,* syncytiotrophoblast; *UE,* uterine epithelium.

erals, and vitamins, plus antibodies, lymphocytes, and monocytes. They are secreted in an apocrine and merocrine manner by tubuloalveolar adenomeres that are organized into a variable number of lobes depending on the species. The body of the gland is encased in a fibroelastic capsule of connective tissue, and the secretory portion is held together by a stroma of loose connective tissue.

SECRETORY UNIT

The alveoli and associated secretory tubules that comprise the secretory units of the mammary gland consist of cuboidal epithelial cells that vary in height according to their state of activity (Figure 19-29). Each lobe undergoes a secretory cycle whereby the secretory cells increase their height while milk is being

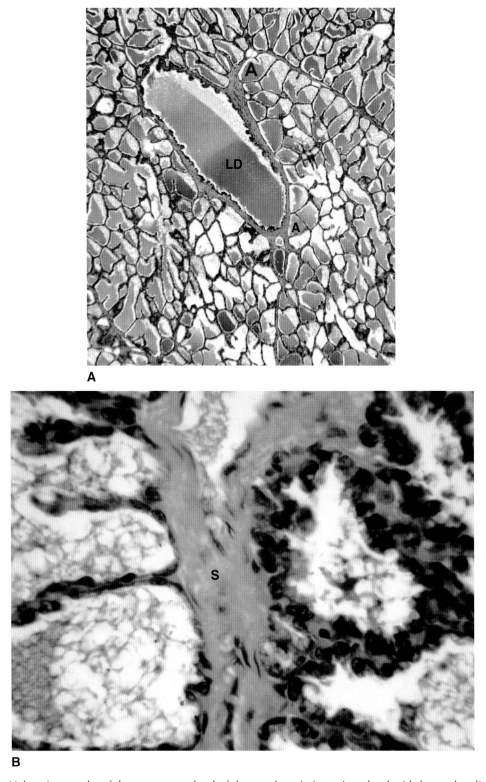

A

B

Figure 19-29. Light micrographs of the mammary gland of the monkey. **A,** Lactating gland with large alveoli *(A)* and lobular duct *(LD)* filled with milk (Hematoxylin and eosin [H&E] stain; ×20). **B,** Separated by an interlobular septum *(S)*, the lobule of the left contains inactive secretory cells, while those on the right contain cells that are actively secreting (H&E stain; ×250).

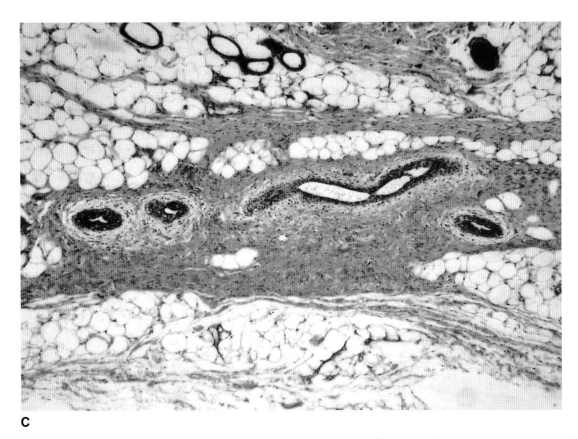

C

Figure 19-29, cont'd C, Nonlactating gland with the presence of lobular and lactiferous ducts among dense connective and adipose tissues (H&E stain; ×20).

released into the lumen of their secretory unit. As the lumen becomes full, the secretory cells wind down in activity and decrease in height. The activity of the lobules varies along the secretory cycle so that the amount of milk secretion and the morphology of the secretory cells differ from one area to another, but are consistent within a lobule.

The secretory cells release lipid in an apocrine manner so that some cell membrane and adjacent cytoplasm is deposited along with lipid droplets. Protein and carbohydrate substances, however, are exocytosed in a merocrine manner.

In addition to the secretory cells, **myoepithelial cells** line the secretory units. These cells are responsive to the pituitary's release of **oxytocin** and will cause the milk-filled lumens of the tubuloalveoli to be squeezed and forced into the duct system, a process referred to as **milk letdown.**

DUCTS

Each lobe has its own **lactiferous duct,** which can dilate as it collects milk to form a sinus that is con-

fluent with the teat sinus or cistern. In the cow, a number of lobar ducts empty into a **lactiferous sinus** that forms a common cavity for each quarter of the udder. The lactiferous ducts drain lobar ducts, which then drain lobular ducts. The lobular ducts in turn drain intralobular ducts. The intralobular ducts and the proximal portion of the lobular ducts are lined by a simple cuboidal to columnar epithelium. As the lobular ducts join the lobar ducts, the lining becomes a bilayered cuboidal epithelium, which further lines the lactiferous sinus. The lobular and lobar ducts possess longitudinally oriented smooth muscle.

TEAT

The lactiferous sinus joins the teat sinus, which then empties into the **papillary duct** or teat canal. In ruminants there is a round fold or annulus of mucosa that extends into the lumen between the sinuses. This portion of the duct system forms the **teat,** or nipple, and leads the milk to the skin. The bilayered epithelium of the lactiferous and teat sinuses becomes transformed within the papillary duct into a stratified squamous epithelium that is keratinized. As a part of this mucosa, bundles of smooth muscle encircle the duct and help hold the milk until it is expressed.

INACTIVE STATE

When active the mammary gland can be thought of as a specialized sweat gland. However, when inactive after a period of lactation, the mammary gland undergoes a process of involution (see Figure 19-29). The parenchyma becomes reduced in amount, especially the secretory units, which consist of simple cuboidal epithelia and comparatively pronounced myoepithelial cells. Interstitial tissue consisting of loose connective tissue, lymphocytes, and plasma cells as well as adipose replace some of it, but overall the volume of the mammary gland is substantially lowered. As the result of a previous period of lactation, there may be dark-staining bodies within the ducts and interstitial tissue that represent concretions of casein and are known as **corpora amylacea.**

AVIAN FEMALE REPRODUCTIVE SYSTEM

The basic design of the avian female reproductive system is not unlike that of mammals. Differences that occur are largely due to the production of offspring that develop beyond the uterus in a nutrient-filled environment that requires the protection of a shell. By the time that a female bird reaches reproductive maturity, only the left ovary and associated oviduct are functional.

OVARY

The avian **ovary** is composed of follicle-laden stalked projections that extend from two lobes. The ovary possesses a diffusely organized medulla and adjacent cortex, which houses the variably developed follicles (Figure 19-30). The avian follicle does not mature into a fluid-filled antrum-bearing entity. Instead, it consists of a single layer of granulosa cells, which surround a primary oocyte that has the capability to expand its cytoplasm with an enormous lipid inclusion, the yolk, to an extremely large size, such as 150 mm or more in diameter in the ostrich; the chicken is approximately one fifth that dimension. As in mammals, surrounding stromal tissue becomes organized into a **theca interna,** which is well vascularized, and a **theca externa**. Before ovulation, a blanched,

vascular-free area, the **stigma,** appears at the site where the follicle will rupture. At ovulation, the first meiosis has already been completed and the secondary oocyte along with the adjacent granulosa cells leaves the follicle. The remaining thecal cell population does not become transformed into any structure that resembles a mammalian corpus luteum.

OVIDUCT

The avian **oviduct** refers to a structure that includes the rest of the female reproductive tract. It consists of an infundibulum, magnum, isthmus, uterus, and vagina, and each component is involved in some capacity in the development and eventual external deposit of the egg. Most of the oviduct possesses an outer serosal lining, consisting of a simple squamous mesothelium overlying a small amount of loose connective tissue. The tunica muscularis of the oviduct gradually increases in size or thickness as the egg moves caudally, being least developed within the infundibulum and most developed within the uterus and vagina, the latter having fairly thick inner circular layers of smooth muscle.

Infundibulum

The ova become fertilized within this portion of the oviduct. As in mammals, the funnel-shaped caudal portion of the **infundibulum** receives the oocyte at ovulation with its ciliated finger-like fimbriae guiding it onto the primary mucosal-submucosal folds. The folds consist of a ciliated pseudostratified columnar epithelium that covers the lamina propria of loose connective tissue with diffusely distributed lymphatic elements (Figure 19-31). The caudal portion of the infundibulum has secondary folds, and the mucus-secreting glandular cells in the epithelium of this region are more numerous than the cranial portion (Figure 19-32).

Magnum

After the eggs have passed through the infundibulum (in less than 30 minutes in the chicken), they move through the next portion of the oviduct, the **magnum,** for a considerably longer period, roughly 3 hours. During that time, **albumen** is supplied for each egg, increasing the overall size of the egg substantially. The mucosal epithelium of the magnum is generally simple columnar, with comparable numbers of mucus-secreting and ciliated cells (Figure 19-33). The lamina

Text continued on p. 483

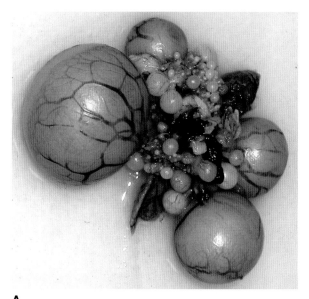

A

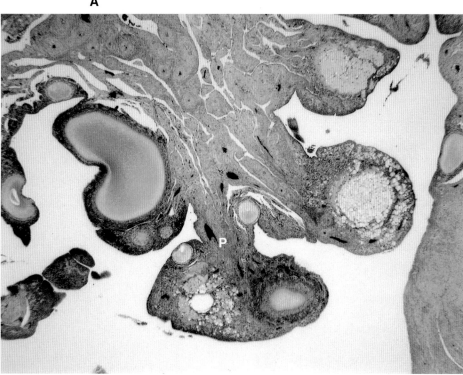

B

Figure 19-30. A, Gross morphology of the avian (chicken) ovary with numerous raised follicles. The large yellow follicles contain secondary oocytes filled with yolk. **B,** Light micrograph of follicles in different stages of development or atresia associated with a peduncle *(P)*. (Hematoxylin and eosin stain; ×20.)

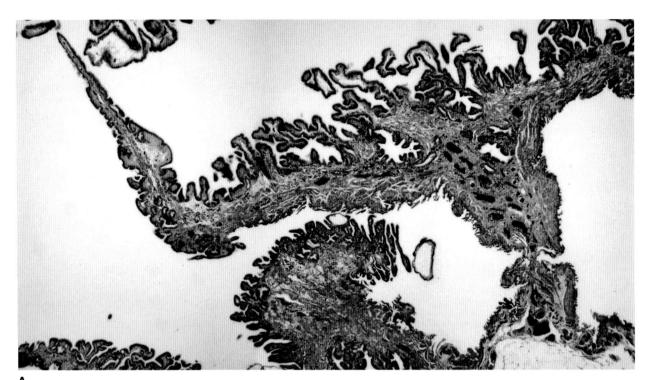

A

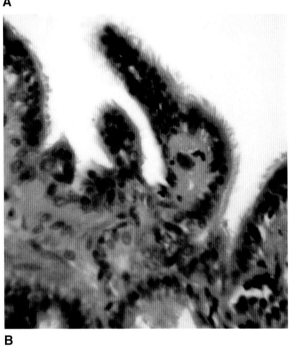

B

Figure 19-31. A, Light micrograph of the fimbriated portion of infundibulum of the chicken. (Hematoxylin and eosin [H&E] stain; ×10.) **B,** Light micrograph of the mucosa with ciliated epithelium along the fimbriated portion of infundibulum. (H&E stain; ×250.)

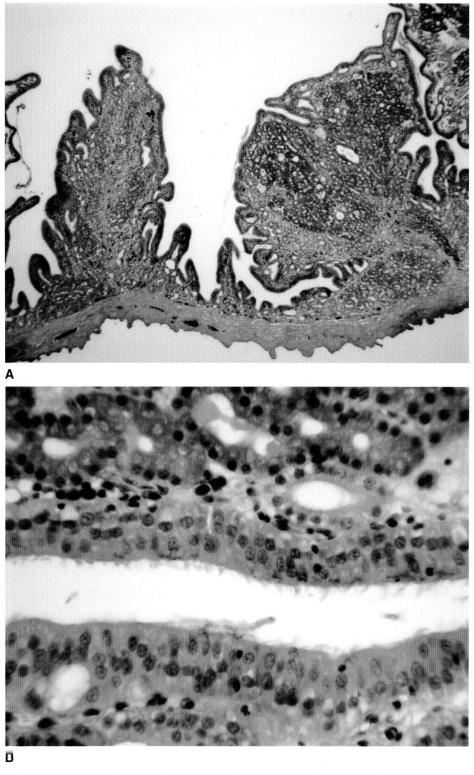

Figure 19-32. A, Light micrograph of the caudal portion of the avian infundibulum, which possesses tubular mucus-secreting glands. (Hematoxylin and eosin [H&E] stain; ×20.) **B,** Light micrograph of the mucosa with ciliated epithelium lining a duct within the caudal portion of the avian (chicken) infundibulum. (H&E stain; ×250.)

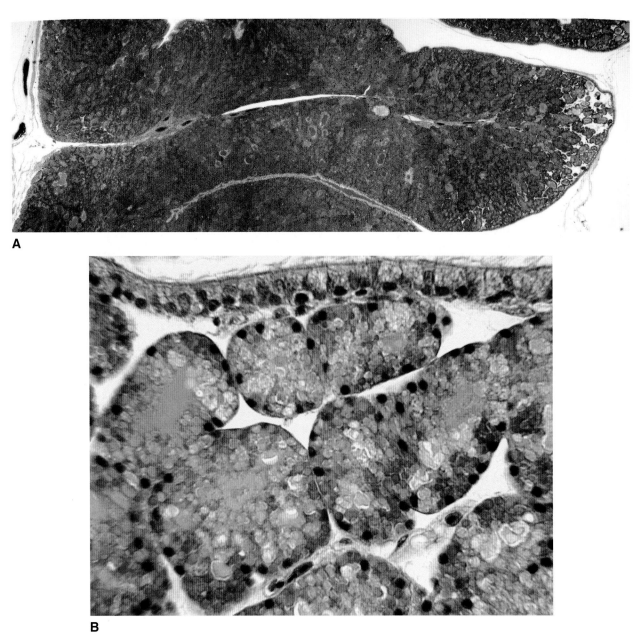

A

B

Figure 19-33. A, Light micrograph of the caudal portion of the magnum of the chicken. (Hematoxylin and eosin [H&E] stain; ×10.) **B,** Mucosa of the magnum filled with branched tubular glands. (H&E stain; ×250.)

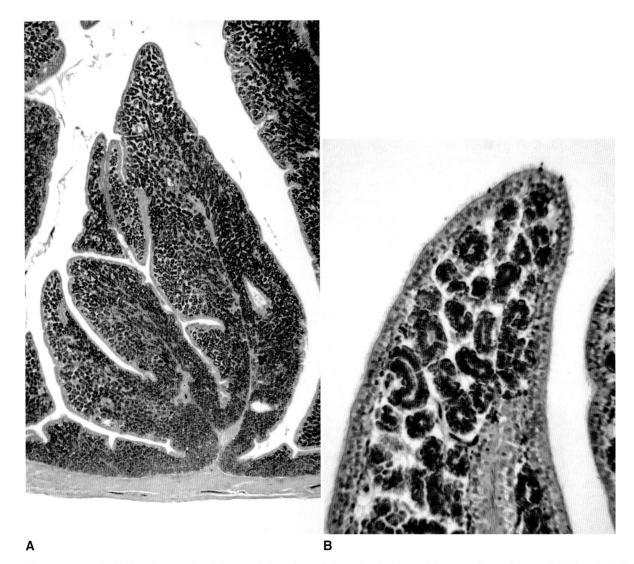

A   **B**

Figure 19-34. A, Light micrograph of the cranial portion of the avian isthmus. (Hematoxylin and eosin [H&E] stain; ×20.) **B,** Light micrograph of the mucosa with ciliated epithelium and adjacent branched tubular glands within the chicken isthmus. (H&E stain; ×250.)

propria contrasts sharply to that of the infundibulum; it is filled with long, tubular glands that can be branched and coiled. The secretory cells of these glands can be cuboidal to columnar. In addition to the glands is a small amount of loose connective tissue with diffuse lymphatic tissue.

Isthmus

In this next portion, the **isthmus,** the egg receives **shell membranes** as it moves along an epithelium largely the same as that occurring in the magnum. Here as well, the propria-submucosa contains numerous tubular glands that are involved in the production

of the shell membranes (Figure 19-34). The transition from the magnum to the isthmus is demarcated by a short glandless region between the two areas.

Uterus

When the egg reaches the **uterus** it spends the greatest amount of time here (around 20 hours in the chicken) as a calcareous shell is formed. For that reason the avian uterus is also called the **shell gland.** The overall thickness of the wall of the uterus is greatest in this portion of the oviduct due not only to an increased thickening of the tunica muscularis but also a greater development of mucosal-submucosal folds within this portion, which are oriented both longitudinally and circularly (Figure 19-35). The folds are lined with a pseudostratified columnar epithelium that is intermittently ciliated and filled with tubular glands that can be both branched and coiled. The secretory cells of these glands are typically granulated and vacuolated.

Vagina

The last portion of the avian oviduct, the vagina, is thick walled but has smaller folds than those of the uterus. The mucosal epithelium is ciliated pseudostratified columnar with nonciliated cells, including occasional goblet cells. The propria-submucosa within these folds lacks glands, consisting of loose connective tissue that is variably populated with cells of defense. The region connecting the vagina and the uterus has sperm-host glands that support the temporary storage of spermatozoa within the avian reproductive tract. These glands are simple tubular and consist of lipid-bearing secretory cells.

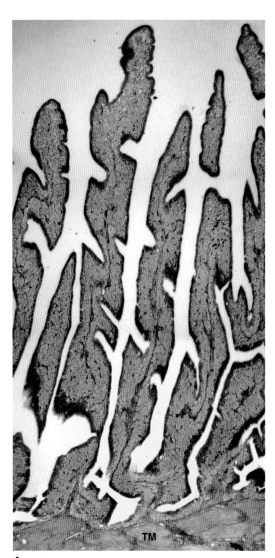

A

Figure 19-35. A, Light micrograph of the uterus of the chicken. *TM,* Tunica muscularis. (Hematoxylin and eosin [H&E] stain; ×10.)

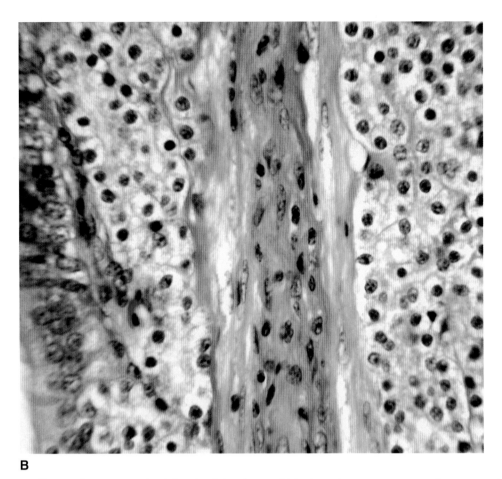

B

Figure 19-35, cont'd B, Light micrograph of the glandular tissue within the avian uterus, surrounding a central core of smooth muscle. (H&E stain; ×250.)

SUGGESTED READINGS

Baker TG: Oogenesis and ovulation. In Austin CR, Short RV, editors: *Reproduction in mammals,* ed 2, Cambridge, UK, 1982, Cambridge University Press.

Benirschke K: Placenta: implantation and development. In Knobil E, Neill JD, editors: *Encyclopedia of reproduction,* vol 3, San Diego, 1998, Academic Press.

Dellmann HD, Carithers JR: *Cytology and microscopic anatomy,* Philadelphia, 1996, Williams & Wilkins.

Duffy DM, Stouffer RL: Luteinizing hormone acts directly at granulosa cells to stimulate periovulatory processes: modulation of luteinizing hormone effects by prostaglandin, *Endrocrine* 22:249, 2003.

Evans AC: Characteristics of ovarian follicle development in domestic animals, *Reprod Domest Anim* 38:240, 2003.

Fawcett DW: *Bloom and Fawcett: a textbook of histology,* ed 11, Philadelphia, 1986, Saunders.

Feldman EC, Nelson RW: *Canine and feline endocrinology and reproduction,* ed 3, St Louis, 2004, Saunders.

Gartner LP, Hiatt JL: *Color textbook of histology,* Philadelphia, 1997, Saunders.

Gosden RG, Brown N, Grant K: Ultrastructural and histochemical investigations of Call-Exner bodies in rabbit Graafian follicles, *J Reprod Fertil* 85:519, 1989.

Gray CA, Bartol FF, Tarleton, BJ, et al: Developmental biology of uterine glands, *Biol Reprod* 65:1311, 2001.

Guraya S: *Biology of ovarian follicles in mammals,* Berlin, 1985, Springer-Verlag.

Kaufmann P, Burton G: Anatomy and genesis of the placenta. In Knobil E, Neill JD, Greenwald GS, Market CL, editors: *The physiology of reproduction,* ed 2, New York, 1994, Raven Press.

Noakes DE: Development of the conceptus. In Noakes DE, Parkinson TJ, England GC, editors: *Arthur's veterinary reproduction and obstetrics,* London, 2001, Saunders.

Rodgers RJ, Irving-Rodgers HF, Van Wezel IL: Extracellular matrix in ovarian follicles, *Mol Cell Endocrinol* 163:73, 2000.

Steven DH: *Comparative placentation,* New York, 1975, Academic Press.

Sturkie PD, Mueller WJ: Reproduction in the female and egg production. In Sturkie PD, editor: *Avian physiology,* ed 4, New York, 1986, Springer-Verlag.

Sunderland SJ, Crowe MA, Boland MP, et al: Selection, dominance and atresia of follicles during oestrous cycle in heifers, *J Reprod Fertil* 101:547, 1994.

Van Wezel IL, Irving-Rodgers HF, Ninomiya Y, Rodgers RJ: Ultrastructure and composition of Call-Exner bodies in bovine follicles, *Cell Tissue Res* 296:385, 1999.

Wenzel JG, Odendhal S: The mammalian rete ovarii: a literature review, *Cornell Vet* 75:411, 1985.

Eye and Ear

KEY CHARACTERISTICS

- Systems designed for vision, audition, and vestibulation.
- For the eye, global structure is designed to refract and focus direct and indirect light onto photon-detecting neurons (photoreceptors) as a part of a nervous coat that transmits the signal to the brain for processing.
- For the ear, a canal system is designed to transmit and amplify sound waves that are transferred to electrical impulses by cells that detect mechanical motion and are then sent to the brain for processing. Within this system, changes in head and body motion are similarly acknowledged and transferred.

EYE

The principal means by which most animals are made aware of their surroundings as well as changes in these surroundings, is the reflection or emission of light toward them by external objects and the reception of this light by the special organ, the eye. This organ perceives light adequately because it consists of a variety of tissues assembled into components that are able to transmit and refract light to specialized cells called photoreceptors that convert light energy into an electrical stimulus that is sent back to the visual cortex. Although vision begins in the eyes of domestic species, eyes do not actually see. Seeing is a function of higher centers located in the brain.

The eye is composed of three basic layers or coats. The outer coat is the **fibrous tunic,** which is further divided into the cornea and sclera (Figure 20-1). The fibrous tunic gives the eye a constant shape and form that is imperative for a functional visual system. In addition the anterior portion of the fibrous tunic—the cornea—is transparent, enabling light to pass through, and shaped in a manner that makes it a powerful lens which refracts (bends) light rays centrally towards the visual axis of the eye.

The second and middle layer is the **uvea** (a Greek term meaning grape), also called the **vascular tunic,** or coat. The uvea is divided into the choroid, the ciliary body, and the iris. The choroid, located in the posterior half of the eye is found between the sclera and the retina. The basic functions of the choroid are to provide nourishment to the highly metabolic retina and modify internal light reflection and scatter because it is either heavily pigmented or reflective. The uvea continues anteriorly as the ciliary body, whose functions include lenticular accommodation through its musculature as well as the attachment of the lens, and the production and outflow of aqueous humor, a fluid that flows through the anterior segment.

The most anterior portion of the vascular tunic—the iris—extends from the ciliary body centrally just anterior to the surface of the lens. The iris is heavily pigmented and contains muscles that change the shape of the iris and the central "hole" within the iris—the pupil. In this manner, the iris is able to control the amount of light that enters the posterior segment to stimulate the retina.

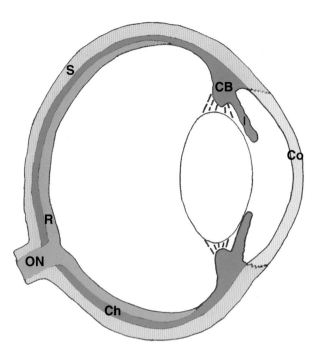

Figure 20-1. Schematic diagram of the three tunics of the eye. The fibrous tunic is salmon (*S,* sclera) and beige (*Co,* cornea). The vascular tunic (*CB,* ciliary body; *Ch,* choroid; *I,* iris) is blue, and the nervous tunic (*ON,* optic nerve; *R,* retina) is green.

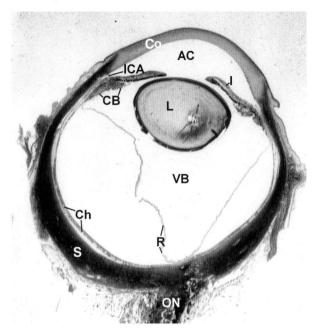

Figure 20-2. Light micrograph of the sheep eye. *AC,* Anterior chamber; *Ch,* choroid; *Co,* cornea; *CB,* ciliary body; *I,* iris; *L,* lens; *ON,* optic nerve; *R,* retina; *S,* sclera; *VB,* vitreous body. (Hematoxylin and eosin stain; ×2.)

The third and most central layer is the **nervous tunic,** or coat, which is made up of the retina and associated optic nerve. Briefly, the retina contains light-sensitive cells, photoreceptors that, after a series of intermediate modifying processes, transmit impulses to the brain via the optic nerve.

Two additional ocular systems are the intraocular fluids and the crystalline lens. The intraocular fluids include the vitreous and aqueous humors, which collectively create a transparent medium for light transmission as well as keep the fibrous tunic normally distended by maintaining a safe level of internal pressure within the eye through the production and removal of these fluids, especially aqueous humor. The crystalline lens acts as a fine-focusing mechanism.

CORNEA

The cornea is the transparent anterior one fifth or so of the fibrous tunic of the globe, which supports the intraocular contents, refracts light (because of its curvature and the principle that light bends when moving air to a liquid medium), and transmits light through its transparency (Figure 20-2).

On microscopic examination, the cornea of animals consists of four and sometimes five layers:

anterior epithelium; the anterior lamina of the cornea, also known as Bowman's layer, stroma, or substantia propria; posterior lamina, also known as Descemet's membrane; and endothelium (posterior epithelium) listed from outside inward (Table 20-1).

The anterior epithelium covers the anterior corneal surface (Figure 20-3, *A*). It consists of nonkeratinized stratified squamous epithelium of uniform thickness approximately 25 to 40μm thick in the domestic carnivore and two to four times thicker in larger domesticated species. The epithelium consists of a single cell layer of columnar basal cells that lie on a thin basement membrane, two or three layers of polyhedral (wing) cells, and two to many layers of nonkeratinized squamous cells, depending on the species. Corneal epithelium is thicker at the periphery of the cornea than it is in the center; however, with the junction of the bulbar conjunctiva it abruptly thins, and pigmented cells are observed. Occasional lymphocytes may be seen from time to time interspersed within the basal cell layer. Unsheathed nerve endings of sensory nerves also exist throughout much of the inner portion of the epithelium.

The **anterior lamina** is not formed in most animals, occurring in avian and human cornea as well as some cetaceans and the giraffe (Figure 20-3, *B*). Though it is considered part of the corneal stroma,

TABLE 20-1 Morphological and Functional Characteristics of Ocular Components Among Domestic Species

OCULAR COMPONENT	MORPHOLOGY	FUNCTIONAL ACTIVITY	SPECIES VARIATIONS
Cornea	Highly organized, avascular, dense regular connective tissue; stroma lined anteriorly by nonkeratinizing stratified squamous epithelium and posteriorly by simple squamous epithelium that forms continually growing basement membrane (posterior lamina)	Transmits and refracts light; provides portion of protective housing for ocular contents	Anterior lamina (Bowman's layer) in primates, cetaceans, giraffes, and birds
Limbus	Dense connective tissue become irregular, variably pigmented, and vascularized; anteriorly lined by nonkeratinizing stratified squamous epithelium and posteriorly by the outer portion of the iridocorneal angle	Houses collecting vessels for aqueous humor outflow and possesses highly regenerative epithelium for wound healing	
Sclera	Outer portion (episclera) of thin loose connective tissue; sclera proper: dense irregular connective tissue with little vasculature and some pigmentation next to the outer choroid (lamina fusca)	Provides most of protective housing for ocular contents	In nonmammals, scleral proper consists of hyaline cartilage ending anteriorly next to an adjacent ring of bony plates—scleral ossicles
Iris	Loosely wound fibrous highly vascularized stroma with melanocytes and other pigmentary cells distributed in species-specific patterns; anteriorly lined by fibrocytes and posteriorly lined by pigmented epithelium; two sets of smooth muscle: dilator, lying next to posterior pigmented epithelium, and sphincter lying next to the pupil	Anterior portion of the black box; lets in and controls amount of light striking the retina by varying size of its pupil	Large herbivores possess pigmented pupillary ridge especially along the dorsal margin—granula iridica; shape of pupil varies with round prevalent shapes (birds, dog, pig), vertical slit (cat), and horizontally oval (large herbivores); muscles are skeletal in nonmammals
Ciliary body	Internally, vascular sinusoids within bilayered epithelial-lined folds (pars plicata); externally, bundles of smooth muscle often interspersed with melanocytes, extending posteriorly (pars plana); anteriorly, cleft or sinus and cellularly lined filtering meshwork for aqueous humor drainage	Continuation of the black box; produces and removes aqueous humor and generates intraocular pressure (IOP); provides lenticular accommodation	Development of iridocorneal angle and ciliary body musculature is inversely proportional; in nonmammals ciliary body musculature is skeletal
Choroid	Highly pigmented vascular region divided into nonvascularized outermost region of loose connective tissue (suprachoroidea); layer of large often anastomosing veins and intermittent arteries; and medium-sized arterioles and venules that lead from the large vessels to a single-layered capillary belt (choriocapillaris)	Major portion of the black box; provides oxygen and nourishment for the outer retina; reflective region (tapetum) enhances vision during twilight and nocturnal periods; site of uveoscleral outflow	In ungulate species, within dorsal layer of medium-sized vessels is highly organized dense connective tissue (tapetum fibrosum), whereas in carnivores this layer consists of reflective cells (tapetum cellulosum) with organized rodlets; diurnal species lack tapeta
Lens	Epithelial ball, typically biconvex shape, consisting of long tubular cells (lens fibers) and anterior simple cuboidal to squamous epithelium that contributes anteriorly to the basement membrane (capsule) and forms new lens fibers peripherally (at lens equator) with older, compressed fibers pushed centrally within the lens (nucleus)	Provides further refraction of light transmitted to the retina—fine tuning for visual resolution	Nonmammalian lenses possess radially positioned lens fibers at the equator for enhanced lenticular deformation during accommodation; especially developed in raptors

Continued

TABLE 20-1   **Morphological and Functional Characteristics of Ocular Components Among Domestic Species—cont'd**

OCULAR COMPONENT	MORPHOLOGY	FUNCTIONAL ACTIVITY	SPECIES VARIATIONS
Vitreous humor	Extremely loose connective tissue consisting of outer region (cortex) of scattered collagen (type II) concentrated mostly along the pars plicata, pars plana, hyaloideo-lenticular capsule, inner limiting membrane, and optic nerve head, and a diffuse layer of fibrocyte-like cells (hyalocytes) near inner retina; and inner (central) region of fewer cells and collagen	Provides transparent medium for light to strike the retina; along with aqueous humor maintains ocular shape and retinal position	Some variations with regard to collagen density; central region of ungulate species often has higher concentrations of collagen and is more gelatinous
Retina	Nervous tissue (neurosensory portion) arranged into nine layers housing three orders of neurons; outermost order of neurons is avascular and consists of photoreceptors, rods, and cones, with modified processes to detect photons of light with the processes attached to a pigmented epithelium, which firmly attaches the retina to the choroid	Acknowledges the presence of light and transforms light energy into electrical signal that is transmitted to the central nervous system for visual interpretation	Numerous variations with regard to the density of neurons that comprise the three different orders; degree of retinal vasculature varies among domestic species, being little vascularized (paurangiotic) in the horse, vascularized along the horizontal plane (merangiotic) in the rabbit, well vascularized (holangiotic) in ruminants and carnivores, and nonvascularized (anangiotic) in birds (chicken)

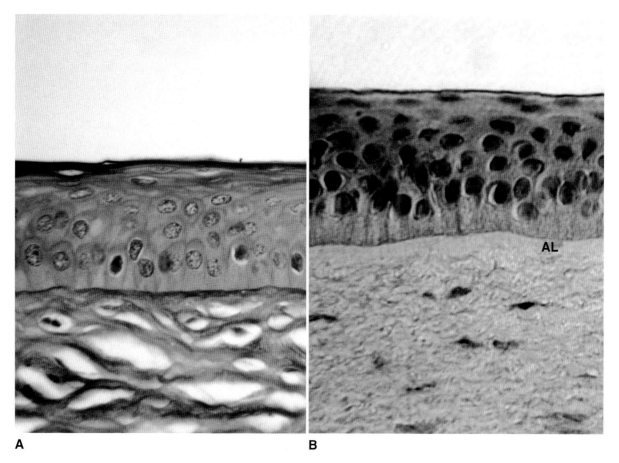

A   B

Figure 20-3. A, Light micrograph of the anterior epithelium of the canine cornea. (Periodic acid–Schiff stain; ×400.) **B,** Light micrograph of the anterior epithelium and anterior lamina *(AL)* of the avian (chicken) cornea. (Hematoxylin and eosin stain; ×400.)

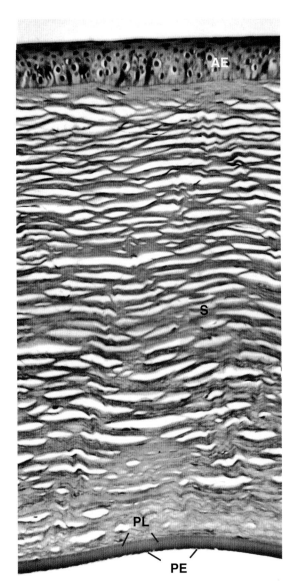

Figure 20-4. Light micrograph of a canine cornea. *AE,* Anterior epithelium; *S,* stroma; *PE,* posterior endothelium; *PL,* posterior lamina. (Periodic acid–Schiff stain; ×100.)

it is formed by the anterior epithelium and is 10 to 15 μm thick (and greater in deep-diving whales), acellular, and composed of small highly organized collagen fibrils. It is not elastic but is fairly tough and when destroyed is replaced by scar tissue.

The corneal stroma is also called the **substantia propria** because it comprises 90% of the thickness of the cornea in most species (Figure 20-4). It is very ligamentous-like, consisting of transparent lamellae of dense regular connective tissue. The lamellae lie in sheets and split easily into planes. Between the lamellae are fixed cells called stromal cells or **keratocytes.** It is the fibrous extensions of these cells that help delineate the stromal lamellae. They have thin nuclei, ill-defined borders, and delicate cell membranes.

These cells can be transformed into fibroblasts when deep corneal injury has occurred and may form scar tissue that is not transparent. Wandering cells are usually leukocytes that have migrated from the limbus, often after trauma. These cells are able to migrate to the center of the cornea in the bovine eye within 30 minutes after injury.

Precise organization of corneal stroma is the most important factor in maintaining corneal clarity. The bulk of corneal stroma is composed of thin evenly positioned collagen fibrils that are organized as lamellae and run the full diameter of the cornea. This special arrangement of stroma permits light entering the eye to pass through the cornea without scatter.

Collagen fibrils, along with proteoglycans and glycoproteins, make up 15% to 25% of the corneal stroma and act as the principal support structure of the cornea. These collagen fibrils form the matrix for a unique population of proteoglycans within the corneal stroma. The cornea is 75% to 85% water and is relatively dehydrated when compared to other tissues. This state of dehydration is referred to as deturgescence and is produced by the endothelium and epithelium.

The **posterior lamina,** Descemet's membrane, is a homogeneous acellular membrane that is 10 to 15 μm thick in the dog and up to 30 μm thick in the horse. It is eosinophilic when stained with hematoxylin and eosin and with periodic acid–Schiff (PAS) it stains brightly (Figure 20-5; see also Figure 3-27). Lying on the posterior surface of the stroma, this layer is a true basement membrane that is formed by the endothelium and continues to thicken slowly throughout the life of the individual as long as the endothelium remains healthy. The posterior lamina ends at the apex of the trabecular meshwork in the limbal region.

The **posterior epithelium,** or endothelial cell layer, also referred to as the **corneal endothelium,** is a single layer of flattened and hexagonally arranged cells that is continuous with the iridocorneal angle of the anterior chamber (see Figure 20-5). Ultrastructural studies reveal the cells are laterally attached to each other by highly convoluted interdigitations (see Figure 3-4). In terms of its function, the corneal endothelium is the most important layer of the cornea because it actively maintains corneal transparency.

The presence of blood vessels in the cornea more centrally than at the limbus is an indication of corneal disease in most instances. The condition producing the vascularization may be local or generalized.

LIMBUS

The limbus, about 1 mm wide in the dog and the cat and up to 5 mm in large herbivores, is the transition

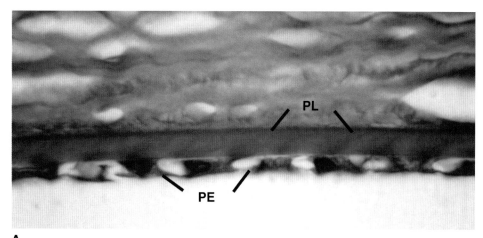

A

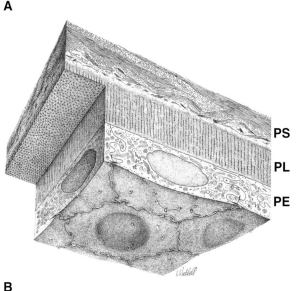

B

Figure 20-5. A, Light micrograph of the posterior lamina *(PL)* and posterior endothelium *(PE)* in the feline cornea. (Hematoxylin and eosin stain; ×400.) **B,** Illustration of the PL and PE. *PS,* Posterior stroma. *(Modified from Hogan MJ, Alvarado JA, Weddell JE:* Histology of the human eye, *Philadelphia, 1971, Saunders.)*

zone between the cornea and the sclera-conjunctiva (Figure 20-6, A; see also Figure 20-2). At this point the sclera is pigmented to varying degrees. Microscopically, the epithelium is thicker than the adjacent corneal epithelium, with closely packed small basal cells that have scanty cytoplasm. The **limbal epithelium** can be stem cells for the regeneration of the corneal anterior epithelium when needed.

The stroma of the limbus loses the regular arrangement characteristic of the cornea and takes on the woven appearance of dense irregular connective tissue. Numerous blood vessels, which represent the anastomosing branches of the anterior ciliary arteries, occur within the outer stroma. Both anterior and posterior laminae of the cornea end in this area. However, the corneal endothelium extends as a thin fibroblastic cell layer onto the pectinate ligament and trabecular meshwork of the iridocorneal angle.

SCLERA

The **sclera** forms the opaque posterior three quarters to five sixths of the fibrous tunic (see Figure 20-2). Anatomically this component of the eye consists of three regions or layers. The inner surface is called the **lamina fusca** and is brown due to the adherent suprachoroidal pigment. This surface forms an outer boundary of a potential space that is lined internally by the suprachoroidea of the outer choroid. The bulk of the sclera is called the **sclera proper.** The histologic structure of the sclera proper is comparable to the dermis of the integument, consisting of dense irregular connective tissue. The sclera contains a considerable amount of elastic fibers that are interlaced among the collagen fibers. The collagen fibers, fibrocytes and occasional melanocytes are arranged meridionally, obliquely, and radially in an irregular fashion. The

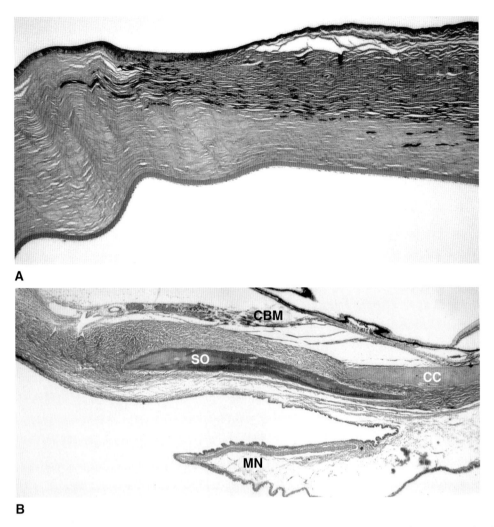

A

B

Figure 20-6. A, Light micrograph of the equine limbus. (Masson trichrome stain; ×20.) **B,** Light micrograph of the scleral ossicle *(SO)* in a chicken. *CC,* Cartilage cup; *CBM,* ciliary body musculature; *MN,* membrana nictitans (third eyelid). (Masson trichrome stain; ×20.)

individual collagen fibrils of the sclera differ from those of the cornea in that the fibrils possess a great deal of variation in their diameters. The sclera is also more hydrated than the cornea and contains larger blood vessels; its rigidity provides the resistance to intraocular fluid tension. The outermost region of the sclera is called the **episclera,** which consists of loose connective tissue that anteriorly blends with the connective tissue of the bulbar conjunctiva and posteriorly with an ocular fascia known as *Tenon's capsule.* The episclera is fairly vascular; the nerve supply is from the ciliary nerves and has very few endings in this portion of the eye.

Besides dense connective tissue, the sclera can be composed of cartilage, as in birds (see Table 20-1). When cartilage is found in the sclera, it usually forms a complete cup that extends to a ring of bony plates or **scleral ossicles** (Figure 20-6, *B*). Ossicles of the

sclera are located anteriorly underneath or external to the ciliary body. Although birds and reptiles possess this structure, the ossicle is believed to have originated from fish and were eventually passed on to amphibia. Birds with perhaps the greatest range of accommodation such as the kingfisher and other diving birds have larger and potentially more powerful ossicles than those species that tend to be more confined to land. Owls and hawks have "used" them to produce elongated and cone-shaped eyes that have resulted in remarkable differences in the radii of curvatures between the cornea and globe. In a functional sense, ossicles are believed to have been devised for retaining ocular rigidity.

The scleral thickness varies considerably among species and in different areas of the globe, but is thinnest near the equator, especially behind (posterior to) the insertions of the extraocular muscles. At the

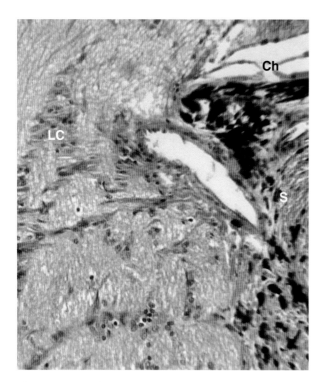

Figure 20-7. Light micrograph of a portion of lamina cribrosa *(LC)* in the canine optic nerve. *S,* Sclera; *Ch,* choroid. (Hematoxylin and eosin stain; ×300.)

point where the optic nerve passes through the sclera it becomes sievelike and is known as the **scleral lamina cribrosa** (Figure 20-7). Abnormal tension in this region due to glaucoma results in the disruption of axoplasmic flow in individual nerve fibers of the optic nerve.

UVEA

The choroid, ciliary body, and iris form the uveal coat or uvea (see Figures 20-1 and 20-2). Unlike the fibrous coat, it is highly vascular and usually pigmented. The choroid and ciliary body are attached to the internal surface of the sclera. The iris originates from the anterior portion of the ciliary body and extends centrally to form a diaphragm in front of the lens. The iris and ciliary body are collectively termed the anterior uvea. The choroid is designated as the posterior uvea.

IRIS

The iris is a diaphragm that is derived from the neural crest, mesoderm, and neuroectoderm and extends centrally from the ciliary body to cover the anterior surface of the lens except for a central opening—the **pupil.** The shape of the moderately dilated pupil varies throughout vertebrates. In mammals it is round in primates, dogs, and pigs; vertical when constricted in the cat; and oval in a horizontal plane in herbivores (horse, oxen, sheep, and goats). Along the upper edge of the pupil in herbivores are several round black masses. They vary in size and are called **granula iridica,** or **corpora nigra.** Similar smaller masses exist on the lower edge of the pupil.

Iridal color varies considerably among individuals as well as various breeds or species of animals, depending on the amount of pigmentation of the iridal stroma. The iris consists of an anterior stroma and a posterior bilayered epithelium. The stroma is covered anteriorly by a layer of fibroblastic cells continuous with the inner iridocorneal angle. The iris stroma is composed of interwoven bundles of fine collagenous fibers, many chromatophores including melanocytes, and fibroblasts. The stroma is loosely arranged except around blood vessels and nerves where it forms dense sheaths, particularly in porcine eyes. Color variation of the iris is partly due to the degree of vascularization along with the amount of pigmentation (Figure 20-8). The chromatophores and fibroblasts can be evenly distributed throughout the stroma of the iris or concentrated as in the canine iris, which often contains a dense band of melanocytes in the posterior stroma anterior to the dilator muscle.

In the stroma near the pupil a flat band of thin circular bundles of smooth muscle forms the **iridal sphincter muscle** or **iridal constrictor muscle.** The sphincter muscle, which is innervated parasympathetically by the oculomotor nerve, is responsible for reducing the size of the pupil (Figure 20-9). Opposing the sphincter muscle is the **iridal dilator muscle,** which consists of a single layer of smooth muscle fibers in the posterior iridal stroma extending from the iris sphincter to the iris periphery. These fibers contain pigment around their nuclei and lie adjacent to the posterior pigmented epithelium of the iris (Figure 20-10). The dilator muscle is innervated sympathetically and when contracted opens the pupil. Both sphincter and dilator muscles arise from the neural ectoderm. In avian species these intrinsic iris muscles are striated. In some birds such as the cormorant, the sphincter and dilator muscles are striated as well as smooth. The posterior iridal surface is covered by two layers of pigmented epithelium continuous with the epithelium of the ciliary body. The anterior layer actually comprises the dilator muscle fibers while the posterior layer—the **posterior pigmented epithelium**—is densely pigmented, and may extend centrally to form the granula iridica.

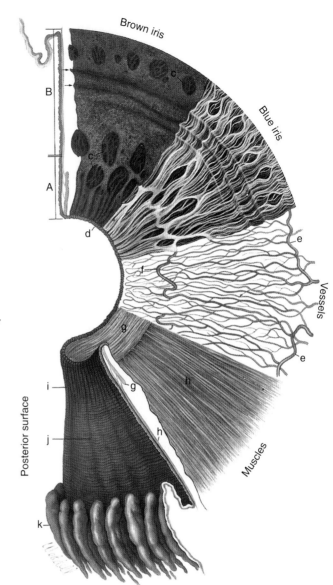

Figure 20-8. Diagram of the pigmentation and vasculature of the mammalian iris and how these two ingredients are responsible for iridal color. *(From Hogan MJ, Alvarado JA, Weddell JE: Histology of the human eye, Philadelphia, 1971, Saunders.)*

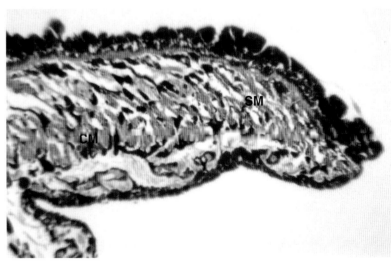

Figure 20-9. Light micrograph of the iridal sphincter muscle *(SM)* in the dog. (Hematoxylin and eosin stain; ×100.)

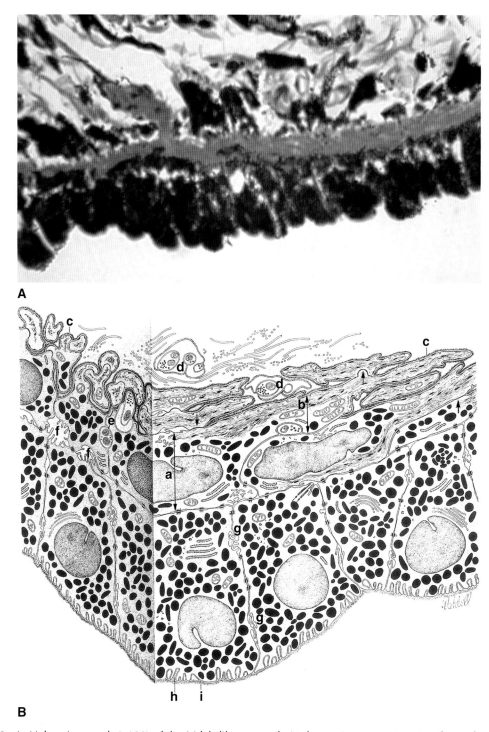

A

B

Figure 20-10. A, Light micrograph (×100) of the iridal dilator muscle in the canine eye. (Hematoxylin and eosin stain, ×250.) **B,** Illustration reveals the overlapping *(b)* organization of the single layer of the iridal dilator muscle and its apical *(a)* attachment to the posterior pigmented epithelium of the iris. *c,* Basal lamina of the muscle cells; *d,* nearby sheathed nerve ending; *e,* unsheathed nerve ending; *f,* intercellular canals; *g,* lateral interdigitations; *h,* basal infoldings; *i,* basal lamina of pigmented epithelium. *(From Hogan MJ, Alvarado JA, Weddell JE: Histology of the human eye, Philadelphia, 1971, Saunders.)*

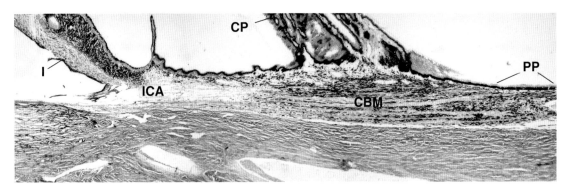

Figure 20-11. Light micrograph of the canine ciliary body. *CBM,* Ciliary body musculature; *CP,* ciliary process; *I,* iridal base; *ICA,* iridocorneal angle; *PP,* pars plana. (Masson trichrome stain; ×10.)

At the iris root (peripherally) in most species is an annular major arterial circle from which many vessels of the iris, which are directed spirally toward the pupil, are derived. The arteries attenuate into capillary beds as they spread throughout the iris stroma.

CILIARY BODY

The ciliary body is an anterior continuation of the choroid, and joins with the iris. The ciliary body is divided into a broad anterior zone, the **pars plicata,** and a narrower posterior zone, the **pars plana** (Figure 20-11; see also Figure 20-2). The inner surface of the anterior zone is composed of radially arranged folds called the **ciliary processes** (70-100) depending on the species (around 75-76 in the dog). Each process possesses a central core of stroma and blood vessels covered by a double layer of epithelium (Figure 20-12). The main mass of the ciliary body, exclusive of the ciliary processes, consists of the smooth ciliary muscles and melanocytes. The flat posterior portion of ciliary body, the pars plana, consists of a thin vascular stroma with two layers of overlying epithelium and extends from the posterior extent of the ciliary process to the junction with the retina at the ora ciliaris retinae. The width of the pars plana varies as the retina extends more anteriorly in the inferior and medial quadrant in most species. The pars plana is therefore wider superiorly and laterally. The lenticular zonules arise from the ciliary body epithelial cells and pass anteriorly in the valleys between the ciliary processes onto the lens equator. Minor species variations occur.

The ciliary body has a variety of functions including aqueous humor production; aqueous humor removal; secretion of hyaluronic acid of the vitreous; lens attachment and its accommodation; and constitution of the blood-aqueous barrier.

Ciliary Process and Aqueous Humor Production

The ciliary process is the structure that produces aqueous humor and varies considerably among domestic species in size, shape, and number. Aqueous humor is the fluid that fills the anterior and posterior chambers of the eye and supplies nutrients to the lens and the cornea; provides a continuously flowing stream into which surrounding tissues can discharge metabolic waste products; creates intraocular pressure by means of its formation and drainage, which maintains ocular rigidity so that the globe is distended to its proper form; and forms an optimal environment for light transmission. The bilayered epithelium of the ciliary process forms aqueous humor as blood plasma passes first through the fenestrated capillaries and venules and adjoining stroma of a scant amount of loose connective tissue (see Figure 20-12). This epithelium consists of an outer pigmented layer and an inner nonpigmented layer that are generally both cuboidal, though columnar in the horse. The two layers are tightly attached to each other and form the blood-aqueous barrier essential for a clear medium to transmit light. Normal aqueous humor is then produced across this barrier through diffusion, ultrafiltration, and active formation.

Iridocorneal Angle and Aqueous Humor Removal

As a component of aqueous humor dynamics, the iridocorneal angle plays a vital role in the removal of aqueous humor from the eye. The **iridocorneal angle,** also referred to as the **filtration** or **chamber angle,** varies greatly in size and organization (Figure 20-13). Among domestic species, animals with large eyes and

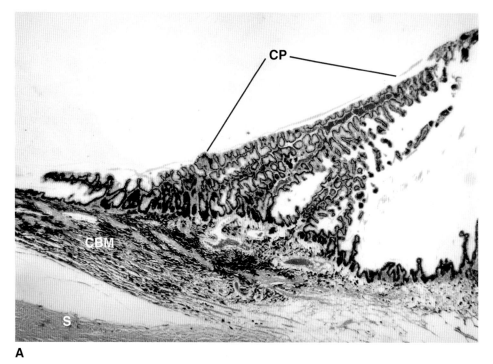

A

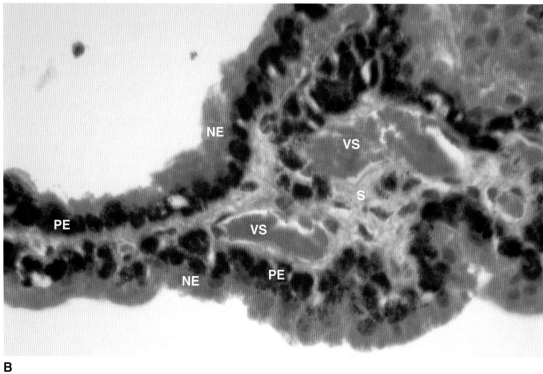

B

Figure 20-12. **A,** Light micrograph of the ciliary process *(CP)* in the dog. *CBM,* Ciliary body musculature; *S,* sclera. (Hematoxylin and eosin stain; ×20.) **B,** Close-up of a portion of a ciliary process of a deer. *NE,* Nonpigmented epithelium; *PE,* pigmented epithelium; *S,* stroma; *VS,* vascular sinusoid. (Masson trichrome stain; ×250.)

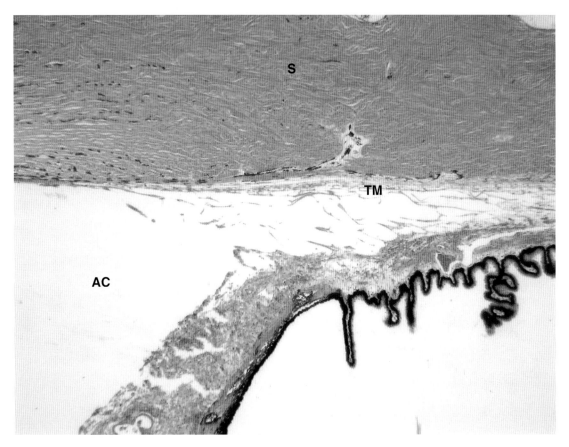

Figure 20-13. Light micrograph of the iridocorneal angle in the cat. *AC,* Anterior chamber; *S,* sclera; *TM,* trabecular meshwork. (Hematoxylin and eosin stain; ×20.)

correspondingly large anterior chambers possess well-developed iridocorneal angles including robust pectinate ligaments and large ciliary (cilioscleral) clefts (sinus) to facilitate large amounts of aqueous humor.

The iridocorneal angle is formed by the junction of the corneoscleral tunic and the iris base. It extends into the anterior ciliary body as a recession—the **cilioscleral sinus,** or cleft. The pectinate ligaments span the cilioscleral sinus anteriorly from the usually pigmented corneoscleral junction to the root of the iris. Behind the pectinate ligament and within the cilioscleral sinus is a matrix of neural crest tissue, the **trabecular meshwork.** Trabecular meshwork consists of crisscrossing collagen cords covered by a unique endothelium known as trabecular cells. As aqueous humor leaves the anterior chamber, it passes through the collagenous pillars of the **pectinate ligament,** which help anchor the anterior base of the iris to the limbus, and the large spaces (spaces of Fontana) between the big trabeculae of the uveal trabecular meshwork. Most of the aqueous humor then enters

and percolates through the corneoscleral trabecular meshwork, which acts as a coarse filter and then enters adjacent outflow vessels (Figure 20-14).

Trabecular meshwork in the cilioscleral sinus appears to be anterior tendinous extensions of ciliary body musculature. This musculature is poorly developed in most domestic animals, thus creating a proportionally larger sinus than found in humans. Adjacent to the meshwork are aqueous humor–collecting channels, which, in turn, empty into the scleral venous plexus and then the vortex veins. The aqueous-collecting channels are collectively referred to as the **angular aqueous plexus** in most species, being an **angular aqueous sinus** (canal of Schlemm) in humans and other primates as well as in many rodents. It is the movement of the aqueous humor through this narrow region that accounts for much of the resistance to outflow. The aqueous humor then flows into a network of veins called the intrascleral plexus before exiting via the subconjunctival venous system anteriorly or the vortex venous system posteriorly.

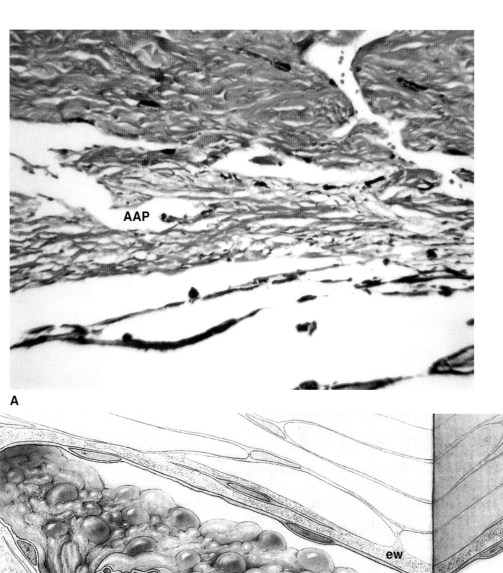

A

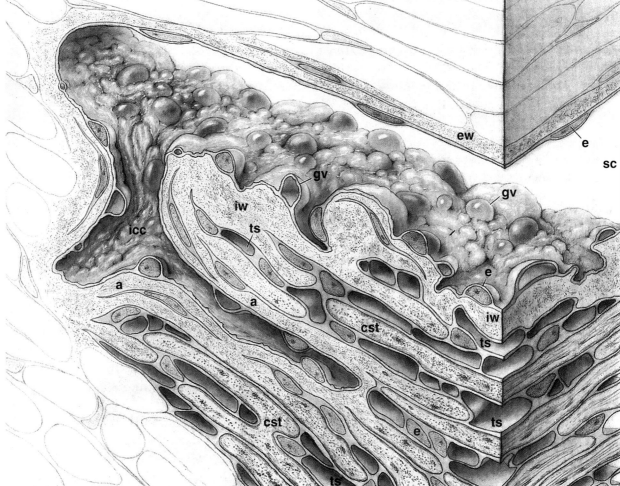

B

Alternate Routes of Aqueous Humor Outflow

In addition to removal by specific veins along the outer boundary of the corneoscleral trabecular meshwork, aqueous humor can leave the eye by additional alternate routes, also known as *unconventional outflow*, whereas removal of aqueous humor by veins along the outer angle is referred to as *conventional outflow*. The largest amount of aqueous humor to leave the eye in an unconventional manner is along a pathway referred to as the **uveoscleral route.** In this instance, aqueous humor moves exteroposteriorly through the length of the iridocorneal angle to the external lining of the ciliary musculature and suprachoroidal space along the outermost choroid.

The Ciliary Body Musculature

The muscle of the ciliary body in most domestic mammals consists of smooth muscle fibers that run primarily along the meridional plane, and is less developed in most herbivorous animals than dogs and cats (see Table 20-1). However, in the pig the anterior portion of the ciliary body musculature is oriented not unlike that occurring in most primates. In the dog and cat, the muscle fibers, which are meridional in direction, form inner and outer leaves that partially embrace the iridocorneal angle. When ciliary body musculature is involved in lenticular accommodation, it also influences aqueous humor outflow.

Lenticular Accommodation

The ciliary body and its processes provide a base on which lenticular zonules are attached. These zonules attach to the outer portions of the lens and hold it in place. Contractions of ciliary body muscle alter the tension of these zonules, which then change the shape of the lens due to the inherent elasticity of the lens capsule. The lens moves slightly forward and rounds up posteriorly and together alter the degree to which light is refracted—this is accommodation. Among domestic species the cat and pig have the most developed musculature for this purpose.

In birds and other nonmammalian animals the ciliary body musculature is composed of skeletal muscle cells that are mostly meridionally oriented. At least two distinct bundles of muscle are positioned in this region of the avian eye: an anterior bundle arises near the margin of the cornea; and a posterior bundle, which in raptors such as the eagle and hawk is well developed and sometimes referred to as two muscles, which will cause the ciliary body to push against the lens and squeeze it.

CHOROID

The posterior uvea (choroid) is composed of blood vessels (mainly thin-walled veins) and pigmented support tissues (Figure 20-15). It is the main source of nutrition for the outer layers of the retina, particularly the photoreceptors, that lie immediately internal to it. The anterior margin of the choroid joins the ciliary body along a junction known as the **ora ciliaris retinae.** Besides providing oxygen and nutrients for the outer retina, the choroid serves as a black box of sorts due to the abundance of melanocytes that usually reside there.

The choroid is composed of four layers: the suprachoroidea, large vessel layer, medium-sized vessel layer, and choriocapillaris (see Figure 20-15).

Suprachoroidea

The suprachoroidea is the outermost choroidal layer, lying adjacent and loosely attached to the sclera, and consists of an avascular membrane of elastic, heavily pigmented connective tissue forming loose lamellae. It has been demonstrated in a variety of species that aqueous humor will exit the eye along this membrane, diffusing through the sclera, in addition to flowing out of the eye through the angular aqueous plexus.

Figure 20-14. A, Light micrograph (×100) of the angular aqueous plexus *(AAP)* of the canine iridocorneal angle. (Hematoxylin and eosin stain.) **B,** Illustration of the trabecular meshwork and outflow vessel, angular aqueous sinus (AAS) in the human iridocorneal angle. *a,* Portion of the internal wall along the angular aqueous sinus; *cst,* corneoscleral trabeculae; *e,* endothelial cells; *ew,* external wall of the AAS; *gv,* giant vacuoles; *icc,* internal collecting channel of the AAS; *iw,* internal wall along the AAS; *sc,* AAP (Schlemm's canal); *ts,* intertrabecular spaces. *(From Hogan MJ, Alvarado JA, Weddell JE:* Histology of the human eye, *Philadelphia, 1971, Saunders.)*

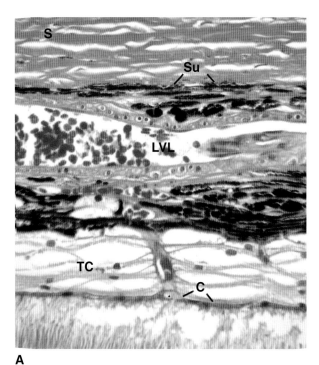

A

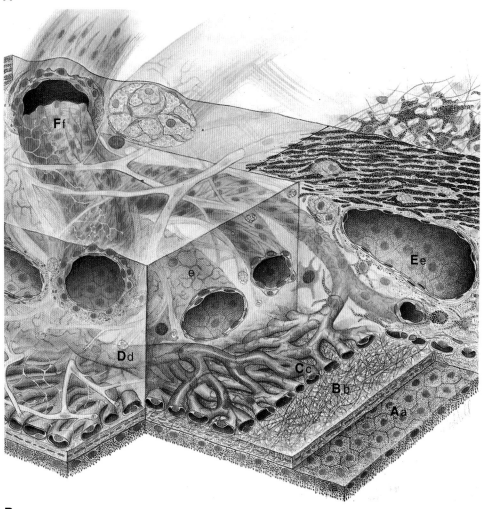

B

Figure 20-15. **A,** Light micrograph of the canine choroid. *C,* Choriocapillaris; *LVL,* large vessel layer; *S,* sclera; *Su,* suprachoroidea; *TC,* tapetum cellulosum. (Hematoxylin and eosin stain; ×250.) **B,** Illustration of the vascular components of the mammalian choroid. *Aa,* Retinal pigment epithelium; *Bb,* Bruch's membrane; *Cc,* choriocapillaris; *Dd,* venule of the middle-sized vessel layer; *Ee,* vein of the large vessel layer; *Ff,* artery of the large vessel layer. *(From Hogan MJ, Alvarado JA, Weddell JE:* Histology of the human eye, *Philadelphia, 1971, Saunders.)*

Large Vessel Layer

Immediately internal to the suprachoroidea is a vascular plexus of large vessels consisting mostly of anastomosing veins embedded in loose connective tissue containing numerous melanocytes.

Medium-Sized Vessel Layer

Internal to the large vessel layer is a layer of medium-sized vessels and fine reticular connective tissue. This forms a continuous vascular membrane in primates, squirrels, and pigs, whereas in dogs, cats, horses, and ruminants the pigmented portion of the elastic reticular vascular membrane is replaced dorsally by a layer of reflective tissue, the **tapetum lucidum.**

Tapetum Lucidum. This layer forms the dorsal or superior portion of medium-sized layer and is composed of regularly arranged collagenous fibers **(tapetum fibrosum)** in herbivores and specific polyhedral cells **(iridocytes, tapetum cellulosum)** containing reflecting crystals in carnivores (Figure 20-16). It reflects light that has passed through the retina to restimulate the retinal photoreceptor cells. The tapetum is responsible for the eyeshine seen at night when animals face a light, and for the variable background color of the ocular fundus (background of the eye as viewed by light projected inside the eye). Animals without a tapetum, such as squirrels, pigs, and birds, are usually diurnal.

Choriocapillaris

The **choriocapillaris** forms the innermost layer of choroidal vessels, consisting of a thin layer of fenestrated capillaries (see Figure 20-15). This capillary sheet is separated from the retinal pigmented epithelium by a membrane complex, **complexus basalis,** most often referred to as **Bruch's membrane,** which tightly connects the choriocapillaris with the outermost layer of the retina, the retinal pigment epithelium.

CRYSTALLINE LENS

The lens is a "fine-tuning" refractive structure that serves to fine focus images on the retina for acute vision (see Figure 20-2). It is held in place by the specialized ligaments called **zonules** arising from ciliary epithelium and attaching to the lens capsule at the lens equator. The lens is largely biconvex in most species with the degree of convexity changing during accommodation due to elasticity of the capsule and

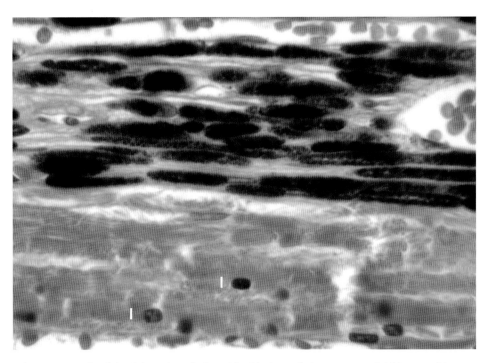

Figure 20-16. Light micrograph of the feline dorsal choroid with the cellular tapetum. *I,* Iridocyte. (Hematoxylin and eosin stain; ×400.)

pliability of lens substance. Some animals, including members of the rodent family and marine mammals, however, possess a round lens. In these animals the ciliary musculature is either poorly developed or practically nonexistent and as a result has no accommodative ability. The round lens provides a greater range of focus, especially when the iris constricts its pupil to a small hole.

The lens is totally epithelial, containing no pigment or blood vessels that would decrease transparency. The lens is held in place by numerous zonules that extend from the ciliary body processes to the equatorial region of the lens. The lens is also held in place to a minor extent by the vitreous humor and the support of the iris.

The lens is completely enclosed within a thick PAS-positive elastic capsule. The adult canine **lens capsule** is 12 to 15 μm thick at the equator, 50 to 70 μm anteriorly, and only 2 to 4 μm thick posteriorly (Figure 20-17). Inside the anterior capsule is the single layer of **lens epithelial cells.** These cells produce the capsule, which is the basement membrane for these cells. The cells are squamous to cuboidal centrally and become columnar near the equator, elongating into slender, highly elongated **lens fibers** that appear hexagonal in cross section (Figure 20-18). New fibers are formed externally at the equator throughout life. As they mature they form small ball-and-socket interdigitations along their lateral surfaces, making these cells tightly adherent to one another as well as to the previous inner layer of forming lens fibers. The outer fibers are the most recently formed and all of the lens fibers curve from one surface of the lens to the other (anterior and posterior) with their tips meeting at an anteroposterior junction that takes the shape of an upright Y on the anterior surface and an inverted Y on the posterior surface. This junction is called the **suture line** and is frequently visible in the normal lens

and accentuated in cataractous lenses. The most recently formed lens fibers extend anteriorly under the anterior epithelium and posteriorly under the lens capsule toward the ever-expanding suture. These fibers comprise the region known as the lens bow due to the arrangement of nuclei in these cells (Figure 20-19). In addition to the cellular interdigitations, the cell membranes possess many gap junctions or nexi, which in avian (chicken) lenses can comprise up to 65% of the lens fiber cell membrane, making these cells quite electronically coupled and contribute to the maintenance of the lens's overall structural integrity.

As each lens fiber attains it full predetermined length and completes its development, the cell's nucleus undergoes degeneration with a concomitant loss of mitochondria, rough endoplasmic reticulum, Golgi apparatus, and other organelles and in fact appears to become senescent. The adult lens then consists of lens fibers formed chronologically throughout life. The oldest portion of the lens, which is formed embryonically, is in the center and is known as the embryonic nucleus. Extending outwardly, the fetal nucleus, adult nucleus, and cortex are encountered (see Figure 20-19). These portions can be further divided into inner and outer portions, such as the inner cortex or the outer adult nucleus.

In birds, lenticular accommodation is dependent on the ability of the lens to change shape even more than in mammals. The avian lens is much softer and more flexible than that of mammalians and consequently is allowed to be readily deformed during the contraction of the ciliary body musculature. As the musculature contracts, the ciliary body pushes against the equatorial region of the lens. As an evolutionary adaptation to this activity, the avian lens has an annular pad or "ringwulst," consisting of lens fibers that are relatively enlarged and arranged radially

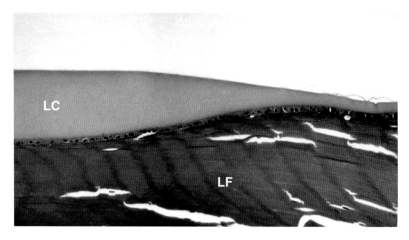

Figure 20-17. Light micrograph of the lens capsule *(LC)* near the equator of the lens where it broadens anteriorly. *LF,* Lens fibers. (Hematoxylin and eosin stain; ×100.)

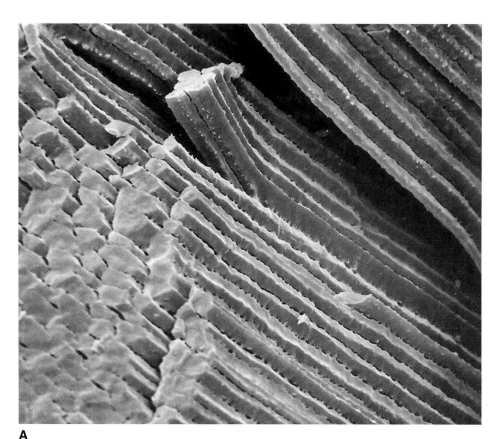

Figure 20-18. Scanning electron micrographic views of young lens fibers oriented obliquely in the canine lens. (**A,** ×800; **B,** ×2000.)

A

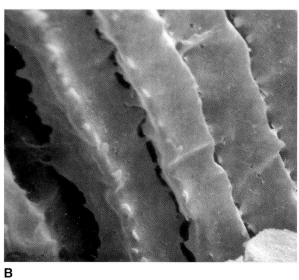

B

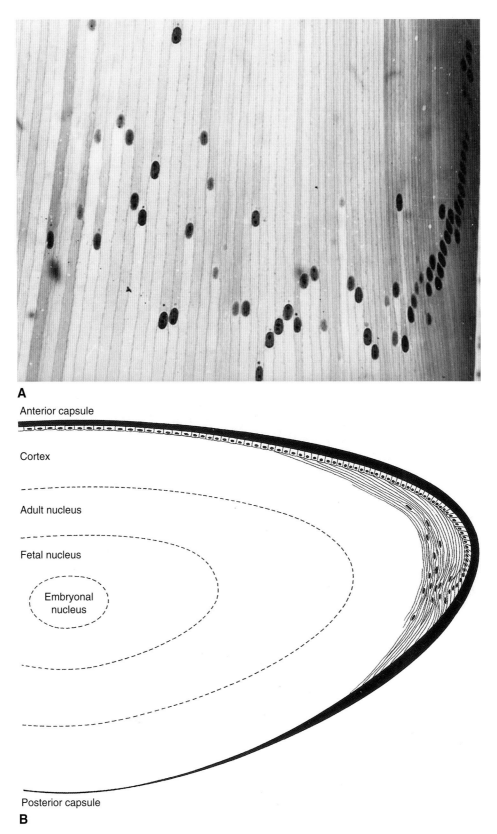

A

Anterior capsule

Cortex

Adult nucleus

Fetal nucleus

Embryonal nucleus

Posterior capsule

B

Figure 20-19. A, Light micrograph of the lens bow region of the canine lens. (Plastic section, toluidine blue; ×250.) **B,** Diagram of the mammalian lens and the different regions. *(Hogan MJ, Alvarado JA, Weddell JE: Histology of the human eye, Philadelphia, 1971, Saunders.)*

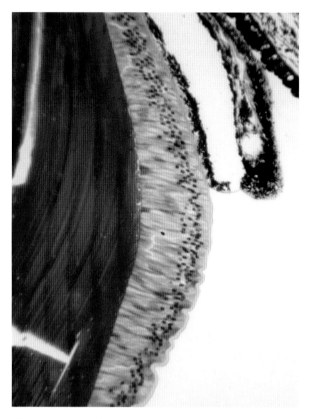

Figure 20-20. Light micrograph of the lens equator in the chicken. (Masson trichrome stain; ×15.)

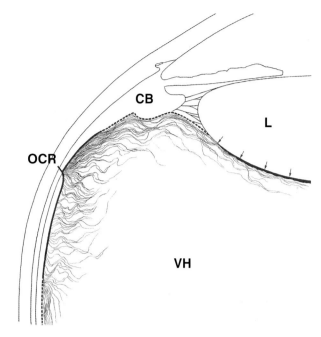

Figure 20-21. Diagram of the vitreous humor *(VH)* in the mammalian eye, with the greatest concentration of collagen along the ciliary body *(CB)*, especially at the ora ciliaris retinae *(OCR)*, and to a lesser extent along the inner face of the retina and posterior capsule *(arrows)* of the lens *(L)*. *(Modified from Hogan MJ, Alvarado JA, Weddell JE:* Histology of the human eye, *Philadelphia, 1971, Saunders.)*

instead of concentrically (Figure 20-20). The size of the pad appears to be directly related to the degree of accommodative ability.

VITREOUS HUMOR

The **vitreous humor,** also called the **vitreous body,** occupies up to four fifths of the volume of the globe, transmits light, fills the central space to maintain the globe's shape, and helps maintain the retina in its normal attached position.

The vitreous encircles a remnant of the hyaloid artery from the embryonic eye called the **hyaloid canal** or Cloquet's canal, which extends from the optic disk to the posterior pole of the lens. In most domestic animals, remnants of this artery normally regress just before or after birth. The hyaloideo-lenticular ligament is a remnant of the artery that attaches the vitreous to the posterior lens capsule in most domestic animals and has surgical implications when removing a cataractous lens. The vitreous is clear, allowing light to reach the retina. Nutrients can diffuse transvitre-

ally from the ciliary body to the retina. The vitreous is 99% water. Collagen and hyaluronic acid (HA) comprise most of the remaining 1%, with collagen supplying what little vitreous framework there is (Figure 20-21). Nearly all visible light is transmitted through the normal vitreous. The collagen content is highest where the vitreous is a gel. The proportion of gel to liquid vitreous varies among domestic species. The collagen network is embedded in the internal limiting membrane of the retina, which produces part of the adult vitreous. Thus, vitreal contraction or the formation of inflammatory bands in the vitreous creates tension on the retina, which can tear or detach the retina. It is generally accepted that collagen turnover is quite slow and perhaps nonexistent in primates, dogs, and other animals, which have vitreous bodies that liquefy with age. The normal vitreous cells, the hyalocytes, may have some responsibility for the production of HA and have phagocytic activities as well. They are not abundant and generally lie 20 to 50 μm away from the basal lamina of the inner limiting membrane, forming a single layer of fairly evenly scattered cells. The exclusion of other cells and large particles is essential to maintain transparency. Except for the collagen and HA, the composition of the vitreous is similar to aqueous humor.

Although essentially invisible, the vitreous humor consists of two principal regions: peripheral and central. The peripheral portion lies next to the retina and is called the cortex, which includes the collagen fibrils that connect to the basal lamina of the Muller and glial cells of the retina. The hyalocytes also reside in this region. The central portion is further subdivided into retrolental (hyaloid canal) and intermediate zones.

RETINA

Being derivatives of the forebrain, the retina and its associated optic nerve are morphologically and physiologically similar to the brain. The function of the retina, as a direct extension of the brain, is to receive light stimuli from the external environment and transmit this data accurately to the brain, which is interpreted there to become vision. The visual process begins with the **photoreceptor cells** of the retina, which comprise a complex layer of specialized cells: **rods** and **cones** (Figure 20-22). These cells contain photopigments that change on exposure to light to produce chemical energy that is converted to electrical energy and ultimately transmitted to the visual cortex of the brain. Once photoreceptors are stimulated by light, they transmit a nervous impulse that is received and modified in various ways by cells whose nuclei are in the inner nuclear layer. The modified message is then transferred to ganglion cells, whose axons form the nerve fiber layer and extend through the optic nerve to the brain (lateral geniculate and cortex). Because many ocular syndromes are associated with loss of function of one or more of these visual pathways, it is important to understand the anatomical, physiological, and embryological relationships of the visual pathways before studying disorders of this system.

RETINAL ORGANIZATION

Ten identifiable layers in the retina are usually considered from outside inward in the following order (see Figure 20-22): the retinal pigment epithelium; neurosensory retina; and visual cell layer, outer limiting membrane, outer nuclear layer, outer plexiform layer, inner nuclear layer, inner plexiform layer, ganglion cell layer, nerve fiber layer, and inner limiting membrane.

RETINAL PIGMENTED EPITHELIUM (RPE)

This layer is derived from the outer layer of the optic cup and consists of a layer of flat polygonal cells adjacent to the choroid. It is more adherent to the choroid than to the rest of the retinal tissue through its attachment to the choriocapillaris by way of Bruch's membrane. The potential space between this layer and the sensory layer is where most retinal detachments occur. The cells are usually densely pigmented but are devoid of pigment overlying the choroid that contains the tapetum. This permits light to pass through, hit the tapetum, and then reflect back to the light-sensitive receptors. The pigment epithelial cells are important in nutrient transport from the choriocapillaris to the outer layers of the retina. They send cytoplasmic processes inward to surround the visual receptors to insulate them from bright light and increase their individual sensitivity. They also phagocytize outer segments of photoreceptors as they are continually shed during normal outer segment renewal.

Visual Cell Layer

This layer, also known as the rod and cone layer, consists of the dendritic processes of the photoreceptors, which are modified to be light sensitive. They are packed closely together side by side and arranged radially to receive incoming light (Figure 20-23; see also Figure 20-22). These processes react to the stimulation of light and initiate the mechanism of vision mentioned previously. The rods' outer segments are slender and are more sensitive to light than cones, being effective in low illumination. The rods provide for detection of shapes and motion, being the type of vision referred to as **scotopic** vision. Rods are inactivated by constant bright light, and thus are well suited for twilight and night vision. The cones' outer segments are slightly less slender and much less sensitive to light, being useful for vision during daylight—**photopic vision.** Cones can rapidly adapt to repeated stimuli and are sensitive to a range of light waves and therefore provide color vision, which creates enhanced resolution and visual acuity.

External Limiting Membrane

This layer is composed of extensions of Muller's fibers. These are supporting cells that extend through the retina. The tips of these extensions form a sievelike membrane through which the rods and cones extend and gain support.

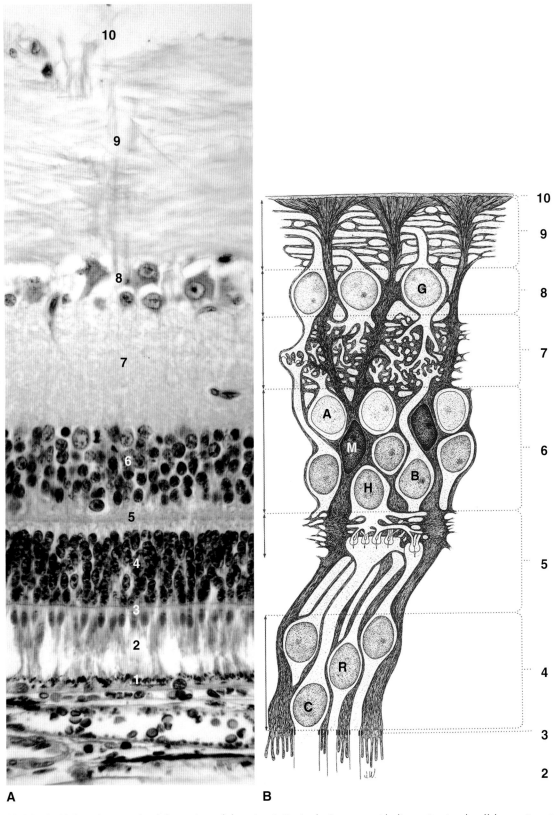

Figure 20-22. A, Light micrograph of the retina of the pig. *1,* Retinal pigment epithelium; *2,* visual cell layer; *3,* external limiting membrane; *4,* outer nuclear layer; *5,* outer plexiform layer; *6,* inner nuclear layer; *7,* inner plexiform layer; *8,* ganglion cell layer; *9,* nerve fiber layer; *10,* internal limiting membrane. (Hematoxylin and eosin stain; ×100.) **B,** Illustration of the 10 layers of the mammalian retina. *A,* Amacrine cell; *B,* Bipolar cell; *C,* cone photoreceptor; *G,* ganglion cell; *H,* horizontal cell; *M,* Muller cell; *R,* rod photoreceptor. *(Hogan MJ, Alvarado JA, Weddell JE:* Histology of the human eye, *Philadelphia, 1971, Saunders.)*

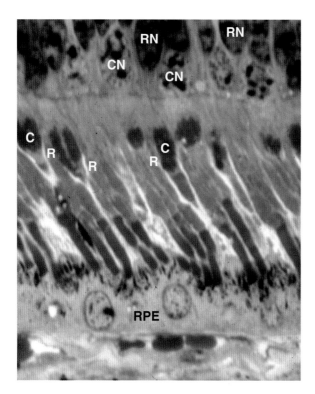

Figure 20-23. Light micrograph of the visual cell layer of the pig. *C,* Cone inner segment; *CN,* cone nuclei; *R,* rod inner segment; *RN,* rod nuclei; *RPE,* retinal pigment epithelium. (Hematoxylin and eosin stain; ×250.)

Outer Nuclear Layer

This layer consists of the nuclei of the rods and cones and is usually 12 to 15 rows thick centrally and thinner peripherally in the dog. Cone nuclei are located nearest the external limiting membrane (see Figure 20-23). They are larger, oval, and stain lighter than rod nuclei, which are smaller, darker, and much more numerous in most species. In animals with greater photopic vision, such as diurnal birds, squirrels, pigs, and ferrets, the number of rows are usually fewer at the area centralis due to fewer rods.

Outer Plexiform Layer

This layer consists of the terminal arborization of rod and cone cell axons mixed with the dendrites of cells of the inner nuclear layer, principally bipolar cells and horizontal cells.

Inner Nuclear Layer

Nuclei of bipolar, amacrine, horizontal, and Muller's cells are located in this layer (see Figure 20-22).

Muller's cells tend to have more cytoplasm and lie in the middle to outer portion of the layer. These serve as supportive cells for the retina. **Horizontal cells** interconnect photoreceptors to other photoreceptors. Typically their dendrites synapse to cones, whereas their axons synapse to rods. **Bipolar cells** and **amacrine cells** transmit the visual signal from rods and cones to the ganglion cells. However, the amacrine cells along with the horizontal cells provide feedback inhibition and consequently are involved in modification and integration of stimuli. The bipolar cells form the principal connection between the visual cell layer and the ganglion cell layer. In domestic species, the inner nuclear layer is usually two to five rows thick except at the area centralis, where it is thicker.

Inner Plexiform Layer

This layer is formed by a multitude of synapses that occur between the axons of the inner nuclear layer cells, the bipolar and amacrine cells, and the dendrites and cell bodies of the ganglion cells. It is best developed in cone-rich retina (i.e., diurnal species).

Ganglion Cell Layer

This layer contains ganglion cells, usually of three different types, plus neuroglial cells and retinal blood vessels. The neurons form a single row of cells with well-defined nuclei, nucleoli, and Nissl's granules except at the area of central vision known as the *area centralis,* where it may be two or three cell layers thick.

Nerve Fiber Layer

This layer is composed of axons of ganglion cells that have turned at right angles to course near the posterior pole where the optic nerve exits. While enveloped by neuroglial cells and/or the inner tips of Muller's cells, the nerve fibers lack myelin sheaths. Large retinal vessels, which arise from the short posterior ciliary arteries as in the dog, occur in the nerve fiber, ganglion cell, and inner plexiform layers with capillaries passing into the inner nuclear and plexiform layers.

Inner Limiting Membrane

This is both a cell membrane and a basement membrane composed of the fused terminations of Muller's cell fibers and has an intimate association with the outer vitreous humor.

THE MACULA, AREA CENTRALIS

This area of the retina is approximately related to the center of the visual field. It is more sensitive to detail vision (clarity) than the rest of the retina. The macula, when present, is easy to identify ophthalmoscopically. It is an area free of large retinal vessels and is more reflective; it has high cone density to the point at which only cones may be found. That area is referred to as the fovea, found in primates and birds. The retinas of most domestic species do not have maculas with foveas, but instead a region called the area centralis. The cone population is most dense in the area centralis, although a completely rod-free area cannot be identified. This is true for many species that do not have well defined photopic vision, such as most domestic species. Cones occur less frequently in the peripheral retina, which is dominated by rod photoreceptors, providing scotopic vision. In domestic animals the area centralis exists dorsolaterally to the optic disk.

THE OPTIC NERVE

Ganglion cell axons leave near the posterior pole and form the optic nerve head, optic papilla, or optic disk. From here they pass through the choroid and sclera and into the orbit. The optic nerve is formed by ganglion cell axons, glial cells, and septae that arise from the pial sheath. The nerve fibers of the disk are medullated (myelinated) in most species. The lamina cribrosa is a sievelike structure formed by a series of thin scleral and glial trabeculae (see Figure 20-7). When leaving the eye, the optic nerve fibers are myelinated and enclosed within a dural sheath continuous with that of the brain. The supportive tissue of the nerve is made of neuroglial elements that are dense at the optic nerve head.

Immediately surrounding the nerve is a thin pial sheath composed of thin, dense connective tissue. From the pia, thin vascular septae invade the nerve, separating the nerve fibers into bundles. The blood vessels carried by the septae come from the pia and are the major supply to the nerve. The pial arteries arise from the posterior ciliary arteries. The longitudinal fibers of the dura blend with the sclera.

OCULAR ADNEXA

Structures associated with the eye that specifically support and protect the eye include the bones and other forms of connective tissue that form the orbit, the fossa in which it lies; fascia associated with the orbit including the periorbita (primarily periosteum of the orbital bones), fascia bulbi or Tenon's capsule (loose connective tissue lining the globe posterior to the conjunctiva) and fascial sheaths of the extraocular muscles; the extraocular skeletal muscles that reposition the eye within its orbit; orbital adipose tissue; the lacrimal gland; the superior and inferior palpebrae (the upper and lower eyelids); and the membrana nictitans (third eyelid).

LACRIMAL GLAND

The **lacrimal gland** is a diamond-shaped gland located in the dorsolateral aspect of the globe lying within the periorbita—15 to 20 small ducts open from it into the superior conjunctival fornix. Histologically, the gland is a serous tubuloalveolar compound type. Its function is the production of the aqueous portion of tears. The innervation of the lacrimal gland involves the lacrimal (branch of the fifth cranial nerve [CN V]), sympathetic, and parasympathetic nerves.

THE EYELIDS

The eyelids consist of dorsal and ventral folds of thin skin continuous with the facial skin. The free edges of the superior and inferior eyelids meet to form the **lateral** and **medial canthi.** The opening formed by the free edges of the eyelids is the **palpebral fissure.** Closure of the fissure is caused by the contraction of the **orbicularis oculi muscle** located deep in the lids around the palpebral fissure. Opening or parting of the fissure is by relaxation of the orbicularis oculi and contraction of the **levator palpebrae superioris,** which inserts on the orbicularis oculi muscle and is located posteriorly within the superior eyelid only. The free margin of the eyelid may contain a row of cilia or lashes that are directed away from the anterior surface of the cornea. The cat lacks these lashes but has accessory hairs to catch dust and small debris. In most domestic species, the lower eyelids lack lashes.

The inner surface of each eyelid is lined with a mucous membrane, the **palpebral conjunctiva.** Posteriorly, the **bulbar conjunctiva** reflects onto the globe and is a part of the outer eye.

Near the posterior surface of the eyelid margin are the **tarsal glands (meibomian glands)** (Figure 20-24). Each gland forms a parallel row of holocrine acini which are arranged in vertical columns and open into a central duct that opens close to the lid margin. The glands are sebaceous and contained in a fibrous connective tissue bed—the **tarsal plate**—in the posterior

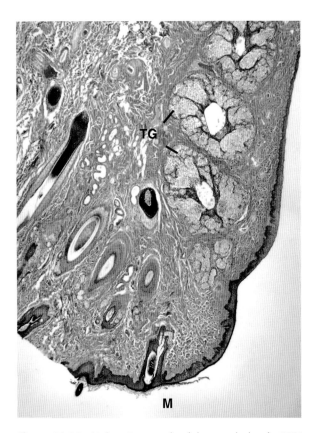

Figure 20-24. Light micrograph of the tarsal glands *(TG)* near the margin *(M)* of the upper eyelid of the dog. (Hematoxylin and eosin stain; ×20.)

eyelid stroma. In addition to the tarsal glands are accessory lacrimal glands that contribute to the pre-ocular film. These glands are usually serous and often associated with lymphoid tissue within the palpebral conjunctiva.

CONJUNCTIVA

The conjunctiva is the most exposed of all mucous membranes. Its primary functions are to prevent desiccation of the cornea, increase mobility of the eyelids and globe, and provide a barrier against microorganisms and foreign bodies. It is a thin, transparent mucous membrane that lines the posterior surface of the lids (palpebral conjunctiva) and is reflected forward on the eyeball (bulbar conjunctiva), becoming continuous anteriorly with the epithelium of the cornea. Ventrally an additional fold is formed by the reflection of the conjunctiva over the nictitating membrane. These reflections of the conjunctiva form the conjunctival sac. All parts of the conjunctiva are continuous, but for description it is divided into the palpebral, bulbar, and fornix conjunctiva.

The conjunctiva contains epithelial cells, within which are goblet cells that are most numerous in the fornix (conjunctival sac). Other intraepithelial glands secrete a mucous fluid that is more viscous than the lacrimal fluid.

The substantia propria of the conjunctiva is composed of two layers, a superficial adenoid layer, which in the dog and cat contains lymphatic follicles and glands, and a deep fibrous layer. The nerves and vessels of the conjunctiva are in the fibrous layer. The arteries of the conjunctiva arise from the anterior ciliary arteries, which are branches of the external ophthalmic artery.

THE THIRD EYELID

The **third eyelid,** or **nictitating membrane,** is a large fold of conjunctiva that protrudes from the inferior medial canthus over the anterior surface of the globe. It is supported by a T-shaped cartilaginous plate in which the horizontal portion is parallel with the free edge of the membrane (Figure 20-25). It is rich in elastic tissue, and the cartilage itself can be elastic in the cat, horse, and pig. Its free edge is usually pigmented in the young adult except in the light-pigmented individuals and the cat. The stroma of the nictitans consists of glandular and lymphoid tissue enveloped by fibrous connective tissue. The anterior surface is lined by nonkeratinized stratified squamous epithelium. The glandular tissue forms the **gland of the third eyelid,** or **nictitans gland,** which envelops the caudal end of the cartilaginous shaft. As in the lymphoid tissue, most of the gland lies near the bulbar surface. In most species of domestic animals it secretes a serous fluid except the pig in which the secretion is mostly mucoid. Although it can be serous, in many species it is mixed and can be considered a compound tubuloalveolar seromucoid gland.

Posteriorly, extra amounts of glandular tissue occur posterior to the third eyelid in a variety of animals including the cow, rabbit, and pig. This tissue is known as Harder's gland and histologically appears to be an extension of the nictitans gland but is deeply seated in the orbit.

EAR

Audition, or hearing, is provided by the special organ, the ear. This sense is fundamental to the lives of domestic species, making each individual keenly aware of the surrounding environment. Balance or

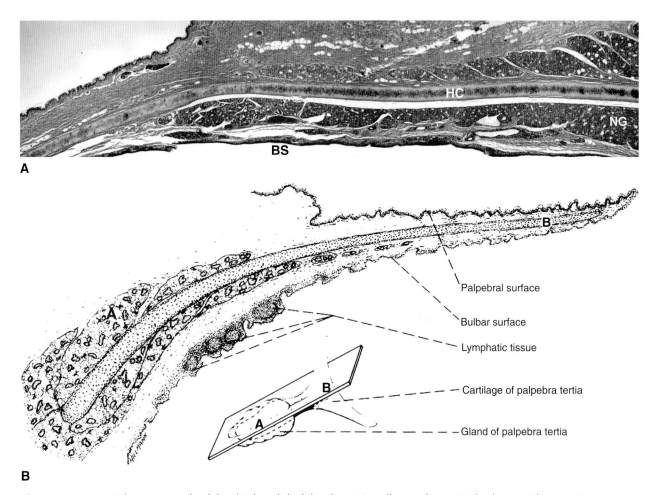

A

B

Palpebral surface

Bulbar surface

Lymphatic tissue

Cartilage of palpebra tertia

Gland of palpebra tertia

Figure 20-25. A, Light micrograph of the third eyelid of the dog. *BS,* Bulbar surface; *HC,* hyaline cartilage; *NG,* nictitating gland. (Hematoxylin and eosin stain; ×8.) **B,** Illustration of the third eyelid of the dog. *(From Evans H, Christensen G: Miller's anatomy of the dog,* ed 2, Philadelphia, 1979, Saunders.)

vestibulation is also provided by the ear, specifically the semicircular canals of the inner ear. As in sight, the comprehension of sound and balance is performed in the higher centers of the brain and highly integrated with vision at that level.

The ear is composed of three regions: the (outer) **external ear,** the **middle ear** (tympanic cavity), and (inner) **internal ear** (Figure 20-26). The external ear functions primarily to receive sound waves which are transmitted by its innermost component, the tympanic membrane, to the middle ear as mechanical vibrations. The middle ear amplifies the mechanical vibrations to the inner ear, which then transfers the sound energy into electrical signals within the auditory portion, the cochlea. The cochlea sends these signals to the auditory cortex by way of the acoustic nerve (CN VIII).

EXTERNAL EAR

The external ear consists of an auricle and external auditory canal, ending at the external surface of the tympanic membrane. The **auricle,** or **pinna,** is composed of a plate of elastic cartilage that varies considerably in shape and size among domestic animals and is covered by thin skin with hair follicles and associated sebaceous and sweat glands. The auricle leads to an irregularly shaped **external auditory canal,** also known as the external auditory meatus, that is lined by thin skin containing small hair follicles and associated sebaceous glands and modified sweat glands called **ceruminous glands** (Figure 20-27). These glands empty a waxy substance either directly to the surface of the skin or to hair follicles. This substance

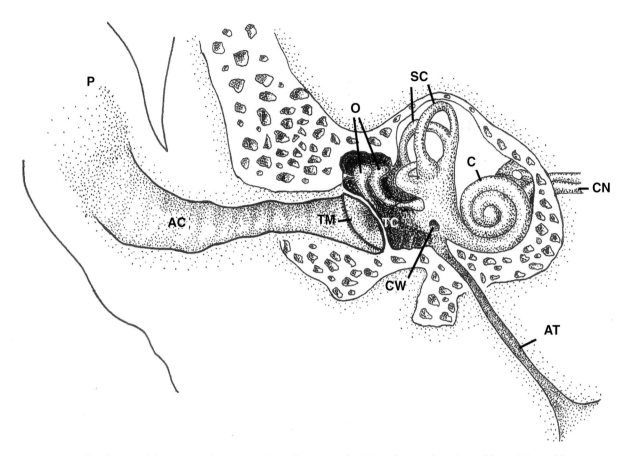

Figure 20-26. Illustration of the mammalian ear. *AC,* Auditory canal; *AT,* auditory tube; *C,* cochlea; *CN,* cochlear nerve; *CW,* cochlear window; *O,* ossicles; *P,* pinna; *SC,* semicircular canal; *TC,* tympanic cavity; *TM,* tympanic membrane.

combined with sebum secretions forms **cerumen,** more commonly referred to as ear wax, which helps moisten and protect the external auditory canal and the tympanic membrane. Most of the external auditory canal is surrounded and protected by the bone and ends internally with the tympanic membrane.

MIDDLE EAR

The **middle ear** consists of a tympanic membrane, tympanic cavity, and auditory ossicles. The **tympanic membrane,** or **tympanum** (eardrum), forms a thin partition between the external auditory canal and the tympanic cavity (see Figure 20-27). This partition is composed of a thin layer of mesodermally derived dense connective tissue, lined externally by a thin epidermis of ectodermal origin and internally by a simple squamous to cuboidal epithelium of endodermal origin. Sound that travels through the external auditory canal causes the tympanum to vibrate. The vibrations are passed on to the bones of the middle ear, and

in this way sound waves are transformed into mechanical energy.

The **tympanic cavity** is an air-filled space that contains the auditory ossicles and is open to the auditory tube (see Figure 20-26). The cavity is lined by a simple squamous or cuboidal epithelium except at the orifice of the auditory tube, where the epithelium becomes pseudostratified columnar.

The **auditory tube** interconnects the nasopharynx with the tympanic cavity and is lined by a respiratory-like epithelium, consisting of a ciliated pseudostratified columnar epithelium with goblet cells. The adjacent loose connective tissue merges with the periosteum of surrounding bone, but less so with the perichondrium of hyaline cartilage, which exists nasopharyngeally as an incomplete collar. In this area, the connective tissue enlarges to house mixed glands and lymphoid tissue. In the act of swallowing or yawning, the pharyngeal orifice of the tube expands and opens, which, in turn, allows air pressure within the tympanic cavity to be equalized with that within the external auditory canal.

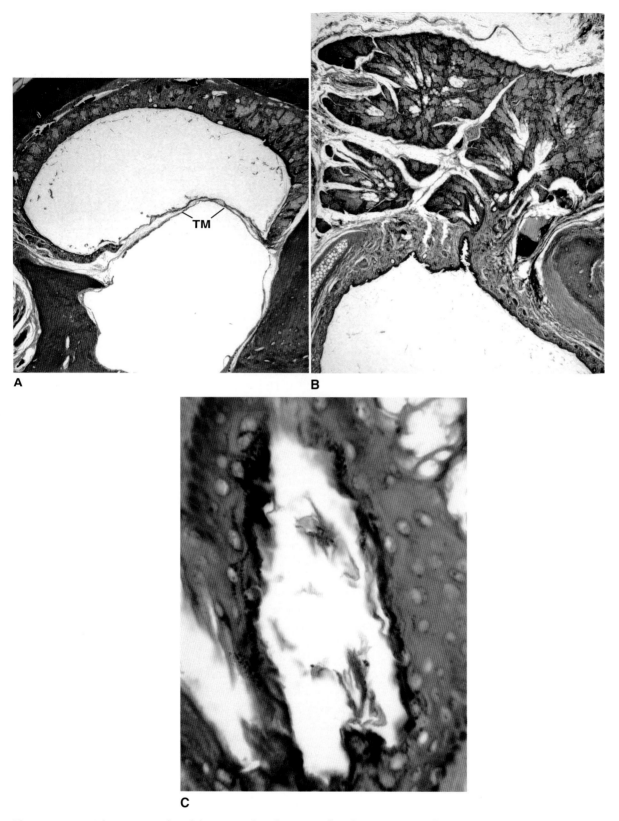

Figure 20-27. Light micrographs of the external auditory canal and tympanic membrane *(TM)* and associated ceruminous gland with waxy secretion within the duct in the rat. (Hematoxylin and eosin stain; **A** and **B,** ×10; **C,** ×250.)

Along the auditory tube of the horse, toward the nasopharynx is a ventral outpocketing—the **guttaral pouch.** Its formation is due to the absence of hyaline cartilage in this region, consisting of the same histological features occurring along the rest of the auditory tube as it approaches the nasopharyngeal opening.

The **auditory ossicles** of the middle ear consist of a series of three small bones that transfer sound from the external ear to the internal ear (Figure 20-28; see also Figure 20-26). The first of these small bones is the **malleus,** or hammer. One process of the malleus is firmly attached to the tympanic membrane, whereas the other process is joined with the next ossicle, the **incus** (also called the anvil) by a synovial joint. The incus is joined to the third ossicle (the **stapes,** or stirrup) by a similar synovial joint. Whereas one portion of the stapes is associated with the incus, the other is attached to the oval window of the internal ear. As ligaments hold these three bones in position, a pair of skeletal muscles, the **tensor tympani** and **stapedius,** helps control movement of the tympanum and ossicles.

INTERNAL EAR

The inner or **internal ear** consists of a bony labyrinth that forms a base plate for a membranous labyrinth to be suspended.

BONY LABYRINTH

The bony labyrinth comprises three regions: the semicircular canals, the vestibule, and the cochlea (Figure 20-29). Each component has an endosteal lining separated from the membranous labyrinth by the **perilymphatic space** filled with a cerebrospinal fluid–like clear watery liquid known as the **perilymph.** The perilymph originates from the subarachnoid space of the nearby meninges by way of the cochlear canaliculus. The **semicircular canals** are three curved tubular bodies positioned at right angles to one another, lying dorsally and caudally to the vestibule (Figure 20-29).

The **vestibule** forms the small central area between the anteriorly positioned cochlea and posteriorly positioned semicircular canals (see Figure 20-29). The lateral portion of the vestibule lies next to the middle ear and has a window (vestibular window) that is associated with the footplate of the stapes.

The **cochlea** consists of a bony tube—the **spiral canal**—that, as the name implies, is shaped spirally in a manner similar to a snail's shell. The amount of spiraling around a central bony column—the modiolus—varies among domestic species, ranging from approximately 3 times in the cat to $4^{1}/_{2}$ times in the cow. By comparison, the amount of spiraling in the human is only $2^{1}/_{2}$ times. The modiolus holds the cochlear nerve, and branches project from the nerve into an osseous or bony shelf within the spiral canal called the **osseous spiral lamina.**

MEMBRANOUS LABYRINTH

The membranous labyrinth lies within the bony labyrinth and consists primarily of interconnecting epithelial tissues that form the saccule, utricle, semicircular ducts, cochlear duct, and endolymphatic system. Within the membranous labyrinth is a viscous plasma-like liquid—the **endolymph**—that freely circulates throughout each component.

Saccule and Utricle

Within the vestibule are two recesses along its medial wall that hold the **saccule** and **utricle** (see Figure 20-29). The saccule and utricle form the **endolymphatic duct,** which blindly ends in the **endolymphatic sac.** In addition, the saccule joins the duct of the cochlea by the small duct, **ductus reuniens.** The membranous walls of the saccule and utricle consist of an internal simple epithelium that is either squamous or cuboidal and an external layer of connective tissue that is associated with the perilymphatic tissue. Within the membranous labyrinth of the saccule and the utricle are sensory regions with specific receptors that are able to orient the body with regard to gravity and changes in the rate of motion (acceleration, deceleration). These regions are called maculae—the **macula of the saccule (macula sacculi)** and the **macula of the utricle (macula utriculi)**—though they tend to be more oval or kidney shaped **(macula utriculi)** or hook shaped **(macula sacculi)** than round as the term macula would imply. They are positioned perpendicularly to one another; the macula of the saccule is located along the floor and the macula of the utricle lies along the lateral wall.

Both maculae possess thickened epithelia that contain two types of **neuroepithelial cells** also referred to as hair cells that are attached to loose connective tissue. **Type I hair cell** has a rounded base enveloped by an afferent nerve fiber in a cup-shaped manner (Figure 20-30). The apical portion of type I is narrowed, holding a single kinocilium and 40 to 100 stereocilia that are aligned in rows of specific lengths—the longest lies closest to the kinocilium. The stereocilia are true long microvilli, possessing cores of actin filaments that become firmly anchored at their base

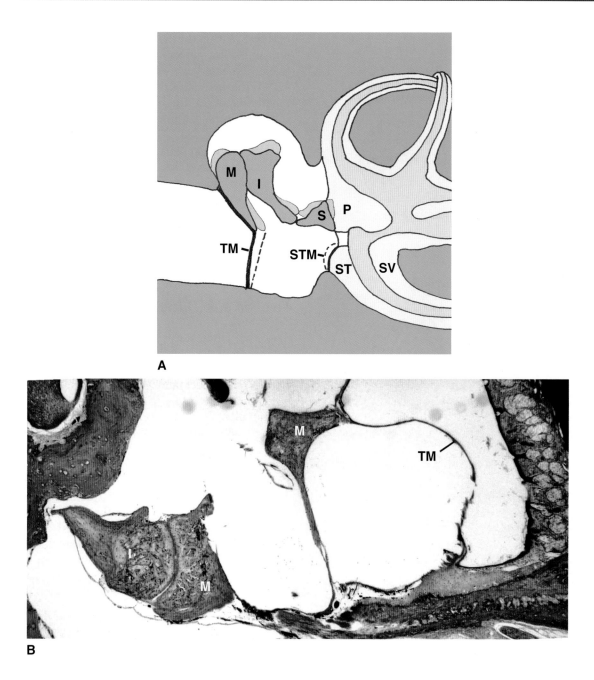

Figure 20-28. A, Diagram of the three ossicles (*I*, incus; *M*, malleus; *S*, stapes) of middle ear. The lighter shade of the bones shows their repositioning after a sound wave hits the tympanic membrane *(TM)*. Dotted lines indicate movement of the TM and secondary tympanic membrane *(STM)* resulting from a sound wave. *P,* Perilymph; *ST,* scala tympani; *SV,* scala vestibuli. **B,** Light micrograph of the two ossicles, the malleus *(M)* and the incus *(I)* of the middle ear of the rat. *TM,* Tympanic membrane. (Hematoxylin and eosin stain; ×10.)

within a terminal web of more actin filaments called the **cuticular plate** (see Figure 3-20). As a result, the basal portion of each stereocilium is rigid, allowing flexibility and bending to occur from the neck region on. The **type II hair cell** has a more columnar-shaped body than that of type I and is not embraced by an afferent nerve in a cup-shaped manner as in the case of type I hair cells. Instead, the base of type II hair cells forms synaptic junctions with numerous afferent fibers. The presence and arrangement of the kinocilium and neighboring stereocilia in the type II hair cell are identical to those of type I hair cells. Cytoplasmically, both types of cells possess a well-developed Golgi apparatus with numerous vesicles (see Figure

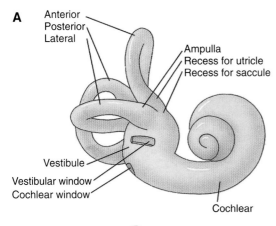

A

Anterior
Posterior
Lateral

Ampulla
Recess for utricle
Recess for saccule

Vestibule

Vestibular window
Cochlear window

Cochlear

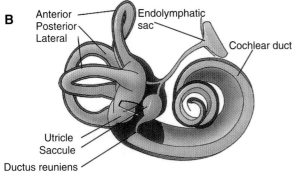

B

Anterior
Posterior
Lateral

Endolymphatic
sac

Cochlear duct

Utricle
Saccule

Ductus reuniens

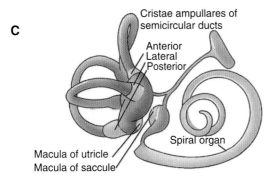

C

Cristae ampullares of
semicircular ducts

Anterior
Lateral
Posterior

Spiral organ

Macula of utricle
Macula of saccule

Figure 20-29. Diagram of the labyrinth system of the inner ear. **A,** Bony labyrinth. **B,** Membranous labyrinth within the bony labyrinth. **C,** Membranous labyrinth with sensory portion in yellow. *(Modified from Gartner LP, Hiatt JL: Color textbook of histology, Philadelphia, 1997, Saunders.)*

20-30). Both types of hair cells are surrounded by supporting cells (sustentacular cells) that form junctional complexes to one another, including the hair cells. Neither type of hair cell reaches the basal lamina formed by these supporting cells.

The kinocilia and stereocilia of the neuroepithelial cells are immersed in a gel-like body of glycoprotein called the **otolithic (statoconial) membrane.** On the surface of the membrane lies a bed of calcium carbonate crystals referred to as **otoliths (statoconia)** (Figure 20-31). Orientation of the kinocilium and adjacent stereocilia among the hair cells differs between the two

maculae. Within the macula of the utricle, the kinocilium and tallest stereocilia are directed toward a curvilinear center known as the **striola.** By comparison, within the macula of the utricle, the kinocilium and tallest stereocilia are directed away from the center. In each instance, movement in any direction is adequately detected.

The nonreceptive epithelium surrounding the maculae consists of light and dark cells that have scattered small microvilli. The dark cells have smooth and coated vesicles, lipid droplets, and numerous mitochondria often associated with basal infoldings. The function of both cells remains unknown, though it is possible that they may have a role in endolymph dynamics.

Semicircular Ducts

Three semicircular ducts emanate from the utricle as extensions of the membranous labyrinth that lines the semicircular canals (see Figure 20-29). The connection of each duct and canal with the utricle and vestibule, respectively, is dilated and referred to as an **ampulla.** Each membranous ampulla contains a sensory region—the **crista ampullaris**—comprised of both supporting and neuroepithelial hair cells that are morphologically identical to those of the two maculae. However, rather than be associated with a disk-shaped area, the supporting and neuroepithelial hair cells lie on a ridge of connective tissue that together project into the lumen of the membranous ampulla. As in the maculae of the saccule and utricle, the stereocilia and kinocilia of the two types of hair cells are embedded in a gelatinous glycoprotein called the **cupula.** Otoliths or any other kind of crystalline material are not associated with the cupula, which extends to the opposite side of the ampulla.

VESTIBULATION

Collectively, the maculae of the saccule and utricle and the cristae ampullares of the semicircular ducts function as the **vestibular apparatus,** which is essential for balance, especially during locomotion. During linear movement, such as moving directly ahead or backward, the head motion initiates endolymph displacement, which, in turn, causes repositioning of the otoliths and the otolithic membrane. With concomitant bending of the stereocilia, a transduction of the physical action to an electrophysiological action that produces an electrical impulse occurs and is transferred by the synaptic junctions of the hair cells to associated afferent nerve fibers, which then transmit

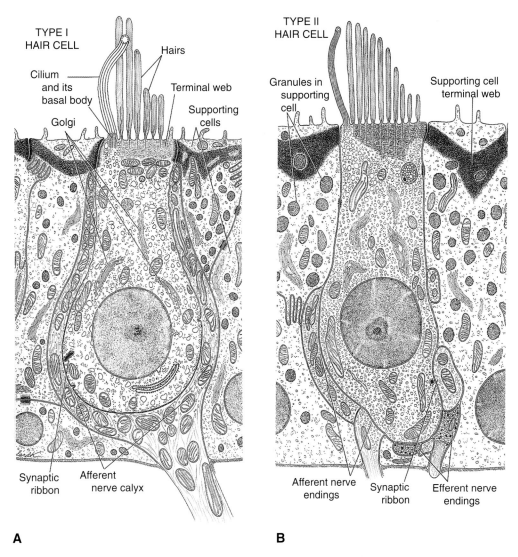

TYPE I HAIR CELL

Cilium and its basal body

Golgi

Hairs

Terminal web

Supporting cells

Synaptic ribbon

Afferent nerve calyx

A

TYPE II HAIR CELL

Granules in supporting cell

Supporting cell terminal web

Afferent nerve endings

Synaptic ribbon

Efferent nerve endings

B

Figure 20-30. Illustration of the vestibular hair cells: type I **(A)** and type II **(B)**. *(From Fawcett DW: Bloom and Fawcett: a textbook of histology, ed 11, Philadelphia, 1986, Saunders.)*

the signal to the vestibular center of the central nervous system.

Circular movements that involve the head are detected by the cristae ampullares within the ampullae of the semicircular canals. As the head rotates, the endolymph within the semicircular ducts pushes against the cupula of each crista ampullaris, which acts much like a sail of a boat as it billows while deflecting endolymph that pushes against it. The movement of the cupula results in the flexion of the stereocilia of the neuroepithelial hair cells within that region, which, in turn, results in the production of electrical impulses that are then transferred to associated afferent nerve fibers for subsequent transmission of the signal to the central nervous system.

ORGAN OF CORTI

The **organ of Corti,** or the **spiral organ,** is the sensory body for audition and lies within that portion of the membranous labyrinth known as the cochlear duct. The **cochlear duct** (also known as the **scala media**) is formed in the spiral canal of the bony cochlea (Figure 20-32; see also Figure 20-29). Two sides of this duct are embraced by perilymph-filled compartments. The compartment above the duct is called the **scala vestibuli** and the two areas are separated by the **vestibular membrane,** which forms the roof of the scala media, or cochlear duct. The compartment below the duct is called the **scala tympani;**

the scala tympani and the scala media are separated by the **basilar membrane,** which forms the floor of the cochlear duct and the foundation for the auditory apparatus to rest on.

The vestibular membrane is formed by two adjoining simple squamous epithelia that connect one to another by their basal laminae. The outer epithelium

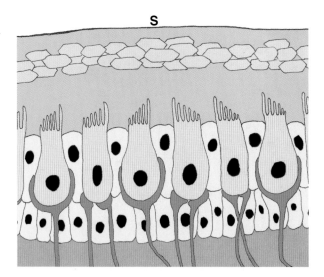

Figure 20-31. Diagram of the hair cells and the orientation of their cilia within the otolithic membrane of the macula of the saccule centered toward the striola *(S)*.

is a portion of the lining of the scala vestibuli, whereas the inner epithelium is a portion of the lining for the scala media. Each epithelium is tightly sealed by the zonula adherens.

The basilar membrane consists of a simple squamous epithelium, which faces the scala tympani, and a small amount of collagen that thickens as the membrane spirals from the cochlear window toward the end of the cochlea, the **helicotrema,** where the scala vestibuli and scala tympani openly connect.

The lateral side of the scala media is composed of a stratified cuboidal to columnar epithelium—the **stria vascularis**—that overlies a truncated layer of loose connective tissue called the **spiral ligament** (Figure 20-33). The stria vascularis possesses **intraepithelial capillaries,** a feature rarely encountered among epithelia throughout the body. The epithelium contributes to endolymph formation and maintains ion composition. The stria vascularis consists of three cell types: marginal, intermediate, and basal. The **marginal cell** has numerous microvilli along its apical surface and contains within its cytoplasm many mitochondria (which are often within deep basal infoldings) and small vesicles. The **intermediate cell** contains far fewer mitochondria and forms many cell processes that interdigitate with other intermediate cells and marginal cells. The **basal cell** also possesses many cell processes that interdigitate with marginal and inter-

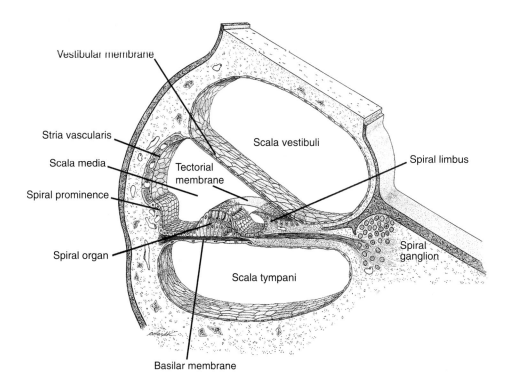

Figure 20-32. Illustration of a portion of the cochlea. *(Modified from Fawcett DW: Bloom and Fawcett: a textbook of histology, ed 11, Philadelphia, 1986, Saunders.)*

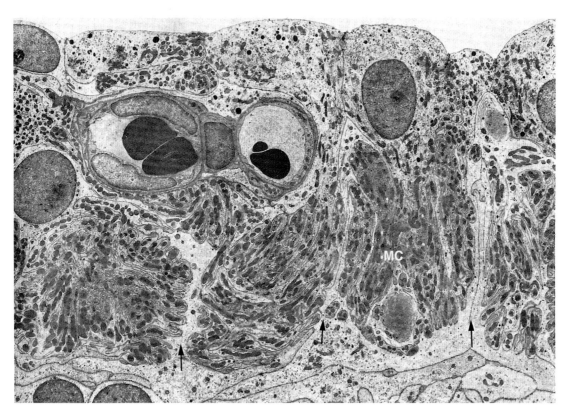

Figure 20-33. Transmission electron micrograph of the stria vascularis of the cat. Large arrows point to intraepithelial capillaries; small arrows point to branched ascending processes of basal cells that partially surround marginal cells *(MC).* *(Modified from Fawcett DW:* Bloom and Fawcett: a textbook of histology, *ed 11, Philadelphia, 1986, Saunders.)*

mediate cells. When interdigitating with marginal cells, these processes isolate the marginal cells from the base of the epithelium in a cuplike manner.

On the other side of the scala media where the basilar and vestibular membranes come to their closest proximity, is a connective tissue called the **limbus of the spiral lamina (spiral limbus)** that extends from the periosteum of the spiral lamina into the scala media (see Figure 20-32). A portion of the upper limbus protrudes farther into the scala media to contribute to the formation of the **internal spiral tunnel.** This protrusion is the **vestibular lip,** which has a rim of epithelial cells called the **interdental cells.** The interdental cells secrete a thick proteoglycan-laden body—the **tectorial membrane**—that lies on the neurosensory cells of the spiral organ. At the lower portion or base of the limbus is another protrusion— the **tympanic lip**—that merges with the basilar membrane. Branches of the cochlear division of the acoustic nerve repeatedly penetrate the lip from the region of the modiolus, connecting with sensory cells of the spiral organ of Corti (Figure 20-34).

The sensory cells of the spiral organ lie on the basilar membrane and are supported by a variety of cells. The sensory cells are referred to as hair cells, or more specifically the **neuroepithelial hair cells of the spiral organ (cochlear hair cells).** Throughout the length of the cochlea, these cells are able to transduce impulses for audition, forming two groups based on their location (see Figure 20-34). One group constitutes the **inner hair cells** that form a single row and morphologically have a strong resemblance to type I cells of the vestibular labyrinth, being fairly short cells with a rounded base and a narrowed neck region. And as in the type I cells, the rounded base is enveloped in a cuplike manner by an efferent nerve ending and afferent nerve endings. The apical modifications consist of 50 or more stereocilia arranged in rows of increasing height on the surface in the shape of a V or W. None of the stereocilia become immersed in the overlying tectorial membrane, which is responsible for causing the stereocilia to move and initiate an electric impulse during a sound-generating event. The adult inner hair cell does not possess a true kinocilium though the presence of a basal body occurs next to the apical cell membrane. Surrounding a centrally placed nucleus, the cytoplasm is filled with rough and smooth endoplasmic reticulum, vesicles, and mitochondria. The inner hair cells are nearly fully lined and supported by inner phalangeal cells.

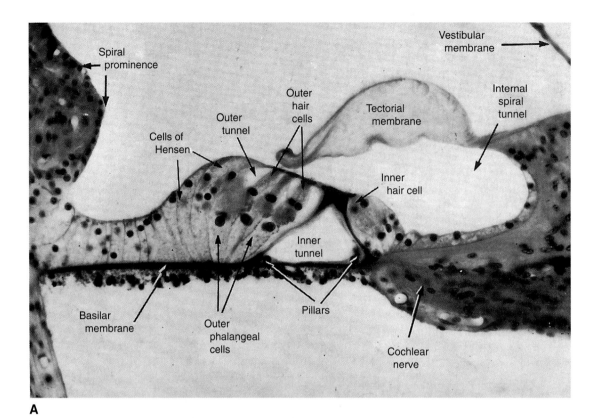

A

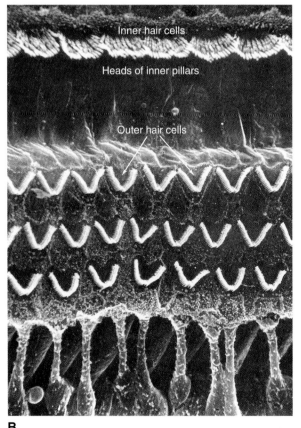

B

Figure 20-34. A, Light micrograph (approximately ×250) of the spiral organ of the cat. **B,** Scanning electron micrograph of the spiral organ from the direction of the tectorial membrane. *(From Fawcett DW:* Bloom and Fawcett: a textbook of histology, *ed 11, Philadelphia, 1986, Saunders.)*

The second group constitutes the **outer hair cells,** which are more elongated than the inner hair cells and form typically three rows along the outer portion of the spiral organ (see Figures 20-32 and 20-34). The nucleus of each cell is positioned basally, and the cytoplasm is filled with rough endoplasmic reticulum (rER) and mitochondria, which also are concentrated basally. The apical modifications again are only stereocilia, which number up to 100 and are arranged in rows of increasing height in the shape of Ws. The tips of the tallest stereocilia are immersed in the tectorial membrane. The base of these cells forms afferent and efferent synaptic junctions. The outer hair cells are supported for most of their lengths by outer phalangeal cells.

SUPPORTING CELLS OF THE SPIRAL ORGAN

The hair cells of the spiral organ are supported by a variety of cells including the phalangeal cells previously mentioned, pillar cells, border cells, outer limiting cells (cells of Hensen, and cells of Claudius and Boettcher) (see Figure 20-34).

The phalangeal cells are tall columnar cells that are attached either directly to the basilar membrane, as in the case of the outer phalangeal cells, or to the tympanic lip that leads to the basilar membrane, as in the case of the inner phalangeal cells. Whereas both inner and outer phalangeal cells line the cochlear hair cells, the outer phalangeal cells form concaved apices that cradle the outer hair cells; just their lateral portions become apical processes that extend to the free surface. Each process contains numerous microfilaments and microtubules that give additional rigidity to the sensory cells. In inner phalangeal cells, similar processes support the inner hair cells. These processes expand and attach to the hair cells by junctional complexes. The cytoskeletal component associated with their attachment among the hair cells and the phalangeal cells results in the **reticular lamina,** which provides rigidity of the apical portions of the hair cells.

Pillar cells consist of outer and inner groups or lines of elongated cells that form an **inner tunnel** as they extend from the basilar membrane to the apices of the outer hair cells (outer pillar cells) and the inner phalangeal cells (inner pillar cells) (see Figure 20-34). Both groups of pillar cells have cytoplasm heavily laden with cytoskeletal elements (filaments and microtubules) that course the length of the cell in bundles and fan out apically as the outer and inner cells contact each other, creating a platelike roof between the inner and outer hair cells. The bases of both groups of pillar cells house their nuclei as they flatten out in a manner similar to their apices.

External to the outer hair cells lies another group of supporting cells that continue along the basilar membrane before joining the spiral prominence. These cells include the taller **cells of Hensen,** which delineate the outer boundary of the spiral organ, and the shorter **cells of Claudius,** which lie on another group of small cells, the **cells of Boettcher.** The roles of these cells are not well delineated.

AUDITION (HEARING)

The function of the cochlear portion of the inner ear is to receive an auditory signal, a sound wave, and transduce the signal into electrical impulses that are transmitted by afferent nerve fibers to the auditory center in the central nervous system (CNS), where hearing occurs. Sounds consist of alternating waves of compressed air that are initially received by the pinna and auditory canal of the outer ear. On reaching the end of the canal, each wave pushes against the tympanic membrane, which in tandem with the three small bones of the middle ear, converts the sound wave into mechanical energy (see Figure 20-28). As each wave hits the tympanic membrane and associated ossicles, the innermost ossicle, the stapes, pushes against the vestibular window, resulting in the immediate compression of the perilymph, lying next to the window. Because liquid cannot by itself become compressed, the force against the perilymph becomes transported spirally up the scala vestibuli within the cochlea to its end at the **helicotrema,** where the scala vestibuli meets open ended with the scala tympani. From that point, the pressure wave within the perilymph of the scala tympani pushes against the basilar membrane as it spirals to the base of the cochlea, where the impulse last pushes against the secondary tympanic membrane covering the cochlear window (round window) and any residual energy is released.

When the pressure wave within the scala tympani pushes against the basilar membrane, the spiral organ moves against the tectorial membrane, which results in the shearing motion of the hair cells' stereocilia, the tallest of which are embedded in the tectorial membrane. The shift in positioning of the stereocilia initiates depolarization within the hair cell, which triggers synaptic activity at the base of the hair cell with adjacent afferent nerve endings. Sound waves at low amplitudes will affect only the outer hair cells because none of the stereocilia of the inner hair cells are immersed in the tectorial membrane. However, as amplitudes increase, the inner hair cells become activated. Much of the hearing process is still not fully understood. It has been known for some time that as the basilar membrane shortens toward the apex of the cochlea, its sensitivity to vibration frequency varies due to the change in the distortion of the basilar membrane along the cochlear tract. However, efferent input to the hair cells may also play a role in how hair cells respond to varying frequencies in conjunction with their position within the cochlea.

SUGGESTED READINGS

Braekevelt CR: The retinal epithelial fine structure in the domestic cat, *Anat Histol Embryol* 9:58, 1990.

Duke-Elder S: *The eye in evolution,* vol 1, London, 1958, Henry Kimpton.

Evans H, Christensen G: *Miller's anatomy of the dog,* ed 2, Philadelphia, 1979, Saunders.

Fawcett DW: *Bloom and Fawcett: a textbook of histology,* ed 11, Philadelphia, 1986, Saunders.

Gartner LP, Hiatt JL: *Color textbook of histology,* Philadelphia, 1997, Saunders.

Goycoolea MV, Carpenter AM, Muchow D: Ultrastructural studies of the round-window membrane of the cat, *Arch Otolaryngol Head Neck Surg* 113:617, 1987.

Hogan MJ, Alvarado JA, Weddell JE: *Histology of the human eye,* Philadelphia, 1971, Saunders.

Kirikae I: *The structure and function of the middle ear,* Tokyo, 1960, University of Tokyo Press.

Klinke R: Physiology of hearing. In Schmidt RF, editor: *Fundamentals of sensory physiology,* New York, 1978, Springer-Verlag.

Ollivier FJ, Samuelson, DA, Brooks DE, et al: Comparative morphology of the tapetum lucidum (among selected species), *Vet Ophthalmol* 7:11, 2004.

Prince JH, Diesen CD, Eglitis I: *Anatomy and histology of the eye and orbit in domestic animals,* Springfield, Ill, 1960, Charles C Thomas.

Raphael Y, Altschuler RA: Structure and innervation of the cochlea, *Brain Res Bull* 60:397, 2003.

Samuelson DA: A reevaluation of the comparative anatomy of the Eutherian iridocorneal angle and associated ciliary body musculature, *Vet Comp Ophthalmol* 6:153, 1996.

Samuelson DA, Gelatt KN: The aging iridocorneal angle and glaucoma. In Mohr U, editor: *Pathobiology of the aging dog,* Ames, Iowa, 1998, Iowa State University Press.

Tachibana M: Sound needs sound melanocytes to be heard, *Pigment Cell Res* 12:344, 1999.

Wysocki J: Dimensions of the vestibular and tympanic scalae of the cochlea in selected mammals, *Hear Res* 161:1, 2001.

Index

Page numbers followed by f indicate figures; t, tables.